Pharmacological Management of Neurological and Psychiatric Disorders

CONTENTS

CONTRIBUTORS

Stanley H. Appel, M.D.
Professor and Chairman, Department of Neurology
Baylor College of Medicine
Houston, Texas
CHAPTER 10

Robert W. Buchanan, M.D.
Associate Professor, and Director, Outpatient
  Program
Maryland Psychiatric Research Center
Baltimore, Maryland
CHAPTER 2

William T. Carpenter, Jr., M.D.
Professor of Psychiatry and Pharmacology
Director, Maryland Psychiatric Research Center
Baltimore, Maryland
CHAPTER 2

Robert R. Conley, M.D.
Assistant Professor, and Director, Treatment
  Resistant Unit
Maryland Psychiatric Research Center
Baltimore, Maryland
CHAPTER 2

Joseph T. Coyle, M.D.
Professor and Chair, Department of Psychiatry
Harvard Medical School
Boston, Massachusetts
CHAPTER 1

F. Michael Cutrer, M.D.
Director, Headache Unit
Massachusetts General Hospital
Assistant Professor of Neurology
Harvard Medical School
Boston, Massachusetts
CHAPTER 16

Kenneth L. Davis, M.D.
Esther and Joseph Klingenstein Professor
Mount Sinai School of Medicine
Chairman, Department of Psychiatry
Mount Sinai Medical Center
New York, New York
CHAPTER 9

S. J. Enna, Ph.D.
Professor and Chair, Department of Pharmacology,
  Toxicology, and Therapeutics
University of Kansas Medical Center
Kansas City, Kansas
CHAPTER 1

Robert S. Fisher, M.D., Ph.D.
Chief, Epilepsy Center, Barrow Neurological Institute
Professor of Clinical Neurology
University of Arizona
Phoenix, Arizona
CHAPTER 14

Wayne K. Goodman, M.D.
Professor, Department of Psychiatry
University of Florida School of Medicine
Gainesville, Florida
CHAPTER 6

Jack M. Gorman, M.D.
Professor of Psychiatry, Department of Psychiatry
Columbia University
New York, New York
CHAPTER 3

M. A. Grados, M.D.
Instructor, Department of Psychiatry
Johns Hopkins University School of Medicine
Baltimore, Maryland
CHAPTER 5

Joseph Grun, B.S.
Research Assistant, Child Psychiatry Research Center
College of Physicians and Surgeons of Columbia
    University
New York, New York
CHAPTER 3

Joseph B. Guarnaccia, M.D.
Assistant Professor, Department of Neurology
Yale University School of Medicine
Director, Yale MS Clinic
New Haven, Connecticut
CHAPTER 12

D. M. Kaplan, M.D.
Postdoctoral Fellow, Department of Psychiatry
Johns Hopkins University School of Medicine
Baltimore, Maryland
CHAPTER 5

Jeffrey E. Kelsey, M.D., Ph.D.
Assistant Professor
Department of Psychiatry and Behavioral Sciences
Emory University School of Medicine
Atlanta, Georgia
CHAPTER 4

Michael A. Moskowitz, M.D.
Director, Stroke and Neurovascular Regulation
Massachusetts General Hospital
Professor of Neurology
Harvard Medical School
Boston, Massachusetts
CHAPTER 16

Tanya Murphy, M.D.
Assistant Professor of Child Psychiatry
Department of Psychiatry
University of Florida College of Medicine
Gainesville, Florida
CHAPTER 6

Charles B. Nemeroff, M.D., Ph.D.
Reunette W. Harris Professor and Chairman
Department of Psychiatry and Behavioral Sciences
Emory University School of Medicine
Atlanta, Georgia
CHAPTER 4

Charles P. O'Brien, M.D., Ph.D.
Chief of Psychiatry
Veterans Administration Medical Center
Professor and Vice-Chairman of Psychiatry
University of Pennsylvania
Philadelphia, Pennsylvania
CHAPTER 8

Gavril W. Pasternak, M.D., Ph.D.
Member, Memorial Sloan-Kettering Cancer Center
Professor of Neurology and Neuroscience and
    Pharmacology
Cornell University Medical College
New York, New York
CHAPTER 13

Richard Payne, M.D.
Professor, Department of Neurology
M.D. Anderson Cancer Center
Houston, Texas
CHAPTER 13

John B. Penney, Jr., M.D.
Department of Neurology
Harvard Medical School
Massachusetts General Hospital
Boston, Massachusetts
CHAPTER 11

Daniel S. Pine, M.D.
Assistant Professor of Clinical Psychiatry
Child Psychiatry Research Center
College of Physicians and Surgeons of Columbia
    University
New York, New York
CHAPTER 3

Allan L. Reiss, M.D.
Professor, Department of Psychiatry and Behavioral
    Sciences
Stanford University School of Medicine
Stanford, California
CHAPTER 5

Steven C. Samuels, M.D.
Assistant Professor, Department of Psychiatry
Mount Sinai School of Medicine
Director, Outpatient Geriatric Psychiatry Program
Mount Sinai Medical Center
New York, New York
CHAPTER 9

Timothy L. Vollmer, M.D.
Associate Professor, Department of Neurology
Director, Neuroimmunology
Yale University School of Medicine
New Haven, Connecticut
CHAPTER 12

James J. Vornov, M.D., Ph.D.
Assistant Professor, Departments of Neurology and
    Neuroscience
Johns Hopkins University
Baltimore, Maryland
CHAPTER 15

Christian Waeber, Ph.D.
Instructor in Surgery,
Harvard Medical School
Massachusetts General Hospital,
Boston, Massachusetts
CHAPTER 16

Stephen G. Waxman, M.D., Ph.D.
Professor and Chairman, Department of Neurology
Yale University School of Medicine
New Haven, Connecticut
Director, PVA/EPVA Research Center
VA Connecticut
West Haven, Connecticut
CHAPTER 12

Andrew Winokur, M.D., Ph.D.
Professor, Department of Psychiatry
Dartmouth-Hitchcock Medical Center
Lebanon, New Hampshire
CHAPTER 7

Anne B. Young, M.D., Ph.D.
Julieanne Dorn Professor of Neurology
Harvard Medical School
Chief, Neurology Service
Massachusetts General Hospital
Boston, Massachusetts
CHAPTER 11

PREFACE

Healthcare is undergoing formidable changes in the manner in which clinical services are provided, as well as in the knowledge base that informs medical practice. Until recently, the diagnosis and treatment of mental disorders were considered to be largely the province of psychiatrists and allied mental health professionals, and neurologic disorders were often viewed as the arcane and untreatable realm of neurology. These assumptions were eclipsed by a transformation in the structure of healthcare services that shifted the burden of diagnosis and initial treatment to the primary care physician. Fortunately, rapid advances in neuroscience and neuropsychopharmacology now offer the opportunity to treat effectively more of these disorders than ever before with drugs possessing better efficacy and greater specificity than earlier agents.

The purpose of this volume is to make accessible to the primary care physician, as well as physicians in training, the advances in diagnosis and pharmacologic treatment of neurologic and psychiatric disorders. Given the lifetime prevalence of these disorders, patients with psychiatric and neurologic disabilities are a significant component of a primary care physician's practice, making an understanding of the fundamental principles of diagnosis and treatment essential for dealing appropriately with these patients. With current knowledge and treatment modalities, primary care physicians are now empowered to identify patients suffering from these conditions and to provide the first tier of treatment.

The text is divided into 16 chapters, all written by experts in the field. Emphasis is placed on addressing the more common neurologic, psychiatric, and substance abuse disorders that a primary care physician is likely to encounter in practice. A brief review of the diagnostic features and the current understanding of the pathophysiology of each disorder precedes a discussion of its pharmacologic management. More subtle details are presented in smaller print to facilitate a rapid review of the essential features of diagnosis and treatment. Diagnostic decision trees and treatment algorithms facilitate decision making in the clinical setting. The volume is extensively cross-referenced with *Goodman and Gilman's The Pharmacological Basis of Therapeutics* to guide interested readers to more detailed, basic information on the pharmacologic features of each drug.

Given their prevalence and debilitating effects, the underdiagnosis and inadequate treatment of neurologic and psychiatric disorders are a major public health problem.

We hope that this volume will provide the practicing physician with a greater under-standing of each disorder and its pharmacologic management, furnishing a comprehen-sive and user-friendly means to identify these conditions more confidently, initiate treatment, and—when necessary—refer patients to appropriate specialists.

S. J. Enna, Ph.D.
J. T. Coyle, M.D.

January, 1998

OVERVIEW OF NEUROPSYCHOPHARMACOLOGY

Joseph T. Coyle and S. J. Enna

Psychiatric, neurologic, and substance abuse disorders are among the most common, costly, and debilitating conditions that confront the primary care physician. The last decade has witnessed remarkable advances in understanding the pathophysiology and treatment of many of these disorders. This chapter reviews the neuroscientific foundations that inform current strategies for the treatment of these disorders. Basic principles of pharmacodynamics and pharmacokinetics of neuropsychotropic medications are discussed as these play a critical role in drug choice and dosing.

OUTMODED ASSUMPTIONS AND NEW REALITIES

In the recent past, patients with obvious mental illness were referred to psychiatrists or allied mental health professionals for diagnosis and treatment. As psychotherapy was accepted as the nearly universal intervention for the management of mental illness, primary care physicians generally viewed these conditions as beyond their realm of responsibility. With the possible exception of Parkinson's disease and epilepsy, the list of effective treatments for neurologic disorders was brief and the prognosis pessimistic. Therefore, neurologic disorders were also not considered to be the responsibility of primary care physicians.

These assumptions were rendered obsolete by advances in neurology and psychiatry and changes in health care management. Because capitated contracts and HMO arrangements provide disincentives for referral to specialists, as well as liabilities for inappropriate provision of clinical services, there is an increasing movement to "carve out" mental health services from primary medical care as if these two sectors represent easily separable entities. To the contrary, many common neurologic and psychiatric disorders can be managed by the primary care physician. For those patients requiring specialized treatment by psychiatrists, neurologists, and allied mental health professionals, their optimal management necessitates that the primary care physician be knowledgeable about treatment modalities to obviate untoward complications.

It is well documented that medical education has not been very effective in training primary care physicians to identify common psychiatric conditions such as major depressive disorder. Epidemiologic studies indicate that only half of the individuals suffering from an episode of major depressive disorder are diagnosed, with only half of these receiving appropriate pharmacologic treatment (Eisenberg, 1992). Not only does untreated major depressive disorder bear the risk of suicide, it also significantly impairs job performance and social relations (Spitzer et al., 1995). Furthermore, it is increasingly apparent that depression seriously complicates the management and outcomes of medical illness. For example, patients with diabetic retinopathy are much more likely to have a history of a mental disorder, predominantly depression, than diabetics without this condition. Likewise, patients hospitalized for myocardial infarction who have a co-existing depression are much more likely to die in the following 6 months as compared to those without depression (Frasure-Smith et al., 1993). A study of patients ultimately diagnosed for panic disorder demonstrated the recurrent, inappropriate use of medical and emergency services costing thousands of dollars in the year prior to diagnosis. Similarly, studies on elderly depressed patients indicate a much higher utilization of medical services than age-matched controls who were not depressed. Thus, in the context of capitated healthcare, underdiagnosis and inadequate treatment of common mental disorders has a direct, adverse impact on total healthcare costs regardless of whether or not mental health services are included (Strum and Wells, 1995).

Substance abuse disorders have also been generally neglected in primary care. Cultural bias led to the erroneous belief that opioid and cocaine abuse are largely restricted to inner-city minorities whereas, in fact, the majority of abusers are white (Eisenhandler and Drucker, 1993). Indeed, individuals rarely report abuse of substances or ethanol, or minimize it on superficial questioning. Nevertheless, the abuse of ethanol, which has a lifetime prevalence of approximately 20%, represents a major cause of medical morbidity, accidents, and intrafamilial trauma. Substance abuse in general is associated with increased frequency of suicide attempts and in risk-taking behaviors that result in sexually transmitted diseases such as hepatitis and HIV. Aside from the stigma of substance abuse, clinicians often express little interest in treating these patients because of the mistaken belief they are highly resistant to treatment. However, recent clinical and basic research has transformed this perspective on substance abuse by proving it is amenable to therapy, albeit many patients relapse in the early stages of treatment (McLellan et al., 1993). Furthermore, an emerging pharmacology that addresses craving, a common cause of relapse, holds promise for augmenting the traditional 12-step approach.

Vigilance for the early identification of neurologic disorders has traditionally not been high because few effective treatments were available except for epilepsy and Parkinson's disease. In fact, it has long been assumed that neurodegenerative disorders that increase in prevalence with age such as Alzheimer's disease (AD) and amyotrophic lateral sclerosis (ALS), as well as catastrophic damage to the brain caused by ischemia and stroke, were untreatable because dead neurons do not regenerate. However, advances in refining the understanding of the processes regulating neuronal cell death offer real opportunities for delaying, if not preventing, neuronal degeneration in several of these disorders. In fact, recent positive experience with thrombolytics indicate that the same sense of urgency for transporting patients with impending heart attack to the emergency room should be applied to those suffering from cerebral ischemia and early stages of stroke.

The costs to society of central nervous system disorders, including mental illness, substance abuse, and neurologic conditions, are immense in terms of direct care costs, lost wages, and associated expenses. It was established that in 1991 alone these costs exceeded $400 billion. Although the burden of diagnosis and, to a significant extent, management of individuals with central nervous system disorders falls increasingly on the shoulders of the primary care physician, the increasing availability of a broad range of less toxic, but more effective, therapeutic agents means these conditions can be managed with greater confidence. Even when patients are referred to specialists for treatment, the primary care physician, as the "case manager," needs to be familiar with the characteristics, course, and treatments of these disorders to oversee effectively the care of patients in their panels.

Evidence is emerging for many central nervous system disorders that early, effective pharmacologic intervention may slow the progression, or reduce the long-term severity in conditions such as manic depressive illness, schizophrenia, and Parkinson's disease. Preclinical studies suggest that early intervention may also positively influence the course of AD and ALS. Thus, a high diagnostic sensitivity, as opposed to "watchful waiting," becomes increasingly important for reducing adverse outcomes and the aggregate cost of care for those with mental, substance abuse, and neurologic disorders.

Advances fostered by neuroscience research have transformed the understanding of the basic pathologic mechanisms, and accordingly the treatment interventions, for an expanding number of neurologic, psychiatric, and substance abuse disorders. Appreciating these developments is essential for organizing strategies for diagnosis and treatment, and prepares the clinician for the increasingly rapid introduction of new diagnostic methods and therapies.

It is not the purpose of this chapter to provide an in-depth review of the scientific underpinnings of the treatment of neurologic and psychiatric disorders. Interested readers may obtain preclinical information from *Goodman and Gilman's The Pharmacological Basis of Therapeutics* (Hardman et al., 1996). Rather, this offering is intended to provide a context for understanding the pharmacotherapy of psychiatric and neurologic disorders as detailed in the present volume.

NEUROPSYCHOPHARMACOLOGY

Early History

Since prehistoric times humankind has ingested substances for the purpose of altering central nervous system activity. Until the mid-nineteenth century, centrally active agents were found only in crude extracts of plants or animal tissues, or were incidentally synthesized during the fermentation of fruits or grains. Although many of these substances were administered as therapeutics, more often they were used to alter the sensorium for recreational or ceremonial purposes. Examples include extracts of opium, ethyl alcohol, belladonna, mescaline, and psilocybin. Although the analgesic and sedative properties of opium were undoubtedly appreciated, as were the anxiolytic, euphoric, and hypnotic actions of ethanol, responses to these and other natural product extracts were highly variable, and sometimes fatal, since the quantity of active substance varied with the preparation.

Developments in chemistry in the nineteenth century dramatically altered the availability and utility of these and other centrally active substances. In particular, the ability to purify and chemically identify active ingredients made it possible to characterize systematically their beneficial and toxic effects. As chemists developed the means to synthesize new compounds de novo, they were able to prepare derivatives of the naturally occurring agents, some of which were more potent than the parent compound. With these capabilities, it became possible to utilize these drugs in a rational and consistent manner to alter central nervous system function for their therapeutic benefits, although recreational use and abuse remains popular to this day.

Although opium has been used for at least 6000 years, it was not until 1803 that morphine was first isolated, 1832 before codeine was characterized, and 1848 before papaverine was purified from the seed capsules of the poppy plant *Papaver somniferum.* Although nitrous oxide was first synthetized in 1776, and its anesthetic properties noted in 1799, its utility as a general anesthetic was not fully appreciated until 1844. Soon thereafter came ether (1846), chloroform (1847), trichloroethylene (1864), ethylene (1865), and cyclopropane (1882), reflecting the maturation of the field of medicinal chemistry. Other relevant discoveries of note during the nineteenth century include physostigmine, which was isolated from the Calabar bean in 1864 and first used to treat myasthenia gravis in 1932. Mescaline, the active principal of peyote, was isolated in 1896, centuries after it was first employed for its hallucinogenic properties. Likewise, cocaine was isolated in the 1880s, with the purified substance used by Sigmund Freud to treat morphine addicts. Of particular relevance to neuropsychopharmacologists was the use of bromide salts, beginning in 1857, as sedatives and anticonvulsants, since this represents one of the earliest attempts to treat anxiety and epilepsy in a rational manner. The barbiturates were developed during the latter half of the nineteenth century and their sedative, hypnotic, and anticonvulsant actions noted. Indeed, since then some 2500 barbiturates have been synthesized and tested, although only a few were ever widely used. Phenobarbital, one of the more popular members of this class, was originally synthesized in 1912. Other sedative/hypnotic agents discovered during this time were chloral hydrate (1869) and paraldehyde (1882), both of which are still used clinically, some 30 years after the discovery of the benzodiazepines, and 100 years following the barbiturates.

With the availability of purified substances, physiologists and biochemists utilized these new tools to define more precisely fundamental biological systems. These studies provided valuable information on the mechanism of action of these agents that, in turn, was used by chemists to design and synthesize additional compounds. The value of this type of research for developing powerful and selective therapeutic agents led to the establishment of pharmacology as an independent discipline a century ago.

As the chemical, biological, and medical sciences matured in the early twentieth century, a host of new drugs were developed for treating a variety of disorders. Although significant advances were made in relieving pain and inflammation, in preventing and treating infections, in managing cardiovascular, pulmonary, and renal dysfunction, there was little progress in identifying agents capable of attenuating selectively the symptoms of neurological and psychiatric disorders. Indeed, research into these conditions was limited because of the difficulties associated with studying human behavior and an organ as complex as the brain, and the uncertainty about whether mental illness was the result of a biological dysfunction.

With the growing dominance of psychoanalysis in the first half of the twentieth century, pharmacologic treatment of mental disorders was discouraged in favor of psychotherapy. When medical treatment was attempted, common practice at the time included restraints, hydrotherapy, surgery (prefrontal lobotomy), and electrical and drug-induced convulsive therapy. Drug treatment of central nervous system disorders was limited to sedatives and hypnotics, in particular barbiturates and bromides, to induce a nonselective sedation. Those who suffered from less obvious, but in some cases no less severe, forms of mental illness such as anxiety disorders or endogenous depression, went undiagnosed and untreated, except for self-medication, which usually entailed the use of alcohol or opioids. Although some medications, such as atropine, physostigmine, and barbitu-

rates were available to reduce the symptoms associated with Parkinson's disease, myasthenia gravis, and epilepsy, respectively, in general neurological disorders were poorly managed. This reflected, in part, the paucity of knowledge on the fundamental biology of the central nervous system.

Emergence of Neuropsychopharmacology

The mid-twentieth century marked the beginning of clinical psychopharmacology. Thus, in 1949 Cade first described the efficacy of lithium salts in the treatment of mania and in 1952 Delay and his colleagues demonstrated the utility of chlorpromazine for treating psychosis (Cade, 1949; Delay et al., 1952). Unlike the barbiturates and other sedative/ hypnotics, chlorpromazine, which was originally developed to potentiate the action of general anesthetics, selectivity attenuates many of the symptoms of schizophrenia without striking sedation. Soon thereafter Kline discovered that reserpine, a natural product obtained from *Rauwolfia serpentina*, was effective in treating schizophrenic patients (Kline, 1954). Extracts of *R. serpentina* had been used for centuries in India to treat a host of conditions, including hypertension and mental illness. However, it was not until 1954 that reserpine itself was isolated and purified and therefore available for controlled clinical studies. In the late 1950s the selective antidepressant properties of certain antihistamines, now referred to as the tricyclic antidepressants, and of the antitubercular drugs isoniazid and iproniazid, subsequently shown to be monoamine oxidase inhibitors, were noted (Kuhn, 1958). Thus, by 1960, psychopharmacology was firmly established as a field and the notion that mental illness was caused by a correctable biological abnormality was beginning to be accepted.

With the discovery of drugs that selectively relieved the symptoms of schizophrenia and affective illness, pharmacologists were able to define more precisely the biochemical systems involved in these conditions. Brodie and his associates at the National Institutes of Health were the first to discover that reserpine depletes norepinephrine, dopamine, serotonin, and histamine from brain and other tissues (Brodie et al., 1957). Since reserpine is effective in reducing the symptoms of psychosis, but causes depression when administered to mentally healthy individuals, these investigators inferred that schizophrenia is caused by an overabundance of one or more of these neurotransmitters, whereas depression was the consequence of an underactivity in one or more of these systems. Using indirect methods, Carlsson proposed that the phenothiazine antipsychotics, such as chlorpromazine, inhibit dopamine receptors in brain, a theory that has proven accurate over the years (Carlsson and Lindqvist, 1963). Studies by Axelrod and his colleagues at the National Institutes of Health characterized the manner in which monoamines are synthesized, stored, and released from nerve terminals (Axelrod, 1959). These findings led to the discovery that the tricyclic antidepressants inhibit monoamine neurotransmitter reuptake into these terminals, and that isoniazid inhibits monoamine oxidase, an enzyme responsible for the catabolism of these substances. Both of these actions result in the prolongation of neurotransmitter action in the central nervous system. The importance and clinical relevance of these discoveries was evident when new compounds displaying these same actions proved to be clinically effective. Thus rational drug design for developing agents to treat neurological and psychiatric illness came into being.

Throughout the 1960s research in psychopharmacology focused on presynaptic processes, including the identification of neurotransmitters, neurotransmitter reuptake systems, and the enzymes responsible for synthesizing and degrading transmitter agents. Studies such as these revealed that amphetamine causes the release, and inhibits the reuptake, of monoamines, in particular dopamine. It was also during this decade that L-dopa was developed for the treatment of Parkinson's disease (Hornykiewicz, 1973). The benzodiazepines were discovered, which revolutionized the treatment of anxiety, sleep disorders, and epilepsy (Zbinden and Randall, 1967). Neuroscience research during these years revealed that GABA, glycine, and glutamic acid serve as neurotransmitters in brain.

Although it was clear from many elegant electrophysiologic studies that some drugs useful for treating neurological and psychiatric disorders exert their effects on postsynaptic receptors, the lack of a simple biochemical technique to study such interactions hindered work on postsynaptic processes. The situation changed in the early 1970s with the popularization of receptor binding techniques by Snyder and his associates at Johns Hopkins (Yamamura et al., 1985). This simple procedure made possible the direct examination of drug interactions at pre- and postsynaptic receptor sites (Creese et al., 1978). Subsequent studies revealed that, as proposed earlier by Carlsson, antipsychotic potency of drugs used to treat schizophrenia correlated precisely with their affinity for dopamine D-2 receptor. Receptor binding studies revealed that although tricyclic antidepressants inhibit neurotransmitter reuptake, they are also potent antagonists at histamine, cholinergic muscarinic, serotonin, and α-adrenergic receptors, explaining, in part, their side effect profile. Binding studies characterized the receptors for opioids, benzodiazepines, and antiparkinson drugs.

Ascendance of Molecular Strategies

Biochemical, behavioral, and electrophysiologic techniques have developed to a point where it is possible to use approaches designed to determine drug mechanisms of action as screening procedures for discovering new agents. These studies also established that individual neurotransmitters act at multiple, molecularly distinct receptor sites. This suggests the possibility of designing and developing more selective neurotransmitter receptor agonists and antagonists that may be safer than current drugs. Indeed, this notion of developing receptor subtype selective compounds is a driving force in drug discovery today. Evidence of the benefit of this approach is the development of fluoxetine and other selective serotonin reuptake inhibitors (SSRI) that, because of their greater safety profile, have virtually supplanted the use of the tricyclic antidepressants and monoamine oxidase inhibitors for the treatment of depression.

Currently, neuroscientists increasingly employ the tools of molecular biology to address many issues of importance to the neuropsychopharmacologist. The isolation and cloning of genes encoding proteins that participate in neuronal structure and function is accelerating rapidly. Results from these studies, for example, have demonstrated unequivocally the existence of molecularly and pharmacologically distinct receptors for virtually all known neurotransmitters. The ability to express neurotransmitter receptor subtypes individually in cell cultures through transfection has facilitated the development of drugs that interact selectivity and potently with these sites (Tallman and Dahl, 1994). The design and development of sumatriptan, a new drug for the treatment of migraine headache, olanzepine, a new antipsychotic, and zolpidem, a new hypnotic, were aided using this approach. The ability to study neuronal function at the molecular level has also provided new insights into the manner in which neurons adapt when chronically exposed to drugs.

Current neuropsychotropic drug development is increasingly taking advantage of the advances in human molecular genetics that is defining gene alleles responsible for an expanding number of neurologic and psychiatric disorders. For example, mutations responsible for Huntington's disease, ALS, AD, and myotonic dystrophy have been identified, and molecular mechanisms have been extensively characterized. Convincing linkage to genes on chromosome 18 have been developed for manic depressive disorder (Berretini et al., 1994), and an allelic variant of the dopamine D-4 receptor has been associated with attention deficit hyperactivity disorder.

The ability to isolate human gene alleles responsible for brain disorders provides powerful new methods for characterizing the pathophysiology of these disorders and for developing drugs that specifically address these mechanisms. For example, early strategies for treating senile dementia focused on poorly understood enhancers of cerebral function known as nootropics. With the cloning of the gene for amyloid precursor protein (APP), the source of amyloid peptide in the senile plaque, the diagnostic stigma of AD, the processing of APP can be studied in experimental models. Furthermore, the mutant APP gene responsible for early-onset AD has been inserted into the mouse genome through transgenic methods, resulting in mice that develop senile plaques containing human amyloid. It is certain that, as they are identified, human genes responsible for psychiatric disorders including manic depressive illness, schizophrenia, or obsessive-compulsive disorder, for example, will similarly be inserted into the mouse genome to provide animal models for drug development (Holsboer, 1997).

NEUROSCIENCE

The Neuron

The neuron is a highly specialized cell both anatomically and biochemically, responsible for signal transduction and information processing (Fig. 1-1). Unlike many other cell types, such as hepatocytes, after maturation neurons do not undergo replacement by cell division after maturation. This apparent irreplaceability has obvious clinical implications when dealing with a damaged central nervous system, and underlines the importance of early interventions to prevent neuronal death.

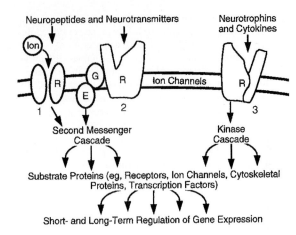

Figure 1–1. Schematic representation of the three major classes of receptors: (1) represents the ligand gated ionic channels; (2) represents the G-protein (G) coupled receptors that activate intracellular metabolic alterations through second messenger systems; (3) represents the tyrosine kinase receptors that mediate the actions of neurotrophins and cytokines through activation of transcription factors.

Neurons consist of four structural components: (1) the cell body, or perikaryon, which contains the nucleus and protein synthetic machinery; (2) the dendrites, the receptive extensions of the neuronal cell body; (3) the axon, which extends from the cell body to innervate other neurons; and (4) the terminal bouton, which forms the synapse for chemical communication with other neurons. Protein synthesis, which is directed by genes contained within the nuclear DNA, takes place primarily in the perikaryon, which supports the structure and function of the entire cell. Protein synthesis occurs by a process of transcription, in which the DNA serves as a template for the synthesis of messenger RNA (mRNA). The mRNA is then processed and exported out of the nucleus to the rough endoplasmic reticulum around the nucleus where the message is translated into protein by ribosomal read-out. Recent data indicate that some mRNA is transported into the dendrites to direct protein synthesis there.

The axon, a membranous tubular extension from the neuronal cell body, conducts electrical impulses to the nerve terminals. Neurons project one axon that branches to varying degrees, depending on the number of neurons on which it makes synaptic contacts. Some neurons have highly restrictive fields of innervation, which are required for very precise communication, whereas others, such as the components of the reticular core aminergic neurons, have extremely diffuse and divergent axonal arbors, contacting literally hundreds of millions of neurons (Coyle, 1986).

The synapse is a specialized structure that serves the purpose of information transduction from one neuron to another. It is comprised of the synaptic bouton at the end of an axon and the adjacent receptive field on the dendrite or neuronal perikaryon of a neighboring neuron. Communication between neurons is mediated primarily by chemical neurotransmitters released by the presynaptic terminal bouton. The neurotransmitters activate receptors on the postsynaptic neuron, which translate the encoded message (see Fig. 1-1). For some neurotransmitters, such as norepinephrine, their synthesis is regulated locally within the presynaptic terminal bouton. Neuropeptides, on the other hand, are synthesized by mRNA-dependent processes within the perikaryon and then transported to the terminal bouton for storage and release.

The excitable nature of the neuronal membrane is a critical feature that permits the cell to integrate information like a transistor. The membrane maintains a voltage gradient between the interior of the neuron and the extracellular fluid, selectively permitting the flow of ions into and out of the cell. Ion distribution across the neuronal membrane is regulated by at least two processes. One of these is the ion "pumps" contained within the membrane that are powered by cellular energy (ATP), and that extrude two sodium ions for each potassium ion that enters. This yields a negative voltage potential of 70mV across the neuronal membrane at rest. When the neuronal membrane is depolarized by activation of sodium ion channels, an action potential generated at the axon hillock proceeds in an anterograde fashion as voltage-dependent sodium channels, the second type of ion-regulating mechanism, successively open like a row of falling dominoes. Other types of ion

channels that play a significant role in modulating neuronal excitability are potassium channels and calcium channels, many of which are the targets of drug action.

Neuronal dendrites and cell bodies are constantly summating excitatory and inhibitory inputs to determine whether the neuron generates an action potential. The influence over this decision is not random, but rather reflects the fact that excitatory terminals are generally concentrated at the distal end of dendrites, whereas inhibitory inputs are located primarily at the proximal end of dendrites and around the perikaryon. This anatomic distribution dictates that inhibitory inputs play the predominant role in determining whether a neuron generates an action potential, which is an all-or-none process. Thus, once adequate depolarization occurs at the axon hillock, an action potential is generated.

Neurotransmitters

The primary process whereby information is conveyed from the presynaptic nerve terminal to the target cell, which may be another neuron, glial cell, or a muscle, is by chemical neurotransmission. The mechanisms of action, as well as side effects, of most drugs used to treat central nervous system disorders are related to their ability to alter neurotransmitter effects in brain (Cooper et al., 1991). Thus, knowledge of the basic principles of chemical neurotransmission, and of the major classes of neurotransmitters, provides a context for understanding the therapeutic actions of most centrally active agents. The dopamine neuron is considered in the following as a model for explicating these processes (Fig. 1-2) and for demonstrating how neurotransmission can be pharmacologically manipulated to influence brain function.

The perikarya of the major dopaminergic neuronal systems are located in the *substantia nigra*, a midbrain region so named because of its pigmentation with neuromelanin, and in the ventral medial tegmental area. The nigral neurons provide a dense innervation to the caudate and putamen, with approximately 15% of the synaptic terminals in these two regions being dopaminergic. The ventral tegmental

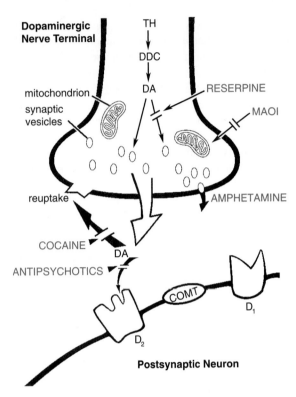

Figure 1–2. *Schematic representation of the dopaminergic synapse. The critical components of the dopaminergic synapse and sites of action of drugs that alter dopaminergic neurotransmission are shown. TH, tyrosine hydroxylase; DDC, dopa decarboxylase; DA, dopamine; MAOI, monoamine oxidase inhibitors; COMT, catechol-o-methyltransferase.*

dopamine neurons terminate in the nucleus accumbens, a reward center, the frontal cortex, cingulate cortex, and hippocampal formation.

Dopamine is synthesized from L-tyrosine, an amino acid devoid of neurophysiologic effects. Tyrosine hydroxylase converts tyrosine to L-dopa (dihydroxyphenylalanine). L-Dopa, through the action of dopa-decarboxylase, a cytosolic enzyme that, like tyrosine, is concentrated in the nerve terminal, is converted to dopamine. Following its synthesis, dopamine is transported into storage vesicles that protect it from enzymatic degradation by monoamine oxidase (MAO) and mediate its release into the syn-

aptic space on depolarization of the terminal bouton. Dopamine levels remain relatively constant in the terminals despite marked changes in neuronal activity, reflecting the tight regulation of its synthesis. Thus, tyrosine hydroxylase is subject to end product inhibition, with excess dopamine inhibiting further synthesis during periods of low neuronal activity. This enzyme inhibition decreases when dopamine is released, thereby enhancing the production of the neurotransmitter. During periods of high neuronal activity, tyrosine hydroxylase is phosphorylated, increasing its affinity for a pteridine cofactor, thereby increasing the efficiency of dopamine synthesis (Nose et al., 1985). With prolonged increases in dopaminergic neuronal activity, the neuron compensates by synthesizing more tyrosine hydroxylase in the perikaryon (enzyme induction), which is then transported down the axons to the terminals.

Regulation of dopamine synthesis at the tyrosine hydroxylase step explains why L-dopa rather than L-tyrosine is effective in the treatment of Parkinson's disease. Because of the feedback inhibition of tyrosine hydroxylase, exogenous L-tyrosine has little influence over dopamine synthesis, whereas dopadecarboxylase, a high-velocity enzyme, is not subject to such inhibition. Thus, administered L-dopa that crosses through the blood-brain barrier into the dopaminergic terminal is rapidly converted to dopamine, increasing the stores of neurotransmitter in the reduced number of dopaminergic terminals characteristic of Parkinson's disease.

Dopamine is enzymatically inactivated by two processes. The first is by MAO, an enzyme located on the exterior membrane of mitochondria in the nerve terminal, which catalyzes the deamination of the transmitter. There are two separate genetic forms of monoamine oxidase: MAO-A, which preferentially catabolizes norepinephrine, serotonin, and dopamine, and MAO-B, which has much broader substrate specificity that includes the biogenic amines and phenethylamines. Inhibitors of MAO are used to enhance dopamine function in Parkinson's disease as well as to increase levels of brain norepinephrine and serotonin in the treatment of depression. Located on the extracellular surface of neurons and glia is catechol-o-methyltransferase, which inactivates dopamine by methylating one of its hydroxyl groups. Together, or individually, deamination and O-methylation inactivate dopamine, transforming it to metabolites having no affinity for dopamine receptors.

Enzymatic degradation is not the primary means for terminating the action of dopamine in the synapse. Rather, this role is played by the active reuptake mechanism on the nerve terminal. The reuptake process, which is driven by the sodium gradient across the neuronal membrane, is mediated by a specific transporter protein that carries dopamine from the extracellular space to the cytosol. The dopamine transporter is a member of a family of related genes that encode for specific neurotransmitter transporters, including those for norepinephrine, serotonin, glutamate, and GABA.

The dopamine transporter is the site of action of cocaine, amphetamine, and methylphenidate (Pacholczyk et al., 1991). By inhibiting the binding of dopamine to the transporter, these drugs increase the extracellular levels of the neurotransmitter prolonging and enhancing activation of dopamine receptors. Studies indicate that the euphoriant and addictive properties of cocaine and other stimulants are a direct function of their ability to increase the postsynaptic action of dopamine by inhibiting its reuptake into neurons in the nucleus accumbens.

The postsynaptic actions of dopamine are mediated by a family of receptors (see Fig. 1-1). These are produced by genes encoding receptors whose intracellular responses are mediated by G proteins. (G refers to the fact that the protein binds guanine nucleotides.) Several different G proteins have been characterized by molecular techniques (Simon et al., 1991). The D-1 and D-5 dopamine receptors couple with Gs, the G protein that activates adenylate cyclase to produce cyclic AMP, an intracellular second messenger. In contrast, the dopamine D-2, D-3, and D-4 receptors couple to Gi, which inhibits adenylate cyclase and the synthesis of cyclic AMP. Both the D-1 and D-2 receptors are broadly expressed in brain regions receiving dopaminergic innervation, whereas dopamine D-3, D-4, and D-5 receptors are found primarily in corticolimbic regions of the brain.

The dopamine D-2 receptor is potently inhibited by antipsychotics such as chlorpromazine, haloperi-dol, and olanzapine, that are used to treat schizophrenia and related psychotic disorders. Conversely, bromocrytine, pergolide, and lisuride stimulate dopamine D-2 receptors and are used to attenuate the symptoms of Parkinson's disease. There is a compelling, significant correlation between the clinical potency of antipsychotic drugs and their affinity for the D-2 receptor (Creese et al., 1976). This mechanism of action also accounts for their tendency to cause extrapyramidal side effects such as parkinsonian symptoms and dystonic reactions. Thus, by blocking dopamine D-2 receptors in the caudate-putamen, these drugs mimic the dopamine deficiency characteristic of Parkinson's disease. Prolonged use of conventional antipsychotics may also produce tardive dyskinesia, a movement disorder that is sometimes irreversible. Brain imaging studies with positron emission tomography indicate that blockade of more than 70% of the dopamine D-2 receptors by antipsychotics is associated with a therapeutic response in psychosis. Because they are localized in the limbic system and cortex, it is thought that dopamine D-3 and/or D-4 receptors, for which typical antipsychotics, and especially the atypical agent clozapine, also have high affinity, and therefore might mediate some of their antipsychotic effects.

Similar mechanisms for the regulation of synthesis, release, and inactivation apply, to a variable degree, to other classical neurotransmitters such as norepinephrine, epinephrine, serotonin, acetylcholine, and histamine, with the receptors mediating their effects being primarily G-protein linked (Table 1-1). Two notable exceptions to this generalization are the nicotinic acetylcholine and 5-HT$_3$ serotonin receptors, both of which are ligand-gated ion channels that pass sodium and, to a lesser degree, calcium.

Amino Acid Transmitters

The amino acid neurotransmitters warrant discussion, not only because they violate the principle that neurotransmitters are synthesized from inactive precursors, but also because they play such an important role in central nervous system disorders. Thus, glutamate appears to be the predominant excitatory neurotransmitter in brain, being utilized in approximately

Table 1-1

Classical Neurotransmitters

Neurotransmitter	Drugs	Indicator	Mechanism
Dopamine	Neuroleptics	Psychosis	D-2 Receptor antagonists
	Stimulants	Attention deficit disorder Narcolepsy	Uptake inhibitors
	Bromocriptine, etc.	Parkinson's disease	D-2 Receptor agonists
Norepinephrine	Antidepressants	Depression, Attention deficit disorder	Uptake inhibitors
Serotonin	Antidepressants	Depression, Panic disorder, Obsessive-compulsive disorder	Uptake inhibitors
Acetylcholine	Cognition enhancers	Alzheimer's disease	Inhibit acetylcholinesterase
	Benztropine, etc.	Parkinsonism	Muscarinic receptor antagonist
Glycine	Strychnine		Receptor antagonist
GABA	Benzodiazepines	Sedation, Anxiety, Muscle relaxation	GABA-A Receptor modulator
	Barbiturates	Epilepsy, Anesthesia	GABA-A Receptor modulator
	Baclofen	Spasticity	GABA-B Receptor agonist
	GABApentin	Epilepsy	GABA Uptake inhibitor
Glutamate	Ketamine	Anesthesia	NMDA Receptor antagonist

40% of all synapses. Both of these amino acids are present in plasma and are important precursors for protein synthesis, a characteristic that would seem incompatible with the role of a neurotransmitter that must exert highly restricted physiologic actions. However, very active and selective transport processes and catabolic enzymes maintain these amino acid neurotransmitters at extremely low concentrations in the extracellular space in brain. For example, in certain brain regions the intracellular concentration of glutamate reaches 5 mM, whereas the concentration in spinal fluid is approximately 0.5 μm, yielding an intracellular-to-extracellular gradient of 10,000.

Glutamate.   As the major excitatory neurons in brain, glutamate-containing neurons are broadly distributed throughout the central nervous system. Included are primary sensory afferents, the climbing fibers innervating the cerebellum, granule cells of the cerebellum, ascending and descending excitatory pathways, excitatory thalamic projections to the cerebral cortex, and cortical pyramidal neurons. Glutamate is sequestered in storage vesicles in the nerve terminal from which it is released into the intrasynaptic space on terminal bouton depolarization. The action of glutamate is terminated by membrane transporters located on glutamatergic neurons and glia, thereby restricting the action of this neurotransmitter to the immediate perisynaptic area. Because these transporters are driven by the sodium gradient across neuronal and glial membranes, under circumstances of energy failure, such as following a stroke or during anoxia, the sodium gradient is dissipated, resulting in a massive release of glutamate into the extracellular space.

The postsynaptic actions of glutamate are mediated by two classes of receptors (see Fig. 1-1): glutamate gated ion channels (iGluRs) and metabotropic receptors (mGluRs), the latter of which are linked to G protein–dependent second messenger systems (Schoepp and Conn, 1993). The glutamate gated ion channels are further subdivided into N-methyl-D-aspartate (NMDA) receptors, which are voltage-dependent cation channels, and the AMPA/kainate voltage-independent cation channels. The genes encoding these proteins, which combine as subunits to form the NMDA and AMPA/KA channels, have been cloned, revealing a significant diversity in their biophysical and pharmacologic characteristics (Seeberg, 1993).

Glutamate acting at AMPA/KA receptors is the primary cause of excitatory postsynaptic potentials. The NMDA receptors at normal resting membrane potential (-70 mV) are inactive because Mg^{2+} blocks the channel. Following neuronal depolarization by activation of AMPA/KA receptors, the Mg^{2+} is removed and the NMDA receptors are then activated by glutamate. Although NMDA receptors also contribute to depolarization by increasing the flow of sodium ions, the channels associated with this receptor are sufficiently large to allow Ca^{2+} entry into the cell as well. This ion, in turn, activates a variety of intracellular systems including nitric oxide synthetase, which generates nitric oxide (NO) from arginine. Nitric oxide is a gaseous molecule that diffuses through cell membranes and interacts with a variety of adjacent cells. One target of nitric oxide is guanylate cyclase, which when activated catalyzes the synthesis of cyclic GMP, another second messenger. Thus, activation of NMDA receptors exerts direct excitatory effects on individual neurons as well as a more widespread metabolic effect on surrounding neurons and their processes by stimulating the production of NO.

NMDA receptors play a critical role in a form of synaptic plasticity, known as long-term potentiation, that is intimately related to memory. This phenomenon, first described in the hippocampus, a brain structure essential for memory formation, reflects a use-dependent alteration in synaptic efficacy (Bliss and Collinridge, 1993). Long-term potentiation has been demonstrated when presynaptic glutamatergic terminals are electrically stimulated and responses from the postsynaptic neuron recorded. With low levels of presynaptic stimulation, a proportional postsynaptic excitatory response is measured. However, if the presynaptic axon is stimulated at high velocity, such as 100 mHz, the efficacy of synaptic transmission is irreversibly enhanced such that the previous level of presynaptic stimulation results in a much more robust postsynaptic excitatory response. Thus, under these circumstances the response to this specific input is markedly accentuated in a use-dependent manner.

It is not surprising, therefore, that drugs that block the NMDA receptor channel, such as phencyclidine (PCP, "angel dust") and ketamine, are dissociative anesthetics that impair memory. Moreover, at subanesthetic doses these drugs exhibit striking psychotomimetic properties. Thus, PCP and ketamine produce in normal individuals the full range of symptoms of schizophrenia including delusions, thought disorder, negative symptoms, and frontal lobe cognitive impairment. These effects prompted the hypothesis that the symptoms of schizophrenia may result from a reduction in the activity of corticolimbic NMDA receptors (Olney and Farber, 1995).

Persistent activation of glutamate-gated ion channels results in a type of neuronal degeneration known as "excitotoxicity." This was originally observed by Olney (1969) who demonstrated that the administration of monosodium glutamate to neonatal rats causes a selective degeneration of neurons in the arcuate nucleus, whereas axons passing through this area, and the surrounding glia, were spared. Subsequent studies revealed a significant correlation between the neurotoxic properties and excitatory effects of substances that stimulate glutamate receptors. Massive activation of glutamate-gated ion channels causes a rapid necrosis of neurons, resulting from an overwhelming influx of Na^+, H_2O, and Ca^{2+}. Recent studies demonstrated that moderate, persistent activation of glutamate-gated ion channels causes a delayed form of neuronal degeneration with the characteristics of apoptosis or programmed cell death (Simonian and Coyle, 1996). Oxidative stress, with cumulative damage to the neuronal DNA, appears to be an important mediator of the form of glutamate neurotoxicity that triggers apoptosis.

Because dysregulation of glutamatergic neurotransmission is implicated in a broad range of neurodegenerative disorders, the pharmaceutical industry has invested heavily in research directed toward the development of drugs that interfere with excitotoxic phenomena. This includes the design of glutamate receptor antagonists, glutamate receptor modulators, and inhibitors of events that occur following glutamate receptor function that contribute to oxidative stress and apoptotic neuronal death. It is likely that such drugs will soon be introduced into the clinic offering the possibility of treating disorders that heretofore were thought to be untreatable. Thus, anoxia and ischemia resulting from local or global hypoperfusion as a consequence of thromboembolic events, cardiac arrest, or drowning result in the loss of oxygen to the brain parenchyma and in the consequent failure of oxidative metabolism of glucose, the primary source of ATP in brain (Choi and Rothman, 1990). Since the transport processes maintaining low extracellular glutamate levels in brain are energy dependent, the fall in ATP causes a reversal of the glutamate transport gradient, resulting in high concentrations of the transmitter in the extracellular space. This leads to a massive activation of glutamate receptors and neuronal degeneration. Although the core area of zero blood flow becomes rapidly necrotic, a large surrounding penumbra of impaired oxygenation utilization exhibits a more delayed neuronal degeneration. Depending on the brain region and type of insult, this delayed degeneration may be mediated by AMPA/KA receptors and/or NMDA receptors. Accordingly, it seems plausible that rapid intervention with a combination of thrombolytics and glutamate receptor antagonists will become the standard of care for stroke patients. Furthermore, it is likely that drugs acting on glutamate receptor systems, or which influence its downstream mediators, will be used prophylacticly in procedures where there is a high risk of brain embolic events or hypoperfusion, such as open heart surgery.

Huntington's disease is a hereditary neurodegenerative disorder characterized by choreoathetotic movements, psychiatric symptoms, and a progressive dementia. The mutation in Huntington's disease, which is transmitted as an autosomal dominant, involves the expansion of a CAG trinucleotide repeat that results in a marked increase in the glutamine residues in the protein huntingtin (MacDonald and Gusella, 1996). The neuropathology of Huntington's disease is reproduced in experimental animals by the intrastriatal injection of NMDA receptor agonists. Such lesions faithfully recreate the very selective pattern of neuronal degeneration characteristic of Huntington's disease. Although the precise mechanism of neuronal degeneration in Huntington's disease remains unclear, it appears the mutant huntingtin sensitizes neurons to NMDA receptor-mediated toxicity. Given the role of oxidative stress in this process, it is noteworthy that clinical trials have demonstrated that vitamin E, a membrane free radical scavenger, slows the progress of Huntington's disease when it is administered early in the course of the disorder.

ALS is an age-related disorder characterized by a progressive degeneration of motor neurons and of pyramidal cells in the motor cortex. Tissue culture studies demonstrate that persistent, low-level activation of glutamate receptors causes a selective degeneration of motor neurons by a process that is prevented by AMPA/KA receptor antagonists. Clinical studies show that glutamate levels in the CSF are elevated in patients suffering from ALS. Furthermore, in the hereditary or familial forms of ALS (FALS), a number of mutations in the gene encoding for superoxide dismutase, the main enzymatic protectant against oxidative stress, have been identified (Deng et al., 1993). As oxidative stress is an intermediate step in delayed glutamate receptor–induced neuronal degeneration, this finding supports the hypothesis that glutamate-related excitotoxic phenomena might be central to the disorder. Consistent with this inference are the results of post-mortem studies indicating a reduction in the expression of glutamate transporters in those who suffered with the "sporadic" form of ALS.

As for AD, there is compelling evidence that amyloid aggregates in senile plaques are the proximate cause of the neuronal degeneration responsible for this condition (Sandbrink et al., 1996). Amyloid precursor protein (APP), a cell surface glycoprotein normally expressed in brain and other tissues, is degraded by two pathways, one of which yields amyloid peptide. Mutations in the APP gene associated with familial early-onset AD favor the degradation pathway that generates amyloid peptide. In addition, more common mutations in two genes encoded on chromosome 14 and chromosome 1, known as presinilin 1 and 2, respectively, favor a catabolic route for APP that generates amyloid peptide. It has been demonstrated that aggregated amyloid sensitizes neurons to glutamate-induced excitotoxicity and generates reactive oxygen species that may potentiate glutamate toxicity because of the sensitivity of glutamate transporters to oxidative damage. Consistent with this is the finding that centrally active antioxidants such as aspirin, estrogen, and vitamin E appear to slow the progression, or delay the onset, of AD.

γ-Aminobutyric acid. Cells that utilize γ-aminobutyric acid (GABA) as a neurotransmitter are the primary inhibitory neurons in brain. Indeed, it is estimated that approximately 40% of synapses in the brain are GABAergic. Thus, GABAergic neurons are widespread in brain and include inhibitory interneurons in corticolimbic areas, output neurons from the caudate and putamen, Purkinje cells in the cerebellum, and local circuit inhibitory neurons in the spinal cord. Because GABAergic neurons play a dominant role in restraining neuronal activity, GABA receptor antagonists cause generalized seizures. Furthermore, the distribution of GABAergic synaptic inputs reinforces this inhibitory role because they are concentrated on the proximal dendrites and cell bodies. Thus, GABAergic inputs determine whether local depolarization by glutamate is sufficient to generate an action potential.

The synthesis of GABA is catalyzed by glutamate decarboxylase, which converts glutamate to GABA in the cytoplasm of the terminal bouton. Following its production, GABA is accumulated into storage vesicles that are critical to synaptic release and that protect it from degradation by GABA-transaminase, an enzyme localized to the outer mitochondrial membrane. The GABA released into the synaptic space following terminal depolarization is inactivated primarily by a sodium-dependent, high-affinity transport process that reaccumulates the neurotransmitter in the presynaptic terminal.

The postsynaptic effects of GABA are mediated by two classes of receptors: the GABA-gated ion channels (GABA-A) and those linked to G proteins (GABA-B). The GABA-B receptors are the site of action of baclofen, a muscle relaxant used to treat spasticity. The GABA-A receptors appear to be the major site of action of several classes of centrally active drugs. Thus, activation of these receptor ionophore complexes by GABA or GABA-A receptor agonists results in the opening of channels through which chloride flows, resulting in neuronal hyperpolarization. Hyperpolarization moves the voltage differential across the membrane lower, diminishing the glutamatergic excitatory drive and raising the threshold for the generation of action potentials.

A family of genes has been characterized that encode for the polypeptides that combine to form the heteromeric GABA-gated ion channels (Levitan et al., 1988). There is considerable heterogeneity in the pharmacologic and biophysical characteristics of these GABA receptors. An important allosteric site on some GABA-gated ion channels is the benzodiazepine receptor. By binding to this site, benzodiazepines enhance the sensitivity of the receptor to GABA. Thus, benzodiazepine receptor agonists are indirect modulators of GABA receptor function in that they require the presence of GABA to exert their hypnotic, anxiolytic, muscle relaxant, and anticonvulsant effects.

Given the primary role of GABA in regulating neuronal excitability, it is not surprising that a number of antiepileptic agents influence GABAergic transmission. Barbiturates, including phenobarbital, appear to prolong GABA-A receptor channel opening, enhancing the response to the neurotransmitter. GABApentin, a newer antiepileptic, influences the uptake of GABA, prolonging its synaptic action.

Neuropeptides

Over the last two decades an expanding number of neuropeptide signaling molecules have been identified in brain (Hokfelt, 1991). Unlike conventional neurotransmitters, which are synthesized by enzymatic processes located within the terminal bouton, neuropeptides are produced within the neuronal cell body. The synthesis of neuropeptides, which are small proteins, is directed by mRNA transcribed from nuclear DNA. Thus, the neuropeptide content within the terminal bouton depends entirely on the synthesis, processing, and transport of the substance from the cell body. Accordingly, neuropeptide-containing neurons may be less rapidly responsive to prolonged increases in the release of neurotransmitter than is the case for monoamines or amino acids because of the delay between the synthesis of the neuropeptide in the cell body and its transport to the axon terminals.

An intriguing aspect of neuropeptide synthesis is that a single gene often directs the production of multiple neuropeptides, and the types of peptides produced from a single gene may vary in different neuronal cell types. This diversity is imparted after transcription of the gene that encodes the peptide precursor. Thus, most genes have their protein coding sequences, called *exons,* interrupted by noncoding sequences, *introns.* When a gene is transcribed, the primary mRNA transcript is co-linear with the DNA and therefore contains both exons and introns. Before the mRNA leaves the nucleus to be translated, the introns are removed and the exons spliced to form the mature mRNA. The diversity of neuropeptides generated by a single gene is owing to the fact that the primary mRNA transcripts of the genes are spliced in alternate ways in different cell types. By including or excluding particular exons in the mature cytoplasmic mRNA, different peptides are produced. Proopiomelacortin (POMC) is a particularly interesting example because it contains a sequences of several active peptides with different biologic functions that are differentially expressed in pituitary cells and neurons. These include beta-lipoprotein, adrenocorticotrophin hormone (ACTH), beta-endorphin, melanocyte stimulating hormone (MSH), and melanocortin. As the number of identified neuropeptides that subserve neurotransmitter function in the brain is increasing steadily, they undoubtedly will be important targets for new centrally active drugs (Table 1-2).

Following their synthesis, neuropeptides are packaged in storage vesicles in which they are transported to the nerve terminal. Until recently it was believed that neurons release only one type of neurotransmitter; however, studies have shown that neuropeptides are co-localized in neurons that use a variety of classical neurotransmitters. Furthermore, neurophysiologic data indicate that neuropeptide release occurs primarily during periods of high presynaptic neuronal activity, whereas other neurotransmitters are released in proportion to the number of presynaptic action potentials. Thus, neuropeptides appear to play a role in modulating the function of other neurotransmitters. Consistent with this hypothesis is the fact that the vast majority of receptors that mediate the action of neuropeptides are linked to G proteins. Furthermore, there is no simple relationship between a given neuropeptide and a particular neurotransmitter. Thus, although some striatal GABAergic neurons also contain enkephalin, others do not. Likewise, dopaminergic neurons in the ventral tegmental area express cholecystokinin, whereas those in the substantia nigra do not. Co-localization of neurotransmitters provides an opportunity for highly complex mixing and matching of neuronal signaling within the synapse, a property that has significant implications for drug actions in brain.

Although neuropeptides, like classical neurotransmitters, subserve a variety of functions in brain, certain dominant effects have obvious clinical importance. For example, enkephalin is a pentapeptide that, along with the larger forms endorphin and dynorphin, activate opioid receptors. A family of genes encode for G protein–coupled opioid receptors. These receptors appears to be particularly important with regard to suppressing the transmission of painful stimuli and are the site of action of morphine and related opioids. Current research is directed at parsing these receptors to identify those that are specific for reducing pain perception as opposed to those involved in the euphoriant and respiratory suppressant effects of opioids. The enkephalin/opioid receptors in the

Table 1-2
Neuropeptides

Neuropeptide	Function
ACTH	Corticosteriod release
Corticotrophin releasing factor (CRF)	Central stress and anxiety circuits
Cholecystokinin	Appetite regulation
Prolactin	Milk ejection
Vasopressin	Obsessional behavior(?)
Enkephalin, endorphin	Pain suppression
Neurotensin	Antipsychotic action(?)
N-Acetyl aspartyl glutamate	Neuroprotection
Substance P	Pain transmission
Galanin	Cognition/memory(?)
Leptin	Body weight
Melanocortin	Body weight

nucleus accumbens appear to be part of the final common pathway of the reinforcing effects of substances of abuse, including heroin, alcohol, and nicotine. Thus, naltrexone, an opioid receptor antagonist, reduces the relapse rate of abstinent alcoholics. Moreover, naloxone, a potent opioid receptor antagonist, is an antidote for opioid overdose, such as with morphine or heroin, although it acts at the receptor that mediates the physiologic effects of endogenous enkephalin.

Several other neuropeptide systems are the targets of drug development. For example, because cholecystokinin plays a major role in regulating appetite, drugs that interact with cholecystokinin receptor subtypes display promise as appetite suppressants for those with morbid obesity. Corticotrophin releasing factor (CRF), a modulator of brain systems that mediate the stress response, is implicated in the pathophysiology of depression and anxiety. Because of this, CRF receptor antagonists are currently being studied as antidepressants and anxiolytics. Vasopressin causes stereotypical and compulsive behaviors when injected into experimental animals, with data indicating its disposition may be altered in obsessive-compulsive disorder. Accordingly, drugs that interfere with vasopressin receptor activation may provide therapeutic benefit in the treatment of this disorder and related conditions.

Trophic Factors

Recently, a new class of signaling polypeptides has been identified in brain. These substances, which have trophic and cytoxic effects on neurons and glia, activate tyrosine kinase receptors (Thoenen, 1995). These receptors (see Fig. 1-1) work through a process of dimerization whereby the ligand on the extracellular surface of the cell membrane unites two transmembrane proteins that together generate an enzymatic response. This results in the phosphorylation of tyrosine residues on intracellular messenger proteins known as transcription factors. In turn, the phosphorylated proteins activate a cascade of metabolic events that alter gene expression. Tyrosine kinase-mediated responses subserve the effects of an growing number of growth factors and cytokines. Beta-

interferon, a drug recently introduced to treat multiple sclerosis, acts through a tyrosine kinase-type receptor.

Thus, the majority of neuropsychotropic medications exert their therapeutic effects by altering the synaptic actions of specific neurotransmitters. The sites of molecular intervention are diverse in the sequence of biochemical events responsible for the synthesis, storage, release, receptor binding, reuptake, and enzymatic degradation of these substances (see Fig. 1-2). Methods for promoting neurotransmitter effects include precursor loading (L-dopa), enhancement of release (amphetamine), inhibition of catabolic enzymes (monoamine oxidase inhibitors), inhibition of reuptake (antidepressants), or direct activation of receptors (morphine). Conversely, strategies for attenuating neurotransmitter effects include depletion of storage vesicles (reserpine), inhibition of release (α-adrenergic receptor agonists) or blockade of postsynaptic receptors (antipsychotics).

Adaptive Responses to Neuropsychotropic Drug Treatment

Pharmacologic treatment of neuropsychiatric disorders, with the possible exception of acute interventions such as the use of diazepam in the treatment of status epilepticus, is associated with adaptive responses to chronic drug administration. Thus, the clinical effects of antidepressants and antipsychotics require several weeks of administration before full efficacy is attained. Treatment of Parkinson's disease with CarbiDopa/L-dopa generally results in loss of efficacy and an increase in side effects over time. Chronic use of opioids to treat pain is characterized by tolerance and the need for escalating doses, and dependency. Recent research has provided new insights into the mechanisms responsible for these adaptive changes.

Plasticity is a fundamental property of the nervous system. Moreover, the adaptive response of the nervous system to chronic pharmacologic treatment is associated with the therapeutic response to neuropsychotropic drugs as well as to their side effects. Although this adaptation occurs at many levels of organization within the cell, it ultimately reflects alterations of gene expression (Hyman and Nestler, 1993).

Many centrally active drugs directly or indirectly exert their effects by altering neurotransmitter receptor function. Thus, antipsychotics block dopamine D-2 receptors, whereas antidepressants potentiate the action of dopamine, norepinephrine, and/or serotonin by inhibiting their reuptake. What has increasingly attracted the attention of neuroscientists are the mechanisms responsible for delays in therapeutic responses. Although much is known about the primary sites of action of neuropsychotropic drugs, it is appreciated these acute effects cannot explain the full range of therapeutic benefits.

Studies with antidepressants provide an example of adaptive mechanisms that may account for delayed therapeutic effects. A peculiar feature of these drugs is their ability to enhance synaptic function for two distinct neurotransmitter systems, norepinephrine and/or serotonin, by inhibiting their neuronal reuptake. Chronic treatment with antidepressants in normal experimental animals results in a delayed, albeit rapid, decrease in β-adrenergic receptor number and function in brain. This implies that antidepressants, counter-intuitively, exert their effects by attenuating central noradrenergic neurotransmission, which is inconsistent with other lines of evidence implicating hypofunction of central noradrenergic activity in the pathophysiology of depression.

Molecular neurobiologic approaches appear to have resolved these apparently conflicting data by defining the long-term impact of chronic antidepressant treatment on neuronal gene expression (Duman et al., 1995). These studies indicate a commonalty between β-adrenergic receptors and subsets of serotonin receptors in affecting the cyclic AMP intracellular signaling pathway (Fig. 1-3). Given the overlap in the pattern of innervation by noradrenergic and serotonergic terminal fibers in corticolimbic regions, this convergence could explain the comparable therapeutic efficacy of norepinephrine and serotonin reuptake inhibitors. Furthermore, these studies revealed an increase in the amount of the cyclic AMP response element binding protein (CREB) that mediates the effects of adrenergic and serotonergic receptor activation of cellular gene expression. Accordingly, in

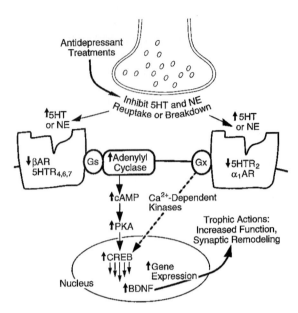

Figure 1–3. *Model of synaptic adaptation of chronic antidepressant treatment. Antidepressants increase the intrasynaptic concentrations of serotonin (5HT) and/or norepinephrine (NE) by inhibiting their reuptake, resulting in a rapid downregulation of β-adrenergic and serotonin receptors as well as α₁-adrenergic receptor. However, chronic treatment with these drugs results in increased levels of cyclic AMP response element binding protein (CREB), a nuclear transcription factor which increases gene expression of brain derived nerve growth factor (BDNF). (Adapted from Duman RS, Henninger GR, Nestler EJ: A molecular and cellular theory of depression.* Arch Gen Psychiatry *1997;54:597–606.)*

spite of β-adrenergic receptor desensitization resulting from chronic drug treatment, the overall impact of antidepressant administration is to persistently enhance the intracellular responses to norepinephrine and serotonin. Finally, activation of the CREB pathway by antidepressant administration induces the expression of brain derived growth factor (BDNF), a peptide that exerts trophic effects on hippocampal neurons. Notably, treatment of rats with BDNF causes behavioral alterations similar to those observed with antidepressants in behavioral models of major depressive disorder. It appears, therefore, that antidepressants may exert functional as well as structural effects on hippocampal and cortical neurons by enhancing BDNF expression.

This example of neuroadaptive consequences to chronic treatment with antidepressants represents only one of the numerous ways in which neuropsychotropic drugs exert their delayed therapeutic effects. A recurring theme from this research is that the therapeutic response often results from drug-induced alterations in gene expression. As advances in molecular genetics reveal the precise molecular pathologies responsible for neurologic and psychiatric disorders, it is likely that drugs will be developed that more directly correct deviant gene expression.

BIOAVAILABILITY

As with all medications, the clinical response to centrally active agents is determined by factors influencing the concentration of the substance at its site of action. Chief among these are the rate and extent of absorption, distribution, metabolism, and excretion. These properties are a function of a host of factors, such as the physicochemical properties of the drug, the dose administered, blood flow at the absorbing surface and target tissue, gastrointestinal motility, the amount of biotransforming enzyme, the number of active metabolites, and hepatic and renal function. These, in turn, vary to some extent, with gender, age, ethnicity, degree of infirmity, and the presence of environmental and other therapeutic agents. Because most neurological and psychiatric conditions are chronic, drugs may be taken for months or years, making it essential the physician has an understanding about the manner in which these factors, which can change over time, influence the therapeutic response.

Reviewed in the following are some general principles pertaining to this issue, with particular emphasis on their importance with respect to drugs used to treat neurological and psychiatric conditions. Readers desiring a more extensive treatment of this topic are urged to consult the relevant chapters in *Goodman and Gilman's The Pharmacological Basis of Therapeutics.*

Absorption and Distribution

Because most neuropsychopharmacological agents are weak acids or bases they exist in both ionized and un-ionized forms depending on their pKa and the pH of their environment. Since the un-ionized form of a drug is more lipophilic, it more readily crosses membrane barriers and penetrates into cells. Lipophilicity is an important, indeed crucial, feature of drugs used to treat central nervous system disorders since the bulk flow of solutes across capillaries is quite limited in brain because of the tight junctions between endothelial cells (blood-brain barrier). Thus, to gain entry into the central nervous system, a drug must be able to diffuse passively from the blood into the tissue or be accumulated by an active, specialized transporter. Examples of the former abound among psychotherapeutic agents, including the antipsychotics, such as haloperidol and clozapine, antidepressants, such as imipramine and fluoxetine, and anxiolytics, such as diazepam and buspirone. L-Dopa is an example of a drug that gains entry into the brain by an active process. In this case, the drug utilizes the transport system responsible for transferring aromatic amino acids from blood into the central nervous system. Although the rate of passive diffusion is controlled primarily by the concentration gradient of the drug on either side of the membrane, the rate of accumulation by an active process is dependent on the availability of the transporter. Thus, dietary substances that utilize the same transporter as L-dopa compete with it for these sites, influencing the concentration of the drug in brain and, ultimately, in the dopamine nerve terminal.

Because of their lipophilic properties, drugs used to influence central nervous system function readily penetrate into highly vascularized organs and tissues, such as the brain. Lipid stores, with their more limited blood flow, accumulate these drugs more slowly, but ultimately in greater concentrations. This is an important principle since the concentration of a lipophilic agent in brain and other vascularized tissue declines much more rapidly than is the case for fat stores that act as depots or reservoirs for the drug. This explains, in part, why traces of antipsychotic metabolites are found in urine weeks after terminating drug therapy. This phenomenon also contributes to the prolonged response to drugs, such as hypnotics, when therapy is halted after several weeks of treatment. Because of this slow clearance the patient may not experience psychological or physiologic withdrawal from the medication until several days after the last dose since the drug is being leeched from lipid stores in quantities sufficient to maintain clinically relevant blood levels.

The extent of ionization also influences the distribution and retention of a drug in tissue. Thus, because approximately 25% of phenobarbital, a weak acid, is excreted unchanged by the kidney, it is possible to enhance its elimination by increasing the pH (alkalinization) of the urine. Conversely, a drug will exit the brain more slowly than it entered if a greater percentage of it is in the ionized, and therefore less lipophilic, form in neuronal and glial tissue than in blood.

Most drugs used to treat pain, psychiatric and neurological conditions are administered orally. This is possible because, as indicated, most are highly lipophilic and therefore readily diffuse through the intestine into the blood and from the blood into brain. Once absorbed from the gastrointestinal tract, drugs pass through the liver before reaching other organs. Because the liver is the primary site for metabolism, some agents are enzymatically inactivated before they have an opportunity to reach the central nervous system (first-pass effect). This rapid metabolism significantly reduces the bioavailability and, in some cases, renders a drug unsuitable for oral administration. Thus, the ergot alkaloids, such as ergotamine, used to treat migraine headache, are extensively metabolized following oral administration, with only a small percentage of an administered dose surviving the first pass through the liver. Likewise, opioids are subject to first-pass metabolism, with up to 75% of the administered dose being biotransformed immediately after absorption from the intestine. Indeed butorphanol, a mixed agonist/antagonist opioid, is almost completely destroyed in this way when given orally. First-pass metabolism was evaded in this instance by preparing a dosage form that is administered intranasally.

The rate of absorption following oral administration can sometimes be erratic, even for very lipid soluble agents. Thus, the presence of food or ancillary effects of the drugs themselves may delay absorption. For example, many tricyclic drugs, such as certain antidepressants and antipsychotics, are potent anticholinergics. As such, they reduce gastrointestinal motility and delay their own absorption.

Other routes of administration used for drugs aimed at modifying central nervous system function include intravenous, intrathecal, intramuscular, and inhalation. The intravenous route is utilized for anticonvulsants, such as diazepam, to terminate an episode of status epilepticus. Analgesics, such as some opioids, or muscle relaxants, such as baclofen, are sometimes administered intrathecally to enhance the desired response while minimizing side effects. Haloperidol decanoate is administered intramuscularly to act as a depot, resulting in prolonged release of this antipsychotic into the circulation. When given in this way, a single injection of haloperidol decanoate will control symptoms for up to 4 weeks in patients who would otherwise be required to take their medication orally on a daily basis. Although inhalation of centrally active agents as a preferred route of administration is limited primarily to volatile and gaseous anesthetics, this route is also widely utilized for substance abuse. Thus, the lungs are the site of absorption for nicotine, cannabinoids, and cocaine when tobacco, marijuana, and crack, respectively, are smoked, and for toluene, kerosene, amyl nitrate, and nitrous oxide vapors when these are inhaled for recreational purposes. As indicated, intranasal administration is used for butorphanol to reduce its rate of metabolism, but it is also commonly used as a route of entry for cocaine.

Following absorption into blood, many neuropsychopharmacological agents are bound to plasma proteins. Acidic drugs, such as barbiturates, bind to albumin, whereas basic ones bind to α_1-acid glycoproteins. Although most lipophilic agents tend to be extensively bound to plasma proteins, this is not always the case. For example, whereas virtually all barbiturates bind to albumin to some extent, with the degree of binding being roughly proportional to lipophilicity, ethosuximide, a lipophilic anticonvulsant, is not bound to plasma proteins to a significant extent.

Drug binding to plasma proteins is important for various reasons. The bound drug is unavailable for diffusing into brain, limiting the amount of active agent that reaches the site of therapeutic action. Moreover, most drugs bind to nonspecific anionic or cationic sites on plasma proteins, making them subject to displacement by other agents, some of which may be chemically and pharmacologically unrelated. For example, barbiturates and salicylates, both weak acids, compete for the same binding sites on albumin. Therefore, it is possible that an arthritic patient receiving high doses of salicylates will have higher circulating levels of the anti-inflammatory agent or of phenobarbital if treated with the barbiturate for seizures. Thus, although total blood levels of either drug may be in the normal therapeutic range, the amount of unbound drug available for exerting a therapeutic or toxic effect may be significantly elevated.

Although the measurement of drug blood levels is useful in monitoring therapy for some central nervous system disorders, in particular epilepsy, it is of limited value in others. Thus, although attempts have been made to match blood levels of commonly used antidepressants and antipsychotics with clinical response, the correlations obtained are imprecise and highly variable. Although the reasons for this are unknown, it is likely they relate to the heterogeneity of the conditions themselves and, in some cases, to the formation of active metabolites, which renders measurement of only the parent compound of little relevance. Nonetheless, these studies have provided ranges that can be utilized to assess whether the drug selected for a particular condition is likely to yield a beneficial response.

Although the number of factors influencing the absorption and distribution, and therefore the bioavailability, of central nervous system active agents is daunting, they are remarkably constant, especially if the patient is receiving only a single medication. Indeed, as newer drugs are developed to maximize the separation between the therapeutically efficacious dose and the dose that induces side effects and toxicities (therapeutic window), fluctuations in blood levels become less troublesome. Nevertheless, an appreciation of the factors that influence absorption and distribution is crucial when undertaking a change in medication or dose, when a predicted therapeutic response is not obtained, or when side effects are intolerable.

Metabolism and Excretion

Once a drug is absorbed and distributes throughout the body, the rate and extent of metabolism and excretion become the critical factors in determining its concentration at the site of action. Metabolism in particular is a crucial variable, especially for lipophilic agents. Thus, lipophilic solutes are extensively reabsorbed by the kidney, limiting their excretion in urine. Indeed, a lipophilic substance that is not made more polar by metabolism would, theoretically, have a half-life of infinity. Thus, because of their lipophilic nature, most central nervous system active agents are metabolized prior to excretion. Exceptions to this rule include lithium ion used to treat bipolar illness and GABApentin, an anticonvulsant, both of which are excreted unchanged in urine.

Although, in general, drug metabolism, or biotransformation, generates less active or inactive metabolites of the parent compound, there are significant exceptions to this rule. Thus, many of the metabolites of some benzodiazepines are pharmacologically active, prolonging the response to these agents even when blood levels of the parent compound have diminished considerably. Primidone, an anticonvulsant used to treat partial and generalized tonic-clonic seizures, is metabolically converted to phenobarbital and phenylethylmalonamide, both of which are effective anticonvulsants. The demethylation of the antidepressants imipramine, amitriptyline, and fluoxetine yields desipramine, nortriptyline, and norfluoxetine, respectively, antidepressants in their own right. In some cases a metabolite may be a more potent therapeutic than the parent compound, as is the glucuronide metabolite of morphine.

Drug metabolism is divided into two major categories: Phase I and Phase II. Phase I metabolism results in the introduction or the exposure of a functional group, such as occurs following hydrolysis of an ester or amide linkage, N- or O-dealkylation, N- or S-oxidation, aromatic, and aliphatic hydroxylation and deamination. These reactions are generally catalyzed by a family of enzymes referred to as the cytochrome P450s. Phase II metabolism entails conjugation by glucuronidation, acetylation, or sulfation of functional groups exposed by Phase I metabolism. Individual drugs commonly undergo more than one type of Phase I transformation, as well as conjugation reactions. In combination, Phase I and Phase II metabolism convert lipophilic drugs to polar metabolites that are more readily excreted in urine.

Although drug metabolizing enzymes are found in virtually all tissues and organs, they are most widely represented and highly concentrated in the liver, making it the major site for biotransformation. As a rule, Phase I enzymes are located on the endoplasmic reticulum, whereas Phase II enzymes are found in the cytosol. When considering the importance of metabolism on the clinical response to drugs, most emphasis is placed on the cytochrome P450 monooxygenase system, enzymes involved in Phase I biotransformations (Wrighton and Stevens, 1992; Parkinson, 1996).

In humans there are a dozen liver microsomal cytochrome P450 enzyme families. The nomenclature applied to this group of enzymes includes, in all cases, the designation CYP to indicate it is a cytochrome P450. A family is defined as a group of enzymes with less than 40% amino acid identity with other families. In general, subfamily members have 55% homology or greater. The CYP designation is followed by a number which indicates the gene family, a letter designating the subfamily, and another number to identify the particular gene encoding this enzyme. Of the four families currently known, CYP1, CYP2, CYP3, and CYP4, only the first three appear to be extensively involved in drug metabolism. The CYP4 family is concerned primarily with metabolism of endogenous agents, although all four groups metabolize endogenous substances, in particular glucocorticoids and fatty acids. Of the various families and subfamilies, CYP2D6 and CYP3A, in particular CYP3A4, appear to be the most important for drug metabolism, with over 50% of drugs biotransformed by these enzymes. Moreover, CYP3A4 is induced by various centrally active drugs, including phenobarbital, phenytoin, and carbamazepine, and is inhibited by macrolide antibiotics and imidazole antimycotics (Table 1-3). Enzyme induction increases the amount of enzyme, enhancing the rate of metabolism, whereas enzyme inhibition decreases the rate and extent of biotransformation. Both of these effects are of particular relevance for drugs used to treat pain, neurological, and psychiatric disorders.

A variety of factors influence cytochrome P450 enzyme activity, thereby influencing the rate of drug biotransformation, drug blood levels, the amount of drug at the active site and, ultimately, the clinical response. Included are environmental agents, drugs, disease, age, gender, and ethnicity. Thus, carbamazepine induces the cytochrome P450 enzymes involved in its metabolism, enhancing its own biotransformation as well as that of any other drug metabolized by these enzymes (Table 1-3). A practical example of this phenomenon is the interaction between glucocorticoids and anticonvulsants, both of which are metabolized by CYP3A4. Thus, a patient experiencing seizures caused by a brain tumor will typically be treated with an anticonvulsant, such as phenytoin, to attenuate the seizures and a corticosteroid to reduce brain edema. Over time, phenytoin will induce CYP3A4 activity to the extent that the rates of metabolism of the glucocorticoid and the anticonvulsant are enhanced, decreasing the blood levels and clinical response to these agents. This necessitates an adjustment in dosage of both, with careful monitoring of blood levels to maximize the therapeutic response while minimizing side effects and toxicity.

The metabolism of a host of psychotherapeutics, including antipsychotics, antidepressants, and anxiolytics, is enhanced by cytochrome P450 enzyme induction. Although many of these drugs themselves do not induce enzyme activity, co-administration with an inducer can dramatically affect their rate of metabolism and therefore their clinical activity. For example, barbiturates enhance the metabolism of chlorpromazine. Likewise, rifampin, an antitubercular agent, increases the biotransformation of diazepam and other drugs, necessitating an increase in the dose of the anxiolytic to a maintain the therapeutic response (Table 1-3).

Some drugs inhibit cytochrome P450 enzymes, increasing their own bioavailability and the circulating levels of any other agent that is biotransformed by that particular enzyme. In so doing, the recommended amount of a centrally active drug may provoke side effects and toxicities normally observed only with much higher doses. Cimetidine, a histamine H_2 receptor antagonist used for treating ulcers, and ketoconazole, a widely used antifungal, inhibit cytochrome P450 catalyzed oxidative drug metabolism, which is an important route of biotransformation for certain centrally active drugs, such as some antipsychotics. Thus, a patient whose psychosis has been well controlled on thioridazine for years may begin to experience antipsychotic side effects when placed on ketoconazole to treat a fungal infection.

Table 1-3

Inducers, Inhibitors, and Substrates of Cytochrome P450 Enzymes Responsible for the Biotransformation of Centrally Active Drugs*

Enzyme	Substrates	Inhibitors	Inducers
CYP1A2	Caffeine, imipramine	α-Naphthoflavone	Cigarette smoke
CYP2A6	Nicotine, valproic acid	Tranylcypromine	Barbiturates
CYP2C8	Carbamazepine	Quercetin	—
CYP2C9	Phenytoin, tetrahydrocannabinol, valproic acid	Sulfinpyrazone	Rifampin
CYP2C19	Citalopram, diazepam, diphenylhydantoin, hexobarbital, imipramine, mephenytoin, mephobarbital	Tranylcypromine	Rifampin
CYP2D6	Amitriptyline, citalopram, clozapine, codeine, deprenyl, desipramine, dextromethorphan, fluoxetine, fluphenazine, haloperidol, imipramine, mianserin, nortriptyline, paroxetine, thioridazine, trifluperidol	Fluoxetine, trifluperiodol	—
CYP2E1	Caffeine, enflurane, isoflurane	Disulfiram	Ethanol
CYP3A4	Carbamazepine, diazepam, imipramine, midazolam, tetrahydrocannabinol, triazolam	Ketoconazole	Carbamazepine, phenobarbital, phenytoin, rifampin, sulfinpyrozone

* Drugs and chemicals listed represent examples of substrates, inducers, and inhibitors for various cytochrome P450 enzymes. As this list is not exhaustive, it should not be used for clinical purposes. Product information provided by the manufacturer must be consulted to assess the potential for drug interactions for any particular agent.

The absence of an example indicates none have been identified for that category.

Other examples of drug-induced cytochrome P450 enzyme inhibition of particular importance when treating neurological and psychiatric conditions are inhibition of the metabolism of carbamazepine by erythromycin and the inhibition of antipsychotic metabolism by SSRIs such as fluoxetine Table 1-3) (Harvey and Preskorn, 1996). In these cases, the blood levels of carbamazepine and the antipsychotic could increase if their dosages, or those of the inhibitors, are not adjusted.

It is now well established that genetic polymorphisms, common gene variants, exist among individuals that can have dramatic effects on their capacity to biotransform certain drugs. For example, the dose of tricyclic antidepressants or SSRIs may need to be adjusted in patients deficient in CYP2D6 since both classes are metabolized by this enzyme and the latter group also inhibits enzyme activity (Table 1-3). Efforts are under way to identify those who may be prone to metabolizing drugs more or less readily than the general population. To this end, tests are conducted to characterize their ability to metabolize certain substances, thereby establishing their phenotype and providing insight into their potential for metabolizing various therapeutic agents.

Drug metabolism is also influenced by age, disease, and gender (Klotz et al., 1975). For example, hepatic dysfunction can dramatically alter the blood levels and clinical response to benzodiazepines and opioids. In these cases, liver disease decreases the metabolism of these agents, increasing the circulating levels of active compound and the likelihood for side effects. With age there is a decrease in drug biotransformation owing, in part, to decreases in hepatic blood flow and cytochrome P450 activity. This explains why the elderly are more sensitive to the effects of anxiolytics and hypnotics, virtually all of which are metabolized to some extent by cytochrome P450 enzymes. Likewise, some drugs are metabolized to a greater or lesser extent in one gender or ethnic group than another, sometimes necessitating an adjustment in dosage.

Because drug blood levels vary with the rate of metabolism, dramatic changes can occur even in the absence of enzyme induction or inhibition if the enzymatic process responsible for biotransformation is limited. This is exemplified by the metabolism of phenytoin, an anticonvulsant. At low blood levels, a constant fraction of phenytoin is biotransformed and eliminated per unit of time (first-order kinetics). However, even a small increase in dose may saturate the metabolic process to the extent that a constant amount, rather than a constant fraction, of the drug is metabolized and excreted with further increases in dose (zero-order kinetics). This results in a substantial increase in the circulating levels of the drug far out of proportion to the increase in dosage, thereby enhancing the likelihood for side effects and toxicity. Since a change from first-order to zero-order metabolism can occur in the absence of any other medication, or modification in the physical state of the patient, the reason for the abrupt shift in tolerability to the drug may not be readily apparent.

As for excretion, the vast majority of centrally active drugs are eliminated by the kidneys. As a consequence, any condition that might compromise renal blood flow, or the ability of the kidney to transfer solutes from the blood into the glomerular filtrate, will delay drug excretion. Since most centrally active drugs are extensively metabolized to inactive products, a delay in excretion of these metabolites may have little or no clinical consequence. However, significant increases in circulating levels of active drugs may result from compromised renal function in cases where a significant amount of parent compound is excreted unchanged, such as with phenobarbital or

GABA-pentin, or when there are active metabolites, such as with some benzodiazepines and antidepressants.

Side Effects and Toxicities

The more common side effects associated with centrally active drugs are dose-dependent and natural extensions of the pharmacological properties of the agent. In general, older drugs display a greater array of side effects than newer agents since the therapeutic benefit in treating a particular condition was typically discovered empirically and therefore the older agents possess a number of pharmacological properties unrelated to their intended use. Because most newer drugs are customized to target a specific receptor or enzyme, ancillary pharmacological actions, and therefore side effects, are reduced. Examples of this type of progress are provided by the improvement in the side-effect profile of antidepressants with the SSRIs, such as fluoxetine and sertraline, in comparison with tricyclic agents, such as imipramine and amitriptyline. Likewise olanzepine, a new antipsychotic, was designed especially to induce fewer of the neurological side effects commonly associated with older members of this class, such as chlorpromazine and haloperidol. Nonetheless, no drug, no matter how selective it is for the target organ or tissue, is completely devoid of side effects. Rather, the objective in drug development is to widen the separation between the maximally effective dose and the appearance of untoward effects (increase the therapeutic window), thereby reducing or eliminating the incidence of side effects and toxicities that may hinder compliance at best, or be life-threatening at worse.

The tricyclic nature of certain antidepressants (e.g., imipramine and amitriptyline), and antipsychotics (e.g., chlorpromazine and thiothixene), is an example of a chemical structure (pharmacophore) that displays a host of pharmacological actions, many of which are unrelated to the intended therapeutic response. This pharmacophore routinely yields compounds that are potent inhibitors of cholinergic muscarinic, dopamine, serotonin, histamine, α-adrenergic, and sigma receptors in brain and peripheral tissues. In some cases, such as with the tricyclic antidepressants, these compounds are also potent inhibitors of monoamine uptake into nerve terminals. Given this array, the reasons for the more common side effects associated with these drugs can be understood. These include dry mouth, blurred vision, constipation, and urinary retention, all of which are a consequence of the anticholinergic properties. Other common side effects are orthostatic hypotension, which is most likely attributable to α-adrenergic blockade, and sedation, which may be related to their antihistaminic activity.

Although many pharmacological actions and side effects are shared by the tricyclic structure, there are differences among these agents that provide the basis for their therapeutic uses. As indicated in the preceding, those tricyclics that potently inhibit monoamine reuptake are most useful as antidepressants, whereas the tricyclic antipsychotics are less effective in inhibiting neurotransmitter uptake but more potent than the antidepressants as dopamine receptor antagonists. Although this latter property is believed to account for antipsychotic efficacy, dopamine receptor blockade is also responsible for the neurological side effects associated with the antipsychotics. Indeed, the neurological side effects associated with conventional antipsychotics, in particular tardive dyskinesia, are the major limitations for their use. These side effects are the result of dopamine receptor blockade in the caudate-putamen, brain regions presumably unassociated with the illness since they are not observed in all patients displaying a positive therapeutic response. The neurological syndromes associated with the use of conventional tricyclic and heterocyclic antipsychotics, the latter represented by haloperidol, molindone, and pimozide, include acute dystonia, akathesia, parkinsonism, neuroleptic malignant syndrome, and tardive dyskinesia (Tarsy and Baldessarini, 1986). It should be noted that the incidence of these side effects and toxicities varies with the individual agent, route of administration, and patient; the elderly are particularly prone to tardive dyskinesia, especially of the irreversible variety.

Although for decades it was believed that neurological side effects were an inherent property of antipsychotics because of the importance of dopamine receptor blockade in attenuating the symptoms of psychosis, the discovery of clozapine altered this notion (Baldessarini and Frankenburg, 1991). Thus, clozapine was found to be an effective antipsychotic while being devoid of the extrapyramidal side effects associated with conventional antipsychotics. Moreover, although clozapine is a dopamine receptor antagonist, it is generally less potent in this regard than conventional antipsychotics, especially in relation to its potency as an inhibitor of other neurotransmitter receptor systems in brain. Unfortunately, agranulocytosis, a potentially fatal toxicity that appears to be unrelated to its mechanism of therapeutic action, limits the use of clozapine.

The improved clinical profile of clozapine led to the design and development of olanzepine, which was recently approved for use in the United States. Although olanzepine blocks dopamine D-2 receptors like conventional antipsychotics, its potent antagonism of 5-HT$_2$ receptors markedly reduces the risk for extrapyramidal side effects. Unlike clozapine, olanzepine does not appear to cause potentially fatal blood dyscrasias. This example illustrates the feasibility of designing safer drugs by targeting more selectively the site of therapeutic action while reducing the affinity of the drug for unrelated sites responsible for side effects.

This principle is also illustrated with antidepressants. The SSRIs, including fluoxetine, sertraline, and paroxetine, were designed to potently block serotonin reuptake like the tricyclic antidepressants, but without the anticholinergic, antihistaminic, and α-adrenergic blocking properties of these other drugs (Kasper et al., 1994). Moreover, by eliminating the tricyclic structure of the pharmacophore, which impairs cardiac conduction, the SSRIs do not display the cardiotoxic effects of the tricyclic antidepressants. Indeed, the cardiotoxic effects of tricyclic antidepresants account for the high lethality with overdoses, a serious risk for the suicidally depressed patient. The clinical success of the SSRIs validate this strategy. Side effects associated with the SSRIs include nausea and vomiting, which may be owing to activation of serotonin systems in various regions of the central nervous system.

Drugs that broadly enhance GABA receptor function, such as benzodiazepines, provide an additional example of this principle. Thus, the most common side effects associated with benzodiazepines, such as diazepam, are ataxia, an increase in reaction time, confusion, and impairment of motor and mental function, all of which are the result of their central nervous system depressant properties. The discovery that the benzodiazepines interact with select components of the GABA receptor-channel, and that there are several distinct molecular forms of GABA receptors, permitted development of safer and more selective anxiolytics and hypnotics with fewer, or at least different, side effects (Enna, 1993). This reasoning led to the development of zolpidem, a hypnotic that is chemically unrelated to the benzodiazepines but that acts at a subgroup of benzodiazepine sites located on a distinct subpopulation of GABA receptors in brain. Unlike the benzodiazepine hypnotics, such as flurazepam, zolpidem has little effect on the normal stages of sleep and tolerance develops more slowly, if at all, to its hypnotic effects. As for side effects, zolpidem appears to be less prone than the benzodiazepines to produce daytime sedation and dizziness (Hoehns and Perry, 1993).

Given the variety of opioid receptors located throughout the body, it is not surprising that opioid drugs display a number of side effects. Indeed, some of those encountered when using these drugs as analgesics, such as constipation, are therapeutic effects when they are used in a different context such as diarrhea. Common side effects associated with the use of opioids as analgesics are respiratory depression, nausea, vomiting, dysphoria, mental clouding, constipation, urinary retention, and hypotension. Each of these can be traced to activation of one or more opioid receptor subtype, making it conceivable that more selective opioids could be developed that induce analgesia while having less of an effect on other systems (Clark et al., 1989).

Other centrally active drugs displaying dose-dependent side effects related to their basic mechanism of action include

L-dopa, bromocriptine, and pergolide, one indirect and two direct-acting dopamine receptor agonists used to treat Parkinson's disease. The use of these agents is associated with nausea and vomiting because of direct stimulation of dopamine receptors in the chemoreceptor trigger zone in brain. Hallucinations and confusion are also common side effects associated with the three antiparkinson drugs, most likely because of their ability to stimulate dopamine receptors in the cerebral cortex. Ergotamine, a nonselective monoamine receptor agonist used to treat migraine, causes numbness and tingling of the digits, which is most likely caused by vasoconstriction in the extremities. This side effect is not observed with sumatriptan, which was designed specifically for the treatment of migraine headache. Given its selectivity as an agonist at certain serotonin receptor subtypes, sumatriptan does not display the panolopy of side effects associated with the pharmacologically less discriminating ergot alkaloids. In general, side effects associated with sumatriptan are minor, including feelings of warmth, paresthesia, and a sense of heaviness in the head. More troublesome is its potential to cause coronary vasospasm, limiting its use in patients with ischemic heart disease. Nonetheless, the development of sumatriptan is another example of how rational drug design based on an understanding of the underlying neurobiological mechanisms associated with the disorder yields safer therapeutics.

Not all side effects of centrally active drugs, however, are related to their known pharmacological actions making it difficult, if not impossible, to design with any degree of precision new agents devoid of these actions. Examples include blood dyscrasias associated with the use of some anticonvulsants, and more benign effects such as hirsutism and gingival hyperplasia encountered with phenytoin, an anticonvulsant. Moreover, some centrally active drugs, such as carbamazepine, induce hypersensitivity reactions, such as exfoliative dermatitis and eosinophilia, which are difficult to predict and may be life-threatening. Given the lack of information on the molecular mechanisms responsible for these types of side effects and toxicities, they are difficult to eliminate using rational drug design. Inasmuch as some of these effects are dose-dependent, it is possible the underlying mechanism of action will be identified in the future.

The foregoing is not intended as a comprehensive review of the side effects and toxicities associated with all drugs described in this volume. Rather, the examples shown are for illustrative purposes. More detailed information concerning the untoward effects of these and other drugs used to treat pain, neurological, and psychiatric conditions is contained in the relevant chapters.

For additional information on the issues discussed in this chapter see chapters 1, 2, 3, and 12 in *Goodman and Gilman's The Pharmacological Basis of Therapeutics* (Ninth Edition), McGraw-Hill, New York, 1996.

REFERENCES

Axelrod J: Metabolism of epinephrine and other sympathemimetic amines. *Physiol Rev* 1959;39:751–776.

Baldessarini RJ, Frankenburg FR: Clozapine a novel antipsychotic agent. *N Engl J Med* 1991;324:746–754.

Berretini W, Ferraro TN, Goldin LR, et al.: Chromosome 18 DNA markers and manic-depressive illness: evidence for a susceptibility. *Proc Natl Acad Sci USA* 1994;91:5918–5921.

Bliss TVP, Collinridge GL: A synaptic model of memory: long term potentiation in the hippocampus. *Nature* 1993;361:31–36.

Brodie B B, Olin J, Kuntzman FG, Shore PA: Possible interrelationship between release of brain norepinephrine and serotonin by reserpine. Ann *NY Acad Sci* 1957;125:1293–1294.

Cade JF: Lithium salts in the treatment of psychotic excitement. *Med J Aust* 1949;2:349–352.

Carlsson A, Lindqvist M: Effect of chlorpromazine and haloperidol on formation of 3-methoxytyramine and normetanephrine in mouse brain. *Acta Pharmacol Toxicol* 1963;20:140–144.

Choi DW, Rothman SM: The role of glutamate neurotoxicity in hypoxic-ischemic neuronal death. *Annu Rev Neurosci* 1990;13:171–182.

Clark JA, Liu L, Price M, et al.: Kappa opiate receptor multiplicity: evidence for two U50,488-sensitive kappa 1 subtypes and a novel kappa 3 subtype. *J Pharmacol Exp Ther* 1989;251:461–468.

Cooper JR, Bloom FE, Roth RH: *The Biochemical Basis of Neuropharmacology,* 6th ed. New York: Oxford University Press, 1991.

Coyle JT: Aminergic projections from the reticular core, in

Asbury A, McKhann G, McDonald W (eds): *Diseases of the Nervous System.* Philadelphia: W.B. Saunders, 1986, pp. 880–889.

Creese I, Burt DR, Snyder SH: Dopamine receptor binding predicts clinical and pharmacological potencies of antischizophrenic drugs. *Science* 1976;192:481–483.

Creese I, Burt DR, Snyder SH: Biochemical actions of neuroleptic drugs: focus on the dopamine receptor, in Iversen LL, Iversen SD, Snyder SH (eds): *Handbook of Psychopharmacology,* vol. 10. New York: Plenum Press, 1978, pp. 37–89.

Delay J, Deniker P, Harl JM: Utilisation en therapeutique psychiatrique d'une phenothiazine d'action centrale elective. *Annis Med Psychol* 1952;110:112–117.

Deng H, Henati A, Tainer J, et al.: Amyotrophic lateral sclerosis and structural defects in Cu$_1$Zn superoxide dismutase. *Science* 1993;261:1047–1051.

Duman RS, Henninger GR, Nestler EJ: A molecular and cellular theory of depression. *Arch Gen Psychiatry* 1997;54:579–606.

Eisenberg L: Treating depression and anxiety in primary care. *N Engl J Med* 1992;326:1080–1084.

Eisenhandler J, Drucker E: Opiate dependency among subscribers of a New York area private insurance plan. *JAMA* 1993;269:2890–2891.

Enna SJ: GABA-A subunits in the mediation of selective drug action. *Curr Opin Neurol Neurosurg* 1993;6:597–601.

Frasure-Smith N, Lesperance F, Talajic M: Depression following myocardial infarction. *JAMA* 1993;270:1819–1825.

Hardman JG, Limbird LE, Molinoff PB, et al. (eds): *Goodman and Gilman's The Pharmacological Basis of Therapeutics,* 9th ed. New York: McGraw-Hill, 1996.

Harvey AT and Preskorn SH: Cytochrome P450 enzymes: interpretation of their interactions with selective serononin reuptake inhibitors. Part I. *J Clin Psychopharm* 1996;16:273–285.

Hoehns JD, Perry DJ: Zolpidem: a nonbenzodiazepine hypnotic for treatment of insomnia. *Clin Pharmacol* 1993;12:814–828.

Hokfelt T: Neuropeptides in perspective: the last ten years. *Neuron* 1991;7:867–879.

Holsboer F: Transgenic mouse models: new tools for psychiatric research. *Neuroscientist* 1997;3:328–336.

Hornykiewicz O: Parkinson's disease: from brain homogenates to treatment. *Fed Proc* 1973;32:183–190.

Hyman SE, Nestler EJ: *The Molecular Foundations of Psychiatry,* Washington, DC: American Psychiatric Press, 1993.

Kasper S, Hoflich G, Scholl H-P, Moller H-J: Safety and antidepressant efficacy of selective serotonin re-uptake inhibitors. *Hum Psychopharmacol Clin Exp* 1994;9:1–12.

Kline NS: Use of *Rauwolfia serpentina* Benth in neuropsychiatric conditions. *Ann NY Acad Sci* 1954;49:107–132.

Klotz U, Avant GR, Hoyumpa A, Schenker S, Wilkinson GR: The effects of age and liver disease on the disposition and elimination of diazepam in adult man. *J Clin Invest* 1975;55:347–359.

Kuhn R: The treatment of depressive states with G22355 (imipramine hydrochloride). *Am J Psychiatry* 1958;115:459–464.

Levitan ES, Schofield PR, Burt DR, et al.: Structural and functional basis for GABA-A receptor heterogeneity. *Nature* 1988;335:76–79.

MacDonald ME, Gusella J: Huntington's Disease: translating a CAG repeat into a pathogenic mechanism. *Curr Opin Neurobiol* 1996;6:638–643.

McLellan AT, Arndt E, Metzger DS, Woody G, O'Brien CP: The effects of psychosocial services in substance abuse treatment. *JAMA* 1993;269:1953–1959.

Olney JW: Brain lesions, obesity and other disturbances in mice treated with monosodium glutamate. *Science* 1969;164:719–721.

Olney JW, Farber NB: Glutamate receptor dysfunction and schizophrenia. *Arch Gen Psychiatry* 1995;52:998–1007.

Pacholczyk T, Blakely RD, Amara SG: Expression cloning of a cocaine-and-antidepressant-sensitive human noradrenaline transporter. *Nature* 1991:350:350–354.

Parkinson A: Biotransformation of xenobiotics, in Klaassen C (ed), *Casarett & Doull's Toxicology, The Basic Science of Poisons,* 5th ed. New York, McGraw-Hill, 1996, pp 113–186.

Sandbrink R, Hartman T, Masters C, Beyreuther K: Genes contributing to Alzheimer's Disease. *Mol Psychiatry* 1996;1:27–40.

Simonian N, Coyle JT: Oxidative stress in neurodegenerative diseases. *Annu Rev Pharmacol Toxicol* 1996;36:83–106.

Schoepp D, Conn DJ: Metabotropic glutamate receptors in brain function and pathology. *Trends Pharmacol Sci* 1993;14:13–17.

Seeberg PH: The molecular biology of mammalian glutamate receptor channels. *Trends Neurosci* 1993;16:359–366.

Simon MI, Strathmann MP, Gautam N: Diversity of G proteins in signal transduction. *Science* 1991, 252:802–808.

Spitzer RL, Kroenke K, Linzer M, et al.: Health-related quality of life in primary care patients with mental disorders. *JAMA* 1995;274:1511–1517.

Strum R, Wells KB: How can care of depression become more cost effective? *JAMA* 1995;273:51–58.

Tallman JF, Dahl SG: New drug design in psychopharmacology. The impact of molecular biology, in Bloom FE, Kupfer DJ (eds); *Psychopharmacology: The Fourth Generation of Progress.* New York: Raven Press, 1994, pp. 1861–1874.

Tarsy D, Baldessarini RJ: Movement disorders induced by psychotherapeutic agents. Clinical features, pathophysiology, and management, in Shah NS, Donald AG (eds): *Movement Disorders.* New York: Plenum Press, 1986, pp. 365–389.

Thoenen H: Neurotropins and neuronal plasticity. *Science* 1995;270:593–598.

Wrighton SA, Stevens JC: The human hepatic cytochromes P450 involved in drug metabolism. *Crit Rev Toxicol* 1992;22:1–21.

Yamamura HI, Enna SJ, Kuhar MJ (eds): *Neurotransmitter Receptor Binding,* 2nd ed. New York: Raven Press, 1985.

Zbinden G, Randall LO: Pharmacology of benzodiazepines: laboratory and clinical correlations. *Adv Pharmacol* 1967;5:213–291.

SCHIZOPHRENIA

William T. Carpenter, Jr., Robert R. Conley, and Robert W. Buchanan

The aim of this chapter is to provide a general description of schizophrenia, its pathophysiology and treatment. Differential diagnosis is discussed with special note of the different aspects of the disease requiring therapeutic attention. Following this background information, there is a general discussion of antipsychotic medication, the pharmacotherapy of acute psychosis, continuation therapy, considerations when patients are treatment resistant, and some special therapeutic issues.

Schizophrenia is a leading public health problem worldwide, affecting about 0.85% of the population (lifetime prevalence). It is often marked by diminished drive and emotion during childhood, followed by a break with reality in which perception and/or ideation deviate substantially from the individual's cultural norm, usually expressed as false beliefs and auditory hallucinations. Visual and somatic hallucinations are also common as are disorganization of thought and behavior. The psychosis, or break with reality, usually emerges between age 17 and 30 in males and age 20 and 40 in females, with the course and outcome varying considerably between individuals. Some (perhaps 15–25%) recover from their first episode and may not become psychotic again by the 5-year follow-up, although this figure is lower from a lifetime perspective. Others (perhaps 5–10%) remain substantially psychotic without remission for many years. Most patients, however, do improve from the initial episode, continue to manifest some symptoms, and remain vulnerable to periodic exacerbation of psychotic symptoms.

In general, while the severity of psychosis plateaus within 5 to 10 years of the first episode, diminished drive and emotion may worsen over a longer period. This apparent progression in the illness is often the consequence of the primary impairments associated with schizophrenia. These include lost relationships, lost jobs, lost educational opportunities, lower expectations of self and from others, high likelihood of remaining single and unemployed, and vulnerability to stress-induced symptom exacerbation which may lead to a progressively poorer functional outcome. Furthermore, schizophrenia remains highly stigmatizing, and societal reaction limits what patients can accomplish. While late in life there is a tendency toward decreased intensity of symptoms and improvement in function, this does not compensate for years of lost experience and opportunity.

The original concept of dementia praecox (and therefore, schizophrenia) as an early-onset, progressive, neurodegenerative disease with a deteriorated endpoint is no longer viable. The more recent hypothesis of schizophrenia as a neurodevelopmental disorder with progression occurring early rather than throughout life fits better with clinical observations. A neurodevelopmental theory of schizophrenia is attractive from an etiologic vantage. Thus, the best established risk factors for schizophrenia are winter birth, genetics, and complications of pregnancy and delivery. These risk factors likely impair brain development, creating an early vulnerability to the illness. Observations of children at high genetic risk, such as offspring of a mother with schizophrenia, reveal motor, cognitive, and affective disturbances well in advance of the onset of psychosis. There is debate whether the disease progresses during childhood and adolescent years to the point of expression of psychosis or whether the early vulnerability is stable until the increased psychological demands associated with approaching adulthood challenge adaptation beyond the threshold in susceptible people. These are not mutually exclusive theories, since both can account for the early manifestation of subtle features and later manifestations of overt psychosis. However, once illness is fully established at the psychotic level, there is little evidence from neuroimaging, cognitive, postmortem, or clinical observation to suggest further progression.

Schizophrenia has lifelong negative consequences for most patients, and progressive slipping downward in life may occur because of an interaction between the ill individual and society. This can be understood at a very basic level when one considers the difficulty in maintaining an occupation if psychosis has interrupted work and social functioning. Employers and fellow workers will consider such an individual to be impaired and friends and family believe that lower expectations are appropriate. Unemployment rates average 80% among schizophrenic individuals although a substantial proportion of patients are capable of some occupational performance. This is made clear in the study of sociocentric cultures in developing countries where schizophrenics can maintain their social and occupational niche in a putatively less stressful environment. In these cultures, the course of the illness appears more benign. Thorough reviews of the etiology and neurobiology of schizophrenia are available (Carpenter and Buchanan, 1994; Waddington, 1994).

Schizophrenia is usually discussed as though it were a single disease entity. However, it is actually a clinical syndrome, with more than one etiology that may eventually be described within the context of a syndrome. The single-disease paradigm emerged at the turn of this century when Emil Kraepelin proposed that paranoia, hebephrenia, and catatonia were not distinct disease entities but rather manifestations of dementia praecox (Kraepelin, 1919). He also made the significant distinction between this form of mental illness and the "manic-depressive insanities." This was possible after the discovery of the "syphilitic insanities" had removed a large number of

patients from the general group of the mentally ill. The discovery of the etiology, treatment, and prevention of the neurosyphilis was, of course, one of the major triumphs of medical research, and led to the hope in psychiatry that the causes of major psychiatric disorders could be identified.

Eugen Bleuler (1950) put forward a new term, schizophrenia, to replace dementia praecox and argued that the fundamental psychopathology shared by all was dissociations within the thought processes and between thoughts and emotion. The term "schizophrenia" was coined to capture this concept and has been the most persevering influence on concepts of this syndrome. The traditional subtypes (e.g., hebephrenic, paranoid, catatonic, simple), with later additions such as schizoaffective and latent schizophrenic, have been maintained for descriptive purposes, although the terminology has shifted somewhat in the DSM-III and DSM-IV renditions of the official American nomenclature. However, these subtypes have not proved useful for the development of differential treatments or etiologic and pathophysiologic studies of this condition.

It has long been noted that as a diagnostic group patients with schizophrenia manifest substantial clinical heterogeneity with respect to pattern of onset, actual symptoms manifested, course of these symptoms, treatment response, and ultimate outcome. In 1974, an alternative paradigm was proposed (Strauss et al., 1974) based on cross-sectional and longitudinal observations of the relative independence between positive psychotic symptoms, negative symptoms, and interpersonal dysfunction. The hypothesis was that these symptom groups were not manifestations of the same underlying pathophysiology but rather each represented its own domain of psychopathology. Correlations of clinical manifestations within each domain over time were high, whereas correlations of manifestations across domains within an individual at any point in time were low, and across time were negligible. This view has been verified in numerous studies with one significant modification. Hallucinations and delusions are closely associated with, but are distinguished from, the other components of positive psychotic symptomatology (i.e., disorganization of thought and behavior). It is now commonly accepted that the key symptomatic domains of schizophrenia are reality distortion, disorganization of thought and behavior, negative symptoms, and cognitive impairment. Negative symptoms include reduced emotional experience and expression, poverty of speech, and low social drive. Kraepelin had earlier described this domain as "a weakening of the wellsprings of volition" (p. 74). Distinctions among domains are crucially important in considering pharmacotherapy. Other clinical manifestations relevant from a clinical management standpoint are depression, anxiety, hostility and aggression, and suicidal behavior.

For many years treatment studies focused on psychotic symptoms or variables closely related to psychosis such as time to discharge or time to psychotic relapse. With the growing appreciation of the relative independence of the various symptom clusters, more explicit evaluation of treatment response within each cluster has now become the standard. This work reveals little or no efficacy of standard antipsychotic therapy for the domains of cognitive impairment or negative symptoms. These two domains account for much of the long-term morbidity and reduced quality of life associated with this illness. Clarification of these therapeutic limitations has focused attention on the development of new drugs for treating these aspects of schizophrenia.

PATHOPHYSIOLOGY

The introduction of psychotropic medications, and the development of highly sensitive assays to measure biochemical processes in brain, provided an important link between central nervous system function and psychiatric disorders. The knowledge acquired from defining the mechanisms of action of these medications generated several hypotheses about the role of specific neurotransmitters in psychosis and schizophrenia. These theories have involved dopamine, noradrenaline, serotonin, acetylcholine, glutamic acid, several neuromodulatory peptides and/or their receptors. The dopamine hypothesis of schizophrenia has been the dominant pathophysiologic theory about the etiology of schizophrenia for over a quarter of a century.

Dopamine and Schizophrenia

Stimulants, including cocaine, amphetamine and methylphenidate activate the dopaminergic system in the brain. Abuse of stimulants can induce a paranoid psychosis that mimics the positive symptoms of schizophrenia. Persons suffering from schizophrenia will experience an exacerbation of their psychosis when given stimulants. Conversely, substantial evidence supports the notion that typical antipsychotic medications act by blocking dopamine receptors. First, most typical antipsychotic medications have a propensity to cause extrapyramidal side effects, which also occur under conditions of loss of brain dopaminergic neurons as in Parkinson's disease. Second, receptor binding studies have demonstrated a highly compelling correlation between the clinical potency of typical antipsychotic drugs and their affinity for the dopamine D2 receptor. Furthermore, while antipsychotic drugs interact with a variety of other neurotransmitter receptors such as muscarinic, α-adrenergic, histaminergic and serotonergic, none of these interactions correlate with antipsychotic efficacy. Thus, the symptoms of schizophrenia are hypothesized to result from excessive stimulation of dopamine receptors, presumably in cortico-limbic regions of the brain.

An important limitation of the dopamine hypothesis of schizophrenia is that manipulation of dopamine function affects primarily positive symptoms and has little effect on negative symptoms and cognitive impairments. Furthermore, it has been difficult to develop evidence of a primary defect in dopaminergic neurotransmission in schizophrenia as clinical studies assessing brain dopamine function have yielded variable results (Carlsson et al., 1997; Knable and Weinberger, 1997). Studies of dopamine and its metabolites in blood, urine and spinal fluid have been inconclusive as these are large compartments where any alterations related to localized dopaminergic dysfunction in schizophrenia would be diluted considerably.

An increased number of dopamine receptors in the caudate nucleus of brains of schizophrenics also supports the dopamine hypothesis, although these findings are inconsistent and may be a result of the disease rather than a cause. A more informative approach for assessing abnormal dopamine metabolism in schizophrenics is to utilize dopamine D2 receptor-specific ligands to determine the extent of binding at these sites. The comparison of pre- and post-infusion receptor occupancy provides an index of the rates of dopamine release and reuptake. Two recent PET studies utilizing this methodology have provided the first direct evidence supporting the hyperdopoaminergic hypothesis of schizophrenia (Breier et al., 1997; Laruelle et al., 1996).

The potential also exists to determine dopamine and dopamine metabolite concentrations in postmortem tissue. However, because cellular components break down following death, true tissue concentrations are often difficult to assess. Furthermore, antipsychotic drug administration may confound postmortem biochemistry. Despite these methodological limitations, postmortem studies have revealed differences between the brains of schizophrenics and suitable controls. For example, increased concentrations of dopamine have been found in the left amygdala (a limbic system structure) in the postmortem brains of schizophrenics. This finding has been replicated and, since it is lateralized, is unlikely to be an artifact. There has also been a report of an increase in dopamine D2 postsynaptic receptors in postmortem brain tissue of patients whose medical records indicated a diagnosis of schizophrenia but did not reveal antipsychotic drug use. These results suggest that the increase in receptor number is not secondary to drug treatment. There have also been reports of increases in dopamine D4 receptor number in certain brain areas independent of antipsychotic use.

A vexing twist of the dopamine hypothesis is associated with the avolitional/anhedonic pathology of schizophrenia. As described in the following, this negative symptom complex appears to be independent of the positive psychotic symptoms. Interestingly, negative symptoms may actually improve with dopamine receptor agonists, whereas dopamine receptor antagonists induce these symptoms in humans and model them in laboratory animals (Lieberman, 1987; Buchanan et al., 1996). Thus, although increased levels of dopamine, present in the anterior cingulate and other limbic structures, may be partly responsible for the positive symptoms associated with psychosis, negative symptoms may be a result of reduced dopamine function in the prefrontal cortex. From this perspective antipsychotic medications aimed at treating both hyperdopaminergia and hypodopaminergia in separate brain areas may be difficult to design.

The Glutamatergic Hypothesis

Glutamate is the major excitalory neurotransmitter in the brain. Interest in the possible role of glutamate in the pathophysiology of schizophrenia has emerged from an increased understanding of the N-methyl-*d*-aspartate (NMDA) receptor complex, a major subtype of glutamate receptor. Recently studies have begun to define the interactions between glutamatergic, dopaminergic, and GABAergic systems in brains, and have shown that the acute and chronic effects of phencyclidine (PCP), a psychotomimetic, noncompetitively blocks the ion channel of the NMDA receptor. Acute administration of PCP produces a syndrome that mimics the positive, negative and cognitive symptoms of schizophrenia. Moreover, early reports of long-lasting exacerbation of psychosis in patients with schizophrenia supports the use of PCP as a mimic for psychosis. Chronic administration of PCP produces a hypodopaminergic state in the prefrontal cortex, a state that has been argued to cause negative symptoms. Moreover, PCP and its chemical analog, ketamine, both attenuate glutamatergic transmission. In addition to the observation of schizophrenia-like symptomatology in humans abusing PCP, ketamine has been used in normal human volunteers to produce mild transitory manifestations of positive, negative and cognitive symptoms of schizophrenia. As with PCP, the perceptual distortions seem most characteristic of ketamine. Thus, glutamatergic deficiency produces symptoms similar to those seen in a hyperdopaminergic state and possibly those present in schizophrenics. Additionally, the existence of dopamine-inhibiting glutamatergic neurons through NMDA receptors, either directly or through an interaction with GABAergic neurons, may explain the relationship between glutamatergic pathways and the dopamine theory of schizophrenia. These considerations support a hypoglutamatergic hypothesis for schizophrenia and predict a therapeutic effect for compounds that activate the NMDA receptor complex.

Development of drugs aimed at stimulating the glutamate system is difficult since excessive glutamatergic activity is neurotoxic. However, activation of the NMDA receptor complex through the glycine site with either glycine itself or *d*-cycloserine has been reported to alleviate negative symptoms in schizophrenic patients and provides the best current example of a possible pharmacotherapy based on the glutamatergic hypothesis of schizophrenia.

The glutamatergic hypothesis exemplifies a major transition that has recently occurred in defining biochemical abnormalities in schizophrenia. Prior to this transition, the discovery of antipsychotics was empirical and neurochemical abnormalities defined on the basis of the mechanism of action of these agents. With the ever-increasing knowledge of the neural organization of the brain, and the characteristics of neurotransmitters, it is now possible to postulate a pathophysiological theory first and then attempt to develop new drugs based on the theory. Because there is now a broader range of hypotheses on the pathophysiology of schizophrenia, there is optimism that treatment with new therapies will be developed more rapidly in the future.

Other Neurotransmitter and Neuromodulatory Hypotheses

The rich innervation of the frontal cortex and limbic system with serotonergic neurons, the modulatory effect of these neurons on dopaminergic neurons, and the involvement of these pathways in the regulation of a broad range of complex functions has led several investigators to posit a pathophysiological role for serotonin in schizophrenia. Of current interest is the hypothesis positing a serotonin excess as being responsible for positive and negative symptoms. The robust serotonin receptor antagonist activity of clozapine and other new-generation antipsychotics, coupled with clozapine's demonstrated effectiveness for positive symptoms in chronic patients resistant to typical antipsychotics, have contributed to this hypothesis. However, several studies have raised questions about the efficacy of serotonin receptor antagonists in relieving negative symptoms secondary to psychosis, depression, or drug side effects. These drugs have not been documented as therapeutics for primary negative symptoms which define core deficit pathology. Emphasis on the putative therapeutic role of serotonin antagonists (especially at the 5HT2a receptor) has played a significant role in the development of new-generation antipsychotics. The major therapeutic advantage of the combined dopamine D2/5-HT2 receptor antagonists appears to be a reduction in extrapyramidal side effects rather than superior efficacy. This advantage, however, may result in better patient compliance and, therefore, more effective treatment.

There have also been hypotheses implicating norepinephrine in the psychopathology of schizophrenia. Anhedonia, that is, the impaired capacity for emotional gratification and the decreased ability to experience pleasure, has long been noted to be a prominent feature of schizophrenia. While abnormality within the norepinephrine reward system could account for this negative symptom, biochemical and pharmacological data in support of this notion are inconclusive. As with the dopamine and serotonin hypotheses, both a noradrenergic excess and deficiency theory have been postulated.

Integrative Hypotheses

Comprehensive models that integrate both neuroanatomical and biochemical hypotheses are the future trend in schizophrenia research. The theory considering the neurotransmitters involved in the connections among cerebral cortical, basal ganglia, and thalamic structures that comprise the basal ganglia-thalamo-cortical neural circuit is an example of this approach. The cerebral cortex, through glutamate projections from the cortex to the basal ganglia, facilitates the performance of selected behaviors while inhibiting others. The excitatory glutamatergic neurons terminate on GABAergic and cholinergic interneurons that, in turn, suppress the activity of dopaminergic and other neurons. The elucidation of the neuroanatomy and biochemistry of cortical circuiting involved in this model has served as a starting point for designing new hypotheses on the pathophysiology of schizophrenia. These models also provide a framework for identifying potential neurotransmitter targets for drug development, as well as providing explanations for some observed effects of drugs, such as PCP, in schizophrenic patients (Olney and Ferber, 1995; Tamminga, 1998).

The current neuroanatomical model has been proposed by Kinan and Lieberman (1996) to explain the response to atypical antipsychotics, such as clozapine, as compared to conventional drugs, such as haloperidol. In this model, the fact that clozapine has very specific effects on the limbic system without altering striatal neuronal activity contrasts with the very prominent effects of typical antipsychotics on striatal neuronal function. Other antipsychotics with similar activity, such as olanzepine, may also be superior to traditional antipsychotics (Conley, 1994). The newer antipsychotics, such as risperidone and sertindole, are not quite as limbic selective as clozapine although they do have benefits in that they produce fewer neurologic side effects at effective doses compared to traditional antipsychotics (Conley et al., 1997). This, and other, hypotheses will be further tested as more agents with a pharmacologic and clinical profile similar to clozapine become available.

THE PRESENTING PATIENT

Ms. Smith is an 18-year-old first-year student at a local college who currently lives at home with her parents. When she was a child, she was shy and decidedly uncomfortable in unfamiliar surroundings. As a teenager, she was known to be a loner with antisocial tendencies. She claimed her shyness was a result of her peers not liking her and conspiring against her. Recently, she decided with her parents to seek psychiatric help.

The first step of this evaluation is a careful drug use and abuse history, as a drug use syndrome can frequently present in young adults as a psychotic disorder. It is also important to decide if persistent delusional thinking intrudes into her thoughts. The clinician should decide if her suspicions are a false belief or whether they merely represent severe suspiciousness at the extreme range of normal. The clinician must also consider an affective disorder presenting with psychotic features. Therefore, her mood also must be carefully evaluated.

Ms. Smith reports that she does not feel depressed but does feel very suspicious that people at college are conspiring against her. She frequently hears the voices of people, such as several of her professors commenting on her thoughts and actions. She clearly describes these voices as emanating from various points in the room. The voices intrude into her thoughts and prevent her from concentrating on her schoolwork. Ms. Smith feels that even if she did her best in school she would still fail in her classes because her professors are conspiring against her. She says that she has been having these experiences for at least the past 2 months. While she remembers feeling suspicious about her friends and teachers in high school, they were "never as bad as now." Ms. Smith is guarded and somewhat withdrawn during the interview and she frequently asks to see her parents to ensure that they have not left the waiting room.

On further historical examination it is discovered that Ms. Smith has had a marked deterioration in her school performance over the past 2 or 3 years. While she had been a bright student, although shy and socially withdrawn, maintaining a B + to A − average, through her first year in high school, her grades deteriorated markedly in her senior year. Although she was able to graduate from high school, her initial plans, which were to attend a nationally ranked college, had to be changed because of her grades. Together with her family, Ms. Smith decided to attend a local college. Again, although she was not happy with this choice, she does not describe any symptoms consistent with an affective disorder. She also denies any recent drug use although she reports that she occasionally experimented with marijuana and will occasionally drink socially.

Paranoid schizophrenia, first episode, is the diagnosis most consistent with Ms. Smith's current symptomatic presentation. She should have a complete physical examination and other diagnostic tests including a complete screen for drugs of abuse and a general chemistry screen, a complete blood count, and a pregnancy test. Although this patient denies current drug use, it is very important to definitively rule out drug use as a possible cause of her disorder. It is also important to rule out any metabolic abnormalities as possible contributing factors and to know the pregnancy status before prescribing psychoactive drugs. In this case the physical exam was normal as were all laboratory evaluations and the pregnancy test negative. These findings help confirm the initial diagnostic impression.

With pharmacologic treatment and support, Ms. Smith can function on an acceptable, although suboptimal, level. She should now have 1 to 2 years of stable pharmacologic treatment, during which time she should be evaluated for response and persistence of symptoms, before a decision is made regarding long-term therapy.

There are many variations on this story. Some patients may be very asocial and eccentric throughout their development, whereas others may tell of friendly voices distracting them for years. Some will have conspicuous disorganization of thought and behavior leaving little doubt that mental illness is present, whereas others hide an inner world of perceptual distortions and delusions. A sensitivity to the possibility of psychotic illness may lead to earlier detection and treatment, although the prodromal signs of the illness are often observed during adolescence and early adulthood independent of schizophrenia. Diagnosis and intervention are, therefore, difficult and uncertain until evidence of psychosis is detected.

DIFFERENTIAL DIAGNOSIS

The first objective in diagnosing psychosis is to identify a cause. When cause is known, treatment and prevention can be most specific. To reinforce the importance of accurate diagnosis, consider the treatment implications of distinguishing delusions caused by temporal lobe epilepsy from those induced by amphetamine, from delusions manifest during a manic phase of affective disorder or from those associated with schizophrenia. Each responds to different medications. The logic and hierarchy of differential diagnosis is contained in the *Diagnostic and Statistical Manual* (4th ed) of the American Psychiatric Association (DSM-IV). Following the rules depicted in Figure 2-1, psychosis should first be attributed to physiological effects of a general medical condition when plausible, and next to substance abuse. If these are excluded, then the clinician should determine if an affective disorder could adequately account for the disease manifestations. If not, depending on the presence of associated features, either schizophrenia or a schizophrenia-like disorder is diagnosed. While each class of psychotic illness has specific treatment modalities, psychosis tends to respond to antipsychotic drugs regardless of the cause.

A diagnosis of schizophrenia identifies a group of patients for whom certain types of drugs are prescribed. However, specific treatment decisions are often based not on diagnosis alone but rather on particular target symptoms and their pattern of manifestation.

Although reality distortion and disorganization are distinctive, they respond to the same medications. In this case, drugs that inhibit dopamine D2 receptors are efficacious in reducing both reality distortion and disorganization symptoms. This justifies the common practice of joining these two symptom complexes together in a discussion of antipsychotic therapy.

Pathophysiologic theories for negative symptoms of schizophrenia involve hypodopaminergic function in the prefrontal cortex rather than hyperdopaminergic function in limbic regions that are involved with psychosis. This raises the concern that drugs effective in treating psychosis would aggravate negative symptoms. While dopamine receptor agonists tend to improve negative symptoms, they exacerbate positive

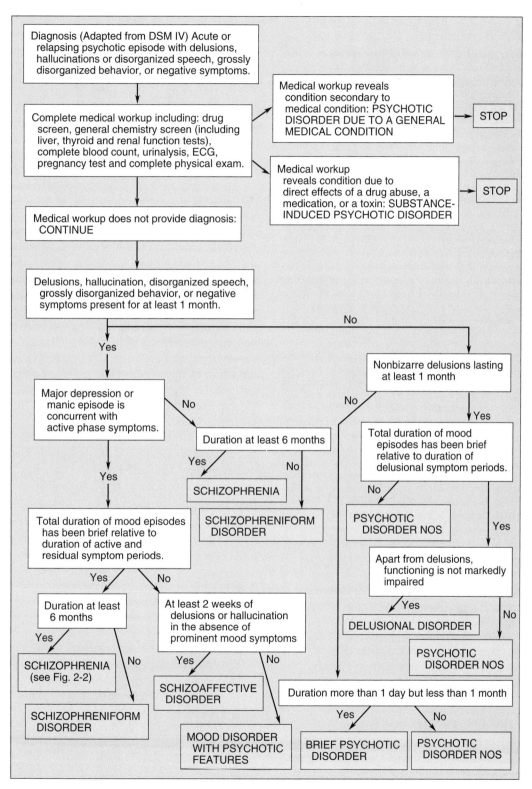

Figure 2–1. Decision tree for the diagnosis and treatment of psychotic disorders.

symptoms. Conceptually, the negative symptoms of schizophrenia refer to an enduring trait pathology that represents long-standing impairments in the general area of volition and affect. Considered in this regard, there is as yet no established treatment for these primary manifestations of the disease. There is evidence, however, that atypical antipsychotics may affect the clinical presentation of negative symptoms as shown by their ability to improve negative symptom ratings in clinical trials. Rating scales, such as the SANS, BPRS, and PANSS, include items such as impersistence at work and school, diminished social contact, and emotional withdrawal. These may be viewed as general pathology measures that tend to improve when the person becomes less psychotic, may be caused by antipsychotic side effects (e.g., bradykinesia, sedation), and may be secondary to depression (e.g., anhedonia). For example, a patient with severe paranoid delusions responding to an antipsychotic drug would naturally become more gregarious, less guarded, and have a greater range of emotional expression as the intensity of the paranoia subsides. This is viewed as a change in secondary negative symptoms rather than a fundamental alteration in the volitional or affective component of the illness.

Many tests of cognitive functioning relating to attention and information processing are of neuroanatomic relevance and show low performance in persons with schizophrenia. These cognitive dysfunctions do not have an immediate relationship to symptom manifestations and tend to remain stable despite substantial improvement in psychotic symptoms. Together with primary negative symptoms, this aspect of the illness appears to account for much long-term functional disability and diminished quality of life. The fact that traditional antipsychotic drugs do not affect these core components of the illness may explain why the long-term morbidity of schizophrenia remains so prominent despite the robust effectiveness of antipsychotic drugs in reducing psychotic symptoms and preventing relapse.

PHARMACOTHERAPEUTICS

Antipsychotics are the primary drug class used to treat schizophrenia (Kane, 1996). These medications are divided into three major categories: conventional antipsychotics, clozapine, and atypical antipsychotics. The pharmacological properties, including side effects, associated with each of these categories is described in the following.

Conventional Antipsychotics

The modern era of the pharmacological management of schizophrenia began in 1952 with the discovery that chlorpromazine possessed antipsychotic properties (Delay and Deniker, 1952). The demonstration of the therapeutic efficacy of chlorpromazine in large multicenter double-blind placebo-controlled trials led to the development of additional compounds for the treatment of schizophrenia. These agents, referred to as conventional or traditional antipsychotics, or neuroleptics, are divided into five chemical classes (Table 2-1).

Mechanism of action.   Antipsychotic medications, with the exception of clozapine, exhibit a compelling correlation between their clinical potency in reducing psychotic symptoms and blockade of dopamine D2 receptors (Carlsson and Lindqvist, 1963; Creese et al., 1976; Seeman et al., 1976). The dopamine D2 receptors are located in the basal ganglia, the nucleus accumbens and the frontal cortex where they play a central role in regulating the flow of information between the cerebral cortex and thalamus. Thus, conventional antipsychotics may help restore the homeostasis of this system (Tamminga, in press). At the cellular level, conventional antipsychotics are thought to exert their therapeutic effect through depolarization blockade of both nigrostriatal (A9) and mesolimbic (A10) dopaminergic neurons (Grace et al., 1997). However, since the therapeutic response occurs before depolarization blockade, this effect may prevent tolerance to these drugs. The observation that dopamine agonists, such as amphetamine, methylphenidate, and L-dopa, induce a paranoid psychosis similar in some ways to that observed in schiz-

Table 2-1
Classes of Conventional Antipsychotics

Phenothiazines
    Aliphatic (e.g., chlorpromazine)
    Piperazine (e.g., perphenazine, trifluoperazine, fluphenazine)
    Piperidine (e.g., thioridazine)
Butryophenones (e.g., haloperidol)
Thioxanthenes (e.g., thiothixene)
Dibenzoxazepines (e.g., loxapine)
Dihydroindolones (e.g., molindone).

ophrenia, provides further support for the proposition that the dopamine system plays a central role in the action of antipsychotics. However, the inability to demonstrate a consistent relationship between dopamine metabolism and the response to antipsychotics, as well as the significant number of schizophrenic patients who do not respond to conventional antipsychotics, suggest that dopaminergic activity is only one factor involved in the pathophysiology of schizophrenia.

Conventional antipsychotics also have varying degrees of activity at serotonin 5HT-1c and 5HT-2a, muscarinic, and α- and β-adrenergic receptors, as well as at dopamine D1, D3, and D4 receptors. Indeed, clozapine, and the newer antipsychotics, have higher affinities for some of these other receptors than for the dopamine D2 site.

Side effects. The major side effects of conventional antipsychotics are listed in Table 2-2. Conventional antipsychotics exhibit a broad range of side effects, with high-potency agents, such as fluphenazine and haloperidol more likely to produce extrapyramidal symptoms, and low-potency agents, including chlorpromazine and thioridazine, more likely to produce sedation and orthostatic hypotension.

The side effect profile of a particular drug is related to its pharmacological profile. Thus, those that are highly anticholinergic are more likely to cause blurred vision, constipation, dry mouth, and/or urinary retention; whereas sedation is more common with drugs with significant antihistaminic properties, and orthostatic hypotension is seen more often with drugs that block α_1-adrenergic receptors. Typically, tolerance develops to the antihistaminic and α_1-adrenergic blockade. The anticholinergic, noradrenergic, and/or dopaminergic blocking actions of these drugs may cause a broad array of alterations in sexual function, including amenorrhea or dysmenorrhea, anorgasmia, loss of lubrication, galactorrhea, breast tenderness or enlargement, and an inability to maintain an erection. Sexual side effects are due to the anticholinergic and adrenergic blocking properties of these drugs, whereas one of the adverse consequences of dopaminergic blockade is an increase in prolactin secretion.

Table 2-2

Major Side Effects of Conventional Antipsychotics

Central nervous system
  Altered thermoregulation
  Extrapyramidal
  Neuroleptic malignant syndrome
  Sedation
  Seizures
  Tardive dyskinesia
Cardiovascular
  ECG changes
  Orthostatic hypotension
  Tachycardia
  Torsade de pointes
Dermatological
  Allergic reactions
  Skin photosensitivity
Endocrine
  Amenorrhea
  Galactorrhea
  Sexual dysfunction
  Weight gain
Gastrointestinal
  Cholestatic jaundice
  Constipation
Hematological
  Agranulocytosis
  Leukopenia
Ophthalmological
  Blurred vision
  Retinitis pigmentosa
Urinary
  Urinary retention

The most problematic side effects associated with conventional antipsychotics involve the motor system. These effects are probably the most common cause of noncompliance. The three major motor system side effects of conventional antipsychotics are extrapyramidal symptoms, tardive dyskinesia, and neuroleptic malignant syndrome.

Extrapyramidal symptoms. Extrapyramidal symptoms (EPS) include parkinsonian motor abnormalities, dystonia, and akathisia. Parkinsonian symptoms, which are thought to be secondary to dopamine D2 receptor blockade in the basal ganglia, include mask-like facies, akinesia, tremor at rest, and rigidity. These symptoms occur early in treatment and tend to persist if left untreated. It is important to differentiate these effects from the negative symptoms of the disorder as they may be confused with emotional withdrawal, blunted affect, and apathy. Parkinsonian symptoms may be treated with either anticholinergic agents such as benztropine mesylate or trihexyphenidyl, by decreasing the dose of the conventional antipsychotic, or by changing to one of the newer antipsychotics.

Dystonic reactions most commonly present as acute contractions of the face, neck, or torso musculature, such as torticollis, oculogyric crisis, and opisthotonos. As with parkinsonian symptoms, acute dystonic reactions typically occur within the first few days of treatment. They are usually rapidly responsive to intramuscular injections of either diphenhydramine or benztropine mesylate. Tardive dystonia usually affects the neck, and, in contrast to acute dystonia, is less responsive to anticholinergics.

Akathisia is characterized by either the subjective experience of inner restlessness and the need to move (e.g., pacing). It too usually appears early in the course of therapy. Although it is somewhat related to other extrapyramidal symptoms, it often appears independently from these. Akathisia may be very troublesome and can be associated with violence, with case reports of patients attempting suicide in an effort to alleviate their distress.

Tardive dyskinesia. Tardive dyskinesia (TD) is characterized by involuntary muscle movements, most commonly associated with the mouth and tongue, although any muscle group may be affected. The incidence of TD is approximately 3 to 5% per year over the initial 8 years of treatment (Kane, 1995). It is estimated that 20 to 25% of young and middle-aged patients treated with conventional antipsychotics develop at least mild TD symptoms with the prevalence higher in older patients (Kane et al., 1983). Tardive dyskinesia is usually a consequence of long-term conventional antipsychotic medication, with duration of treatment as the primary risk factor for its development. However, there are documented cases of TD schizophrenic patients independent of exposure to conventional antipsychotics (Fenton et al., 1994). The incidence of TD is greater in older women and may be more common in patients with affective disorders. It has been argued that TD is caused by an increase in the number of striatal dopamine receptors, although γ-aminobutyric acid and other neurotransmitters have been implicated as well. The severity of TD is variable, with the majority of cases being mild. Severe cases of TD may be disabling and are less likely to be reversible.

Although a variety of treatments have been proposed for TD, there are no consistently effective therapies. It has been proposed that vitamin E may be modestly effective in treating this condition. Whereas the most appropriate treatment may be to lower the dose of conventional antipsychotic, this is not always possible. Accordingly, persistent moderate to severe TD may be an indication for a trial of clozapine.

Neuroleptic malignant syndrome. Neuroleptic malignant syndrome (NMS) is a rare and potentially fatal complication of antipsychotic treatment. It is characterized by muscle rigidity, hyperthermia, autonomic dysregulation, and mental status changes (Gratz et al., 1992). Neuroleptic malignant syndrome is associated with an elevated white blood cell count and an increase in serum creatinine phosphokinase (CPK). The condition may lead to rhabdomyolysis and acute renal failure. Risk factors for NMS are underlying medical illnesses, including infection, dehydration, physical exhaustion, extremes of age, and rapid changes in antipsychotic dosage. The incidence of NMS has been estimated at 0.5% to 1.0%. While the pathophysiology is unknown, it has been hypothesized to be secondary to excessive dopamine receptor blockade or dopamine deprivation. The differential diagnosis of NMS includes heatstroke, lethal catatonia, and malignant hyperthermia.

Neuroleptic malignant syndrome is an acute medical emergency. Patients should be immediately hospitalized and supported with IV fluids. All antipsychotic medications should be stopped. In some cases treatment with dopamine agonists such as bromocriptine or amantadine, or muscle relaxants such as dantrolene are helpful, although the efficacy of these agents has not been systematically studied. The most important treatment for NMS is adequate hydration and secondary medical support. Antipsychotic treatment should not be reinitiated for at least 2 weeks after the resolution of the NMS episode, with either gradual dosing of a low-potency agent or a new-generation drug with low EPS liability. These patients should have regular monitoring of their vital signs, WBC and CPK.

Toxicity. Conventional antipsychotics are relatively nonlethal. The manifestations of overdosage are largely dependent on the antiadrenergic and anticholinergic properties of the particular agent (Table 2-3). Since most conventional antipsychotics are also potent antiemetics, overdoses should be treated with gastric lavage, rather than emetics. Hypotension is usually the manifestation of α_1-adrenergic receptor blockade and is optimally treated with dopamine or norepinephrine administration. Patients who develop cardiac abnormalities should be treated with lidocaine. Conventional antipsychotics with long half-lives may require cardiac monitoring for several days after an overdose is consumed.

Clozapine

Clozapine, a dibenzodiazepine, was first synthesized in 1959. It was introduced into the European market in the 1960s (Hippius, 1989) and almost immediately thought to be more effective than conventional anti-

Table 2-3
Manifestations of Overdosage

Severe EPS, including dystonia, severe rigidity, and sedation

Mydriatic pupils; DTRs are decreased

Tachycardia (low-potency agents); hypotension (α-adrenergic receptor blockade, in the face of unopposed β-adrenergic receptors)

EEG: diffuse slowing and low voltage; seizures (low-potency agents)

Prolongation of the QT interval; atypical ventricular tachycardia (torsade de pointes), with secondary heart block or ventricular fibrillation

psychotics (Davis and Casper, 1977). However, in 1975, eight patients died in southwestern Finland from infections secondary to clozapine-induced agranulocytosis. These deaths led to the withdrawal of clozapine from unrestricted usage, with use permitted only for selected treatment-resistant patients. The successful use of clozapine in these patients led to a large multicenter study in the United States to examine whether it was more effective than conventional antipsychotics for treatment-resistant patients (Kane et al., 1988). The successful outcome of this study led to the approval of clozapine by the Food and Drug Administration in 1990. It is approved for the treatment of patients whose positive symptoms do not adequately respond to conventional antipsychotic therapy, either because of ineffective therapy or because conventional therapy cannot be continued because of intolerable side effects. Clozapine is the only drug with demonstrated superior efficacy to conventional antipsychotics in rigorously defined treatment-resistant schizophrenia (Christison et al., 1991; Barnes and McEvedy, 1996). Clozapine is also effective in reducing symptoms of hostility and violence (Mallya et al., 1992; Breier et al., 1994; Wilson, 1992), tardive dyskinesia (Tamminga et al., 1994), and the risk of suicide (Meltzer and Okayli, 1995).

Mechanism of action. Clozapine modifies the activity of a number of neurotransmitter systems (Mel-

tzer et al., 1989). Clozapine is an antagonist of both the D1 and D2 dopamine receptors in the brain. However, in contrast to conventional antipsychotics, clozapine has a higher affinity for the D1 than the D2 sites, and has its highest affinity for the dopamine D4 receptor. Clozapine is also a potent serotonin antagonist, with higher affinity for the 5HT2a receptor than for any of the dopamine receptors. Clozapine is also an antagonist at serotonin 5HT2c, 5HT6, and 5HT7 receptors, noradrenergic (α-1 and α-2), cholinergic (nicotine and muscarinic) and histaminergic (H1) receptors.

There are several other properties that distinguish clozapine from conventional antipsychotics. In laboratory animals clozapine does not cause catalepsy, block apomorphine- and/or amphetamine-induced stereotyped behaviors, elevate serum prolactin, or cause dopamine receptor supersensitivity (Fitton and Heel, 1990). Moreover, clozapine only induces depolarization blockade in A10 dopamine neurons, an observation that is consistent with the pattern of clozapine-induced c-*fos* activation (Robertson et al., 1994). Clozapine activates c-*fos* expression, a new marker of cellular activity, in the nucleus accumbens, ventral striatum, anterior cingulate, and medial prefrontal cortex. In contrast, haloperidol also activates c-*fos* expression in regions that receive projections from A9 dopamine neurons, such as the dorsal striatum. However, it is still not known which of these pharmacological properties is associated with its superior efficacy.

Side effects. Despite the superior efficacy of clozapine it is used sparingly because of its side effect profile, even though it may be safer than other antipsychotics in some respects. In contrast to traditional antipsychotics, clozapine has a very low incidence of acute or chronic motor side effects. Indeed, there are no known cases of acute dystonic reactions, with parkinsonian symptoms and akathisia being rare with clozapine therapy. In addition, it is believed clozapine may not cause TD, although there have been several equivocal case reports. Moreover, extended clozapine treatment has actually been associated with decreased TD (Tamminga et al., 1994) and clozapine has also been used to treat patients with tardive dystonia and intractable akathisia. Clozapine may also be less likely to cause NMS and should be considered as an alternative therapy for patients with a previous history of this reaction.

However, clozapine is associated with a number of serious side effects, the most serious of which is agranulocytosis, which occurs in 0.25% to 1.0% of treated patients. The peak incidence of agranulocytosis is within the first 4 to 18 weeks of treatment, although cases have been observed after more than 1 year of therapy. The onset of agranulocytosis may be either precipitous or gradual. The condition may be more common in older women and in people on other myelosuppressive drugs. The mechanism of clozapine-induced agranulocytosis is unknown, with direct toxic, immune, and/or combined toxic/immune mechanisms having been postulated. There are unreplicated data suggesting an association between HLA haplotypes and an increased risk for agranulocytosis. Alternatively, the clozapine metabolite, norclozapine, may be toxic to bone marrow cells. The FDA currently requires weekly white blood cell monitoring, with specific guidelines for the management of clozapine-induced abnormalities of bone marrow function. Since the vulnerability period is greatest in the first 6 months, a change in these guidelines for chronic treatment is anticipated. Further, patients should not be simultaneously treated with other drugs that are known to suppress the bone marrow, such as carbamazepine. If the white blood cell count is below 2000/mm^3, with a granulocyte count below 1000/mm^3, clozapine must be discontinued at once and the patient hospitalized in protective isolation. During hospitalization the white cell count differential should be monitored at least every other day. Filgastrim, a granulocyte-colony stimulating factor, may be used to stimulate granulocyte regeneration. Patients who develop agranulocytosis should not be rechallenged with clozapine. There is no evidence of cross-reactivity between clozapine and other drugs that cause agranulocytosis.

The other major side effects associated with clozapine are sedation, hypersalivation and a weight gain which is superimposed on any weight gain from previous antipsychotic treatment; other side effects include tachycardia, orthostatic hypotension, and seizures. The risk of grand mal seizures is relatively high (up to 10%) with clozapine which may also cause myoclonic and atonic activity. Myoclonic jerks frequently presage the development of grand mal seizures. Electroencephalographic changes and seizures appear to be dosage-related, with the risk for seizures markedly increased at doses greater than 600 mg/day. The occurrence of a seizure is not a contraindication for continued clozapine treatment. Rather, patients who experience a seizure should have their dosage reduced to 50% of the last dose that did not cause seizures, with consideration given to instituting antiepileptic drug therapy such as valproic acid. Carbamazepine should not be used for this purpose because of its association with agranulocytosis.

Toxicity. Clozapine overdose is associated with altered mental status including somnolence to coma, anticholinergic toxicity (tachycardia, delirium), seizures, respiratory depression, hypotension, and EPS. Fatalities have been reported with doses greater than 2500 mg.

New Generation Antipsychotics

The discovery of clozapine, with its superior efficacy and benign EPS side effect profile, has led to the development of a new generation of antipsychotics. These drugs mimic one or more of the pharmacological characteristics of clozapine in an attempt to reproduce its efficacy, lower the EPS liability and agranulocytosis. While this new generation of drugs has actually surpassed clozapine with respect to safety, including a decreased incidence of EPS, to date, none has been shown to be as efficacious as clozapine (Conley, 1997). These new drugs are often referred to as atypical antipsychotics because of their decreased likelihood for producing EPS.

Risperidone. Risperidone was approved for use as an antipsychotic in 1994. A benzisoxazol derivative, risperidone has a high affinity for 5HT2a and dopamine D2 receptors, being markedly more potent as an antagonist of the former than the latter. Risperidone is also a potent antagonist at the α_1-adrenergic and histamine H1 receptors, with modest activity at the α_2-adrenergic receptor. It lacks significant activity at the dopamine D1 and cholinergic receptors. Like conventional antipsychotics, risperidone produces depolarization blockade in both A9 and A10 neurons, and causes catalepsy at high doses and dystonia in laboratory animal models.

These preclinical characteristics are reflected in the EPS side effect profile of risperidone. Parkinsonian side effects occur in a dose-related manner, becoming pronounced with doses equal to or greater than 10 mg/day. There are case reports of both TD and NMS with risperidone, although the relative risk of TD compared to conventional antipsychotics has not been clearly established. Other side effects include nausea, vomiting, agitation, anxiety, insomnia, sedation, an increase in prolactin secretion, and weight gain. However, in general, risperidone is relatively well tolerated.

Risperidone overdose is characterized by somnolence, seizures, prolonged QT and widened QRS, hypotension, and EPS. Fatalities have been associated with risperidone overdose.

Olanzapine. Olanzapine was approved for the treatment of schizophrenia in 1996. It has a receptor binding profile very similar to clozapine, with high affinity as an antagonist at dopamine (both D1 and D2 receptors), serotonin (5HT2a, 5HT2c, 5HT6), adrenergic (α-1), histamine (H1), and muscarinic (M1) receptors. In contrast to clozapine, olanzapine has relatively little activity at the same 5HT-, α-2, and other cholinergic receptors. Similar to clozapine, risperidone, and other atypical antipsychotics, olanzapine has higher affinity for the 5HT2a than dopamine D2 receptors. Like clozapine it produces depolarization blockade in A10, but not A9, dopamine neurons, and, in laboratory animal models, causes catalepsy and dystonia only at high doses (Tamminga and Kane, 1997).

As would be predicted from its preclinical profile, olanzapine treatment is not associated with significant EPS across a broad dosage range. The relationship among olanzapine treatment, TD and NMS has not been established. In addition, olanzapine has minimal effects on the plasma levels of prolactin, and does not appear to produce any cardiac side effects including tachycardia. Olanzapine does cause somnolence, dizziness, dry mouth, constipation, and moderate weight gain.

Olanzapine overdose is associated with sedation, anticholinergic toxicity, including tachycardia, delirium, seizures, hypotension, and EPS. There has been insufficient experience with olanzapine to determine its lethality.

Quetiapine. Quetiapine has low affinity as an antagonist at dopamine D1 and D2 receptors and serotonin 5HT2a and 5HT1c sites, although it has a relatively higher affinity for the 5HT2a than the D2 receptor. It also has some affinity for α_1- and α_2-adrenergic receptors, but is not an anticholinergic. Quetiapine does not cause c-*fos* activation in the dorsal striatum, nor does it cause catalepsy or dystonia in laboratory animals at clinically relevant doses.

Quetiapine is not associated with significant EPS, including akathisia. It does, however, produce sedation, somnolence, headache, reversible elevation of hepatic transaminases, and weight gain. Its use does not cause an elevation of plasma prolactin.

Ziprasidone. Ziprasidone is under FDA review. Ziprasidone has a relatively unique profile as a neurotransmitter receptor antagonist. In addition to being a potent 5HT2a and D2 dopamine receptor antagonist, ziprasidone is a potent inhibitor of norepinephrine and serotonin reuptake. While ziprasidone causes depolarization blockade of both A10 and A9 dopamine neurons, it only causes catalepsy at high doses. Ziprasidone use is not associated with EPS.

There are a host of potential new antipsychotics still in the early stages of development. This next generation promises to include drugs with novel mechanisms of action (e.g., partial agonist at glycine sites on the NMDA receptor complex) for different target symptoms (e.g., negative symptoms).

Initial Treatment of an Acute Psychotic Episode

If the psychotic episode is the first, or the patient has not been treated with an antipsychotic for longer than 1 year, treatment should commence with a new-generation antipsychotic. The current choices are risperidone, olanzapine, quetiapine, and possibly sertindole. The recommended doses are for risperidone, 1 to 4 mg given in a once-daily dose at night, increasing no higher than 6 mg. Olanzapine treatment begins at 10 mg given as a once-daily dose at night, increasing to 20 to 25 mg within the first week. Sertindole is administered at 12 mg on day 1, and increased to 20 to 24 mg given as a once-daily dose at night. For quetiapine, the beginning dose is 75 mg titrating to 150 to 300 mg twice daily (total daily dose of 300–600 mg).

The initial therapy is continued for 3 weeks. If the patient has a good response with no complications, medication should be maintained for 6 months to 1 year. At that time the need for antipsychotic medication should be reevaluated. During this time, the diagnosis of the patient should become clearer with new cases, whereas chronic schizophrenia will probably need long-term maintenance medication.

If the patient has a history of prior response to a conventional antipsychotic with good tolerance, the prior medication should be resumed. Commonly used conventional antipsychotics that are often well tolerated are haloperidol in a dose range of 5 to 15 mg/day, and fluphenazine, in the dose range of 4 to 15 mg/day. Those who had a history of response to intermediate or low-potency antipsychotics, such as perphenazine or chlorpromazine can be treated with these again. Because of the likelihood of causing extrapyramidal side effects with conventional antipsychotics, these agents should not normally be used as first-line drugs in newly diagnosed patients.

Agitation and insomnia. Quite often patients will experience marked agitation and hostility when they first enter a care setting. This agitation will usually be lessened by a calm, controlled environment. Lorazepam, ½ to 2 mg, may be used as an adjunct anxiolytic and hypnotic to help calm the patient. The use of lorazepam should be limited to the time needed to help the patient maintain control. Most patients respond well to a calm, structured environment and return to control following 1 to 2 days of lorazepam treatment. If the use of short-term benzodiazepines is contraindicated, high-dose antipsychotic medications, such as haloperidol 1 to 5 mg orally or 1 to 2 mg intramuscularly, or droperidol, 1 to 2 mg intramuscularly, may also be used as an adjunct medication to control agitation and hostility. These medications should be considered second line because of their likelihood of producing extrapyramidal side effects, including dystonia. Droperidol should only be used if acute cardiovascular support is available since cardiovascular collapse, while rare, is a potentially fatal side effect of this therapy. As with the benzodiazepine, the time of use of these adjunct medications should be limited to the first day or two of initial care.

A second common complication of an acute psychotic episode is insomnia. The first-line recommended therapy is a benzodiazapine, such as lorazepam. If benzodiazapines are contraindicated, diphenhydramine or chloral hydrate may be used as hypnotics. The use of hypnotics should be time limited since patients usually return to a more normal sleep pattern within 1 to 2 weeks following onset of the acute psychotic episode.

Extrapyramidal symptoms. Some of the most troublesome side effects of antipsychotic medications are extrapyramidal symptoms. These are expressed as both acute and chronic parkinsonian symptoms, akathisia, and dystonia. The occurrence of acute and chronic parkinsonism can be minimized by the use of new generation antipsychotics. Clozapine is the only drug known to be an effective antipsychotic which virtually never causes parkinsonian side effects. This agent is, however, not recommended for first-line antipsychotic therapy because of its potential to induce agranulocytosis. The other new generation antipsychotics (risperidone, olanzapine, sertindole, and quetiapine) all have a markedly reduced tendency to cause extrapyramidal symptoms compared to traditional antipsychotics. Because these drugs can, however, cause parkinsonian symptoms, particularly in higher doses, it is important to carefully adhere to the recommended dose ranges and to monitor the patients. One of the most important hallmarks of the new antipsychotics is the possibility to adequately treat parkinsonian symptoms in most patients by reducing the dose without a loss of antipsychotic efficacy. If a patient experiences parkinsonian symptoms while taking one of these drugs, the symptoms should be treated with a rapidly acting antiparkinsonian agent, such as diphenhydramine or benztropine mesylate, if they are acutely distressing. The use of these medications also lessens the likelihood of an acute dystonic reaction. However, the primary therapy for parkinsonian symptoms in patients on new antipsychotics is dose reduction, with the use of secondary antiparkinsonian medications being time-limited.

Parkinsonian symptoms that present with traditional antipsychotics are more problematic and persistent than with the new antipsychotics. Again, the primary method for treating these symptoms should be dose reduction, which is effective in most cases. Secondary antiparkinsonian medication can also be helpful, with its use limited to the acute situation, if possible. A patient who has been treated chronically with traditional antipsychotics and develops parkinsonism, or other extrapyramidal side effects that are

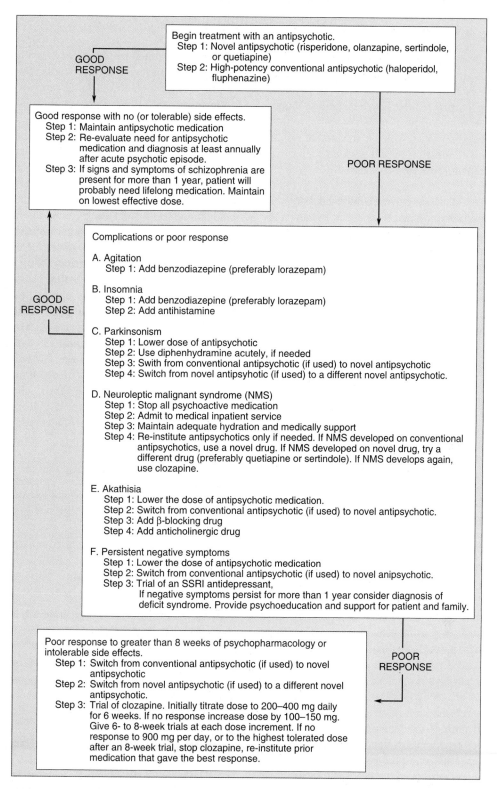

Figure 2–2. *Decision tree for treatment of acute or relapsing psychotic episode.*

refractory to dosage reduction, should be changed to a new antipsychotic medication. This procedure should also be followed if the patient develops refractory parkinsonism on one of the new antipsychotics. If a change from a typical to a new antipsychotic, or from one new antipsychotic to another, is not effective for eliminating chronic parkinsonian symptoms, clozapine should be considered.

Akathisia.   Akathisia may be associated with other extrapyramidal symptoms. It is caused by new antipsychotics as well as conventional agents. The treatment of akathisia is dose reduction of the antipsychotic and the adjunctive use of a β-adrenergic blocking agent. A change from one antipsychotic drug class to another may also reduce this side effect. Clozapine may be effective in reducing akathesia in a patient who fails to respond to other therapy.

Continuation Pharmacotherapy of Schizophrenia

Following reduction of symptoms and the establishment of clinical stability, long-term management must be considered. Treatment during this phase is usually outpatient-based and involves maintaining symptom reduction, preventing relapse, minimizing adverse effects, and maximizing adherence with treatment recommendations. Quality of life and cost-effectiveness become increasingly important in this phase. Crucial to all these goals is the integration of effective psychosocial treatments with pharmacotherapy (Hogarty et al., 1995; Scott and Dixon, 1995; Carpenter, 1996).

Continuous antipsychotic medication has long been established as the optimal approach for most patients suffering from schizophrenia (Carpenter, 1996; Kane, 1996). Controlled studies document that symptom exacerbation occurs at almost three times the rate on placebo as compared to active drug (Baldessarini et al., 1990; Davis et al., 1993). For many years, very substantial doses of antipsychotic were administered during maintenance therapy (600–1200 mg chlorpromazine equivalents). Although reduced in rate, relapse and rehospitalization continued at very significant levels between the 1960s and 1980s. In an effort to increase therapeutic efficacy, very high doses were used. However, controlled studies show no advantage to these high doses (Baldessarini et al., 1988; Baldessarini et al., 1990; Bollini et al., 1994). In fact, the incidence of TD is much greater, as is poor compliance, with high-dose antipsychotic regimens.

Long-acting depot fluphenazine and haloperidol has been developed to address poor compliance. The antipsychotic is linked to the lipid decanoate and is injected intramuscularly. A single injection provides steady blood levels for 4 weeks. A modest advantage has been documented in relapse prevention with depot as compared to oral administration (Davis et al., 1993). Many believe depot antipsychotic treatment is underutilized in the United States.

For maintenance treatment, clinical studies suggest that doses above 375 mg chlorpromazine equivalents are not associated with greater efficacy (Bollini et al., 1994) and that the minimal effective dose for about half of patients is between 50 and 150 mg chlorpromazine equivalents (Baldessarini et al., 1988). Current recommendations for standard maintenance doses are in the range of 300 to 600 mg chlorpromazine equivalents (Baldessarini et al., 1988; Lehman et al., 1998).

An alternative approach to improving the risk/benefit ratio during maintenance treatment was investigated during the past decade. It was hypothesized that a substantial dose reduction in maintenance treatment would decrease adverse effects, increase medication compliance, yet retain most therapeutic effects. The results of these studies are interesting and have changed standard practice (Dixon et al., 1995; Carpenter, 1996; Kane, 1996). With continuous medication, 10% of the standard dose resulted in more relapses but in better social course and a remarkable reduction in drug exposure. Doses representing 20% of the standard dose were associated with more small exacerbations, but these could usually be managed on an outpatient basis with supplemental oral medication. Other aspects of illness, such as negative symptoms, also improved.

Similar effects were observed with patients who were drug free until the first signs of relapse triggered a rapid medication intervention, a more taxing strategy for therapists and patients than continuous medication. The results with this approach were generally not as good as with continuously administered, low-dose medication. In the one study directly comparing standard continuous-dose, low-dose continuous, and targeted medication, the low-dose continuous was as successful in leading to a medication reduction in the long run, and was associated with fewer psychotic symptom exacerbations compared to a targeted medication strategy. Both of these dose reduction approaches reduced medication exposure and diminished negative symptoms compared to standard dose, continuous treatment. However, at the end of the 2-year study there was no psychotic symptom disadvantage to the dose reduction approaches, with more exacerbations encountered compared to the standard dose strategy.

The following guidelines are derived from the preceding work:

1. The optimal long-term treatment is continuous medication for most patients.
2. The dose range of conventional antipsychotic drugs should be much lower than the 600 to 1000 mg chlorpromazine equivalents previously used in standard practice. A range of 200 to 400 mg is now accepted, and most patients will do well in the range of 150 to 300 mg.
3. Depot antipsychotics can assure compliance in patients willing to undergo this treatment. Most information on low-dose, continuous medication has involved depot dosing. If close clinical monitoring is available, 12.5 mg fluphenazine decanoate administered every 2 to 3 weeks, or 25 to 50 mg haloperidol decanoate every 4 weeks, will suffice for most patients. Rapid oral supplementation for a few weeks can be effective for those experiencing periodic symptom exacerbations.
4. Patients who refuse continuous drugs or patients who experience prolonged stability after a single psychotic episode are candidates for a targeted drug approach.
5. Continuing side effects are an indication for dose reduction.
6. Early signs of TD are an indication for targeted drugs, substantial dose reduction, or a change to clozapine.

The preceding guidelines are likely to be modified as data become available from maintenance studies with the new generation antipsychotics. There is already evidence that clozapine is superior in relapse prevention in treatment-resistant, chronic patients (Essock et al., 1996). The relatively benign EPS side effect profiles of the new drugs leads to the hope that medication adherence will increase and greater effectiveness will be achieved in the future. It is not evident that the same efforts at dose reduction will be required to optimize the risk/benefit ratio with the new drugs. On the other hand, it will be interesting to determine the treatment profiles of the new generation drugs in long-term treatment as compared to low-dose conventional drugs. Risperidone, at 4 mg per day, will have decided advantages over haloperidol at 15 to 20 mg per day, although it is less certain that advantages will be seen in comparison to 4 to 6 mg of haloperidol per day or 12.5 mg fluphenazine decanoate every third week. Cost-effectiveness data will no doubt influence the choice as well.

Treatment Resistance

One of the most difficult problems associated with antipsychotic therapy is partial or inadequate response. Historically, drug therapy for treatment-resistant schizophrenia entailed using different dose strategies of conventional antipsychotics or the administration of adjunct agents such as lithium, anticonvulsants, or benzodiazepines. With the development of clozapine, attention has shifted to the use of new antipsychotics for such patients. This shift occurred because of the superior efficacy of clozapine and the fact that new antipsychotics have either significantly fewer side effects or improved efficacy as compared to conventional antipsychotics.

Treatment resistance refers to the continuation of psychosis (reality distortion and disorganization symptoms) and associated features despite receiving what is usually adequate pharmacotherapy.

Conventional Antipsychotic Drugs

Conventional antipsychotics have long been the first-line therapy for treating schizophrenia. These drugs are considered interchangeable in terms of efficacy since in over 100 comparative studies only once was a differential effect observed (Klein and Davis, 1969; Janicak et al., 1993). In controlled trials in patients with drug-resistant symptoms, fewer than 5% responded after changing from one conventional antipsychotic to another (Kane et al., 1988; Breier et al., 1994). The primary reason for selecting one conventional antipsychotic over another is to reduce side effects and to provide different dosing strategies. High-potency drugs, such as haloperidol and fluphenazine, have a significantly greater tendency to induce extrapyramidal side effects although they cause less sedation and postural hypertension than low-potency agents such as chlorpromazine or thioridazine. Haloperidol and fluphenazine are the only two conventional antipsychotics available as injectable depot medication, a formulation that can ensure drug compliance and sometimes optimizes response (see Maintenance section).

The choice of a particular conventional antipsychotic should be influenced by a patient's past response and proneness to side effects. If no clinical improvement is observed after 3 weeks of therapy, patient compliance in taking the medication at the recommended dose should be evaluated by obtaining a blood level. If the patient is compliant, a different drug should be considered if there is no significant improvement following 4 to 8 weeks of therapy.

New Generation Drugs

Novel antipsychotics should be the first considered when conventional drug therapy fails. Four of these, clozapine, risperidone, olanzapine, and quetiapine are reviewed here because they are available for use in the United States.

Clozapine.   Clozapine was approved for the treatment of patients whose symptoms do not respond adequately to conventional antipsychotics either because they were ineffective or because side effects were intolerable. Clozapine remains the only drug with proven efficacy in rigorously defined treatment-resistant schizophrenia (Christison et al., 1991; Barnes and McEvedy, 1996).

Despite the robust clinical response to clozapine (Meltzer et al., 1990; Wilson, 1992; Breier et al., 1993), benefits that translate into improved living situations and decreased cost of care have not always been demonstrated with this agent (Zito et al., 1993), particularly in the first year of use (Essock et al., 1996). Partly this is because clozapine is normally administered to only those who are difficult to treat (and discharge) (Safferman et al., 1991) and is being used by only a subset of clinicians who are comfortable with this agent. Other studies have shown that clozapine is a cost-effective treatment over the long term (Rosenheck et al., 1997).

Slow dose escalation is the optimal strategy for clozapine administration. Patients should be evaluated for response at a dose range of 200 to 600 mg per day. Only those experiencing few side effects should be titrated to doses higher than 600 mg per day. Patients should not be given a higher dose of clozapine if myoclonus occurs, as this may portend the development of seizures (Bak et al., 1995). Patients who respond to clozapine do so within 8 weeks of reaching their optimal dose (Conley et al., 1997).

Risperidone.   Risperidone is an effective treatment for positive symptoms of this disorder (Chouinard et al., 1993; Marder and Meibach, 1994). Moreover, risperidone has also been shown to be equivalent to placebo in the production of EPS at doses at or below 6 mg per day. Doses of 10 mg per day or higher, however, do cause EPS in a dose-dependent fashion. Thus, risperidone may have a very different clinical profile in low versus high doses. There is no evidence that doses above 8 mg per day are more effective, with the optimal dose range appearing to be 2 to 6 mg for most patients.

Despite some indication that risperidone might be more efficacious than haloperidol (Marder and Meibach, 1994), it remains an open question whether it is superior to conventional antipsychotics in patients with well-defined treatment-resistant schizophrenia. Although there have been reports of patients who respond poorly to their medications who improved on risperidone (Chouinard et al., 1994; Keck et al., 1995), these studies were open-labeled, retrospective, or uncontrolled.

The results of one study suggested risperidone is equivalent to clozapine in the treatment of chronic schizophrenics (Klieser et al., 1995). However, in this case the subjects were not categorized on the basis of treatment resistance, and the study was not large enough to adequately test for a differential effect between the drugs.

It appears firmly established that risperidone is usually not effective in treatment-resistant clozapine responders (Lacey et al., 1995; Shore, 1995), although there are reports of its effectiveness in improving the quality of life and reducing hospital stays in drug-responsive patients (Cohen and Underwood, 1994; Lindstrom et al., 1995). As risperidone is a much safer drug than clozapine, and usually better tolerated than traditional antipsychotics, a trial with this agent is warranted to determine whether a patient who responds poorly to conventional antipsychotics will benefit from risperidone before switching to clozapine.

Olanzapine.   With a receptor binding profile similar to clozapine, olanzapine is effective in treatment-responsive schizophrenia (Tolefson et al., 1997). Moreover, olanzapine is less likely to induce extrapyramidal symptoms then traditional agents and it is no different from placebo in the incidence of akathisia. In an open clinical trial it was found that some well-characterized patients with treatment-resistant schizophrenia improved when given olanzapine (Conley et al., 1996), although it did not show superior efficacy in a double-blind trial of such patients, except in anxiety and depression ratings (Conley et al., 1997). Olanzapine was substantially better tolerated than chlorpromazine, with the most effective doses being 15 and 25 mg per day. While olanzapine is also an acceptable choice for patients unresponsive to conventional antipsychotics, it is unlikely a risperidone nonresponder will benefit from this drug.

Quetiapine. Quetiapine has a pharmacological profile that includes high serotonin (5HT1a) receptor affinity relative to its affinity for dopamine receptors. A low-potency compound, the most effective doses for quetiapine are 300 mg to 450 mg per day, similar to clozapine (Arvanitis et al., 1996). A safer medication than conventional agents, there is no difference between placebo and quetiapine in the induction of EPS or akathisia.

The following points summarize considerations when confronting a treatment-resistant patient:

1. Treatment resistance is defined by persistent psychosis and other difficult-to-treat psychopathology.
2. Treatment resistance is a continuum, and refractory patients are the most severely affected.
3. Clozapine has documented superior efficacy as an antipsychotic in treatment-resistant cases.
4. While new-generation drugs have side effect advantages over clozapine and conventional agents, there is as yet no adequate documentation of their superior efficacy in treatment-resistant subjects.

Alternate Therapies

If patients remain refractory to treatment after trials with novel agents, alternate therapies should be considered. These include adjunct medication, reserpine, and ECT. While the evidence for the efficacy of these therapies is limited, they may be of use in certain circumstances.

Lithium. Adjunct lithium therapy is beneficial in some patients with treatment-resistant schizophrenia (Small et al., 1975; Growe et al., 1979; Carmen et al., 1981; Kane and Marder, 1993). A 4-week trial of lithium appears adequate to detect a response. Although patients with affective symptoms are most likely to benefit, others do so as well (Delva and Letemendia, 1986). There are reports that lithium has been useful in reducing hostility in treatment-resistant schizophren-

ics, and thus may be of particular value in some violent patients (Christison et al., 1991).

Published trials of adjunct lithium, although positive, have been conducted with small numbers of patients (Kane, 1996). Therefore, definitive evidence of its benefit as adjunct therapy is lacking (Johns and Thompson, 1995). Lithium should be used with caution in combination with conventional antipsychotics or clozapine because of the possibility of inducing delirium and encephalopathy with these combinations (Barnes and McEvedy, 1996).

Anticonvulsants. Carbamazepine and valproic acid are effective in the treatment of bipolar affective disorder with psychosis (Post, 1990; Freeman et al., 1992), and are often considered as an adjunct therapy in patients with schizophrenia. In this regard, carbamazepine has been used as an adjunct in several controlled trials with schizophrenics. The results of these trials have been consistently positive (Simhandl and Meszaros, 1992), although the patient populations were small. The positive effects reported were modest and usually involved nonspecific improvement in areas such as behavior and social adjustment. Carbamazepine is not an alternative to antipsychotics since it is no better than placebo in preventing relapse (Carpenter et al., 1991).

Carbamazepine must be used with caution because it can cause disorientation, ataxia and agranulocytosis. Moreover, carbamazepine can reduce haloperidol blood levels by as much as 50%. Likewise, valproic acid should be used with caution because of potential hepatotoxicity (PDR, 1996).

Benzodiazepines. There have been several reports on the use of adjunct benzodiazapines in treatment-resistant schizophrenia. The results have been mixed, however, with some double-blind studies showing a treatment effect (Wolkowitz et al., 1986), while others found no benefit with their use (Pato et al., 1989). Because patients with schizophrenia are often irritable and anxious, it is not surprising that benzodiazapines are frequently administered to these individuals. However, these drugs should be used with caution because of the risks of chronic sedation, fatigue, ataxia, dependence and behavioral disinhibition (Pato et al., 1989). There is also a possibility of synergistic toxicity with clozapine and the benzodiazepines (Meltzer et al., 1989). The main role of antianxiety drugs in the treatment of schizophrenia is in the acute management of agitation or in the early treatment of prodromal symptoms (early signs of relapse) in patients who decline antipsychotics.

Antidepressants. Many patients with schizophrenia are depressed during acute episodes and demoralized during the chronic stages of the illness. Indeed, antipsychotic drugs may increase the symptoms of depression. While antidepressants were used sparingly in the past because of concern they might precipitate psychosis, this is not believed to be a significant risk. In general, antidepressants have a very modest effect in most schizophrenic patients and are not an effective treatment for demoralization. Nonetheless, patients with persistent depression or depressive episodes separate from psychosis merit a trial with antidepressants at a minimally effective dose. There is some evidence that clozapine has a positive effect on depressed mood and may reduce suicide rates (Meltzer, 1994).

OTHER THERAPIES

While there are historical studies suggesting that β-adrenergic receptor blockers and reserpine may be useful in the treatment of refractory schizophrenia (Conley et al., 1997), there have been no controlled studies on these agents using the current diagnostic criteria. Thus, there is very limited evidence that long-term therapy with either of these drugs may prove beneficial.

Likewise, there have been no controlled studies of the effectiveness of ECT in treatment-resistant schizophrenics. Before clozapine was available there were some data from uncontrolled trials that ECT was beneficial for treatment-resistant patients (Friedel, 1986), although the effect was most robust in those with a short duration of illness (Small, 1985). Two open trials of ECT with patients who failed to respond to clozapine (Benatov et al., 1996; Remington et al., 1996) found some benefit. However, persistence of effect and the utility of ECT in long-term maintenance have not yet been addressed.

The following principles should help ensure the likelihood of success when initiating antipsychotic drug therapy:

1. Identification of defined target symptoms. Antipsychotics are most effective in treating the positive symptoms of psychosis, including hallucinations, delusions, thought disorder, and bizarre behavior. Newer medications may also be helpful in reducing negative symptoms, such as poor socialization, withdrawal, and affective blunting, particularly if these are secondary to side effects of conventional antipsychotics. Clozapine is particularly effective in hostile, aggressive psychotic patients. Understanding the target symptoms for a specific drug trial allows for greater clarity in defining the success or failure of the therapy.

2. Antipsychotics should be systematically examined at optimal dosages and for a sufficient duration to establish efficacy. This is particularly critical before adjunct drugs are used as these may complicate the clinical situation to the point where defining the optimal drug treatment is not possible. Conventional antipsychotics are generally used at too high a dose, diminishing their effectiveness even for acute treatment because of adverse effects and poor compliance.

3. Consideration should be given to the possibility that medication intolerance, noncompliance, inadequate social support and lack of psychosocial treatment may create the appearance of treatment resistance. These factors should be explored before declaring any particular drug therapy a failure. Although therapeutic dose ranges for most antipsychotics are not well established, blood level measurements may be useful to establish compliance.

4. The utility of a single agent must be fully defined before using multiple drugs. There is tremendous pressure for the clinician to find a therapy that rapidly treats every psychological problem manifest in a patient. It must be remembered, however, that no adjunct agent has ever been conclusively demonstrated to consistently and robustly improve antipsychotic response. Hostility, irritability, insomnia and withdrawal can all be secondary to psychosis and may resolve only after the patient has responded fully to the antipsychotic of choice.

5. Every effort must be made to prevent EPS by the appropriate choice of primary therapy. In this regard the new antipsychotics are effective at doses that do not produce extrapyramidal symptoms in the majority of patients. This property should minimize persistent side effects responsible for therapeutic failure.

6. Maintaining a positive therapeutic attitude. There are more choices than ever of antipsychotics with new drugs appearing annually. Patients should be encouraged to believe there is reason to be optimistic a beneficial therapy will be found, even if they have a history of severe mental illness.

7. Fully utilize psychosocial treatment which, by reducing stress and increasing the patient's and family's understanding of the illness, will enhance significantly the likelihood of a positive therapeutic response.

Because the new antipsychotics being introduced have different mechanisms of action than conventional agents, clinicians must explore fully the possibility of response with each of these drugs in turn in attempting to treat persistently refractory symptoms. To date, clozapine is the only medication with demonstrated efficacy in treatment-resistant subjects. The differential efficacy of new drugs in treatment-resistant schizophrenia will only be established upon completion of well-designed double-blind studies using rigorous entry criteria.

Negative Symptoms

Although most definitions of treatment resistance focus on the persistence of positive symptoms, there has been a growing awareness of the problems associated with persistent negative symptoms. Clozapine, and the novel antipsychotics risperidone, olanzapine, and quetiapine, have all been shown to have superior efficacy to conventional agents in reducing negative symptom ratings in double-blind clinical trials (Kane et al., 1988; Marder and Meibach, 1994; Tollefson et al., 1997; Tamminga et al., in press). There is some controversy, however, as to whether these drugs directly attenuate primary negative symptoms or whether their beneficial effect is secondary to improvement in other symptoms (Meltzer, 1994; Carpenter et al., 1995).

Comorbidity

Depression. Many schizophrenic patients treated with conventional antipsychotics exhibit persistent depression after recovery from the acute exacerbation of their psychosis. These patients should be re-evaluated for extrapyramidal side effects, negative symptoms, and incomplete response to the drug. If these problems are ruled out, post-psychotic depression should be considered and an antidepressant prescribed. The use of an SSRI antidepressant is recommended since they are devoid of the anticholinergic side effects that are characteristic of tricyclic antidepressants which may complicate the care and recovery of the patient. Also, SSRI antidepressants are less lethal in overdose than conventional antidepressants.

Substance abuse. Many patients with chronic schizophrenia and related psychoses suffer from substance abuse. These patients need recognition and therapy. Often they will benefit from 12-step type programs to treat their problem. If so, it is important to integrate pharmacotherapy into the program since it is critical for patients with schizophrenia to continue their medication to remain in remission. Because substance abusing patients have a greater risk for antipsychotic-induced TD, they should be treated with a new antipsychotic medication if possible.

Psychogenic polydipsia. Patients with chronic psychosis frequently suffer from psychogenic polydipsia. This disorder appears to be secondary to a dysregulation of the thirst satiation mechanisms in brain and is often resistant to any type of behavioral intervention. Psychogenic polydipsia is a potentially serious complication since it can result in severe renal and cardiac complications. Optimal therapy with an antipsychotic having limited direct anticholinergic effects is the first step in the first-line management of psychogenic polydipsia. Recommended drugs include risperidone and sertindole. If a patient remains unresponsive, clozapine has been found to be useful in some cases of chronic psychogenic polydipsia, being effective in treating the psychosis as well as in decreasing water intake. Therefore, a switch to clozapine should be considered for patients with persistent psychogenic polydipsia.

Noncompliance. Patients with chronic schizophrenia and related psychoses frequently have difficulties complying with their drug regimen. Thus, because patients with these disorders have limited insight into their problems, they tend to be noncompliant over time. Moreover, antipsychotics induce a number of unpleasant side effects whereas their benefits are subtle and obvious only over the long term. This too discourages compliance. If a patient appears to be noncompliant a careful examination should be performed to identify even minor extrapyramidal symptoms or akathisia. These symptoms are often very troublesome to a patient, even if their clinical appearance is modest on examination. The aggressive management of these conditions will often lead to major improvements in compliance. In this regard, antipsychotic doses will often need to be very carefully titrated to allow for a positive antipsychotic effect, while minimizing side effects. The novel antipsychotics, aside from clozapine, that appear to be least associated with extrapyramidal side effects are sertindole and quetiapine. Olanzapine and risperidone, while causing fewer extrapyramidal side effects than traditional antipsychotics, appear to have some intrinsic liability for causing EPS that needs to be carefully monitored. Risperidone, in particular, is likely to cause motor abnormalities if used in doses greater than 8 mg/day (Marder and Meibach, 1994).

If patients continue to be noncompliant while in the absence of side effects, it may be beneficial to consider the use of a depot antipsychotic. There are currently two depot antipsychotics available in the United States, haloperidol decanoate and fluphenazine decanoate. Haloperidol decanoate is most beneficial in doses of 25 to 100 mg intramuscularly every 4 weeks. While frequently initial doses will need to be somewhat higher, tolerance is best at doses of 100 mg or less. Fluphenazine decanoate appears to be most beneficial at doses between 25 to 50 mg intramuscularly every 3 to 4 weeks. When using depot medications it is important to carefully monitor the patient for extrapyramidal side effects and to establish the minimal effective dose of the drug (Schooler, 1996).

Persistent side effects.   If patients experience persistent bradykinesia or muscle rigidity, the dose of antipsychotic is probably too high and needs to be reduced. If bradykinesia and muscle rigidity persist even after a dose reduction, a switch of drug from one drug class to another is recommended. This is particularly true if patients are being treated with a conventional antipsychotic, in which one of the new novel antipsychotics should be tried. It may take some months for bradykinesia and muscle rigidity to remit fully in patients who have been on conventional antipsychotics for some time, as these drugs persist for months since they are slowly released from sec-

ondary storage areas in the body. Therefore, it is important to make patients aware of the fact that they will need to take the new therapy for several weeks before clinical improvement is seen.

Likewise, patients experiencing persistent akathisia should also undergo a careful evaluation to determine whether the minimal effective dose of the antipsychotic is being used, with a dose reduction often being beneficial in reducing this side effect. If akathisia persists, the addition of propranolol or other β-adrenergic receptor blocking agent is sometimes beneficial. It is sometimes of value to switch to a new drug class, even among the novel antipsychotics. If patients continue to have severe refractory akathisia, treatment with clozapine should be considered.

Patients receiving antipsychotics often experience sexual difficulties such as loss of lubrication or inability to maintain an erection. Female patients may also experience amenorrhea or dysmenorrhea and male patients as well as female patients may experience lactorrhea, breast tenderness, or enlargement. Because antipsychotics that have significant anticholinergic effects cause loss of erectile function and difficulties with lubrication and painful intercourse, minimizing the anticholinergic load should reduce or eliminate these side effects. This is accomplished by decreasing the dose of the antipsychotic or switching to a less anticholinergic agent. Drugs with marked adrenergic receptor blocking activity can also cause changes in sexual function. It has been reported that abnormal ejaculation has been seen with thioridazine (Tamminga et al., 1997) and may be present with other antipsychotics as well. Again, dose reduction or changing to another drug class is indicated if these side effects persist even after a dose reduction. Side effects that appear to be most related to prolactin dysregulation, such as breast enlargement or tenderness, and menstrual irregularities, are associated with antipsychotics that are potent dopamine receptor antagonists and thereby increase prolactin secretion. These problems are seen with conventional antipsychotics, particularly high-potency drugs, as well as with risperidone. While decreasing the dose of the drug can be useful in this case, it will often be necessary to switch to a completely new drug class to abolish this side effect.

For additional information on the drugs discussed in this chapter see chapters 17, 18, and 19 in *Goodman & Gilman's The Pharmacological Basis of Therapeutics* (Ninth Edition), McGraw-Hill, New York, 1996.

REFERENCES

Arvanitis LA, Miller BG, Seroquel Trial Study Group: ICI 204,636, an atypical antipsychotic: results from a multiple fixed-dose, placebo-controlled trial. Presented at the 32nd Annual Meeting of the New Clinical Drug Evaluation Unit, Boca Raton, FL, May 1996.

Arvanitis LA, Miller BG: Multiple fixed doses of "Seroquel" (quetiapine) in patients with acute exacerbation of schizophrenia: a comparison with haloperidol and placebo. Seroquel Trial 13 Study Group. *Biol Psychiatry* 1997;42:233–246.

Bak TH, Bauer M, Schaub RT, et al.: Myoclonus in patients treated with clozapine. *J Clin Psychiatry* 1995;56(9):418–422.

Baldessarini RJ, Cohen BM, Teicher M: Significance of neuroleptic dose and plasma level in the pharmacological treatment of psychoses. *Arch Gen Psychiatry* 1988;45:79-91.

Baldessarini RJ, Cohen BM, Teicher M: Pharmacologic treatment. In Levy ST, Ninan PT, *Schizophrenia: Treatment of Accute Psychotic Episodes;* Washington DC: American Psychiatric Press; 1990; pp. 61-118.

Barnes TRE, McEvedy CJB: Pharmacological treatment strategies in the non-responsive schizophrenic patient. *Intl Clin Psychopharmacol* 1996;11(2):67–71.

Benatov R, Sirota P, Megged S: Neuroleptic-resistant schizophrenia treated with clozapine and ECT. *Convulsive Ther* 1996;12(2):117–121.

Bleuler E, in Zinkin J (trans): *Dementia Praecox; or, the Group of Schizophrenias.* New York: International Universities Press, 1950 (original work published 1911).

Bollini P, Pampallona S, Orza MJ, et al.: Antipsychotic drugs: is more worse? A meta-analysis of the published randomized control trials. *Psychol Med* 1994;24:307–316.

Breier A, Buchanan RW, Irish D, et al.: Clozapine in schizophrenia outpatients, II: Outcome and long-term response patterns. *Hosp Commun Psychiatry* 1993;44:1145–1154.

Breier A, Buchanan RW, Kirkpatrick B, et al.: Clozapine in schizophrenic outpatients: effects of clozapine on positive and negative symptoms in outpatients with schizophrenia. *Am J Psychiatry* 1994;151:20–26.

Breier A, Su T-P, Saunders R, et al.: Schizophrenia is associated with elevated amphetamine-induced synaptic dopamine concentrations: evidence from a novel positron emission tomography method. *Proc Natl Acad Sci USA* 1997;94:2569–2574.

Buchanan RW, Brandes M, Breier A: Treating negative symptoms: pharmacological strategies. In Breier A: *The New Pharmacotherapy of Schizophrenia*, Washington DC: American Psychiatric Press; 179–204.

Carlsson A, Lindqvist M: Effect of chlorpromazine or haloperidol on formation of 3-methoxytyramine and normatanephrine in mouse brain. *Acta Pharmacol Toxicol* 1963;20:140–144.

Carmen JS, Bigelow LB, Wyatt RJ: Lithium combined with neuroleptics in chronic schizophrenic and schizoaffective patients. *J Clin Psychiatry* 1981;42:124–128.

Carpenter WT, Buchanan RW: Schizophrenia. *N Engl J Med* 1994;330:681–690.

Carpenter WT, Conley RR, Buchanan RW, et al.: Patient response and resource management: another view of clozapine treatment of schizophrenia. *Am J Psychiatry* 1995;152:827–832.

Carpenter WT: Maintenance therapy of persons with schizophrenia. *J Clin Psychiatry* 1996;57 (suppl 9):10–18

Carpenter WT, Kurz R, Kirkpatrick B, et al.: Carbamazepine maintenance treatment in outpatient schizophrenics. *Arch Gen Psychiatry* 1991;48:69–72

Chouinard G, Jones BD, Remington G, et al.: A Canadian multicenter placebo-controlled study of fixed doses of risperidone and haloperidol in the treatment of chronic schizophrenic patients. *J Clin Psychopharmacol* 1993;13:25–40.

Chouinard G, Vainer JL, Belanger MC, et al.: Risperidone and clozapine in the treatment of drug-resistant schizophrenia and neuroleptic-induced supersensitivity psychosis. *Prog Neuropsychopharmacol Biol Psychiatry* 1994;18(7):1129–1141.

Christison GW, Kirch DG, Wyatt RJ: When symptoms persist: Choosing among alternative somatic treatments for schizophrenia. *Schizophr Bull* 1991;17:217–245.

Cohen SA, Underwood MT: The use of clozapine in a mentally retarded and aggressive population. *J Clin Psychiatry* 1994;55(10):440–444.

Conley RR, Carpenter WT, Tamminga CA: Time to clozapine response in a standardized trial. *Am J Psychiatry* 1997;154:1243–1247.

Conley RR, Tamminga CA, Bartko J, et al.: Olanzapine vs. chlorpromazine in treatment-resistant schizophrenia. *Am J Psychiatry*, in press.

Creese I, Burt D, Snyder S: Dopamine receptor binding predicts clinical and pharmacological potencies of antischizophrenic drugs. *Science* 1976;192:481–483.

Davis JM, Casper R: Antipsychotic drugs: clinical pharmacology and therapeutic use. *Drugs* 1977;12:260–282.

Davis JM, Janicak PG, Singla A, et al.: Maintenance antipsychotic medication. In Barnes TRE (ed): *Antipsychotic Drugs and Their Side Effects.* New York: Academic Press, 1993; pp. 183–203.

Delnay J, Deniker P: Le traitement des psychoses par une méthode neurolytique dérivée de l'hibernotherapie. In Luxembourg MP (ed): *Congrès des Médecins Aliénistes et Neurologistes de France*. MANF, 1952; pp. 497–502.

Delva NJ, Letemendia FJ: Lithium treatment in schizophrenia and schizoaffective disorders. In Kerr A, Snaith P (eds): *Contemporary Issues in Schizophrenia*. London: Royal College of Psychiatrists, 1986; pp. 381–396.

Essock SM, Hargreaves WA, Dohm FA, et al.: Clozapine eligibility among state hospital patients. *Schizophr Bull* 1996;22(1):15–25.

Fenton WS, Wyatt RJ, McGlashan TH: Risk factors for spontaneous dyskinesia in schizophrenia. *Arch Gen Psychiatry* 1994;51:643–650.

Fitton A, Heel RC: Clozapine: a review of its pharmacological properties and therapeutic use in schizophrenia. *Drugs* 1990;40:722–747.

Freeman TW, Clothier JL, Pazzaglia P, et al.: A double-blind comparison of valproate and lithium in the treatment of acute mania. *Am J Psychiatry* 1992;149:108–111.

Friedel RO: The combined use of neuroleptics and ECT in drug-resistant schizophrenic patients. *Psychopharmacol Bull* 1986;22:928–930.

Grace AA, Bunney BS, Moore H, et al.: Dopamine-cell depolarization block as a model for the therapeutic actions of antipsychotic drugs. *Trends Neurosci* 1997;20:31–37.

Gratz SS, Levinson DF, Simpson GM: The treatment and management of neuroleptic malignant syndrome. *Prog Neuropsychopharmacol Biol Psychiatry* 1992;16:425–443.

Growe GA, Crayton JW, Klass DB, et al.: Lithium in chronic schizophrenia. *Am J Psychiatry* 1979;136:454–455.

Hippius H: The history of clozapine. *Psychopharmacology* 1989;99:S3–S5.

Hogarty GE, Kornblith SJ, Greenwald D, et al.: Personal therapy: a disorder-relevant psychotherapy for schizophrenia. *Schizophr Bull* 1995;21(3):379–393.

Janicak PG, Davis JM, Preskorn SH, et al.: *Principles and Practice of Psychopharmacotherapy*. Baltimore: Williams & Wilkins, 1993; pp. 104–106.

Johns CA, Thompson JW: Adjunctive treatments in schizophrenia: pharmacotherapies and electroconvulsive therapy. *Schizophr Bull* 1995;21:607–619.

Kane JM: Tardive dyskinesia: epidemiological and clinical presentation. In: Bloom FE, Kupfer DJ (eds): *Psychopharmacology: The Fourth Generation of Progress*. New York: Raven Press, 1995; pp. 1485–1495.

Kane JM: Schizophrenia. *N Engl J Med* 1996;334:34–41.

Kane J, Honigfeld G, Singer J, et al.: Clozapine for the treatment-resistant schizophrenic: a double-blind comparison with chlorpromazine. *Arch Gen Psychiatry* 1988;45:789–796.

Kane JM, Marder SR: Psychopharmacologic treatment of schizophrenia. *Schizophr Bull* 1993;2:287–302.

Kane JM, Rifkin A, Woerner M, et al.: Low-dose neuroleptic treatment of outpatient schizophrenics. *Arch Gen Psychiatry* 1983;40:893–896.

Keck PE, Wilson DR, Strakowski SM, et al.: Clinical predictors of acute risperidone response in schizophrenia, schizoaffective disorder, and psychotic mood disorders. *J Clin Psychiatry* 1995;56(10):455–470.

Klieser E, Lehmann E, Kinzler E, et al.: Randomized, double-blind, controlled trial of risperidone vs. clozapine in patients with chronic schizophrenia. *J Clin Psychopharmacol* 1995;Feb 15 (suppl 1):45S–51S.

Klein DF, Davis JM: *Diagnosis and Drug Treatment of Psychiatric Disorders*. Baltimore: Williams & Wilkins, 1969.

Knable MB, Weinberger DR: Dopamine, the prefrontal cortex and schizophrenia. *J Psychopharmacol* 1997;11:123–131.

Kraepelin E, Barclay RE (trans, ed): *Dementia Praecox and Paraphrenia*. Edinburgh: ES Livingstone, 1919.

Lacey RL, Preskorn SH, Jerkovich GS: Is risperidone a substitute for clozapine for patients who do not respond to neuroleptics? (Letter to editor). *Am J Psychiatry* 1995;152(9):1401.

Laruelle M, Abi-Dargham A, van Dyck CH, et al., Single photon emission computerized tomography imaging of amphetamine-induced dopamine release in drug-free schizophrenic subjects. *Proc Natl Acad Sci U S A* 1996;93:9235–9240.

Lehman AF, Steinwachs DM, and the Co-Investigators of the PORT Project: At issue: translating research into practice: The Schizophrenia Patient Outcomes Research Team (PORT) Treatment Recommendations. *Schizophr Bull* 1998;24:1–10

Liberman JA, Kane JM, Alvir J: Provacative tests with psychostimulant drugs in schizophrenia. *Psychopharmacology* 1987;91:415–433.

Lindstrom E, Eriksson B, Hellgren A, et al.: Efficacy and safety of risperidone in the long-term treatment of patients with schizophrenia. *Clin Ther* 1995;17(3):402–412.

Mallya AR, Roos PD, Roebuck-Colgan K: Restraint, seclusion, and clozapine. *J Clin Psychiatry* 1992;53:395–397.

Marder SR, Meibach RC: Risperidone in the treatment of schizophrenia. *Am J Psychiatry* 1994;151:825–835.

Meltzer HY: An overview of the mechanism of clozapine. *J Clin Psychiatry* 1994;55(suppl B):47–52.

Meltzer HY, Bastani B, Yound Kwon K, et al.: A prospective study of clozapine in treatment-resistant schizophrenic patients. I. Preliminary report. *Psychopharmacology* 1989;99:S68–S72.

Meltzer HY, Burnett S, Bastani B, et al.: Effects of six months of clozapine treatment on the quality of life of chronic schizophrenic patients. *Hosp Comm Psychiatry* 1990;41:892–897.

Meltzer HY, Okayli G: Reduction of suicidality during clozapine treatment of neuroleptic-resistant schizophrenia: impact on risk-benefit assessment. *Am J Psychiatry* 1995;152:183–190.

Olney JW, Farber NB. Glutamate receptor dysfunction and schizophrenia. *Arch Gen Psychiatry* 1995;52:998–1007.

Pato CN, Wolkowitz OM, Rapaport M, et al.: Benzodiazepine augmentation of neuroleptic treatment in patients with schizophrenia. *Psychopharmacol Bull* 1989;25:263–266.

Physicians' Desk Reference 1996, 50th Ed. Montvale, NJ: Medical Economics Data, 1996.

Post RM: Non-lithium treatment for bipolar disorder. *J Clin Psychiatry* 1990;51(suppl):9–16.

Remington GJ, Addington D, Collins EJ, et al.: Clozapine: current status and role in the pharmacotherapy of schizophrenia. *Can J Psychiatry* 1996;41(3):161–166.

Robertson GS, Matsumura H, Figiber HC: Induction patterns of neuroleptic-induced Fos-like immunoreactivity as predictors of atypical antipsychotic activity. *J Pharmacol Exp Ther* 1994;271:1058–1066.

Rosenheck R, Cramer J, Waken X, et al., for the Department of Veterans Affairs Cooperative Study Group on Clozapine in Refractory Schizophrenia: A comparison of clozapine and haloperidol in hospitalized patients with refractory schizophrenia. *N Engl J Med* 1997;337(12):809–815.

Safferman A, Lieberman JA, Kane JM, et al.: Update on the clinical efficacy and side effects of clozapine. *Schizophr Bull* 1991;17(2):247–261.

Scott JE, Dixon LB: Psychological interventions for schizophrenia. *Schizophr Bull* 1995;21(4):621–630.

Seeman P, Lee T, Chau-Wong M, et al.: Antipsychotic drug doses and neuroleptic/dopamine receptors. *Nature* 1976;261:717–719.

Shore D: Clinical implications of clozapine discontinuation: report of an NIMH workshop. *Schizophr Bull* 1995;21(2):333–337.

Simhandl C, Masseurs K: The use of carbamazepine in the treatment of schizophrenia and schizoaffective psychosis: a review. *J Psychiatry Neurosci* 1992;17:1–14.

Small JG: Efficacy of electroconvulsive therapy in schizophrenia, mania, and other disorders. I. Schizophrenia. *Convul Ther* 1985;1:263–270.

Small JG, Kellams JJ, Milstein V, et al.: A placebo-controlled study of lithium combined with neuroleptics in chronic schizophrenic patients. *Am J Psychiatry* 1975;132:1315–1317.

Strauss JS, Carpenter WT, Bartko JJ: Towards an understanding of the symptom picture considered characteristic of schizophrenia: its description, precursors, and outcome. *Schizophr Bull* 1974;11:61–69.

Tamminga CA: Schizophrenia and glutamatergic transmission. *Crit Revs Neurobiol* 1998;12:21–36.

Tamminga CA: Principles of the pharmacotherapy of schizophrenia. In Charney D, Nestler E, Bunney S (eds): *Neurobiology of Psychiatric Disorders*, in press.

Tamminga CA, Kane JM: Olanzapine (Zyprexa): characteristics of a new antipsychotic. *Expert Opin Invest Drugs* 1997;6:1743–1752.

Tamminga CA, Mack R, Silber CJ, et al.: Sertindole in the treatment of psychosis in schizophrenia: efficacy and safety. *Int Clin Psychopharmacol* 1997;12 (Suppl 1):S29–S35.

Tamminga CA, Thaker GK, Moran M, et al.: Clozapine in tardive dyskinesia: observations from human and animal model studies. *J Clin Psychiatry* 1994;55:102–106.

Tollefson GD, Beasley CM, Tran PV, et al.: Olanzapine versus haloperidol in the treatment of schizophrenia and schizoaffective disorders: results of an international collaborative trial. *Am J Psychiatry* 1997;154:457–465.

Waddington JL: Schizophrenia: developmental neuroscience and pathobiology. *Lancet* 1993;341:531–536.

Wilson WH: Clinical review of clozapine treatment in a state hospital. *Hosp Commun Psychiatry* 1992;43(7):700–703.

Wolkowitz OM, Pickar D, Doran AR, et al.: Combination alprazolam-neuroleptic treatment of the positive and negative symptoms of schizophrenia. *Am J Psychiatry* 1986;143:85–87.

Zito JM, Volavka J, Craig TJ, et al.: Pharmacoepidemiology of clozapine in 202 inpatients with schizophrenia. *Ann Pharmacother* 1993;27:1262–1269.

C H A P T E R 3

ANXIETY DISORDERS

Daniel S. Pine, Joseph Grun, and Jack M. Gorman

In the clinical literature the term anxiety refers to the presence of fear or apprehension out of proportion to the context of the life situation. Hence, extreme fear or apprehension is considered "clinical anxiety" if it is developmentally inappropriate (e.g., fear of leaving home in a college senior) or if it is inappropriate to an individual's life circumstances (e.g., worries about unemployment in a successful business executive) (Barlow, 1988; Marks, 1988). In the last 30 years of clinical research, the nosology for clinical anxiety disorders has been progressively refined. Although anxiety disorders were broadly conceptualized in the early twentieth century, narrower definitions have arisen, partially stimulated by pharmacological distinctions among the various conditions.

A consensus has emerged that anxiety disorders represent a family of related, but distinct, mental disabilities. This is reflected in the relatively minor changes in the broad categorization of anxiety disorders between the third (DSM-III) and fourth (DSM-IV) editions of the Diagnostic and Statistical Manual of Mental Disorders, *with the DSM-IV specifying nine conditions as primary "anxiety disorders." Included are panic disorder with and without agoraphobia, agoraphobia without panic disorder, specific phobia, social phobia, obsessive-compulsive disorder, posttraumatic stress disorder, acute stress disorder, and generalized anxiety disorder. Discussed in this chapter are treatments for four of these conditions: panic disorder with and without agoraphobia, social phobia, posttraumatic stress disorder, and generalized anxiety disorder. Whereas treatment of obsessive-compulsive disorder is discussed elsewhere in this volume (see Chap. 6), agoraphobia without panic is not considered because this condition is infrequently seen in clinical settings. In addition, neither specific phobia nor acute stress disorder is discussed as there are only minimal data from randomized controlled trials on their pharmacological management. Finally, anxiety disorders can arise as complications of substance abuse or other disorders such as epilepsy or pulmonary disease. The treatment of anxiety secondary to these conditions is more properly considered in the context of the primary condition.*

The aim of this chapter is to provide sufficient information to facilitate the management of anxiety disorders. Effective therapy requires a delineation of presenting signs, diagnostic considerations and an understanding of the complicating features of each disorder. Also required is a thorough knowledge of the medications available for treating these conditions, including the advantages and disadvantages of each. Armed with this knowledge it is possible to effectively manage the vast majority of patients suffering from an anxiety disorder.

CLINICAL FEATURES AND DIAGNOSIS

Panic Disorder with and without Agoraphobia

Presenting symptoms. The key feature of panic disorder is recurrent panic attacks (Pollack and Smoller, 1995). Panic attacks are characterized by abrupt, intense fear, accompanied by at least four autonomic or cognitive symptoms (Table 3-1). The panic attack must develop rapidly, with anxiety that escalates to a crescendo within minutes. Panic attacks typically end abruptly, lasting less than 30 min, although moderate anxiety surrounding the attack can persist for more than an hour.

Three types of panic attacks are described in the *Diagnostic and Statistical Manual of Mental Disorders,* 4th ed. (DSM-IV). The unexpected or spontaneous attack occurs without cue or warning; the situationally bound panic attack occurs with exposure to, or anticipation of, a feared stimulus. Although the situationally predisposed panic attack is more likely to occur when triggered by a stimulus, this is not an absolute requirement. In panic disorder, attacks occur spontaneously, arising without any trigger or environmental cue. The diagnosis of panic disorder requires that at least two spontaneous panic attacks have occurred, at least one of which is associated with concern about additional attacks or changes in behavior that last at least 1 month (Table 3-2).

While patients with panic disorder present with a number of comorbid conditions, there is considerable interest in the relationship between panic disorder and agoraphobia, which is fear or anxiety related to places from which escape might be difficult (Tables 3-2 and 3-4) (Magee et al., 1996). Although there remains considerable controversy on the distinctiveness of agoraphobia separate from panic disorder, the treatment of the former is considered part of the therapy for the latter. The current controversy centers on the frequency with which patients develop agoraphobia in the absence of panic disorder or panic attacks (Eaton et al., 1991) (Table 3-3). This designation is based partly on epidemiological data, in which the prevalence of agoraphobia is considerably higher

Table 3-1
Criteria for a Panic Attack

A discrete period of intense fear or discomfort, in which four (or more) of the following symptoms develop abruptly and reach a peak within 10 min:

1. Palpitations, pounding heart, or accelerated heart rate
2. Sweating
3. Trembling or shaking
4. Sensations of shortness of breath or smothering
5. Feeling of choking
6. Chest pain or discomfort
7. Nausea or abdominal distress
8. Feeling dizzy, unsteady, lightheaded, or faint
9. Derealization (feelings of unreality) or depersonalization (being detached from oneself)
10. Fear of losing control or going crazy
11. Fear of dying
12. Paresthesias
13. Chills or hot flashes

Note: A panic attack is not a codable disorder. Code the specific diagnosis in which the panic attack occurs (e.g., 200.21 Panic Disorder With Agoraphobia).

SOURCE American Psychiatric Association: *Diagnostic and Statistical Manual of Mental Disorders*, 4th ed. Washington, DC, American Psychiatric Association, 1994.

than that of panic disorder. The two conditions are considered together in this chapter because there are questions concerning the validity of these epidemiological data; virtually all patients with agoraphobia suffer from panic attacks, and agoraphobia tends to respond to antipanic treatment. Moreover, even when agoraphobia is present without a history of panic disorder, it is related to the fear of developing panic-like symptoms.

Course. Panic disorder typically has its onset in late adolescence or early adulthood, although cases of childhood-onset and late adulthood-onset have been described (Barlow, 1988; Eaton et al., 1991;

Table 3-2
Criteria for Agoraphobia

A. Anxiety about being in places or situations from which escape might be difficult (or embarrassing) or in which help may not be available in the event of having an unexpected or situationally predisposed panic attack or panic-like symptoms. Agoraphobic fears typically involve characteristic clusters of situations that include being outside the home alone; being in a crowd or standing in a line; being on a bridge; and traveling in a bus, train, or automobile.

   Note: Consider the diagnois of specific phobia if the avoidance is limited to one or only a few specific situations, or social phobia if the avoidance is limited to social situations.

B. The situations are avoided (e.g., travel is restricted) or else are endured with marked distress or with anxiety about having a panic attack or panic-like symptoms, or require the presence of a companion.

C. The anxiety or phobic avoidance is not better accounted for by another mental disorder, such as social phobia (e.g., avoidance limited to social situations because of fear of embarrassment), specific phobia (e.g., avoidance limited to a single situation like elevators), obsessive-compulsive disorder (e.g., avoidance of dirt in someone with an obsession about contamination), posttraumatic stress disorder (e.g., avoidance of stimuli associated with a severe stressor), or separation anxiety disorder (e.g., avoidance of leaving home or relatives).

Note: Agoraphobia is not a codable disorder. Code the specific disorder in which the agoraphobia occurs (e.g., 300.21 Panic Disorder With Agoraphobia or 200.22 Agoraphobia Without History of Panic Disorder)

SOURCE American Psychiatric Association: *Diagnostic and Statistical Manual of Mental Disorders*, 4th ed. Washington, DC, American Psychiatric Association, 1994.

Magee et al., 1996; Marks, 1988). There are only tentative data on the natural course of panic disorder (Otto and Whittal, 1995; Pollack and Smoller, 1995). The best evidence derives from prospective epidemiological research, because both retrospective and clinically based studies are vulnerable to biases that preclude firm conclusions. Research from retrospective or clinical studies suggests that panic disorder tends to exhibit a fluctuating course, with varying levels of persistence throughout life (Pollack and Smoller, 1995; Schweizer et al., 1995). Approximately one-third to one-half of patients are psychiatrically healthy at follow-up, with the majority living relatively normal lives despite fluctuating or recurrent symptoms. Typically, patients with chronic disorders exhibit a pattern of exacerbation and remission rather than continuous disability. Clinicians are most likely to encounter patients either early in the course of the disorder or during a period of exacerbation. Therefore it is crucial to take a thorough history of prior symptoms when evaluating a patient suffering from panic attacks. This examination should focus specifically on prior history of medical evaluations or emergency department visits for unexplained somatic symptoms, and the use of prescribed or illicit substances.

Differential diagnosis. The diagnostic process begins with a careful elicitation of the symptoms described previously, then follows with a consideration of other potential contributors (Fig. 3-1). As with most anxiety disorders, panic disorder is often seen with a number of mental conditions beyond agoraphobia, particularly anxiety and depressive disorders (Eaton et al., 1991; Kendler et al., 1995; Weissman, 1990). Other comorbidities include specific and social phobia, generalized anxiety disorder, major depressive disorder, substance abuse, bipolar disorder, and suicidal behavior (Keck et al., 1993). Although the high degree of comorbidity partially reflects referral bias, comorbidity with anxiety and depressive disorders is also found in epidemiological studies.

Panic disorder with or without agoraphobia must be differentiated from these comorbid conditions. This differentiation begins with a clear documentation of spontaneous panic, which patients describe as arising "out of the blue" or "without warning."

Table 3-3
Criteria for Panic Disorder and Agoraphobia

Criteria for panic disorder without agoraphobia	*Criteria for panic disorder with agoraphobia*	*Criteria for agoraphobia without history of panic disorder*

A. Both (1) and (2)
  1. Recurrent unexpected panic attacks
  2. At least one of the attacks has been followed by 1 month (or more) of one (or more) of the following:
    a. Persistent concern about having additional attacks
    b. Worry about the implications of the attack or its consequences (e.g., losing control, having a heart attack, "going crazy")
    c. A significant change in behavior related to the attacks
B. Absence of agoraphobia.
C. The panic attacks are not due to the direct physiological effects of a substance (drug of abuse, a medication) or a general medical condition (e.g., hyperthyroidism).
D. The panic attacks are not better accounted for by another mental disorder, such as social phobia (e.g., occurring on exposure to feared social
	A. Both (1) and (2)
	  1. Recurrent unexpected panic attacks
	  2. At least one of the attacks has been followed by 1 month (or more) of one (or more) of the following:
	    a. Persistent concern about having additional attacks
	    b. Worry about the implications of the attack or its consequences (e.g., losing control, having a heart attack, "going crazy")
	    c. A significant change in behavior related to the attacks
	B. Presence of agoraphobia.
	C. The panic attacks are not due to the direct physiological effects of a substance (drug of abuse, a medication) or a general medical condition (e.g., hyperthyroidism).
	D. The panic attacks are not better accounted for by another mental disorder, such as social phobia (e.g., occurring on exposure to feared social
		A. The presence of agoraphobia related to fear of developing panic-like symptoms (e.g., dizziness or diarrhea).
		B. Criteria have never been met for panic disorder.
		C. The disturbance is not due to the direct physiological effect of a substance (e.g., a drug of abuse, a medication) or a general medical condition.
		D. If an associated general medical condition is present, the fear described in criterion A is clearly in excess of that usually associated with the condition.

(Continued)

Table 3-3

Criteria for Panic Disorder and Agoraphobia (Continued)

Criteria for panic disorder without agoraphobia	Criteria for panic disorder with agoraphobia	Criteria for agoraphobia without history of panic disorder
situations), specific phobia (e.g., occurring on exposure to a specific phobic situation), obsessive-compulsive disorder (e.g., on exposure to dirt in someone with an obsession about contamination), posttraumatic stress disorder (e.g., on exposure to stimuli associated with a severe stressor), or separation anxiety disorder (e.g., on response to being away from home or close relatives).	situations), specific phobia (e.g., occurring on exposure to a specific phobic situation), obsessive-compulsive disorder (e.g., on exposure to dirt in someone with an obsession about contamination), posttraumatic stress disorder (e.g., on exposure to stimuli associated with a severe stressor), or separation anxiety disorder (e.g., on response to being away from home or close relatives).	

SOURCE American Psychiatric Association: *Diagnostic and Statistical Manual of Mental Disorders*, 4th ed. Washington, DC, American Psychiatric Association, 1994.

Such true spontaneous panic attacks must be differentiated from attacks that are triggered by exposure to a feared situation. For example, an individual with social phobia might suffer a panic attack before a public speaking engagement, an individual with posttraumatic stress disorder might suffer a panic attack during a flashback, and someone with a specific phobia might panic on exposure to the feared object. True spontaneous panic attacks must also not be attributable to prescribed or illicit drugs.

Following the establishment of the existence of spontaneous panic attacks, the frequency and level of distress associated with panic must be documented. Isolated, spontaneous panic attacks occur in many adults, but the diagnosis of panic disorder rests on the presence of multiple, recurrent attacks. To qualify for the diagnosis, a patient must exhibit significant distress related to attacks and express either fear of recurrent attacks or a change in routine to limit the impact of attacks. Differentiation from generalized anxiety disorder can also be difficult. Classically, panic attacks are characterized by their rapid onset and short duration, typically less than 10 to 15 min, in contrast to the anxiety associated with generalized anxiety disorder, which emerges and dissipates more slowly. This distinction can be difficult to make, however, as the anxiety felt with panic attacks may be diffuse and may dissipate slowly. Finally, because anxiety is prominent in many psychiatric disorders, including psychoses and affective illness, distinctions between panic disorder and a multitude of other conditions are difficult. In general, emphasis should be placed on the course of the psychiatric symptoms. For cases of recurrent panic attacks that occur only during the course of another psychiatric syndrome, treatment should be aimed at the primary condition

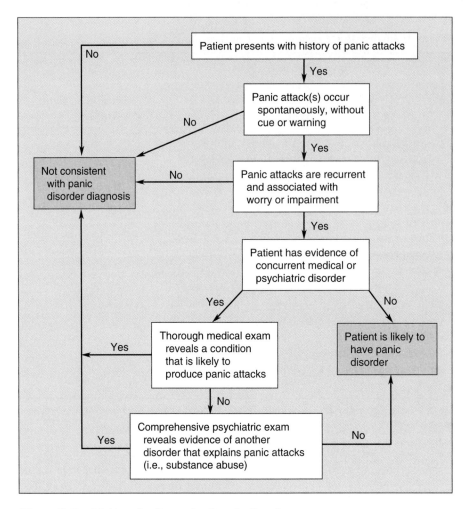

Figure 3–1.   *Making the diagnosis of panic disorder.*

while selecting medications that are also beneficial in panic disorder. For example, panic attacks can develop during major depressive episodes, which generally respond to tricyclic antidepressants, monoamine oxidase inhibitors, or selective serotonin reuptake inhibitors, all of which are effective for panic disorder. In general, panic disorder should be diagnosed only if recurrent panic attacks cannot be attributed to another, concurrent psychiatric condition.

Panic disorder with or without agoraphobia must be differentiated from medical conditions that produce similar symptomatology. Panic attacks are asso-

ciated with a variety of endocrine disorders, including both hypothyroid and hyperthyroid states, hyperparathyroidism, and pheochromocytomas. Episodic hypoglycemia associated with insulinomas can also produce panic-like states, as can primary neuropathological processes. In such patients, a thorough physical examination, including a review of systems, routine blood chemistries, and endocrinological tests, usually provides clues as to the possible presence of an underlying endocrine disorder. Although such conditions can produce symptoms nearly identical with idiopathic panic disorder, it is rare for an endocrine dysfunction to be unaccompanied by other medical symptoms. Similarly, symptoms of panic disorder can result from underlying neuropathological processes, such as seizure disorders, vestibular dysfunction, neoplasms, or the use of prescribed or illicit medications. A thorough medical assessment with attention to signs of neurological illness typically provides clues of an underlying neuropathology. Although electroencephalogram (EEG) or brain imaging procedures are not recommended in all cases, consideration should be given to these procedures, or a neurological consultation, when suggestive medical signs are present. Thus panic attacks associated with auras or postepisode confusion should prompt a neurological examination and EEG, whereas the presence of previously undocumented cognitive deficits or focal neurological findings usually suggest the need for neurological consultation. Disorders of the cardiac and pulmonary systems, including arrhythmias, chronic obstructive pulmonary disease, and asthma, may produce autonomic symptoms and crescendo anxiety that may be difficult to distinguish from panic disorder (Klein, 1993). In these cases, signs of cardiopulmonary disease are usually part of the clinical picture.

Pathophysiology. Although the pathophysiology of panic disorder is not completely understood, more is known about this condition than the others discussed in this chapter. Detailed in the following section are current theories that carry implications for the treatment of panic disorder with or without agoraphobia.

Respiratory-based theories. One theory conceptualizes the spontaneous panic attack as an alarm reaction related to an underlying abnormality in respiratory control (Coplan and Klein, 1996; Klein, 1993; Papp et al., 1993). The suffocation false alarm theory suggests that panic is triggered by cues of suffocation acting on a hypothetical suffocation center. The neuroanatomical model of Gorman et al. (1996) suggests that the panic attack originates in the hyperactive brain stem loci, as reflected in abnormal ventilatory, noradrenergic, and serotonergic profiles in panic patients. With this model other aspects of the disorder are thought to be related to other brain regions. For example, anticipatory anxiety is believed to be associated with limbic areas of the brain, such as the amygdala, and phobic avoidance is thought to originate within the prefrontal cortex.

Respiratory-based theories evolved from a series of well-replicated findings in adults with panic disorder. First, respiratory complaints are a prominent component of the panic attack (Klein, 1993). Second, individuals with respiratory illnesses that produce dyspnea exhibit more panic-like symptoms than individuals with illnesses that do not produce dyspnea. Third, adults with panic disorder consistently exhibit heightened anxiety in response to challenges with agents that stimulate the respiratory system, such as carbon dioxide, sodium lactate, and doxapram, a carotid body stimulant (Coplan and Klein, 1996; Papp et al., 1993). Finally, the heightened anxiety response is mirrored in respiratory physiology, where the panic attack is associated with a marked increase in ventilation (Klein, 1993), and panic disorder is associated with a series of abnormalities in the neural control of breathing, including hyperventilation and "chaotic ventilation" during room-air breathing (Klein, 1993). Although there is considerable disagreement on the extent to which these respiratory findings relate to the severity of anxiety, the fact that such respiratory abnormalities are found during sleep suggests they are not entirely dependent on cognitive factors.

The respiratory model of panic has implications for treatment. Medications effective in blocking respiratory-induced panic are also effective in natural panic, whereas medications effective in generalized anxiety disorder, but not panic disorder, do not block respiratory-induced panic attacks (Coplan and Klein, 1996). There is also evidence of a heritable component to these respiratory abnormalities, with psychiatrically healthy relatives of panic disorder patients exhibiting abnormal responses to carbon dioxide challenge. Given the strength and consistency of these findings, research continues in pursuit of a link between panic disorder and respiratory control.

Autonomic-based theories. It has also been suggested there is a close relationship between the autonomic nervous system and panic disorder. Early research noted an association between heart rate elevations and panic disorder, particularly in the laboratory setting. This was attributed to an interaction between patient status and trait anxiety because such cardiac abnormalities are less consistently found in natural surroundings. More recent research relies on either cardiac indices of parasympathetic-sympathetic interactions, or on biologic responses to noradrenergic challenges. These data suggest that panic disorder arises from a subtle dysfunction in the sympathetic nervous system, the parasympathetic nervous system, or the interplay between the two.

The best evidence for parasympathetic abnormalities in panic disorder comes from measures of heart period variability. Although the results are not always consistent, adults with panic disorder display a reduction in the high-frequency component of the heart period variability power spectrum, indicating a deficient parasympathetic control over the heart (Klein et al., 1995; Yergani et al., 1994, 1992). Perhaps the most consistent finding in the heart period variability literature is the suggestion of an imbalance between the parasympathetic and sympathetic branches, with a predominance in sympathetic outflow (Klein et al., 1995). Panic disorder is associated with an enhanced ratio of low-frequency to high-frequency heart period variability power. This enhanced ratio is particularly evident when sympathetic activity is maximized, such as when standing upright or following the administration of yohimbine. There is also some preliminary evidence that the heart rate elevation during the panic attack is caused by parasympathetic withdrawal (Yergani et al., 1994).

The most significant limitation of this research is that these findings are not specific to panic disorder. Other psychiatric conditions, including major depression and generalized anxiety disorder, also appear to be associated with reduced parasympathetic components of heart period variability.

Another experimental approach uses neuroendocrine challenge to examine the role of the noradrenergic system in panic disorder. The most consistent results are found with clonidine, a selective α_2-adrenergic receptor agonist. Adults with panic disorder consistently exhibit a blunted growth hormone response to clonidine, suggesting a decrease in the sensitivity of the hypothalamic α_2-adrenergic receptors. Inasmuch as this response persists following successful treatment of panic disorder, it may be a trait marker. Panic disorder may also be associated with an enhanced blood pressure and 3-methoxy-4-hydroxyphenylglycol (MHPG) response to clonidine. Moreover, there is evidence of abnormalities in the hypothalamic-pituitary-adrenal (HPA) axis that relate to noradrenergic abnormalities in that panic disorder is associated with an uncoupling of these systems. Data from clonidine challenge tests suggest that noradrenergic abnormalities may be best characterized as dysregulatory, rather than as a relative excess or insufficiency in noradrenergic output. Panic disorder is associated with a more chaotic MHPG response to α_2-adrenergic receptor stimulation, with successful treatment of the condition reestablishing the normal, regular MHPG decline associated with clonidine administration. Adults with panic disorder also exhibit enhanced anxiety responses to challenges with yohimbine, an α_2-adrenergic receptor antagonist that stimulates the locus ceruleus (Goddard and Charney, 1997; Johnson and Lydiard, 1995). These findings, which are consistent with heart period variability data, suggest that panic disorder is associated with an underlying abnormality in the ability to regulate autonomic nervous system function.

The most significant limitation of this research relates to the degree to which findings are specific to panic disorder. Adults with related conditions, such as major depression, generalized anxiety disorder, and social phobia, also exhibit a blunted growth hormone response to clonidine challenge (Abelson et al., 1991; Tancer, 1993). Moreover, adults with posttraumatic stress disorder exhibit an enhanced anxiety response to yohimbine (Bremner et al., 1997), whereas adults with major depression or generalized anxiety disorder exhibit a normal response to yohimbine (Goddard and Charney, 1997).

Serotonin. The best evidence implicating serotonin in panic disorder derives from pharmacological studies. Anecdotally, some investigators suggest that panic disorder patients are particularly susceptible to anxiety upon initiation of therapy with a specific serotonin reuptake inhibitor, a finding that received mixed support with more systematic research (Heninger, 1995; Johnson and Lydiard, 1995).

Although not all experiments yield consistent results, neuroendocrine challenge studies with serotonergic drugs, such as fenfluramine, isapirone, or methchorlophenylpiperazine (mCPP), have suggested abnormalities among patients with panic disorder (Coplan and Klein, 1996; Johnson and Lydiard, 1995). Most prominent is a change in the cortisol response to both fenfluramine and mCPP. Panic disorder is also associated with abnormalities in platelet serotonin-related proteins, although results vary in this regard (Coplan and Klein, 1996; Johnson and Lydiard, 1995). It has also been suggested that there is an association between panic disorder and serotonin autoantibodies (Coplan et al., 1996).

Some research on the role of serotonin in panic disorder emphasizes the interplay between serotonin and other neurotransmitter systems. The serotonergic and noradrenergic systems, in particular, are closely allied, suggesting a relationship between serotonin and autonomic abnormalities in panic disorder. Thus, specific serotonin reuptake inhibitors might influence the symptoms of panic disorder indirectly by modifying the noradrenergic system. Evidence for this includes the finding that fluoxetine, a specific serotonin reuptake inhibitor, normalizes the chaotic nature of the MHPG response to clonidine in panic patients (Coplan and Klein, 1996).

Fear-conditioning theory. Fear-conditioning is an animal model of anxiety where a neutral, conditioned stimulus, such as a light or a tone, is paired to a negative or unconditioned stimulus, such as a shock.

This pairing eventually results in a conditioned stimulus eliciting the behavioral and physiological reactions typically associated with the unconditioned stimulus. The neural circuitry underlying fear-conditioning has been elucidated (Davis, 1992; LeDoux, 1996). This circuit involves neural pathways extending from sensory organs to the thalamus and the central nucleus of the amygdala. The central nucleus also receives cortical projections capable of modifying the subcortical circuit, which is the main neural pathway involved in fear-conditioning. These projection sites include the hippocampal region and prefrontal cortex. Alarm reactions, such as a panic attack, are thought to result from interactions between the amygdala and the brain stem, basal ganglia, hypothalamic, and cortical pathways.

Fear-conditioning theory has been applied to panic disorder (LeDoux, 1996). In this case internal stimuli associated with a panic attack, such as blood pressure elevations or changes in ventilation, are viewed as conditioned stimuli for subsequent panic attacks. Panic disorder is therefore thought to result from activation of the neural pathway subserving conditioned fear as a result of the typical hour-to-hour changes in bodily stimuli. Clinical research suggests the neural structures that mediate fear-conditioning in animals are important in humans as well (Goddard and Charney, 1997). Results from clinical neuroimaging studies are generally consistent with the fear-conditioning theory (Johnson and Lydiard, 1995), with the patient studies showing signs of dysfunction in areas projecting to the amygdala, such as the prefrontal cortex and hippocampal region. The fact that both the respiratory and the physiological responses to carbon dioxide can become "conditioned" in humans is also consistent with the animal model (Van den Bergh et al., 1995). Agoraphobia is also considered to be a form of "conditioned fear," with the panic attack serving as the unconditioned stimulus for the development of such fear (Goddard and Charney, 1997), a conceptualization that is consistent with results from animal-based research. Although the fear-potentiated startle paradigm has been offered as a possible model of the human condition (Davis, 1992; LeDoux, 1996), results with panic disorder patients are inconsistent.

Cognitively based theories. Most theoreticians recognize a strong biological component to the panic attack, but theories differ about what initiates the disorder, with some emphasizing a casual role for cognitive factors.

A number of cognitive factors have been proposed as mediators of panic (Barlow, 1988; Marks, 1988; Otto and Whittal, 1995). Thus, heightened anxiety sensitivity is thought to predispose individuals to panic disorder, because such individuals are more aware of the state of their internal milieu. The best support for this theory derives from the finding that individuals who endorse descriptors of anxiety sensitivity tend to overreport symptoms during anxiety provocation exercises. This theory receives only inconsistent support from research on the relative skill with which patients with panic disorder perceive externally monitored physiological signals, such as heart rate.

A second, related, theory suggests that individuals with panic disorder tend to catastrophize, particularly in situations where they feel out of control. This theory receives support from studies suggesting that manipulations of perceived control influence panic susceptibility during biological challenges.

A number of theories suggest that an individual's experience with separations, particularly during childhood, influence susceptibility to panic (Klein, 1993; Klein, 1995). These theories are supported by the inconsistently replicated observation that childhood difficulties with separation predict panic disorder, and by the observation that the onset of panic disorder is often preceded by adverse social experiences. Moreover, one recent biological challenge study suggested that separation from a "safe" person moderated the response to carbon dioxide. It should be noted that the more recent versions of these cognitively based theories integrate biologically based theories such as those described in the foregoing.

Social Phobia

Presenting symptoms. The term phobia refers to an excessive fear of a specific object, circumstance, or situation (Magee et al., 1996). Phobias are classified by the nature of the feared object or situation.

The DSM-IV recognizes three distinct classes of phobias: agoraphobia, which is closely related to panic disorder; specific phobia, which is not discussed further, as it rarely requires pharmacological intervention; and social phobia (Table 3-4).

The diagnosis of social phobia requires intense anxiety, even to the point of situationally bound panic, upon exposure to social or performance situations where an individual is scrutinized and might be embarrassed. This can involve specific fears about performing certain activities, such as writing, eating, or speaking in front of others, or a vague general fear of embarrassing oneself. The DSM-IV provides a specifier for the diagnosis of social phobia, with

Table 3-4
Criteria for Social Phobia (300.23)

A. A marked or persistent fear of one or more social or performance situations in which the person is exposed to unfamiliar people or to possible scrutiny by others. The individual fears that he or she will act in a way (or show anxiety symptoms) that will be humiliating or embarrassing. **Note:** In children, there must be evidence of the capacity for age-appropriate social relationships with familiar people and the anxiety must occur in peer settings, not just in interactions with adults.

B. Exposure to the feared social situation almost invariably provokes anxiety, which may take the form of a situationally bound or situationally predisposed panic attack. **Note:** In children, the anxiety may be expressed by crying, tantrums, freezing, or shrinking from social situations with unfamiliar people.

C. The person recognizes that the fear is excessive or unreasonable. **Note:** In children, this feature may be absent.

D. The feared social or performance situations are avoided or else are endured with intense anxiety or distress.

E. The avoidance, anxious anticipation, or distress in the feared social or performance situation(s) interferes significantly with the person's normal routine, occupational (academic) functioning, or social activities or relationships, or there is marked distress about having the phobia.

F. In individuals under age 18 years, the duration is at least 6 months.

G. The fear or avoidance is not due to the direct physiological effects of a substance (e.g., a drug of abuse, a medication) or a general medical condition and is not better accounted for by another mental disorder (e.g., panic disorder with or without agoraphobia, separation anxiety disorder, body dysmorphic disorder, a pervasive developmental disorder, or schizoid personality disorder).

H. If a general medical condition or another mental disorder is present, the fear in criterion A is unrelated to it, (e.g., the fear is not of stuttering, trembling in Parkinson's disease, or exhibiting abnormal eating behavior in anorexia nervosa or bulimia nervosa).

Specify as Generalized if the fears include most social situations (also consider the additional diagnosis of avoidant personality disorder)

SOURCE American Psychiatric Association: *Diagnostic and Statistical Manual of Mental Disorders,* 4th ed. Washington, DC, American Psychiatric Association, 1994.

those who fear most situations being considered to suffer from generalized social phobia. Such individuals are fearful of initiating conversations in many situations, fearful about dating or participating in most group activities or social gatherings, and fearful about speaking with authority figures. The diagnosis of social phobia also requires that social fears either interfere with functioning or cause marked distress, that they be recognized by the patient as excessive or irrational, and that social situations are either avoided or are endured with great difficulty.

Many people exhibit some degree of social anxiety or self-consciousness without ever meeting the criteria for social phobia (Davidson et al., 1994). In fact, community studies suggest that approximately one-third of the population believes it is far more anxious than other people in social situations. Such anxiety is considered a sign of social phobia only when it prevents an individual from participating in desired activities or causes marked distress in such activities. Those with the more specific form of social phobia possess fear of particular, circumscribed social situations. For example, extreme anxiety about public speaking that may be sufficient to interfere with job performance is a common type of specific social phobia.

Like other anxiety disorders, social phobia frequently occurs with other mood and anxiety disorders (Magee et al., 1996). The association of social phobia with panic disorder and major depression has received considerable attention. Associations with substance abuse and childhood conduct problems have also been documented (Davidson et al., 1994).

Course. The onset of social phobia is typically in late childhood or early adolescence (Eaton et al., 1991). The generalized form tends to be a chronic condition although, as with the other anxiety disorders, there is limited prospective epidemiological data (Juster and Heimberg, 1995). Both retrospective epidemiological and prospective clinical studies suggest social phobia can profoundly disrupt the life of an individual for many years. This disruption includes negative effects on academic achievement, job performance, and social development.

Differential diagnosis. Patients present with symptoms of social phobia under a variety of circum-

stances. One scenario, often suggestive of the disorder, involves a patient who complains of having difficulty functioning in the work or social environment because of an inability to perform certain tasks. Another scenario, which is less suggestive of the disorder, involves a patient who presents, at the urging of friends or family, with a history of social withdrawal (Fig. 3-2).

As a number of psychiatric conditions are associated with social withdrawal, it is often difficult to diagnose social phobia correctly. Perhaps the most difficult distinction involves the differentiation of social phobia and agoraphobia because both involve fears of situations where people gather. The key distinction between these two centers on the nature of the feared object. Whereas patients with social phobia specifically fear encounters with people, individuals with agoraphobia fear situations from which escape is difficult, but are not particularly afraid of social interchange. Hence, although an individual with agoraphobia might be reassured in the presence of others, provided the physical properties of the location are suitable, an individual with social phobia flees any type of social intercourse.

Difficulty might also be encountered in distinguishing social phobia from the social isolation that accompanies a psychiatric illness, including major depression and the early stages of psychosis. Two factors are essential in making this distinction. First, the individual with social phobia must experience anxiety or fear in social situations, whereas individuals who are alone because of depression or indolent psychosis often isolate themselves for other reasons. Second, with social phobia symptomatology is restricted to the fears of social situations, whereas with other disorders social isolation is accompanied by symptoms not found in social phobia.

Relative to panic disorder, social phobia is less likely to be confused with anxiety resulting from other medical conditions. Anxiety related to a medical disorder tends to be associated with prominent somatic symptoms that occur without particular cues or triggers. Although it is common for patients with social phobia to report somatic symptoms, these symptoms are seen almost exclusively in association with exposure to feared social situations. Nevertheless, as with the diagnosis of panic disorder, a careful medical his-

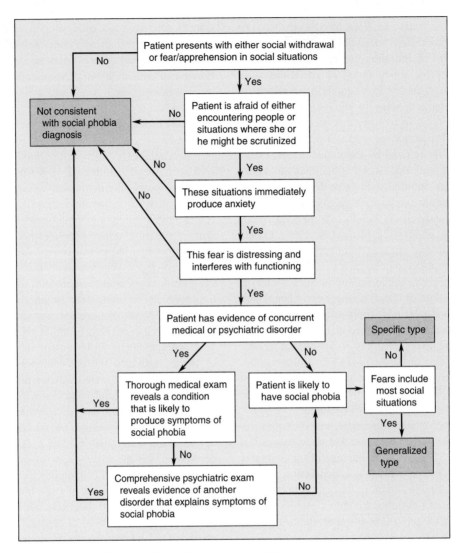

Figure 3–2. *Making the diagnosis of social phobia.*

tory and physical examination should be conducted in all patients with symptoms of social phobia.

Pathophysiology. Compared with panic disorder, considerably less is known about the pathophysiology of social phobia (Rosenbaum et al., 1994); the bulk of research examines biological correlates of panic disorder in patients with social phobia. This research highlights the strong association between panic disorder and social phobia within individuals and their families.

Biological findings with reference to panic disorder. By a number of biological measures, patients with social phobia tend to exhibit profiles that are intermediate between patients with panic disorder and psychiatrically healthy individuals (Tancer, 1993). Thus, patients with social phobia exhibit heightened anxiogenic responses to carbon dioxide relative to healthy individuals, but less extreme responses than those seen with panic disorder (Johnson and Lydiard, 1995; Papp et al., 1993). A blunted growth hormone response to noradrenergic challenge has also been reported in social phobia, the magnitude of which is intermediate between healthy subjects and patients with panic disorder (Tancer, 1993). Whereas autonomic-based theories predict enhanced cardiac reactivity to social challenges, preliminary data suggest the opposite with social phobia, with these patients exhibiting reduced cardiac reactivity to socially challenging situations. Although neuroendocrine challenge experiments provide evidence for serotonergic abnormalities in social phobia, further studies of this type are needed comparing normal individuals to patients with panic disorder, social phobia, and major depression.

Specific findings in social phobia. Family studies and longitudinal research with children suggest a degree of specificity in the transmission of social phobia (Fyer et al., 1995; Pine et al., in press), which may account for the unique aspects of the condition. Indeed, social phobia is an early-onset anxiety disorder, with a median onset in early adolescence or late childhood (Eaton et al., 1991).

Childhood temperament and social phobia. There has been considerable research on the relationship between anxiety disorders and behavioral inhibition to the unfamiliar. This temperamental construct relates to the tendency in childhood to appear reticent in novel environments, particularly in social situations (Biederman et al., 1995; Kagan, 1995). Such children exhibit a long latency before speaking with strangers and show a tendency to refrain from group play and to display limited facial expressions, characteristics that bear a phenotypic resemblance to social phobia. Findings suggest that behavioral inhibition has a strong genetic component, although environmental factors play a role as well. Behavioral inhibition is thought to result from an abnormally low threshold for arousal in the amygdala, although the evidence is indirect (Kagan, 1995). Furthermore, the association between behavioral inhibition and social phobia remains tenuous, because studies were aimed at examining the relationship with panic disorder more than the relationship with social phobia (Biederman et al., 1995). Nevertheless, evidence continues to accumulate suggesting an association between early childhood inhibition and adolescent social phobia.

Brain lateralization. It has been postulated that asymmetries in frontal central nervous system activity relate to behavioral tendencies. Individuals with enhanced frontal activity in the right hemisphere tend to exhibit withdrawal behaviors when confronted with stressors, including the stress of social situations; those with enhanced frontal activity in the left hemisphere tend to exhibit approach behaviors under similar circumstances. Inhibited children also exhibit a pattern of right frontal asymmetry, suggesting a tendency to withdraw (Davidson, 1995). The main limitation of this theory is that it does not specifically apply to social phobia, but rather relates to a broad diathesis for anxiety and depressive disorders.

Posttraumatic Stress Disorder

Presenting symptoms. Both posttraumatic stress disorder (PTSD) and acute stress disorder are characterized by the onset of symptoms immediately after exposure to a traumatic event (Davidson and Foa, 1991). Hence, the patient with PTSD always presents with either new symptoms, or a change in symptoms, that can be referenced to a specific trauma. Although different patients will ascribe different levels of significance to a given event, all patients with PTSD must have symptoms that are related to a trauma. Such a traumatic event normally involves either witnessing or experiencing the threat of death or injury (Table 3-5). Further, the response to the traumatic event must involve intense fear or horror. Such traumatic experiences might include involvement in, or witnessing, a violent accident or crime, combat, assault, kidnapping, or natural disaster; being diagnosed with a life-threatening illness; or experiencing systematic physical or sexual abuse. Only PTSD is discussed in this chapter because there are more extensive data on its pharmacological management. There is evidence of a dose-response relationship between the degree of trauma and the likelihood of PTSD symptoms, with the proximity to, and intensity of, the trauma relating to the probability of developing the condition.

With PTSD, the patient develops symptoms in three domains: reexperiencing the trauma, avoiding stimuli associated with the trauma, and increased autonomic arousal, such as an enhanced startle. Flashbacks, where the individual acts and feels as if the trauma is recurring, are the classic form of reexperiencing. Other forms of reexperiencing include distressing recollections or dreams, and either physiological or psychological stress reactions on exposure to stimuli associated with the traumatic event. An individual must exhibit at least one symptom of reexperiencing to meet the criteria for PTSD. Other symptoms of PTSD include efforts to avoid thoughts or activities related to the trauma, anhedonia, reduced capacity to remember events related to the trauma, blunted affect, feelings of detachment or derealization, and a sense of a foreshortened future. An individual must exhibit at least three of these

Table 3-5
Criteria for Posttraumatic Stress Disorder

A. The person has been exposed to a traumatic event in which both of the following were present:

    1. The person experienced, witnessed, or was confronted with an event that involved actual or threatened death or serious injury, or a threat to the physical integrity of self or others.

    2. The person's response involved intense fear, helplessness, or horror. **Note:** In children this may be expressed instead by disorganized or agitated behavior.

B. The traumatic event is persistently reexperienced in one (or more) of the following ways:

    1. Recurrent and intrusive distressing recollections of the event, including images, thoughts, or perceptions. **Note:** In young children, repetitive play may occur in which themes or aspects of the trauma are expressed.

    2. Recurrent distressing dreams of the event. **Note:** In children, there may be frightening dreams without recognizable content.

    3. Acting or feeling as if the traumatic event were recurring (includes a sense of reliving the experience, illusions, hallucinations, and dissociative flashback episodes, including those that occur on awakening or when intoxicated). **Note:** In young children, trauma-specific reenactment may occur.

    4. Intense psychological distress at exposure to internal or external cues that symbolize or resemble an aspect of the traumatic event.

    5. Physiological reactivity on exposure to internal or external cues that symbolize or resemble an aspect of the traumatic event.

C. Persistent avoidance of stimuli associated with the trauma and numbing of general responsiveness (not present before the trauma), as indicated by three (or more) of the following:

    1. Efforts to avoid thoughts, feelings, or conversations associated with the trauma

    2. Efforts to avoid activities, places, or people that arouse recollections of the trauma

    3. Inability to recall an important aspect of the trauma

    4. Markedly diminished interest or participation in significant activities

    5. Feeling of detachment or estrangement from others

    6. Restricted range of affect (e.g., unable to have loving feelings)

    7. Sense of a foreshortened future (e.g., does not expect to have a career, marriage, children, or a normal life span)

(Continued)

Table 3-5

Criteria for Posttraumatic Stress Disorder (Continued)

D. Persistent symptoms of increased arousal (not present before the trauma), as indicated by two (or more) of the following:

1. Difficulty falling or staying asleep
2. Irritability or outbursts of anger
3. Difficulty concentrating
4. Hypervigilance
5. Exaggerated startle response

E. Duration of the disturbance (symptoms in criteria B, C, D) is more than 1 month.

F. The disturbance causes clinically significant distress or impairment in social, occupational, or other important areas of functioning.

Specify as acute—if duration of symptoms is less than 3 months; chronic—if duration of symptoms is 3 months or more; with delayed onset—if onset of symptoms is at least 6 months after the stressor

SOURCE American Psychiatric Association: *Diagnostic and Statistical Manual of Mental Disorders,* 4th ed.Washington, DC, American Psychiatric Association, 1994.

symptoms to be diagnosed with PTSD. Symptoms of increased arousal, two of which must be present for PTSD, include insomnia, irritability, hypervigilance, and exaggerated startle. The diagnosis of PTSD is made only when these symptoms persist for at least a month, with the diagnosis being acute stress disorder during the interim. The DSM-IV lists three subtypes of PTSD that differentiate among syndromes with varying time courses. Thus, acute PTSD lasts less than 3 months, whereas the chronic form refers to an episode lasting longer than that. Delayed-onset PTSD refers to the situation in which the condition becomes apparent 6 months or more after the patient experiences the traumatic event.

Because individuals often exhibit complex biological and behavioral responses to extreme trauma, other medical and psychiatric conditions may be present in the traumatized patient. Particularly after events involving physical injury, neurological etiologies must be considered for some symptoms. Trau-

matized patients often develop mood disorders, including dysthymia and major depression, other anxiety disorders, such as generalized anxiety disorder or panic disorder, and substance abuse disorders. Research suggests that some psychiatric features of posttraumatic syndromes relate to the state of a patient before the trauma. For example, those with premorbid anxiety or affective syndromes may be more prone to developing posttraumatic symptoms than individuals who were previously free of mental illness. Accordingly, consideration must be given to the premorbid mental state of the traumatized patient to enhance understanding of symptoms that develop following the traumatic event.

Course. The likelihood of developing symptoms as well as the severity and duration of symptoms are proportional to the proximity, duration, and intensity of the trauma (Davidson and Foa, 1991). Thus, many individuals develop acute stress reactions when faced with close, persistent, and intense trauma, and most PTSD patients exhibit features of the acute stress syndrome before developing the condition. However, many patients with acute stress syndromes do not develop PTSD. Moreover, the full syndrome of PTSD exhibits a variable course, which also may relate to the nature of the trauma, with many patients experiencing complete remissions, whereas others display only mild symptoms. Some 10% of patients with PTSD, possibly those with more severe or persistent trauma, exhibit a chronic course. Such individuals often are reexposed to the traumatic event. Patients are often encountered in the wake of a trauma; some, however, might present following an exacerbation of chronic symptoms that worsen following reexposure to the precipitating event.

Differential diagnosis. In diagnosing PTSD care must be taken to exclude other syndromes when evaluating patients presenting after trauma (Fig. 3-3). It is particularly important to recognize treatable medical conditions that may contribute to posttraumatic symptomatology. For example, neurological damage following head injury can contribute to the clinical picture, as can substance abuse or withdrawal syndromes, either in the period immediately after the trauma or weeks later. Medical contributors can usually be detected through a careful history and physi-

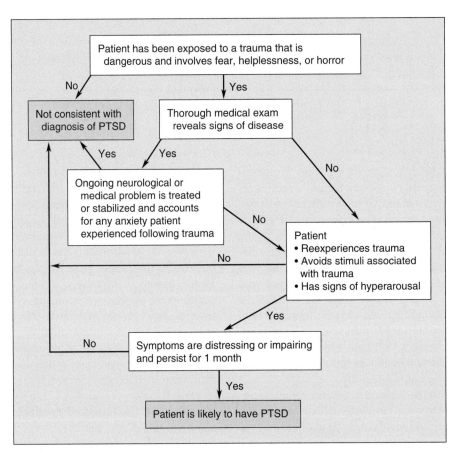

Figure 3–3. Making the diagnosis of posttraumatic stress disorder.

cal examination, with the cognitive examination being integral in making the correct diagnosis. With classical, uncomplicated PTSD, the patient should be alert and fully oriented. If patients show abnormalities on cognitive examination, particularly in the absence of a prior history of cognitive deficits, efforts must be made to exclude underlying medical contributors.

Symptoms of PTSD may be difficult to distinguish from panic disorder or generalized anxiety disorder because all three syndromes are associated with prominent anxiety and autonomic arousal. An important step in diagnosing PTSD is a careful review of the time course of the symptoms as they relate to the traumatic event. Further, PTSD is associated with reexperiencing and avoidance of a trauma, features typically not present in panic or generalized anxiety disorder. Major depression is also frequently a component of PTSD. Although the two syndromes are, in most cases, readily distinguishable phenomenologically, it is important to note the presence of comorbid depression, as this may influence the choice of treatment for PTSD. Furthermore, PTSD must be differentiated from borderline personality disorder, dissociative disorders, and factitious disorders, all of which exhibit phenomenological similarities.

Pathophysiology. Because PTSD is as a behavioral disorder resulting from the direct effects of trauma, there is a wealth of research aimed at examining the effects of traumatic stress on laboratory animals and humans.

Hypothalamic-pituitary-adrenal axis. One of the more consistent findings with PTSD is an abnormality in cortisol regulation (Yehuda et al., 1995). The role of the HPA axis in acute stress has been appreciated for years, and there is a wealth of information on both the acute and the chronic effects of stress on the functioning of this system (Sapolsky, 1997). For example, although acute stress produces elevations in corticotrophin releasing factor (CRF), adrenocorticotropin (ACTH), and cortisol, over time there is a reduction in cortisol release, even in the face of elevated CRF levels.

In contrast to major depressive disorder, which is characterized by a deficiency in the regulation of the HPA axis in humans, there is an enhanced feedback control of this axis with PTSD (Yehuda et al., 1995).

Thus, individuals with PTSD have reduced levels of cortisol, a similar diurnal variation in cortisol, and enhanced

sensitivity of lymphocyte glucocorticoid receptors in comparison with depressed and psychiatrically healthy individuals. Moreover, neuroendocrine challenge tests indicate that PTSD is associated with an enhanced ACTH response to CRF challenge and an enhanced cortisol sensitivity to dexamethasone. These are thought to arise from abnormalities in the hypothalamic or hippocampal regulation of the HPA axis. For example, Sapolsky (1997) suggests that traumatic stress, through effects on cortisol release, affects the hippocampus over time, and quantitative magnetic resonance imaging studies suggest that PTSD is associated with a reduction in hippocampal volume (Bremner et al., 1995).

Autonomic nervous system. Because autonomic overarousal is a key element of PTSD, there has been a great deal of research on the role of the noradrenergic system in this condition. Challenges with yohimbine, an α_2-adrenergic receptor antagonist, reliably elicit flashbacks and paniclike reactions in patients with PTSD (Charney et al., 1993). Positron emission tomography suggests that these effects are due to an increase in the sensitivity of the noradrenergic system (Bremner et al., 1997). These findings may be related to those on the HPA axis, given the interplay between the HPA and noadrenergic systems.

Serotonin. The most direct evidence of a role for serotonin in PTSD is from pharmacological studies in humans. There are also data from animal models to suggest a role for this neurotransmitter in PTSD. For example, the environment can have marked effects on the serotonin system of rodents and nonhuman primates (Azmitia and Whitaker-Azmitia, 1995). Moreover, preliminary data from human studies suggest an association between environmental rearing circumstances and serotonin activity in childhood. There have been few studies directly examining the serotonergic system in PTSD using neuroendocrine challenge, imaging, or target-gene approaches.

Conditioned fear. It has been shown that PTSD closely resembles conditioned fear models of anxiety (LeDoux, 1996). In PTSD, the profound trauma could serve as an unconditioned stimulus, theoretically influencing the amygdala and its associated fear circuits, which could account for flashbacks and a general increase in anxiety. Environmental features related to the trauma, such as the sounds of battle, might serve as conditioned stimuli so that similar sounds elicit the conditioned response, including a flashback and the associated anxiety, through an activation of the amygdala. Through projections from the amygdala to the temporal lobe, the fear circuit could activate memories of traumatic events even without an obvious environmental cue. The most relevant research in this area uses the fear-potentiated startle paradigm. In this test, a conditioned stimulus, such as a light or a tone, is paired with an unconditioned stimulus, such as a shock. An increase in the amplitude of the startle reflex when a conditioned stimulus is presented represents the degree of fear potentiation of the reflex. The neuroanatomical pathway involved in this response is the fear circuit outlined by LeDoux (1996). Although the data are somewhat inconsistent (Grillon et al., 1996; Morgan et al., 1995), there is evidence of an association between PTSD and fear-potentiated startle in humans. Moreover, results from neuroimaging studies implicate components of the nervous system related to fear acquisition in PTSD, particularly the hippocampal formation and other temporal lobe structures, and the amygdala (Bremner et al., 1997; Shin et al., 1997).

Generalized Anxiety Disorder

Presenting symptoms. Generalized anxiety disorder is characterized by frequent, persistent worry and anxiety that is out of proportion to the event or circumstance that is the focus of concern (Table 3-6) (Schweizer, 1995). For example, although college

Table 3-6
Criteria for Generalized Anxiety Disorder

A. Excessive anxiety and worry (apprehensive expectation), occurring more days than not for at least 6 months, about a number of events or activities (such as work or school performance).

B. The person finds it difficult to control the worry.

C. The anxiety and worry are associated with three (or more) of the following six symptoms (with at least some symptoms present for more days than not for the past 6 months). **Note:** Only one item is required in children.

    1. Restlessness or feeling keyed up or on edge
    2. Being easily fatigued
    3. Difficulty concentrating
    4. Irritability
    5. Muscle tension
    6. Sleep disturbance (difficulty falling or staying asleep, or restless, unsatisfying sleep)

D. The focus of the anxiety and worry is not confined to features of an Axis I disorder, for example, the anxiety or worry is not about having a panic attack (as in panic disorder), being embarrassed in public (as in social phobia), being contaminated (as in obsessive-compulsive disorder), being away from home (as in separation anxiety disorder), gaining weight (as in anorexia nervosa), having multiple physical complaints (as in somatization disorder), or having a serious illness (as in hypochondriasis), and the anxiety or worry does not occur exclusively during posttraumatic stress disorder.

E. The anxiety, worry, or physical symptoms cause clinically significant distress or impairment in social, occupational, or other important areas of functioning.

F. The disturbance is not due to the direct physiological effects of a substance (e.g., a drug of abuse, a medication) or a general medical condition (e.g., hypothyroidism) and does not occur exclusively during a mood disorder, a psychotic disorder, or a pervasive developmental disorder.

SOURCE American Psychiatric Association: *Diagnostic and Statistical Manual of Mental Disorders*, 4th ed. Washington, DC, American Psychiatric Association, 1994.

students are often apprehensive about examinations, a student who worries persistently about failure despite consistently obtaining outstanding grades displays a pattern of anxiety typical of generalized anxiety disorder. Patients with generalized anxiety disorder may not acknowledge the excessive nature of their worry but must be bothered by the degree of apprehension, and this pattern must occur frequently for at least 6 months. The patient must find it difficult to control this worry and must report at least three of six somatic or cognitive symptoms. Included are feelings of restlessness, fatigue, muscle tension, or insomnia. It must be appreciated, however, that worry is a common feature of many anxiety disorders. Thus, patients with panic disorder are often apprehensive about panic attacks, patients with social phobia worry about social encounters, and patients with obsessive-compulsive disorder are concerned about their obsessions. The worries in generalized anxiety disorder must go beyond those characteristic of other anxiety disorders. Although children exhibiting these symptoms are also considered to be suffering from generalized anxiety disorder, they are only required to meet one of the six somatic/cognitive symptom criteria to qualify.

Course.   Symptoms of generalized anxiety disorder are often observed in patients presenting to primary care physicians. Typically, such individuals report a history of vague somatic complaints, such as fatigue, muscle aches or tension, and minor sleep difficulties. The lack of prospective epidemiological studies precludes firm conclusions about the course of the condition, with the most complete data coming from retrospective epidemiologically based studies. These studies suggest that generalized anxiety disorder is a chronic condition, as most patients report the presence of symptoms for many years before assessment.

Differential diagnosis.   As with other anxiety disorders, generalized anxiety disorder must be differentiated from other medical and psychiatric conditions (Fig. 3-4). Neurological, endocrinologic, metabolic, and medication-related disorders must be considered as possibilities in the differential diagnosis of generalized anxiety disorder. In addition, commonly co-

occurring anxiety disorders, including panic disorder, phobias, obsessive-compulsive disorder, and PTSD, must also be considered when making a diagnosis. The patient, however, must exhibit the full syndrome of generalized anxiety disorder in the absence of a comorbid anxiety condition. To diagnose generalized anxiety disorder in the presence of other anxiety states, it is most important to document anxiety or worry related to circumstances or topics that are either unrelated, or only minimally related, to other conditions. Hence, proper diagnosis involves documenting the symptoms of generalized anxiety disorder and properly establishing the presence or absence of other anxiety conditions. Because patients with generalized anxiety disorder frequently develop major depression, this condition must also be recognized and distinguished. Again, the key feature to making a correct diagnosis is documenting anxiety or worry that is unrelated to the affective illness.

Pathophysiology.   Of all the anxiety disorders, the least is known about the pathophysiology of generalized anxiety disorder. This lack of information is owing, in part, to the relatively major changes in the conceptualization of the condition over the past 15 years. During this time the definition of generalized anxiety disorder has grown narrower, whereas the definition of panic-related conditions has expanded. The lack of pathophysiologic data might relate to the fact that patients rarely present to psychiatrists for treatment of isolated generalized anxiety. Patients with generalized anxiety disorder usually exhibit comorbid mood or anxiety disorders, even in the epidemiological setting where patients with isolated generalized anxiety disorder are rarely seen. As a result, much of the data on pathophysiology considers the extent to which generalized anxiety disorder can be differentiated from other frequently co-occurring anxiety or mood disorders. Because the strongest comorbidity is found with either major depression or panic disorder, research has been aimed at making distinctions among generalized anxiety, panic, and major depressive disorders.

Family/genetic studies. A series of twin and family studies have considered the distinctiveness of generalized anxiety,

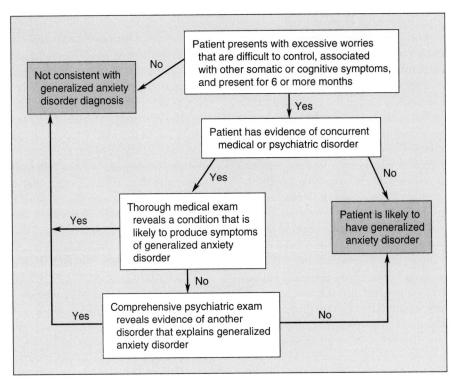

Figure 3–4. *Making the diagnosis of generalized anxiety disorder.*

panic, and major depressive disorders (Fyer et al., 1995; Kendler et al., 1995; Weissman, 1990). Although data are consistent in suggesting that panic disorder is distinguishable from generalized anxiety and major depressive disorders by the pattern of familial transmission, distinctions between generalized anxiety and major depressive disorders are less clear. Based on their study of adult female twins, and a consideration of existing data, Kendler et al. (1995) proposed that generalized anxiety and major depressive disorders may share a common genetic base, becoming distinct by environmental effects. Lesch et al. (1996) found that a polymorphism in the serotonin reuptake transporter predicted scores on neurotocism questionnaires, which shows strong associations with the symptoms of both major depression and generalized anxiety disorder. The results of longitudinal studies with children are consistent with this view (Pine et al., in press). Thus, the associations between childhood generalized anxiety disorder and adult major depression are equally as strong as those between childhood depression and adult generalized anxiety, between childhood and adult generalized anxiety disorder, or between childhood and adult major depression.

Differentiation from panic disorder. A number of studies have compared the biology of panic and generalized anxiety disorders. Although the results indicate some distinctions between the two, most studies revealed that patients with generalized anxiety disorder also differ from psychiatrically healthy individuals on biological correlates of panic disorder. For example, whereas studies comparing the anxiogenic response to respiratory-related challenge agents, such as lactate or carbon dioxide, showed that generalized anxiety disorder patients exhibit more extreme responses than healthy subjects, the response in panic disorder involves more prominent complaints of dyspnea than is the case with generalized anxiety disorder (Coplan and Klein, 1996; Johnson and Lydiard, 1995). The response of generalized anxiety disorder patients is usually characterized by a high degree of anxiety coupled with somatic complaints unrelated to the respiratory system. Moreover, generalized anxiety disorder is associated with a blunted growth hormone response to clonidine challenge, similar to panic disorder and major depression (Abelson et al., 1991), and abnormalities in heart period variability profiles and serotonin are also found with generalized anxiety disorder (Johnson and Lydiard, 1995).

PHARMACOTHERAPEUTICS

Selective Serotonin Reuptake Inhibitors

The selective serotonin reuptake inhibitors (SSRIs) represent a unique class of medication. Before their development in the 1980s, the discovery of new medications for anxiety, as for most psychiatric disorders, resulted from chance clinical observations (Carlsson, 1987). Psychiatric medications developed before the SSRIs typically exerted effects on many neurotransmitter systems. In contrast, the SSRIs were designed to act only on the serotonin reuptake site located presynaptically on serotonergic nerve terminals. The rationale for this approach was provided by the observation that medications that are effective in treating anxiety and depressive disorders all inhibit serotonin reuptake in the brain (Carlsson, 1987).

The efficacy of the SSRIs in treating anxiety and depressive disorder has focused research on the role of serotonin in these conditions. This has led to new animal models of psychiatric disorders and to targeted genetic studies in humans (Lesch et al., 1996). The efficacy of the SSRIs in a host of psychiatric conditions has also stimulated research aimed at defining the neurochemical similarities and differences among the anxiety and depressive disorders. Clinically, the SSRIs are extremely popular because they combine efficacy in an array of conditions with tolerability and safety.

Currently there are four SSRIs approved for use in the United States: fluoxetine, sertraline, paroxetine, and fluvoxamine. A fifth, citalopram, is available in Europe, and a sixth, zimelidine, has been withdrawn since it was associated with cases of Guillain-Barré syndrome. The five SSRIs available in the United States and Europe are discussed as a group, with differences highlighted only if they have an impact on clinical care.

Data from large, randomized, controlled trials demonstrate the efficacy of the SSRIs for the treatment of acute episodes of various anxiety disorders (Boyer, 1995). Beyond the data with obsessive-compulsive disorder discussed elsewhere in this volume, the greatest amount of information on the SSRIs is on panic disorder, where successful results with fluvoxamine, paroxetine, sertraline, and zimelidine have been reported (Boyer, 1995). Although there are few data on direct comparisons of the various SSRIs in panic disorder, all are considered to be equally effective. The major differences among the SSRIs relate to their half-lives and potential for drug-drug interactions. The latter, especially, stem from different effects on hepatic enzymes involved in their metabolism.

There is little published information on the efficacy of the SSRIs in anxiety disorders other than panic. Two of three small-scale studies in social phobia suggest that both fluvoxamine and sertraline are efficacious; study of paroxetine offers less definitive results (Marshall et al., 1996). One study also demonstrated fluoxetine's efficacy in treating PTSD, particularly when it results from trauma in civilians as opposed to veterans (Van der Kolk, 1994). There are no published studies in noncomorbid, generalized anxiety disorder. Despite substantial data on the efficacy of most SSRIs in panic disorder, only paroxetine carries an FDA indication for this condition.

The SSRIs are also effective treatments for major depressive disorder and dysthymia, conditions that often complicate the diagnosis of anxiety disorders (Song et al., 1993; Montgomery et al., 1994). Indeed, controlled clinical trials of SSRIs in anxiety disorders do not always exclude patients with comorbid affective symptoms. As a result it is unclear whether SSRIs are more or less effective in subgroups of anxious patients with and without depression. Further, although the SSRIs prevent relapse in major depression, few studies examined this issue with respect to anxiety disorders. Nevertheless, SSRIs are used over periods of months to years to prevent relapse in patients whose acute anxiety disorders respond to these medications (Schweizer et al., 1995).

There are few studies directly comparing the efficacy of SSRIs with other medications known to be effective in the treatment of anxiety disorders. Clinically, the SSRIs are often chosen over the tricyclic antidepressants, monoamine oxidase inhibitors, and benzodiazepines because of their superior side effect profile, low abuse potential, and safety in overdose (Coplan et al., 1995).

The SSRIs were designed to inhibit the reuptake of serotonin into the presynaptic nerve terminal. Extensive basic research suggests this action is intimately related to their efficacy as antidepressants (Barker and Blakely, 1995; Jacobs and Fornal, 1995). For example, medications known to inhibit serotonin reuptake are effective in animal models of depression. Although data from animal models of anxiety are less consistent, this may be owing to the appropriateness of the animal models (Coplan and Klein, 1996). In particular, there is debate about whether animal tests that use approach-avoidance conflict paradigms are models of panic (Goddard and Charney, 1997).

There is agreement that blockade of serotonin reuptake is responsible for the effects of the SSRIs, but it is unclear as to how this translates into clinical efficacy. Because the therapeutic effects of SSRIs on behavior, in either laboratory animals or humans, are not apparent for many days, the acute effect on serotonin reuptake cannot alone account for their efficacy (Barker and Blakely, 1995). It has been suggested that long-term treatment enhances serotonergic transmission from the raphe to the prefrontal cortex or limbic areas (Coplan et al., 1995). To what extent this is related to the effect of SSRIs on human anxiety or depressive disorders remains unknown.

An advantage of the SSRIs over other medications is their more favorable side effect profile (Preskorn, 1996). Of particular note is the fact that SSRIs have few clinically relevant effects on the cardiovascular system. In contrast, the tricyclic antidepressants have effects on cardiac conduction and blood pressure. The most common side effects of the SSRIs are nervousness or anxiety, which can interfere with sleep, particularly when high doses are administered initially, and headaches. Gastrointestinal effects are also common, including nausea, constipation, anorexia, and loose stools. One of the major complications associated with their use is the high incidence of sexual side effects, which include changes in libido and interference with orgasm in both sexes. Other, less frequently encountered, side effects are urinary retention, increased sweating, visual disturbances,

akathisia, dizziness, fatigue, and effects on motor control. Moreover, as with all antidepressants, SSRIs can precipitate mania. Because there are few direct comparisons of the risk for mania among the various antidepressants, it is unclear whether the SSRIs are safer in this regard than other agents.

There are few absolute contraindications for the use of SSRIs. However, caution must be exercised when prescribing them in combination with other medications. The SSRIs are potent inhibitors of various cytochrome P450 isozymes, a family of hepatic enzymes responsible for the metabolism of many drugs. As a result, blood levels of some medications may increase to toxic levels when they are coadministered with SSRIs. Examples include tricyclic antidepressants coadministered with fluoxetine or sertraline, theophylline or haloperidol when taken with fluvoxamine, and phenytoin when given with fluoxetine (Nemeroff et al., 1996; Preskorn, 1996). With some drugs, such as the tricyclic antidepressants, the two medications can be administered together provided the blood levels of the tricyclic antidepressant are closely monitored. For others, such as the monoamine oxidase inhibitors, combination therapy with SSRIs should be avoided because serious adverse events, such as the serotonin syndrome, can result. In all cases, standard references of drug-drug interactions should be consulted before initiating SSRIs in a patient receiving other medications (Ciraulo et al., 1995; Nemeroff et al., 1996; Preskorn, 1996).

The SSRIs are safe, even at doses five-fold to ten-fold higher than the therapeutic dose. Although overdose in adults has been associated with agitation, vomiting and, rarely, seizures, no deaths have yet been reported as a result of an overdose with an SSRI alone. The only two reported deaths followed an overdose of at least 1800 mg of fluoxetine in combination with other medications.

Azapirones

The azapirones are a class of drugs with a high affinity for the 5HT1A serotonin receptor, which is located on the cell body and terminals of serotonergic neurons, and on the dendrites of postsynaptic neurons adjacent to serotonergic terminals (Coplan et al., 1995; Feighner, 1987). This group includes three agents currently available in either the United States or Europe: buspirone, gepirone, and ipsapirone. In laboratory animal models of anxiety, the azapirones display effects similar to the benzodiazepines, although they are less potent. These effects are believed to result from their partial agonist actions at presynaptic 5HT1A receptors. The azapirones also display efficacy in animal models of depression.

Buspirone is established as an effective treatment for generalized anxiety disorder and is approved for this indication (Feighner, 1987; Rickels et al., 1993, 1988). As with the SSRIs, the beneficial effect of buspirone in generalized anxiety disorder is apparent only after several days of continuous therapy. Buspirone is approximately as effective as the benzodiazepines in the treatment of this condition, although the onset of the therapeutic effect is considerably delayed with buspirone as compared with the benzodiazepines (Rickels et al., 1988). Results from randomized clinical trials suggest that the azapirones may also be effective in the treatment of major depressive disorder, particularly when anxiety is prominent. However, the validity of these findings has been questioned because of the high drop-out rates in some of these studies. One randomized trial found that buspirone reduced anxiety symptoms in detoxified alcoholics who suffered from comorbid generalized anxiety disorder. In contrast with the SSRIs, a number of studies have failed to demonstrate any significant efficacy for the azapirones in panic disorder (Coplan et al., 1995). Although there are data suggesting that azapirones might be beneficial in social phobia, the only controlled trial, which was for specific social phobia, failed to note efficacy (Liebowitz and Marshall, 1995). Clearly, the most conclusive data on azapirones relate to their effectiveness in generalized anxiety disorders, where perhaps their main advantage is their lack of tolerance and abuse potential. This contrasts with the benzodiazepines, the other therapeutic mainstay for this condition.

Although the site of action of the azapirones is known, the manner in which this effect yields clinical benefit is poorly understood. In general, azapirones are partial agonists at 5HT1A receptors at postsynaptic sites, potentially in the hippocampus and prefrontal cortex (Coplan et al., 1995). They also exert actions at autoreceptors located on the cell body of presynaptic serotonergic neurons (Coplan et al., 1995). Because a therapeutic response is not noted for several days after initiation of therapy, these acute actions cannot by themselves account for their efficacy in generalized anxiety disorder. Animal studies suggest that the anxiolytic response to these agents is mediated by an action at presynaptic receptors, and the antidepressant effect is due to their effects on postsynaptic sites (Lucki and Wieland, 1990).

The azapirones are relatively free of side effects. In particular, they lack the abuse liability, tolerance, withdrawal symptoms, and psychomotor and cognitive effects of the benzodiazepines. Unlike the tricyclic antidepressants, they are also devoid of effects on the cardiovascular system. The azapirones have been associated with gastrointestinal upset, headaches, and, occasionally, restlessness, nervousness, and sleep disturbances. These symptoms are rarely severe enough to interfere with their use. As compared with the benzodiazepines, the azapirones cause less drowsiness, cognitive side effects, and fatigue, but they are associated with more nervousness and gastrointestinal complaints. Although there are reports of movement disorders resulting from azapirone treatment, these have been isolated, anecdotal findings.

The azapirones should be used cautiously with monoamine oxidase inhibitors as there are reports of blood pressure elevations associated with this drug combination.

Tricyclic Antidepressants

As with many of the older drugs, the efficacy of the tricyclic antidepressants in anxiety and depressive disorders was discovered by chance. The utility of these agents for depression was noted during trials for psychosis, and their efficacy in anxiety disorders was noted while they were being tested in anxious patients, somewhat haphazardly, along with a variety of other medications (Carlsson, 1987).

The designation of tricyclic antidepressants derives from the fact that these drugs share a common chemical structure, consisting of two benzene rings joined by a seven-membered ring. They are sub-classified according to variations in their chemical structure. Thus, one group consists of tertiary amines (imipramine, amitriptyline, clomipramine, and doxepin) and the other secondary amines (desipramine, nortriptyline, protriptyline, and amoxapine). Two of the secondary amine tricyclics (desipramine and nortiptyline) are demethylated tertiary amines (imipramine and amitriptyline). Because the tertiary amines are metabolized partially by demethylation, treatment with either imipramine or amitriptyline yields both tertiary and secondary amines in the bloodstream. The tricyclic antidepressants were once the drugs of choice for a number of anxiety disorders; they are used less frequently today. The decline in their popularity is owing, in part, to the more favorable side effect profile of newer medications, rather than to a lack of efficacy. Indeed, with respect to efficacy, tricyclics remain an outstanding treatment for a variety of anxiety disorders.

Panic is the most common anxiety disorder treated with tricyclic antidepressants. Beginning with the observation that panic attacks selectively respond to tricyclics, a number of investigators have noted the efficacy of these agents for this condition, either with or without agoraphobia (Klein, 1993). Although early studies focused on imipramine, there are also many controlled clinical trials demonstrating the efficacy of clomipramine, nortriptyline, and other drugs of this class in the treatment of panic disorder (Pollack and Smoller, 1995; Mavissakalian and Perel, 1995; Schweizer et al., 1995). Based on the efficacy of the serotonin reuptake inhibitors, it appears that treatment of panic disorder requires a modification in serotonergic function, which is particularly robust with the tricyclic clomipramine. This is probably an oversimplification, however, because the efficacy of the SSRIs probably also involves their indirect effects on the noradrenergic system (Coplan et al., 1997). Indeed, the fact that panic disorder responds to desipramine, the tricyclic most selective for the noradrenergic system, suggests that modifications of either the serotonergic or noradrenergic system might be sufficient for a therapeutic response.

Klein's initial studies emphasized the pharmacological distinctions between panic disorder, which

responded to tricyclics but not benzodiazepines, and generalized anxiety disorder, which responded to benzodiazepines but not tricyclics. More recently, however, this conclusion has been questioned, with controlled clinical trials demonstrating efficacy for the tricyclic antidepressants in generalized anxiety disorder (Rickels et al., 1993). Hence, the tricyclics are useful for treating generalized anxiety disorder, particularly when there are concerns about the abuse potential of benzodiazepines.

Although there are relatively few controlled clinical trials on the pharmacological management of PTSD, at least four studies have examined the efficacy of tricyclic antidepressants, with mixed results. Amitriptyline was found to have some benefit in one study, another study reported that desipramine is ineffective, and a third found imipramine to be inferior to phenelzine (Marshall et al., 1996). Given the paucity of pharmacotherapeutic research on PTSD, no firm conclusions can be drawn on the role of tricyclic antidepressants in the treatment of this condition. Because of the relative safety and tolerability of the SSRIs, coupled with some suggestive data on their efficacy in PTSD, it has been suggested that a trial with an SSRI be undertaken before attempting to use a tricyclic antidepressant to treat this condition. Moreover, tricyclic antidepressants are not considered a first-line treatment for social phobia, either specific or generalized (Liebowitz and Marshall, 1995), given the solid data on the efficacy of the monamine oxidase inhibitors and SSRIs in the treatment of this condition.

The mechanism of action of the tricyclic antidepressants is not completely understood. Most of the drugs have acute effects on a variety of neurotransmitter pathways, including those associated with the catecholamine, indoleamine, and cholinergic systems. Preclinical research has demonstrated an effect on the reuptake of serotonin and norepinephrine in the brain (Barker and Blakely, 1995). These drugs inhibit these reuptake transporters to varying degrees, with desipramine being relatively selective for the norepinepherine transporter and clomipramine for the serotonin transporter; the others display a mixed affinity for the two sites. As with the SSRIs, the acute effects on neurotransmitter reuptake cannot totally account for the efficacy of the tricyclic antidepressants because their clinical effects are not generally observed until after several days or weeks of continuous administration. This suggests the therapeutic response is due to changes in the brain that occur over time. It has been speculated that the mechanism of action of the tricyclic antidepressants on anxiety may involve gradual changes in serotonergic or catecholaminergic neurotransmission, changes in second messenger pathways, or alterations in gene expression.

Side effects limit the use of tricyclic antidepressants. Most notable is their effect on intracardiac conduction, with dose-related changes in the electrocardiogram (ECG). Included are tachycardias, prolongation of ECG intervals, bundle branch or heart block, and ST- and T-wave changes. There is anecdotal evidence these effects may be more common in children than in adults. Hence, caution must be exercised when prescribing these medications to children. The tricyclic antidepressants also induce orthostatic hypotension by blocking postsynaptic α_1-adrenergic receptors. These actions complicate the use of these drugs, making them far more dangerous in overdose than SSRIs.

Other side effects of the tricyclic antidepressants that are less dangerous, but can affect patient compliance, include anticholinergic actions, particularly common with the tertiary amines, which include drowsiness, lethargy, urinary retention, dry mouth, constipation, blurred vision, and gastrointestinal disturbances. Their antihistaminic effects can exacerbate cognitive complaints, and these drugs can affect sexual functioning, causing anorgasmia, delayed ejaculation, and decreased libido. Like the SSRIs, the tricyclic antidepressants can precipitate manic episodes. Although it is unknown whether particular members of this class are more prone to unmasking mania, data suggest the entire group has this potential.

The most significant contraindications to the use of tricyclic antidepressants involve either underlying cardiac disease or a serious concern with the possibility of overdose, in which case these drugs should be avoided. Narrow-angle glaucoma is a less frequent, but equally troubling, contraindication, because the anticholinergic properties of the tricyclic antidepressants pose a serious danger in such patients. Although they can be used in patients with open-angle glaucoma, an ophthalmologic consultation should be obtained before initiating therapy in such patients. Tricyclic antidepressants should also be very cautiously prescribed in the elderly, even when there is no underlying medical disease, given the possibility of falls due to orthostasis. Care should be taken with children because of potential cardiac toxicity, and with adolescents because the risk of overdose is relatively high in this age group.

Clinicians should be wary of drug-drug interactions when using tricyclic antidepressants. Concomitant use with medications that inhibit cytochrome P450 activity, such as the SSRIs, can result in toxic levels of the tricyclic antidepressants even when they are taken in low doses. Concomitant use of other anticholinergics can cause delirium and severe urinary retention. Also, coadministration with sedative/hypnotic agents, such as the benzodiazepines or antihistamines, or with medications that affect the cardiovascular system, such as neuroleptics or β-adrenergic receptor blockers, can result in central nervous system or cardiac toxicity, even at low doses.

The most serious toxicity associated with the tricyclic antidepressants relates to their effect on cardiac conduction, with high doses producing life-threatening arrhythmias. The difference between a therapeutic and a toxic dose is small (narrow therapeutic window), with an overdose of 1 g being potentially lethal. This amount is usually less than the total taken over the course of a week. Other toxicities include orthostatic hypotension and effects related to their anticholinergic and antihistaminic properties. Toxicity is also a problem when tricyclic antidepressants are prescribed with other medications that affect blood pressure, cholinergic function, and arousal.

Monoamine Oxidase Inhibitors

The therapeutic effects of the monamine oxidase inhibitors (MAOIs) were discovered by accident in the 1950s when iproniazid was used to treat tuberculosis (Carlsson, 1987). Since then the MAOIs have been found to be quite effective in the treatment of a variety of depressive and anxiety disorders (Thase and Rush, 1995). Their ability to produce robust therapeutic responses, even in patients refractory to other medications, has made them a valuable component of the therapeutic armamentarium for treating anxiety disorder. Their use is limited, however, by relatively rare, but potentially fatal, side effects (Murphy et al., 1987).

Monoamine oxidase is one of the major enzymes responsible for the degradation of catecholamines and indoleamines. One isoform, MAO-A, which is located in the gastrointestinal tract, brain, and liver, metabolizes primarily norepinephrine and serotonin, whereas MAO-B, which is located in the brain, liver, and platelets, but not the gastrointestinal tract, metabolizes primarily dopamine, phenylethylamine, and benzylamine (Murphy et al., 1987). Phenelzine and tranylcypromine are nonselective inhibitors of MAO, reducing the activity of both MAO-A and MAO-B. Some have argued that inhibition of MAO-A is more important for the treatment of anxiety and depression, whereas inhibition of MAO-B is more useful in treating Parkinson's disease. Selegiline selectively inhibits MAO-B at low doses, and at high doses it inhibits both forms of the enzyme. Thus, it is thought to be more useful in the treatment of Parkinson's disease than in the treatment of anxiety and depression. Because these medications bind irreversibly to MAO, new enzyme must be synthesized to recover full activity, a process requiring 1 to 2 months off therapy (Murphy et al., 1987). Moclobemide, a newer medication that is not available in the United States, binds reversibly to MAO, with selectivity for MAO-A. Because it is not necessary for new enzyme to be manufactured when reversible inhibitors are used, they provide greater flexibility in the care of refractory patients. Although most research on the treatment of anxiety or depressive disorders has entailed the use of older, nonselective MAOIs, more recent work has focused on the clinical properties of the newer, reversible agents.

The MAOIs are effective in the treatment of panic disorder, social phobia, and PTSD (Liebowitz and Marshall, 1995). Moreover, there is some indication that variants of depression complicated by panic attacks, such as atypical depression, are particularly responsive to MAOIs. The MAOIs are also efficacious in the teatment of social phobia, with at least four large studies showing them to be particularly useful as a therapy for the generalized form of the disorder (Liebowitz and Marshall, 1995).

Because MAO in brain is responsible for the catabolism of biogenic amines, MAOIs inhibit the metabolism of monamine neurotransmitters, increasing their bioavailability and prolonging their actions (Murphy et al., 1987). The relationship between this acute effect and therapeutic efficacy in anxiety disorders is, however, poorly understood. Thus, as is the case with SSRIs and tricyclic antidepressants, the clinical benefits of the MAOIs are not apparent until treatment has continued for days or weeks, even though the enzyme is inhibited with a single dose. A number of theories have been put forth to account for the therapeutic effects of MAOIs. In general it is thought the acute changes in neurotransmitter availability might lead to adaptive changes in gene expression, which, in turn, may affect neurotransmitter receptor number or affinity, or signal transduction systems.

The most serious side effect associated with the use of MAOIs is hypertension resulting from the ingestion of tyramine-containing foods or beverages (cheese reaction). Thus, MAO in the gastrointestinal tract normally degrades tyramine, an agent that induces a pressor response by causing the release of endogenous catecholamines. Tyramine is present in various foods and libations, including cheeses, meats, and wine. In combination with a MAOI, tyramine ingestion can have life-threatening consequences by producing a hypertensive crisis characterized by signs of sympathetic overactivation, such as elevated blood pressure, fever, tremulousness, and diaphoresis (Murphy et al., 1987). This crisis can lead to lethal cardiac arrhythmias and dangerous elevations in blood pressure. Patients taking MAOIs should proceed immediately to an emergency department for care if they develop signs of a hypertensive crisis.

In addition to this rare, but dangerous, side effect, MAOIs have a number of other actions that limit their use. These actions include postural hypotension, insomnia, agitation, somnolence, weight gain, and inhibition of sexual function. As is the case for all antidepressant medications, the MAOIs are capable of precipitating a manic episode in susceptible individuals.

Only patients who can rigorously follow the complicated dietary regimen required for the safe use of MAOIs should use these medications. Hence, patients with organic or cognitive deficits, and patients with poor impulse control, are not good candidates for this therapy. Beyond dietary tyramine, any sympathomimetic medication is capable of precipitating a hypertensive crisis in these patients. Other drugs, such as narcotics, oral hypoglycemics, and L-dopa, can also have dangerous interactions with MAOIs. As with the tricyclic antidepressants, MAOIs should be used with caution in the elderly because of the risk of a fall due to orthostatic hypotension.

The MAOIs are extremely toxic in overdose, although signs and symptoms of toxicity may not develop immediately. Toxic effects include seizures, arrhythmias, rhabdomyolysis, and coagulopathies.

Benzodiazepines

The introduction of the benzodiazepines in the 1960s revolutionized psychopharmacology. The class derives its name from a shared chemical structure, consisting of a benzene ring connected to a seven-member diazepine ring (Enna and Möhler, 1987). The characteristics of the benzodiazepines vary as a result of substitutions on either ring. Before the introduction of the benzodiazepines, the barbiturates were the most frequently prescribed sedative/hypnotics. The benzodiazepines rapidly supplanted the barbiturates, however, because the latter produce severe respiratory depression and, when given chronically, can lead to a dangerous withdrawal syndrome. Because the benzodiazepines are considerably safer, the barbiturates are seldom used today for the routine management of anxiety or insomnia.

Psychiatrists most often prescribed benzodiazepines for their anxiolytic effects, which occur at relatively low doses, or their hypnotic effects. As anxiolytics, benzodiazepines are often classified as high-potency medications, such as clonazepam and alprazolam, and low-potency drugs, such as chloradiazepoxide, diazepam, and most other oral preparations.

The potency of a benzodiazepine should not be confused with either its distribution or elimination half-life (Shader and Greenblatt, 1995). Potency refers to the dose necessary to cause a particular effect; half-life is a measure of the time needed for metabolism and elimination. The distribution half-life refers to the time required for distribution into lipid-rich tissues, such as the brain, and the elimination half-life is the time necessary for metabolism. It should be noted that many benzodiazepines yield clinically active metabolites. In general, the high-potency medications have relatively short distribution and elimination half-lives, although there are low-potency benzodiazepines that possess short half-lives as well. The potency of the medication has implications for clinical utility; there are more extensive data on the use of high-potency medications in the treatment of panic disorder. The half-life has implications with regard to tolerance, abuse, and withdrawal, because agents with more rapid distribution and elimination tend to be more abused (Shader and Greenblatt, 1995; Woods et al., 1992).

A number of randomized, controlled clinical trials have demonstrated the efficacy of low-potency benzodiazepines in the treatment of generalized anxiety disorder (Shader and Greenblatt, 1995). This literature is somewhat difficult to interpret, however, because most of these studies were conducted before the publication of the DSM-IV criteria for this condition. Because the definition of generalized anxiety disorder has undergone significant change, the results of older clinical studies may not provide a clear indication for this condition, at least as it is currently conceptualized. Nevertheless, benzodiazepines appear effective in this condition, regardless of the definition applied to the disorder (Shader and Greenblatt, 1995). For panic, the most complete data are for the two high-potency drugs, clonazepam and alprazolam (Ballenger et al., 1988; Rickels et al., 1988). Three controlled clinical studies examined the use of high-potency benzodiazepines in social phobia. One study found clear superiority of clonazepam over placebo; the others reported either equivocal results or contained methodological flaws that preclude firm conclusions (Liebowitz and Marshall, 1995). One controlled clinical study examined the efficacy of alprazolam in PTSD, finding no specific benefit for this condition (Marshall et al., 1996).

Gamma-aminobutyric acid (GABA) is an important inhibitory neurotransmitter in brain. There are at least two classes of GABA receptors, the GABA-A and GABA-B sites, but the benzodiazepines appear to act only on the former. The GABA-A receptors are a macromolecular complex that includes a binding site for benzodiazepine and a ligand-gated chloride ion channel. The GABA-induced entry of chloride ions into the neuron causes hyperpolarization, increasing the threshold for cell excitation (Enna and Möhler, 1987). Many substances, including the barbiturates, alcohol, and benzodiazepines, exert their effects enhancing GABA-A receptor activity (Shader and Greenblatt, 1995). Benzodiazepines and other medications acting on the GABA-A complex exert their effects at different sites on this receptor. As a result, combining substances such as alcohol and benzodiazepines can produce additive effects, at least, with potentially lethal consequences. In contrast with the tricyclic antidepressants and SSRIs, the beneficial therapeutic effects of benzodiazepines are immediately apparent after a single dose. Therefore, the interaction of the benzodiazepines with the GABA-A receptor is thought to be intimately related to their efficacy. Because benzodiazepine binding sites are located throughout the brain, the neural pathways that mediate anxiolysis are unknown. Recent studies suggest that limbic structures, including the septo-hippocampal complex, or the amygdala and associated structures, are important for mediating conditioned fear (LeDoux, 1996).

In contrast with the tricyclic antidepressants and MAOIs, the benzodiazepines have little effect on the cardiovascular system, making them excellent therapies for a host of medical disorders with concomitant anxiety. Although benzodiazepines cause respiratory depression at moderate doses, this effect is less dramatic than with other sedative/hypnotic agents. The most common side effects of the benzodiazepines relate to their central nervous system depressant properties. These include fatigue, drowsiness, and difficulty concentrating, particularly with higher doses. Benzodiazepines also impair cognitive abilities, including memory and learning, and cause

ataxia (Schweizer et al., 1995). Although benzodiazepine use has been associated with exacerbation of major depressive disorder, the high-potency members of this group have been shown to improve depressive symptoms. Particularly in children and individuals with organic brain syndromes, benzodiazepines are liable to produce disinhibition, characterized by rage, agitation, and increased impulsivity. Perhaps the major clinical concern is the risk of physical dependence and withdrawal (Woods et al., 1992). Thus, as with all central nervous system depressants, there is a potential for abuse with the benzodiazepines.

Benzodiazepines should be given with extreme caution, if at all, to individuals with a history of substance abuse (Woods et al., 1992). An underlying cognitive deficit or organic brain disease is also a relative contraindication, because these drugs can produce behavioral disinhibition and exacerbate cognitive deficits in such patients (Schweizer et al., 1995). As many benzodiazepines yield active metabolites that accumulate in patients with compromised liver function, care should be exercised with the elderly, even if there is no evidence of cognitive decline. Similar caveats apply to individuals with lung disease given the respiratory depressant effects of these medications. Extreme caution should be employed in combining benzodiazepines with other central nervous system depressants, such as alcohol or barbiturates, because this could lead to fatal respiratory depression, even with low doses of each agent (Schweizer et al., 1995; Woods et al., 1992).

Compared with the tricyclic antidepressants and the MAOIs, the benzodiazepines are relatively safe in overdose when taken alone, although they can be lethal when ingested with other central nervous system depressants.

Other Medications

Although the medications described in the foregoing are the main treatments for anxiety disorders, others are occasionally used to treat these conditions.

β-Adrenergic receptor blockers. Although β-adrenergic receptor blockers have been used to treat a number of psychiatric disorders, they are not approved for any of these conditions. These medications appear to have little efficacy in either panic disorder or generalized anxiety disorder. There has been interest in their use for PTSD, but there are no definitive data suggesting they are of clinical benefit in this condition. Perhaps the only established role for β-adrenergic receptor blockers is in treating performance anxiety, a specific form of social phobia. The main advantage of these drugs in this situation, relative to the benzodiazepines, is their minimal effect on cognitive function. For performance anxiety, β-adrenergic receptor blockers are used as a one-time or as-needed medication. With propranolol, the most frequently used medication, a single 10- to 40-mg dose within 1 h of performance is thought to be beneficial. It should be noted, however, that these drugs are of no benefit in the generalized form of social phobia.

α₂-Adrenergic receptor agonists. One model of panic and related anxiety states posits locus ceruleus hyperactivity as an important component of the disorder. Because α₂-adrenergic receptor agonists, such as clonidine, increase the inhibitory tone on the locus caeruleus, they should be of benefit in treating these conditions. This hypothesis was supported by studies on narcotic withdrawal, a condition associated with anxiety and locus ceruleus hyperactivity, where it was found that clonidine is an effective adjuvant treatment. Controlled clinical trials also suggest clonidine may provide some modest benefits in panic disorder, although its side effects limit its utility.

Anticonvulsants. There is a growing interest in the use of anticonvulsants for various psychiatric conditions. Much research in this area centers on the value of carbamazepine and valproic acid in the treatment of bipolar disorder. The use of anticonvulsant therapy for bipolar illness was stimulated by an animal model of epilepsy associated with a neurobiological phenomenon found in bipolar disorder. Preliminary data suggest a role for valproic acid in panic disorder, although more definitive data from randomized clinical trials are needed (Keck et al., 1993). There are also reports of a beneficial effect of valproic acid in posttraumatic stress disorder. At present, however, valproic acid should be considered a third-line agent in the treatment of anxiety disorders. Its use might be consistent in refractory patients with suggestive features of bipolar disorder.

Non-SSRI/tricyclic serotonergic/noradrenergic compounds. Trazodone is a novel antidepressant that activates the serotonin system, possibly through its metabolite *m*-chlorophenylpiperazine. Although trazodone is not a first-line treatment for most anxiety disorders, one randomized trial in generalized anxiety disorder suggested it may have a role in the treatment of this condition (Rickels et al., 1993). Trazodone is without marked effects on cardiac conduction, but can cause orthostatic hypotension. Priapism is a rare, but notable, side effect.

A number of other agents have been developed, or are in the late stages of clinical testing, that share properties with older medications used to treat anxiety disorders (Shader and Greenblatt, 1995). Included is venlafaxine, a mixed serotonin/noradrenaline reuptake inhibitor, which may be beneficial in the treatment of panic disorder, although published data are lacking. Nefazadone, which is structurally related to trazodone, also yields m-chlorophenylpiperazine as a metabolite and therefore may prove beneficial in treating some anxiety disorders. Preliminary data for ritanserin, a potent 5HT2 receptor antagonist, do not suggest marked efficacy in anxiety disorders. Other serotonergic medications with possible beneficial effects in treating anxiety include odansetron, a 5HT3 receptor antagonist, with preliminary data suggesting it may be efficacious in the treatment of generalized anxiety disorder.

Experimental treatments. Basic research on panic disorder has led to novel treatments for this and other anxiety disorders. Based on the hypothesized role of calcium-dependent second messenger pathways in mental illnesses, Benjamin et al. (1995) have administered inositol in an attempt to treat panic disorder, obsessive-compulsive disorder, and major depression. Although there are positive data from one small-scale, controlled clinical trial in panic disorder, this therapy should be considered experimental. Similarly, based partly on the relationship between hyperventilation and brain blood flow in panic disorder patients, trials with calcium channel blockers have been undertaken and have demonstrated some positive effects (Johnson and Lydiard, 1995). Moreover, based on the finding that an infusion of cholecystokinin (CCK) evokes panic attacks in susceptible individuals, CCK receptor antagonists are being developed as potential antipanic or anxiolytic agents (Coplan and Klein, 1996).

CLINICAL PHARMACOLOGY

Described in this section are clinical issues to consider when treating patients with anxiety disorders. Flow charts are provided to facilitate the selection of medications. In addition, dosing regimens for each medication are reviewed (Table 3-7), suggestions made for maximizing the therapeutic benefit, and steps outlined for treating refractory patients. Emphasis is placed on the treatment of patients with acute anxiety. Because most anxiety disorders are chronic or recurrent, however, many patients require continuous care (Rapee and Barlow, 1991). Accordingly, issues relating to the long-term management of anxiety disorders are outlined, with interested readers referred elsewhere for a more comprehensive treatment of this topic (Schweizer et al., 1995).

The first step in providing appropriate care for a patient suffering from anxiety is to conduct a com-

Table 3-7

Selected Medications and Available Dosages (in Capsule or Tablet Form)

Drug	Trade name	Dosage
Benzodiazepines		
Alprazolam	Xanax	0.25, 0.5, 1.0, 2.0 mg
Chlordiazepoxide	Librium	5, 10, 25 mg
Clonazepam	Klonopin	0.5, 1.0, 2.0 mg
Clorazepate	Tranxene	3.75, 7.5, 15 mg
Diazepam	Valium	2, 5, 10 mg
Flurazepam	Dalmane	15, 30 mg
Halazepam	Paxipam	20, 40 mg
Lorazepam	Ativan	0.5, 1.0, 2.0 mg
Oxazepam	Serax	15 mg
Serotonin Reuptake Inhibitors		
Fluoxetine	Prozac	20 mg, 10 mg/5 mL solution
Fluvoxamine	Luvox	25, 50, 100 mg
Paroxetine	Paxil	10, 20, 30, 40 mg
Sertraline	Zoloft	50, 100 mg
Tricyclic Antidepressants		
Desipramine	Norpramine	10, 25, 50, 75, 100, 150 mg
Amitriptyline	Elavil	10, 25, 50, 75, 100, 150 mg
Clomipramine	Anafranil	25, 50, 75 mg
Imipramine	Tofranil	10, 25, 50, 75, 100, 125, 150 mg
Nortriptyline	Pamelor	10, 25, 50, 75 mg
Azapirones		
Buspirone	Buspar	5, 10, 15 mg
Monoamine Oxidase Inhibitors		
Phenelzine	Nardil	15 mg
Tranylcypromine	Parnate	10 mg

prehensive psychiatric and medical assessment. Rational pharmacotherapy can be provided only after the correct diagnosis is made, comorbid psychiatric conditions recognized, and a complete medical assessment performed.

Of paramount importance is the identification of comorbid disorders. For example, it is essential that depression be diagnosed and treated to successfully manage patients with anxiety and affective illness, a common combination. Similarly, anxiety disorders are often complicated by substance abuse, which can alter the course of treatment. Thus, although benzodiazepines might be an appropriate treatment for uncomplicated generalized anxiety disorder, they are ineffective in patients with comorbid generalized anxiety and major depressive disorders, and inappropriate in patients with comorbid generalized anxiety and substance abuse disorders.

Appropriate treatment also requires an understanding of underlying medical factors that may contribute to the presenting clinical picture or complicate treatment. All new patients should undergo a comprehensive physical examination that should attend to signs and symptoms of medical conditions that yield symptoms of anxiety disorders. A careful history of all prior and current medications must be elicited to aid in the choice of therapy. Any suspicion of substance abuse should prompt a toxicology screen. Although a neurological consultation is usually not necessary, any sign of neurological illness should prompt more extensive neurological testing.

Panic Disorder with and without Agoraphobia

After arriving at a diagnosis of panic disorder with or without agoraphobia, and excluding underlying medical illness, an SSRI is usually the drug of choice, although certain clinical features could modify this decision (Fig. 3-5).

In most patients with panic disorder, particularly those with comorbid major depression or a history of substance abuse, SSRIs should always be the initial therapy. The SSRIs must be prescribed at very low doses initially in patients with panic disorder (approximately 5 to 10 mg of fluoxetine, 25 mg of fluvoxamine, 25 mg of sertraline, or 10 mg of paroxetine). The patient must be fully informed of potential side effects, with particular attention to the activating nature of these medications. The sexual side effects of the drugs must also be discussed, as well as their potential for inducing mania. Careful attention must be given to any concurrent medications. The initial dose of the SSRI is usually taken in the morning because of the behavioral activation. Some patients, however, experience drowsiness, in which case the medications should be taken at night.

The dose of an SSRI should be increased gradually, typically once each week, while closely monitoring the patient for increases in anxiety or panic attack frequency as the dose is escalated. After the first few weeks of treatment the dose may be increased more quickly. In patients exhibiting increased anxiety after a dose escalation, consideration should be given to either a slower titration or a reduction in dose. Although blood levels of SSRIs are not clinically useful, it may be important to monitor those of other medications, particularly tricyclic antidepressants, that may be coadministered.

The anxiolytic effect of the SSRIs is usually not apparent before 1 week, and the full effect before many weeks or months of continuous therapy, depending on how quickly the patient tolerates the increase in dose. Effective doses in panic disorder are in the same range as those used for depression, with a low end of approximately 20 mg per day for fluoxetine and paroxetine, 50 mg per day for sertraline, and 150 mg per day for fluvoxamine. The dose of most SSRIs can be administered once daily.

Although there is little evidence of differential efficacy for the SSRIs, there are reasons to select one over another for particular patients. With those taking other medications, the choice should be based on the effect of the SSRI on cytochrome P450; care should be taken to avoid concomitant use of drugs that might be adversely affected. In addition, consideration should be given to the different half-lives of the SSRIs. Thus, for patients likely to exhibit poor compliance, SSRIs with a longer half-life, such as fluoxetine, might be preferable. Although patients sometimes experience withdrawal or rebound anxiety after missing a dose of an SSRI with a short half-life, this rarely occurs with longer-half-life agents. For patients who require additional medications, the shorter-half-life SSRIs may be a better choice. Thus, because of the longer half-life, the blood levels of fluoxetine remain elevated for many weeks after discontinuation of this drug. This complicates the use of other medications, particularly the MAOIs and tricyclic antidepressants, which are often administered to refractory patients.

Two clinical scenarios generally favor the use of high-potency benzodiazepines in panic disorder. First, benzodiazepines are a good choice for patients without comorbid substance abuse or major depression and who require immediate relief from paralyz-

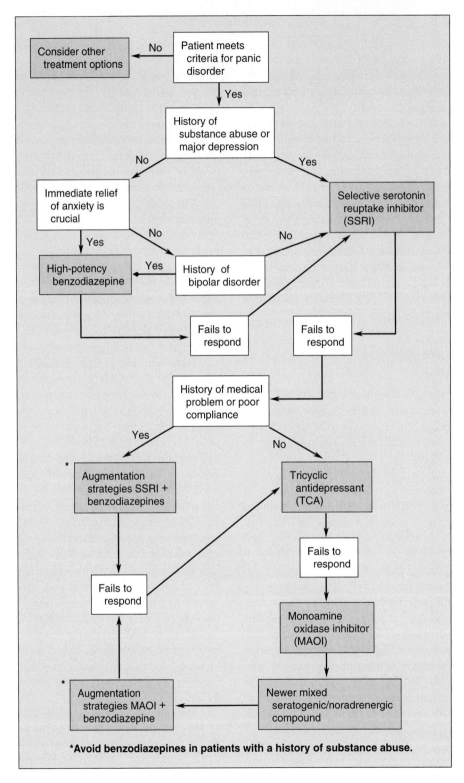

Figure 3–5. *Treating panic disorder.*

ing anxiety because the SSRIs usually require weeks to be effective. Even with those having no history of substance abuse, the risk of *physical dependence* on benzodiazepines must be carefully explained. Because of this risk, benzodiazepines are a second-line treatment for panic disorder. Usually, patients should be started on an SSRI, using a benzodiazepine only in the early stages of treatment for immediate relief of symptoms.

The benzodiazepines are also preferred in patients with a history of *mania*. In contrast with other treatments for panic disorder, the benzodiazepines do not induce mania. Indeed, these drugs may be of therapeutic benefit in this condition.

As with SSRIs, benzodiazepine therapy should begin with low doses. Usually clonazepam is preferred, in part because of the withdrawal anxiety associated with alprazolam. However, there is some anecdotal evidence that exacerbation of depression may be more frequent with clonazepam than with alprazolam. Many patients do well on a clonazepam dose of either 0.25 or 0.50 mg, taken two to three times per day, with an additional dose taken as needed. Doses of up to 2 mg per day are typical in patients with moderately severe panic disorder, although many require larger doses, with 4 mg needed sometimes before full remission is achieved. For alprazolam, a 0.25- or 0.50-mg dose is also used at the start of treatment, and is increased to the 2- to 6-mg range, with some patients requiring as much as 10 mg daily, the upper limit of recommended doses (Lydiard et al., 1992). Because of its short half-life, alprazolam may have to be administered four times a day, with an additional dose as needed.

In patients who respond to initial therapy, medication should be continued for at least 6 months. Some difficulty may be encountered with withdrawal symptoms in tapering the dose of benzodiazepines. In this case, a slower taper is recommended, over periods as long as 1 to 2 months. Alternatively, the implementation of adjunctive psychotherapeutic techniques in the cognitive-behavioral domain may facilitate the withdrawal of benzodiazepines (Barlow, 1988; Otto and Whittal, 1995). In patients who cannot tolerate even a slow taper, consideration should be given to substituting with a benzodiazepine with a longer half-life, or to adding an SSRI, before attempting a taper. In patients who do well, long-term treatment is an option. Many patients, however, prefer to discontinue their medications as soon as possible.

In those who do not respond to SSRIs, a benzodiazepine, a tricyclic antidepressant, or a newer mixed noradrenergic/serotonergic reuptake inhibitor is a good choice for therapy. Particularly with the tricyclic antidepressants, a baseline ECG should be obtained on patients with other medical problems, children, and the elderly to rule out underlying cardiac conduction defects. The patients should also be warned about anticholinergic side effects and orthostatic hypotension. Mixed reuptake inhibitors, such as venlafaxine, should be started at low doses, much like the SSRIs, as they may produce a transient increase in anxiety.

Dosing with a tricyclic antidepressant to treat anxiety can be similar to the regimens typically used for major depression. With panic disorder imipramine therapy begins at 10 mg, taken either once or twice each day, and is increased up to about 200 mg per day, or 1.5 to 3.0 mg/kg per day, with 2.25 mg/kg per day considered optimal. As with the SSRIs, the dose of a tricyclic antidepressant should be increased gradually in the beginning, usually in 10-mg increments once or twice each week. It has been suggested that total blood levels of imipramine and N-desmethylimipramine in the 110- to 140-ng/mL range are optimal (Mavissakalian and Perel, 1995).

Although there are fewer data in panic disorder on dosing regimens for tricyclic antidepressants other than imipramine, the optimal dose and blood levels are probably similar to those for treating depression. These blood levels are 125 ng/mL for desipramine, and between 50 and 150 ng/mL for nortriptyline, the only tricyclic antidepressant with an upper limit to its therapeutic dose range in major depression. For desipramine, typical starting doses are 25 mg per day, increasing to 150 to 200 mg per day, with some patients requiring as much as 300 mg per day. For nortriptyline, typical starting doses are either 10 or 25 mg per day, increasing to 100 to 150 mg per day. Although ECG monitoring is not indicated for most healthy adult patients, the ECG should be followed for children and the elderly during dose titration to ensure that there are no adverse effects on cardiac conduction. It is most prudent to check the ECG before each dose change in these groups.

There are a number of options for treating patients who do not respond to either first-line or second-line therapy. The MAOIs are an excellent choice for panic disorder, although their use is limited by their side effect profile (Buigues and Vallejo, 1988; Murphy et al., 1987). In particular, there must be an appropriate drug-free interval between the use of an SSRI and an MAOI because the combination can precipitate the serotonin syndrome. For the shorter-acting SSRIs, a 2-week minimum is required, with a considerably longer drug-free period, up to 2 months, for the longer-acting agents such as fluoxetine. Typically, MAOI therapy begins at a low dose (15 mg of phenelzine or 10 mg of tranylcypromine), which is increased either once or twice each week. There is some debate about the utility of following platelet MAO levels in major depression because there is evidence that therapeutic effects are evident only with a high degree of inhibition of this enzyme. There is rarely a need for this method in the treatment of anxiety. The MAOIs are usually taken two to three times a day in panic disorder, with typical doses of phenelzine in the 60- to 75-mg-per-day range (or approximately 1 mg/kg), with typical doses of tranlycypromine being 20 to 30 mg per day.

For patients in which MAOI treatment is not advisable, consideration can be given to combining two antipanic medications, a strategy referred to as augmentation. For example, an SSRI can be augmented with a benzodiazepine, and vice versa. The combination of a tricyclic antidepressant with a benzodiazepine is also common. The disadvantages of this approach are that the side effects of each medication may be potentiated when they are used together, and the database supporting the efficacy of this approach is not extensive. For most combinations there is not even a single randomized clinical trial to demonstrate efficacy relative to conventional monotherapy, or to demonstrate the combination of a single agent with psychotherapeutic techniques. Care must be exercised to avoid potentially disastrous drug combinations, such as an SSRI with an MAOI. In lieu of combination therapy, an attempt may be made

with third-line treatments, including calcium channel blockers or anticonvulsants, particularly in patients with bipolar features.

Although most patients are stabilized with one of the preceding regimens, panic disorder can be a chronic or recurrent condition, requiring long-term treatment. Most patients who respond favorably should receive a stable medication regimen for at least 6 months, although it may be continued for a longer period in those who are difficult to stabilize. For those who respond quickly to treatment, an attempt should be made to taper the medication within a year. For virtually all these drugs, a slow taper is advisable to avoid a withdrawal syndrome. Although there are only preliminary data, there is evidence suggesting that adjunctive psychotherapy might be helpful when attempting to taper medications in chronically treated patients (Schweizer et al., 1995).

Social Phobia

As with panic disorder, treatment of social phobia begins with a comprehensive evaluation, with attention to both psychiatric and general medical issues (Fig. 3-6). In particular, the degree of general social phobia must be determined, as the treatment of specific and generalized social phobia is quite different. Most patients suffering from social phobia come under the generalized type; subtypes tend to respond well to nonspecific treatments and are generally mild.

For specific social phobia uncomplicated by any other medical or psychiatric problems, either clonazepam or a β-adrenergic receptor blocker is recommended. Both should be used as needed, taken within an hour of exposure to a feared situation. The main disadvantage of the benzodiazepines, beyond their abuse liability, is their cognitive side effects. Treatment usually begins with very low doses, such as 0.25 mg of clonazepam, increasing to a maximum of about 0.50 to 1 mg. The main disadvantage of β-adrenergic receptor blockers is their effect on the cardiovascular system. Treatment usually begins with a 10- to 20-mg dose of propranolol, increasing to about 40 mg taken 1 h before a performance. For both medications, a test dose should be taken in a

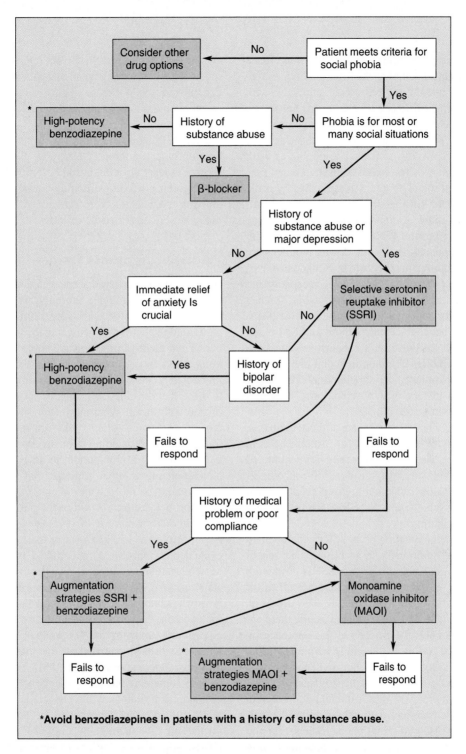

Figure 3–6. *Treating social phobia.*

nonperformance situation to ensure that side effects are no more incapacitating than the phobia.

For the generalized type of social phobia, as with panic disorder, the SSRIs are the drugs of choice. The steps outlined in the foregoing for initiating SSRI treatment for panic disorder, and adjusting the SSRI dose, should be followed for social phobia as well. In particular, low doses should be used initially, particularly when social phobia is complicated by panic attacks or panic disorder. For those who fail to respond to an SSRI, a high-potency benzodiazepine could be added to the SSRI, or a trial initiated with a benzodiazepine alone. Again, dosing regimens are the same as those in panic disorder. Benzodiazepines are most useful with either severe, incapacitating anxiety, where immediate relief is desirable, or when there is a history of bipolar illness. As in panic disorder, use of a benzodiazepine without an SSRI is not recommended for those with concurrent depressive symptoms, which is common in social phobia. Furthermore, benzodiazepines should be avoided in patients with a history of substance abuse, which is also common in social phobia.

For those who respond to one of these regimens, treatment should be continued for 6 months. As in panic disorder, some difficulties may be encountered when attempting to taper the dose of benzodiazepines. A very slow reduction in dose, supplemented with either psychotherapy or SSRIs, can prove valuable in this circumstance.

Beyond augmentation of an SSRI with a benzodiazepine, the addition of an azapirone may benefit patients who respond partially to SSRIs. Although this is a safe, easy combination, there are far fewer data on its efficacy than for MAOIs. The use of an azapirone alone is also an option, although there are few data to support the efficacy of this approach. In general, social phobia is thought to be unresponsive to tricyclic antidepressants. Hence, with patients who fail to respond to either SSRIs, benzodiazepines, or a combination thereof, an MAOI should be considered.

There are excellent data documenting the efficacy of the MAOIs in social phobia (Liebowitz and Marshall, 1995). With cooperative patients having no preexisting contraindications, these agents are an excellent choice. The reversible MAOIs are not yet available in the United States, but experience in Europe suggests they may be an effective treatment for generalized social phobia. The dosing regimen in social phobia is similar to that outlined in the foregoing for panic disorder.

As with panic disorder, social phobia tends to be a chronic condition. Thus, most patients should receive at least a 6-month trial before reducing dosage. Similar procedures should be followed in withdrawing medications from patients with social phobia as described for panic disorder.

Posttraumatic Stress Disorder

As with other anxiety disorders, appropriate treatment of PTSD requires a thorough psychiatric and medical evaluation because a few clinical issues are particularly salient in devising therapy for this condition. First, medical problems are common following traumatic events. This applies both to those occurring immediately, such as neurological compromise, and to those that develop later, such as substance abuse-related withdrawal syndromes. Moreover, it is common to encounter patients who are reexposed to a trauma. Thus, in deciding upon an appropriate treatment for PTSD it is important to assess the risk for reexperiencing trauma, consider that symptomatic patients may be faced with ongoing trauma, and reduce the risk factors for future trauma.

Although a number of pharmacological agents have been tested in PTSD, fewer than 10 have been evaluated in published randomized clinical trials. Moreover, there are no definitive data indicating the superiority of any given agent. A number of drugs, however, have been found to be moderately effective. Included in this group are fluoxetine, phenelzine, alprazolam, amitriptyline, imipramine, and desipramine. No firm statements can be made about the efficacy of these substances in PTSD. For fluoxetine, there is some evidence of greater benefit for victims of noncombat trauma, while phenelzine, perhaps the most studied agent, appears to be more effective for the intrusive than the hyperarousal symptoms of PTSD. Alprazolam appears to have little effect in PTSD beyond reducing anxiety, which is a prominent component of the disorder. As for the tricyclic antidepressants, the results have been mixed. In general, dosing regimens for these agents in the treatment of PTSD are the same as those used in panic disorder, although some patients with PTSD may tolerate more rapid increases in dose.

Because of conflicting data on efficacy, the choice of drug for treating PTSD should draw on the literature covering treatment of other anxiety disorders. Hence, based on their safety, wide therapeutic window, efficacy in a variety of comorbid conditions, and low abuse potential, SSRIs are a reasonable choice for treating PTSD. Benzodiazepines pose problems because of their abuse potential, since patients with PTSD often suffer from comorbid substance abuse. Benzodiazepines are probably most useful in the treatment of severe anxiety associated with PTSD that requires immediate intervention. The tricyclic antidepressants and MAOIs are often attempted after the SSRIs because of their side effects and toxicities. Other medications, including β-adrenergic receptor blockers, anticonvulsants, and α_2-adrenergic receptor agonists, have been used in open trials. There are data suggesting these medications reduce some symptoms, but the results must be viewed with caution until controlled studies are completed. As with social phobia, there are no data from controlled clinical trials on combination therapies for the treatment of PTSD. Many of the combinations used in social phobia or panic disorder, however, have been attempted with PTSD. These include combinations of benzodiazepines with SSRIs, or benzodiazepines with tricyclic antidepressants.

Generalized Anxiety Disorder

The diagnostic approach for establishing generalized anxiety disorder is similar to that taken with other anxiety disorders. With generalized anxiety disorder, however, particular attention must be paid to assessing a variety of other comorbid anxiety and depressive disorders that are frequently found in association with this condition. Symptoms of major depression are very common among patients with generalized anxiety disorder, as are symptoms of panic disorder and social phobia. The pharmacological approach to patients with generalized anxiety

disorder, with or without panic attacks, depressive symptoms, or social phobia, is somewhat different than for patients with isolated generalized anxiety disorder (Fig. 3-7). Thus, SSRIs are an excellent first choice for patients with generalized anxiety disorder who also exhibit signs of major depression, social phobia, or panic attacks.

Relative to other anxiety disorders, there is at least one unique feature in the pharmacological management of generalized anxiety disorder for patients presenting without comorbid anxiety or depression. Thus, there is evidence that azapirones, such as buspirone, are effective medications for either noncomorbid generalized anxiety disorder or generalized anxiety disorder complicated by alcohol or other types of substance abuse. For this reason azapirone should be considered seriously for patients who present with a history of substance abuse or major depressive disorder coupled with generalized anxiety disorder. Some suggest that the azapirones should be the drug of choice in treating naive patients, in light of preliminary evidence that prior benzodiazepine use may produce resistance to azapirones (Thompson, 1996). This opinion remains debatable. The main disadvantage of the azapirones as compared with the benzodiazepines is their delayed onset of action, with as much as a week of continuous therapy required for any relief, and the full effect requiring as long as a month of therapy. Buspirone is typically given in an initial 5-mg dose, taken twice a day, with 5-mg increases two to three times each week. The usual effective dose for buspirone is 30 to 40 mg per day, with some patients requiring as much as 60 mg, taken in two divided doses per day. Although the azapirones may have some efficacy in treating major depression, they are ineffective for panic attacks. Hence, although these medications are a viable option for patients with generalized anxiety disorder, major depression, and substance-use disorders, they should not be used if there is a question of concurrent panic disorder or panic attacks.

A range of benzodiazepines may be employed to treat generalized anxiety disorder (Thompson, 1996). This provides flexibility because there are cases in which one benzodiazepine might be favored over another. With elderly patients it is best to avoid

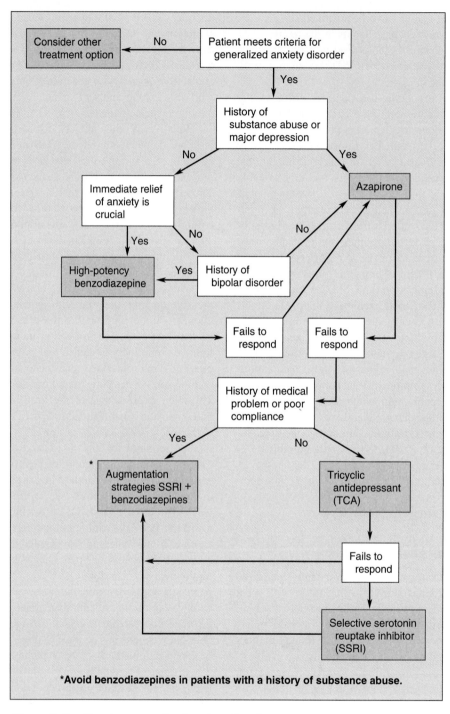

Figure 3-7.   *Treating generalized anxiety disorder.*

benzodiazepines with active metabolites that may accumulate over time, making lorazepam or alprazolam preferable in this circumstance. A typical starting dose for generalized anxiety disorder is 0.5 or 1 mg of lorazepam, or 0.25 mg of alprazolam, taken one to three times per day. For lorazepam, doses can be increased to as much as 6 mg per day, taken in either three or four divided doses. With alprazolam, the dose can be escalated to as much as 10 mg per day, although considerably lower doses are ususaly effective. Although benzodiazepines are frequently used in higher doses, side effects normally preclude administration of amounts beyond these thresholds. In general, doses of benzodiazepines tend to be lower for treating generalized anxiety than panic disorder.

Beyond the azapirones and benzodiazepines, the tricyclic antidepressants are the medications with the most established efficacy in generalized anxiety disorder, having been the subject of two positive randomized clinical trials. Although the side effect profile and delayed onset of action keep the tricyclic antidepressants from being drugs of choice, they are potentially effective in patients who are unresponsive to azapirone and for whom benzodiazepines are contraindicated. The doses of tricyclic antidepressants used for treating generalized anxiety disorder are similar to those used to treat major depression or panic disorder.

Trazodone is another alternative medication for generalized anxiety disorder, with one controlled clinical trial suggesting efficacy for the treatment of this condition (Rickels et al., 1993).

Although the majority of patients with generalized anxiety disorder respond to first- or second-line treatments, refractory patients are encountered. The most common reason for treatment failure relates to the high degree of comorbidity in patients with generalized anxiety disorder, with concurrent depression or anxiety disorder hindering the response to medications. Hence, for patients who fail to respond, there should be a careful reevaluation of the possibility of such comorbid conditions, the results of which may indicate appropriate therapy. For example, in a treatment-resistant patient with evidence of social fears or panic attacks, consideration should be given to prescribing an MAOI. Alternatively, in a patient

with signs of bipolar illness, an anticonvulsant might be appropriate.

Because generalized anxiety disorder tends to be a chronic condition requiring long-term therapy, discontinuation of benzodiazepines can be a problem in the management of this condition (Noyes et al., 1988). Patients usually tolerate a slow taper, where the dose of benzodiazepine is decreased in 25% increments on a weekly basis. The rate of the taper should be adjusted to ensure there is no return of anxiety or withdrawal-related symptoms.

OTHER TREATMENTS

Although the current text is focused on pharmacological approaches to the treatment of anxiety disorders, there has been extensive research on the use of non-pharmacological treatments for anxiety. A number of such treatments have been proposed, including hypnotherapy, exercise training, and psychotherapy (Barlow, 1988; Marks, 1988). Most clinical research in this area focuses on various types of psychotherapy, including supportive psychodynamic, and cognitive behavioral psychotherapies. It is difficult to draw firm conclusions on the efficacy of most psychotherapies. Because anxiety disorders typically exhibit an episodic course, randomized controlled trials are essential for evaluating the efficacy of any treatment in this area. There are many obstacles confronting such randomized controlled trials for psychotherapies, including difficulties in standardizing treatments and in developing suitable control treatments. Among the various psychotherapies used to treat anxiety disorders, the best data on efficacy are found for cognitive behavioral psychotherapy (Juster and Heimberg, 1995; Otto and Whittal, 1995; Shear et al., 1994).

Cognitive behavioral psychotherapy attempts to alleviate anxiety by addressing the cognitive correlates of specific symptoms for a particular patient. Thus, patients are first taught to recognize the abnormal cognitive correlates that accompany their anxiety symptoms; for example, those with panic disorder are taught that they have a tendency to overreact to normal bodily sensations (Barlow, 1988). Similarly, patients with social phobia are taught that they have a tendency to overreact to situations where they feel scrutinized (Juster and Heimberg, 1995). Patients then learn to use techniques such as controlled breathing or progressive muscle relaxation exercises to reduce anxiety. Finally, patients are instructed to expose themselves to anxiety-provoking situations, either by imaging scenarios that increase their anxiety or by actually placing themselves in the feared environment. The degree of challenge is increased in a graded fashion, beginning with mildly anxiety-provoking situations. Patients practice using the newly learned techniques to cope with the anxiety that results from such exposures. For example, patients with panic disorder complicated by agoraphobia might be encouraged to begin their exposure treatment by attending a movie or lecture in a large auditorium before progressing to more anxiety-provoking places such as a subway or elevator. Patients with social phobia might be encouraged to ask a stranger for directions or to order a meal at a restaurant before being challenged by presenting a lecture in front of a small group.

These techniques often reduce anxiety in many patients with social phobia, panic disorder, and obsessive-compulsive disorder (Marks, 1988). Although there are fewer data for other anxiety states, such as posttraumatic stress disorder or generalized anxiety disorder, it has been reported that symptoms of these disorders also respond to psychotherapies. The fact that symptoms improve must, however, be cautiously interpreted because it has not yet been definitively established that the improvement in anxiety symptoms results specifically from the psychotherapeutic intervention. For example, in a randomized controlled trial studying the treatment of panic disorder, Shear and colleagues (1994) compared the efficacy of cognitive behavioral treatments with a nonprescriptive listening therapy. The authors found that both treatments were effective in panic disorder, raising questions about which aspects of psychotherapy are essential for success. Thus, although cognitive behavioral therapy is of benefit in treating anxiety, the mechanisms responsible for improvements in the patient's condition remain incompletely understood.

For additional information on the drugs discussed in this chapter see chapters 10, 17, 18, and 19 in *Goodman & Gilman's The Pharmacological Basis of Therapeutics* (Ninth Edition), McGraw-Hill, New York, 1996.

REFERENCES

Abelson JL, Glitz D, Cameron OG, et al.: Blunted growth hormone response to clonidine in patients with generalized anxiety disorder. *Arch Gen Psych* 1991;48:157–162.

Azmitia EC, Whitaker-Azmitia PM: Anatomy, Cell Biology, and Plasticity of the Serotonergic System: Neuropsychopharmacological Implications for the Actions of Psychotropic Drugs, in Bloom FE, Kupfer DJ (eds): *Psychopharmacology: The Fourth Generation of Progress.* New York, Raven Press, 1995, pp 443–450.

Ballenger J, Burrows G, DuPont R, et al.: Alprazolam in panic disorder and agoraphobia: Results from a multicenter trial, I: Efficacy in short-term treatment. *Arch Gen Psych* 1988;45: 413–422.

Barker EL, Blakely RD: Norepinephrine and Serotonin Transporters: Molecular Targets of Antidepressant Drugs, in Bloom FE, Kupfer DJ (eds): *Psychopharmacology: The Fourth Generation of Progress.* New York, Raven Press, 1995, pp 321–334.

Barlow DH: *Anxiety and Its Disorders: The Nature and Treatment of Anxiety and Panic.* New York, Guilford Press, 1988.

Benjamin J, Levine J, Fux M, et al.: Double-blind placebo-controlled crossover trial of inositol treatment for panic disorder. *Amer J Psych* 1995;152:1084–1086.

Biederman J, Rosenbaum JF, Chaloff J, Kagan J: Behavioral Inhibition As a Risk Factor for Anxiety Disorders, in March J (ed): *Anxiety Disorders in Children and Adolescents.* New York, Guilford Press, 1995, pp 61–81.

Boyer W: Serotonin uptake inhibitors are superior to imipramine and alprazolam in alleviating panic attacks: A meta-analysis. *Intern Clin Psychopharm* 1995;10:45.

Bremner D, Randall P, Scott TM, et al.: MRI-based measurements of hippocampal volume in combat-related posttraumatic stress disorder. *Amer J Psych* 1995;152:973–981.

Bremner JD, Innis RB, Ng CK, et al.: Positron emission tomography measurement of cerebral metabolic correlates of yohimbine administration in combat-related posttraumatic stress disorder. *Arch Gen Psych* 1997;54:246–254.

Buigues J, Vallejo J: Therapeutic response to phenelzine in patients with panic disorder and agoraphobia with panic attacks. *J Clin Psych* 1987;48:55–59.

Carlsson A: Monamines of the Central Nervous System: A Historical Perspective, in Meltzer HY (ed): *Psychopharmacology: The Third Generation of Progress.* New York, Raven Press, 1987, pp 39–48.

Charney DS, Deutch AY, Krystal JH, et al.: Psychobiologic mechanisms of posttraumatic stress disorder. *Arch Gen Psych* 1993;50:294–305.

Ciraulo DA, Shader RI, Greenblatt DJ, Creelman W: *Drug Interactions in Psychiatry,* 2d ed. Baltimore, Williams and Wilkins, 1995.

Coplan JD, Klein DF: Pharmacological Probes in Panic Disorder, in Westenberg HGM, Den Boer, JA, Murphy DL (eds): *Advances in the Neurobiology of Anxiety Disorders.* New York, John Wiley and Sons, 1996, pp 173–196.

Coplan JD, Tamir H, Calaprice D, et al.: Elevation of plasma anti-idiotypic auto-antibodies to the 5-HT receptors in panic disorder. *Proc Amer Col Neuropsychopharm* 1996; 178.

Coplan JD, Wolk SJ, Klein DF: Anxiety and the Serotonin 1A Receptor, in Bloom FE, Kupfer DJ (eds): *Psychopharmacology: The Fourth Generation of Progress.* New York, Raven Press, 1995, pp 1301–1310.

Davidson JRT, Foa EB: Diagnostic issues in posttraumatic stress disorder: Considerations for the DSM-IV. *J Abnorm Psychol* 1991;1900:346.

Davidson JRT, Hughes DC, George LK, Blazer DG: Boundaries of social phobia: Exploring the threshold. *Arch Gen Psych* 1994;51:975–983.

Davidson RJ: Cerebral Asymmetry, Emotion and Affective Style, in Davidson RJ, Hugdahl K (ed): *Brain Asymmetry.* Cambridge, MA, MIT Press, 1995, pp 361–388.

Davis M: The role of the amygdala in fear and anxiety. *Ann Rev Neurosci* 1992;15:353–375.

Eaton WW, Dryman A, Weissman MM: Panic and Phobia, in Robins LN, Regier DA (eds): *Psychiatric Disorders in America: The Epidemiologic Catchment Area Study.* New York, The Free Press, 1991, pp 180–203.

Enna SJ, Möhler H: Gamma Aminobutyric Acid Receptors and Their Association with Benzodiazepine Recognition Sites, in Meltzer HY (ed): *Psychopharmacology: The Third Generation of Progress.* New York, Raven Press, 1987, pp 265–272.

Feighner JP: Buspirone in the long-term treatment of generalized anxiety disorder. *J Clin Psych* 1987;48:3–6.

Fyer AJ, Mannuzza S, Chapman TF, et al.: Specificity in familial aggregation of phobic disorders. *Arch Gen Psych* 1995;52:564–573.

Goddard AW, Charney DS: Toward an integrated neurobiology of panic disorder. *J Clin Psych* 1997;58:4–11.

Gorman JM, Papp LA, Coplan JD: Neuroanatomy and Neurotransmitter Function in Panic Disorder, in Roose SP, Glick RA (eds):

Anxiety as Symptom and Signal. Hillsdale, NJ, The Analytic Press, 1995, pp 39–56.

Grillon C, Morgan CA, Southwick SM, et al.: Baseline startle amplitude and prepulse inhibition in Vietnam veterans with posttraumatic stress disorder. *Psych Res* 1996;64:169–178.

Heninger GR: Indoleamines: The Role of Serotonin in Clinical Disorders, in Bloom FE, Kupfer DJ (eds): *Psycho-pharmacology: The Fourth Generation of Progress.* New York, Raven Press, 1995, pp 471–482.

Jacobs BL, Fornal CA: Serotonin and Behavior: A General Hypothesis, in Bloom FE, Kupfer DJ (eds): *Psycho-pharmacology: The Fourth Generation of Progress.* New York, Raven Press, 1995, pp 461–470.

Johnson MR, Lydiard RB: The neurobiology of anxiety disorders. *Psych Clin N Amer* 1995;18:681–725.

Juster HR, Heimberg RG: Social phobia: Longitudinal course and long-term outcome of cognitive-behavioral treatment. *Psych Clin N Amer* 1995;18:821–843.

Kagan J: *Galen's Prophecy.* New York, Basic Books, 1995.

Keck PE, McElroy SL, Tugrul KC, et al.: Antiepileptic drugs for the treatment of panic disorder. *Neuropsychopharmacology* 1993;27:150–153.

Kendler KS, Walters EE, Neale MC, et al.: The structure of the genetic and environmental risk factors for six major psychiatric disorders in women. *Arch Gen Psych* 1995;52:374–383.

Klein DF: False suffocation alarms, spontaneous panics, and related conditions: An integrative hypothesis. *Arch Gen Psych* 1993;50:306.

Klein E, Cnaani E, Harel T, et al.: Altered heart rate variability in panic disordered patients. *Biol Psych* 1995;37:18–24.

Klein RG: Anxiety Disorders, in Rutter M, Taylor E, Hersov L (eds): *Child and Adolescent Psychiatry: Modern Approaches,* 3d ed. London, Blackwell Scientific Publications, 1995, pp 351-374.

LeDoux J: *The Emotional Brain: The Mysterious Underpinnings of Emotional Life.* New York, Simon and Schuster, 1996.

Lesch KP, Bengel D, Heils A, et al.: Association of anxiety-related traits with a polymorphism in the serotonin transporter gene regulatory region. *Science* 1996;274:1527–1531.

Liebowitz MR, Marshall RD: Pharmacological Treatment of Social Phobia: Clinical Application, in Heimberg RG, Liebowitz MR, Hope DA, Schneier FR (eds): *Social Phobia: Diagnosis, Assessment, and Treatment.* New York, Guilford Press, 1995, pp 366–386.

Lucki I, Wieland S: 5-Hydroxytryptamine 1A receptors and behavioral responses. *Neuropsychopharmacology* 1990;31:481–493.

Lydiard RB, Lesser IM, Ballenger JC, et al.: Fixed dose study of alprazolam 2 mg, alprazolam 6 mg, and placebo in panic disorder. *J Clin Psychopharm* 1992;12:96–103.

Magee WJ, Eaton WW, Wittchen H, et al.: Agoraphobia, simple phobia, and social phobia in the National Comorbidity Survey. *Arch Gen Psych* 1996;53:159–168.

Marks IM: *Fears, Phobias, and Rituals: Panic, Anxiety, and Their Disorders.* Oxford University Press, 1988.

Marshall RD, Stein DJ, Liebowitz MR, Yehuda R: A pharmacotherapy algorithm in the treatment of posttraumatic stress disorder. *Psych Ann* 1996;26:217–226.

Mavissakalian MR, Perel JM: Imipramine treatment of panic disorder with agoraphobia: Dose ranging and plasma level-response relationships. *Amer J Psych* 1995;152:673–682.

Montgomery S, Henry J, McDonald G, et al.: Selective serotonin reuptake inhibitors: Meta-analysis of discontinuation rates. *Int Clin Psychopharm* 1994;9:47.

Morgan CA III, Grillon C, Soutwick SM, et al.: Fear-potentiated startle in posttraumatic stress disorder. *Biol Psych* 1995; 38:378–385.

Murphy DL, Aulakh CS, Garrick NA, Sunderland T: Monamine Oxidase Inhibitors as Antidepressants: Implications for the Mechanism of Action of Antidepressants and the Psychobiology of the Affective Disorders and Some Related Conditions, in Meltzer HY (ed): *Psychopharmacology: The Third Generation of Progress.* New York, Raven Press, 1987, pp 545–552.

Nemeroff CB, DeVane CL, Pollock BG: Newer antidepressants and the cytochrome P450 system. *Amer J Psych* 1996; 153:311–320.

Noyes R, Garvey M, Cook B, Perry P: Benzodiazepine withdrawal: A review of the evidence. *J Clin Psych* 1988;40:382–389.

Otto MW, Whittal ML: Cognitive-behaviour therapy and the longitudinal course of panic disorder. *Psych Clin N Amer* 1995;18:803–820.

Papp LA, Klein DF, Gorman JM: Carbon dioxide hypersensitivity, hyperventilation and panic disorder. *Amer J Psych* 1993; 150:1149–1157.

Pine DS, Cohen P, Gurley D, et al.: The relationship between anxiety and depression in adolescence and early-adulthood. *Arch Gen Psych* (in press).

Pollack MH, Smoller J W: The longitudinal course and outcome of panic disorder. *Psych Clin N Amer* 1995;18:785–801.

Preskorn SH: *Clinical Pharmacology of Selective Serotonin Re-Uptake Inhibitors.* Caddo, OK, Professional Communications, 1996.

Rapee RM, Barlow DH (eds): *Chronic Anxiety.* New York, Guilford Press, 1991.

Rickels K, Downing R, Schweizer E, Hassman H: Antidepressants for the treatment of generalized anxiety disorder: A placebo-controlled comparison of imipramine, trazodone and diazepam. *Arch Gen Psych* 1993;50:884–895.

Rickels K, Schweizer E, Csanalosi I, et al.: Long-term treatment of anxiety and risk of withdrawal. Prospective comparison of clorazepate and buspirone. *Arch Gen Psych* 1988;45:444–450.

Rosenbaum JF, Biederman J, Pollock RA, Hirshfeld DR: The etiology of social phobia. *J Clin Psych* 1994;55:10–16.

Sapolsky RM: Stress, glucocorticoids, and damage to the nervous system: The current state of confusion. *Stress* 1997;1:1–19.

Schweizer E, Rickels K, Uhlenhuth EH: Issues in the Long-term Treatment of Anxiety Disorders, in Bloom FE, Kupfer DJ (eds): *Psychopharmacology: The Fourth Generation of Progress.* New York, Raven Press, 1995, pp 1349–1359.

Schweizer E: Generalized anxiety disorder: Longitudinal course and pharmacologic treatment. *Psych Clin N Amer* 1995;18:843–856.

Shader RI, Greenblatt DJ: The Pharmacotherapy of Acute Anxiety: A Mini-update, in Bloom FE, Kupfer DJ (eds): *Psychopharmacology: The Fourth Generation of Progress.* New York, Raven Press, 1995, pp 1341–1348.

Shear MK, Pilkonis PA, Cloitre M, Leon AC: Cognitive behavioral treatment compared with nonprescriptive treatment in panic disorder. *Arch Gen Psych* 1994;51:395–401.

Shin LM, Kosslyn SM, McNally RJ, et al.: Visual imagery and perception in posttraumatic stress disorder. A positron emission tomographic investigation. *Arch Gen Psych* 1997;54:233–241.

Song F, Freemantle N, Sheldon T, et al.: Selective serotonin reuptake inhibitors: Meta analysis of efficacy and acceptability. *Brit Med J* 1993;306:683.

Tancer ME: Neurobiology of social phobia. *J Clin Psych* 1993;54:26–30.

Thase ME, Rush AJ: Treatment-Resistant Depression, in Bloom FE, Kupfer DJ (eds): *Psychopharmacology: The Fourth Generation of Progress.* New York, Raven Press, 1995, pp 1081–1098.

Thompson PM: Generalized anxiety disorder treatment algorithm. *Psych Ann* 1996;26:227–232.

Van den Bergh O, Kempynck PJ, Van De Woestigne KP, et al.: Respiratory learning and somatic complaints: A conditioning approach using CO_2-enriched air inhalation. *Behav Res Ther* 1995;33:517–527.

Van der Kolk BA, Dreyfuss D, Michaels M, et al.: Fluoxetine in posttraumatic stress disorder. *J Clin Psych* 1994;55:517–522.

Weissman MM: Panic and generalized anxiety: Are they separate disorders? *J Psych Res* 1990;24:157.

Woods JH, Katz JL, Winger G: Benzodiazepines: Use, abuse, and consequences. *Pharm Rev* 1992;44:155–186.

Yehuda R, Boisoneau D, Lowy MT, Giller EL: Dose-response changes in plasma cortisol and lymphocyte glucocorticoid receptors following dexamethasone administration in combat veterans with and without posttraumatic stress disorder. *Arch Gen Psych* 1995;52:583–593.

Yergani VK, Srinivasa K, Balon R, et al.: Lactate sensitivity and cardiac cholinergic function in panic disorder. *Amer J Psych* 1994;151:1226–1228.

AFFECTIVE DISORDERS

Jeffrey E. Kelsey and Charles B. Nemeroff

Affective disorders are a significant source of distress for patients and are commonly seen in a variety of patient care settings. Accurate recognition of these disorders, as well as differentiating one from another, is the cornerstone of successful treatment. A number of different treatments exist for the affective disorders. The clinician must be aware of the differences between approaches, indications, and contraindications for different treatment strategies and the expected course of treatment.

This chapter reviews the clinical presentation, differential diagnosis, and treatment options for the affective disorders. Guidelines and treatment algorithms for clinical decision making regarding initiating, maintaining, and switching treatments are discussed. The biochemical properties of different antidepressants and augmentation strategies are presented so as to make this information clinically useful. Selection of treatment for bipolar affective disorder based on subtype and past response is also reviewed. A discussion of the potential for drug–drug interactions is presented from the perspective of its utility in making clinical decisions.

To be diagnosed as having major depression, the patient must have had one or more episodes of depression, in contrast to the bipolar subtypes, which are characterized by episodes of mania or hypomania in addition to depression or dysthymia. A simplified schematic illustration of the differences between these disorders is shown in Fig. 4-1.

MAJOR DEPRESSION

Major depression is a common affective disorder that can lead to suicide, the ninth leading cause of death in the United States (Table 4-1). It is estimated that approximately 15% of individuals with severe depression commit suicide, including patients with major depression or depression with bipolar disorder. Depression is also an independent risk factor for increased morbidity following myocardial infarction or stroke. Quality of life for individuals with major depression, and even patients with prominent depressive symptoms who do not fulfill criteria for major depression, so-called subsyndromal depression, is markedly decreased compared to healthy individuals and patients with other types of chronic medical disabilities (Wells et al., 1989).

Affective disorders constitute a major source of distress, disability, and dysfunction in this country and remain a significant public health concern. The economic burden of major depression alone exceeds $43 billion per year with $12 billion as treatment costs, $23 billion in absenteeism and lost productivity, $8 billion as a result of early death by suicide, and countless losses secondary to decreased quality of life. The affective disorders consist of major depression, dysthymia, bipolar disorder (manic-depressive illness), cyclothymia, and mood disorders that are related to a medical condition. The relatively high prevalence rates of the affective disorders (Table 4-1) render them an issue of concern for all medical practitioners.

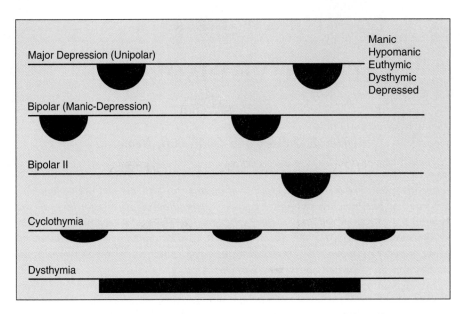

Figure 4–1. *A schematic representation of the differentiation of the affective disorders. Time, in months to years, is represented on the horizontal axis. Relative degrees of change in mood along the degrees of mania, hypomania, euthymia, dysthymia, and depression are shown for each disorder. Individual patients vary significantly with regard to rate of cycling and severity of each episode. Not shown is bipolar affective disorder, mixed episode, which is very common among hospitalized patients.*

The cardinal symptoms of major depression are depressed mood, anhedonia, changes in appetite or sleep, psychomotor agitation or retardation, fatigue or decreased energy, decreased concentration, or increased indecisiveness and recurring thoughts of death or suicide. To diagnose depression at least five or more of these symptoms must be present for 2 weeks or more (Table 4-2). Moreover, to diagnose the condition it is necessary to eliminate other causes for the symptoms such as bereavement, depressogenic medications, or a medical disorder known to be associated with depression. In contrast to what many believe, an individual need not be suicidal to have depression.

While over the last several years the lifetime prevalence for major depression has stabilized, the age of onset for the initial episode has markedly decreased. Depression is a chronic disorder for 50 to 55% of afflicted individuals and at the time of initial presentation there is no way to determine whether the patient will suffer a single episode or more. For those who experience a second episode, the odds for a third are 65 to 75% and are 85–95% for a fourth. The third episode, or second if it is particularly severe, is the time when many clinicians

Table 4-1
The Population Prevalence of Affective Disorders

Major depressive disorder	10–25% females
	5–12% males
Dysthymic disorder	6%
Bipolar affective disorder I	0.4–1.6%
Bipolar affective disorder II	0.5%
Cyclothymic disorder	0.4–1.0%

SOURCE American Psychiatric Association: *Diagnostic and Statistical Manual of Mental Disorders*, 4th ed (DSM-IV). Washington, DC: American Psychiatric Association, 1994.

Table 4-2

The Diagnostic Criteria for an Episode of Major Depression

Five (or more) of the following symptoms have been present during the same 2-week period and represent a change from previous functioning; at least one of the symptoms is either (1) depressed mood or (2) loss of interest or pleasure. (*Note.* Do not include symptoms that are clearly owing to a general medical condition, or mood-incongruent delusions or hallucinations.)

  Depressed mood most of the day, nearly every day, as indicated by either subjective report (e.g., feels sad or empty) or observation made by others (e.g., appears tearful). *Note:* In children and adolescents, can be irritable mood.

  Markedly diminished interest or pleasure in all, or almost all, activities most of the day, nearly every day (as indicated by either subjective account or observation made by others).

  Significant weight loss when not dieting or weight gain (e.g., a change of more than 5% of body weight in a month), or decrease or increase in appetite nearly every day. *Note:* In children, consider failure to make expected weight gains.

  Insomnia or hypersomnia nearly every day. Psychomotor agitation or retardation nearly every day (observable by others, not merely subjective feelings of restlessness or being slowed down).

Fatigue or loss of energy nearly every day.

Feelings of worthlessness or excessive or inappropriate guilt (which may be delusional) nearly every day (not merely self-reproach or guilt about being sick).

Diminished ability to think or concentrate, or indecisiveness, nearly every day (either by subjective account or as observed by others).

Recurrent thoughts of death (not just fear of dying), recurrent suicidal ideation without a specific plan, or a suicide attempt or a specific plan for committing suicide.

The symptoms do not meet criteria for a Mixed Episode.

The symptoms cause clinically significant distress or impairment in social, occupational, or other important areas of functioning.

The symptoms are not owing to the direct physiological effects of a substance (e.g., a drug of abuse, a medication) or a general medical condition (e.g., hypothyroidism).

The symptoms are not better accounted for by bereavement, i.e., after the loss of a loved one, the symptoms persist for longer than 2 months or are characterized by marked functional impairment, morbid preoccupation with worthlessness, suicidal ideation, psychotic symptoms, or psychomotor retardation.

SOURCE American Psychiatric Association: *Diagnostic and Statistical Manual of Mental Disorders,*
  4th ed (DSM-IV). Washington, DC: American Psychiatric Association, 1994.

consider the appropriateness of long-term maintenance therapy.

Large numbers of depressed individuals, especially in general medical practice, will not complain of depression per se, but rather are more likely to generate a complaint based on one of the signs or symptoms. The most common presenting complaints of a first episode of depression are shown in Fig. 4-2 (Baker et al., 1971). These highlight the importance of including depression in the differential diagnosis of a variety of somatic complaints. The onset of depression is often over days or weeks. Because of the insidious nature of the disorder, it is difficult to precisely define the time of onset, with friends, significant others, or family members often noticing problems before the patient.

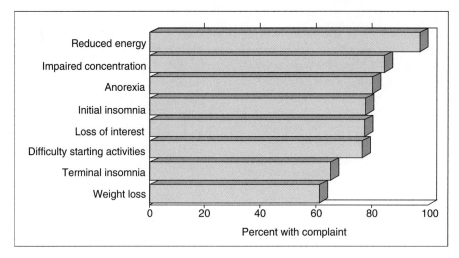

Figure 4–2.   *Symptoms of a first episode of major depression and the percentage of patients who complain of each symptom. Adapted with permission from Baker et al., 1971.*

Presenting a Diagnosis of Depression

There are a number of issues that should be considered when the initial diagnosis of depression is discussed with the patient (Table 4-3). Many who are not in a mental health treatment setting are not aware that they have depression when first diagnosed. They are certainly aware there is a difficulty or problem, but tend to present the symptoms rather than the disorder (see Fig. 4–2.). An understanding of the effect that affective disorders can have on the family or relationships is important in optimizing care. The patient and, if possible, his or her family or support

Table 4-3
Key Points in Discussing the Diagnosis of Major Depression with the Patient

Review signs and symptoms
Depression as a common illness
Medical disorder, not weakness of character
Neurovegetative symptoms predict a potentially good response to antidepressants
Review common side effects of treatment

See text for elaboration.

group should be told that depression is a medical illness, and not weakness of character. Many families are unaware of what has been causing the sometimes frightening changes they see in their loved one, and may be expecting that "more effort" on the part of the patient would produce a positive response. This perspective needs to be addressed with the patient and family. A discussion of likely side effects, but without frightening the patient, is called for, as are strategies to deal with them.

Differential Diagnosis

The differential diagnosis of major depression includes other mood disorders, such as dysthymia and, importantly, bipolar affective disorder (BPAD). Close to 10% of individuals with major depression will develop BPAD, which is not surprising in that the prevalence of BPAD is about 1/10 that of major depression. This is of particular concern in the young adult patient. Other diagnoses to be considered include schizoaffective disorder, schizophrenia, dementia, and drug abuse (both prescribed and illicit), or an underlying medical condition.

The presence of psychotic features with major depression indicates the need for combination therapy with an antidepressant and an antipsychotic or electroconvulsive therapy (ECT). Atypical features, such as increased appetite, often with a craving for carbohydrates or sweets, increased sleep, leaden paralysis of the limbs, anxiety, reversed diurnal mood variation, and heightened rejection sensitivity, point toward the use of medications that enhance serotonergic activity or with monoamine oxidase inhibitors (MAOIs). Melancholic features are characterized by either a loss of pleasure in most activities or a lack of reactivity to what was previously considered pleasurable. Individuals with melancholic features often cannot be "cheered up" even briefly. Other characteristics of major depression with melancholia include a depressed mood that is distinct, diurnal mood variability with depression worse in the morning, early morning awakening, psychomotor slowing or agitation, anorexia or weight loss, and feelings of excessive guilt. Depression with psychotic features may be either mood-congruent with delusions or hallucinations having a content consistent with depressive themes, or mood-incongruent with delusions not related to depressive themes. Catatonic features are characterized by psychomotor disturbances, negativism, or disruption of speech by echolalia or echopraxia. Diagnostic criteria for these subtypes are shown in Tables 4-4 through 4-6.

Dysthymic disorder is a chronically (2 years or longer) depressed mood that is present on more days than not, but that does not fulfill criteria for an episode of major depression.

Some individuals have "double depression," which consists of episodes of major depression superimposed on a baseline of dysthymia. This can pose a problem in determining the extent of the treatment response if the baseline mood is one of dysthymia rather than euthymia. Patients with dysthymic disorder appear chronically sad or "down." When asked the last time they felt well, these patients may have a difficult time recalling. Because such chronic symptoms may become almost part of the person's self-image, the individual with dysthymic disorder may not complain of mood symptoms to the same extent as someone with major depression. In adults, women are two to three times more likely than men to have dysthymic disorder, with the lifetime prevalence rate

Table 4-4

Diagnostic Criteria for Melancholic Features of Major Depressive Episode, in Major Depressive Disorder or in the Most Recent Mood Episode of Major Depressive Episode in Bipolar I Disorder or Bipolar II Disorder

Either of the following, occurring during the most severe period of the current episode:

Loss of pleasure in all, or almost all, activities

Lack of reactivity to usually pleasurable stimuli (does not feel much better, even temporarily, when something good happens)

Three (or more) of the following:

Distinct quality of depressed mood (i.e., the depressed mood is experienced as distinctly different from the kind of feeling experienced after the death of a loved one)

Depression regularly worse in the morning

Early morning awakening (at least 2 hours before the usual time of awakening)

Marked psychomotor retardation or agitation

Significant anorexia or weight loss

Excessive or inappropriate guilt

SOURCE American Psychiatric Association: *Diagnostic and Statistical Manual of Mental Disorders*, 4th ed (DSM-IV). Washington, DC: American Psychiatric Association, 1994.

being about 6%, with a 3% point prevalence. Onset is in childhood to early adulthood. The DSM-IV diagnostic criteria for dysthymic disorder are presented in Table 4-7.

Somatic Treatment of Depression

The use of antidepressants in the treatment of major depression has been documented in placebo-controlled trials involving tens of thousands of patients. The overall response rate for antidepressant medication is typically 55 to 65%. The last decade has witnessed major changes in the pharmacological ar-

Table 4-5

Diagnostic Criteria for Catatonic Features of Major Depressive Episode, Manic Episode or Mixed Episode in Major Depressive Disorder Bipolar I Disorder, or Bipolar II Disorder

The clinical picture is dominated by at least two of the following:

Motoric immobility as evidenced by catalepsy (including waxy flexibility) or stupor

Excessive motor activity (i.e., apparently purposeless and not influenced by external stimuli)

Extreme negativism (an apparently motiveless resistance to all instructions or maintenance of a rigid posture against attempts to be moved) or mutism

Peculiarities of voluntary movement as evidenced by posturing (voluntary assumption of inappropriate or biazarre postures), stereotyped movements, prominent mannerisms, or prominent grimacing

Echolalia or echopraxia

SOURCE American Psychiatric Association: *Diagnostic and Statistical Manual of Mental Disorders*, 4th ed (DSM-IV). Washington, DC: American Psychiatric Association, 1994.

Table 4-6

Diagnostic Criteria for Atypical Features*

Mood reactivity (i.e., mood brightens in response to actual or potential positive events)
Two (or more) of the following features:

Significant weight gain or increase in appetite

Hypersomnia

Leaden paralysis (i.e., heavy, leaden feelings in arms or legs)

Long-standing pattern of interpersonal rejection sensitivity (not limited to episodes of mood disturbance) that results in significant social or occupational impairment

Criteria are not met for With Melancholic Feature or With Catatonic Features during the same episode.

* Can be applied when these features predominate during the most recent 2 weeks of a Major Depressive Episode in Major Depressive Disorder or in Bipolar I Disorder or Bipolar II Disorder when the Major Depressive Episode is the most recent type of mood episode, or when these features predominate during the most recent 2 years of Dysthymic Disorder.

SOURCE American Psychiatric Association: *Diagnostic and Statistical Manual of Mental Disorders*, 4th ed (DSM-IV). Washington, DC: American Psychiatric Association, 1994.

mamentarium available for treating depression. In particular, there have been significant advances in the safety and tolerability of the drugs used to treat this condition.

During the early twentieth century "shock" therapy, such as insulin-induced hypoglycemia or injection of horse serum, was the treatment of choice for major depression. Electroconvulsive therapy (ECT) was introduced in the 1930s and represented a significant advance in the field. Indeed, even today ECT is a very safe and extremely effective treatment for major depression. It should be seriously considered among treatment options for severe depression, depression with psychotic features, mixed bipolar disorder, or depression that is immediately life-threatening owing to suicidality or a failure to adequately maintain nutrition and fluid balance as a result of the affective disorder.

While stimulants such as *d*-amphetamine and methylphenidate were employed as antidepressants in the 1940s and 1950s, their use was limited by the complications associated with such agents. Stimulants do, however, have a role as augmentation agents, or as single-line therapy in the medically ill or geriatric patient, although controlled studies on the efficacy of this therapy are lacking. The mid-1950s saw a major advance in the pharmacotherapy of major depression with the serendipitous observation that iproniazid, a monoamine oxidase inhibitor (MAOI) being used to treat tuberculosis, also had mood elevating properties. This was followed by the observation that imipramine (Tofranil), a drug studied as a potential alternative to chlorpromazine (Thorazine), an antipsychotic, is devoid of antipsychotic properties, but is effective as an antidepressant. Imipramine was introduced for this purpose in the United States in 1958. The next several years witnessed the introduction of a series of new tricyclic antidepressants (TCAs) that were more similar than different in their pharmacological and clinical properties. Secondary TCAs such as desipramine (Norpramin), a metabolite of imipramine, and nortriptyline (Pamelor), a metabolite of amitriptyline (Elavil), while somewhat safer in terms of side effects than the tertiary TCAs, still displayed a troubling side effect of their own. In 1982, trazodone (Desyrel) was approved and

Table 4-7

Diagnostic Criteria for Dysthymic Disorder

Depressed mood for most of the day, for more days than not, as indicated either by subjective account or by observation by others, for at least 2 years. (*Note:* In children and adolescents, mood can be irritable and duration must be at least 1 year.)	Depressive Disorder, In Partial Remission. *Note:* There may have been a previous Major Depressive Episode provided there was full remission (no significant signs or symptoms for 2 months) before development of the Dysthymic Disorder. In addition, after the initial 2 years (1 year in children or adolescents) of Dysthymic Disorder, there may be superimposed episodes of Major Depressive Disorder, in which case both diagnoses may be given when the criteria are met for a Major Depressive Episode.
Presence, while depressed, of two (or more) of the following:	
Poor appetite or overeating	There has never been a Manic Episode, a Mixed Episode, or a Hypomanic Episode, and criteria have never been met for Cyclothymic Disorder.
Insomnia or hypersomnia	
Low energy or fatigue	
Low self-esteem	
Poor concentration or difficulty making decisions	The disturbance does not occur exclusively during the course of a chronic Psychotic Disorder, such as Schizophrenia or Delusional Disorder.
Feelings of hopelessness	
During the 2-year period (1 for children or adolescents) of the disturbance, the person has never been without the symptoms in the criteria above for more than 2 months at a time.	The symptoms are not owing to the direct physiological effects of a substance (e.g., a drug of abuse, a medication) or a general medical condition (e.g., hypothyroidism).
No Major Depressive Episode has been present during the first 2 years of the disturbance (1 year for children and adolescents): i.e., the disturbance is not better accounted for by chronic Major Depressive Disorder, or Major	The symptoms cause clinically significant distress or impairment in social, occupational, or other important areas of functioning.

SOURCE American Psychiatric Association: *Diagnostic and Statistical Manual of Mental Disorders,* 4th ed (DSM-IV). Washington, DC: American Psychiatric Association, 1994.

widely prescribed until the serotonin selective reuptake inhibitors (SSRIs) appeared with the introduction of fluoxetine (Prozac) in 1988. Fluoxetine was the first SSRI to be approved by the Food and Drug Administration (FDA) with an indication for treating depression. Fluvoxamine (Luvox) had, however, been introduced in Switzerland 5 years earlier. The SSRIs revolutionized the treatment of major depression because they have markedly fewer side effects, a much improved safety profile, and an easier dose titration than the TCAs and MAOIs.

The SSRIs have become an integral part of American culture and have raised interesting questions about their use. These drugs have helped to make the public more aware of the biological basis of severe psychiatric disorders and, for many, decreased the stigma associated with receiving treatment. At the same time, some have questioned whether the prescribing

of antidepressants has become too commonplace and whether pharmacological interventions are inappropriately replacing other approaches for the treatment of mental disabilities.

Sertraline (Zoloft) was approved by the FDA 4 years after fluoxetine, with paroxetine (Paxil) following in 1993. Both of these agents have subsequently received FDA indications for panic disorder and obsessive-compulsive disorder (OCD) in addition to major depression. Fluvoxamine was introduced in the United States with the sole indication for treatment of OCD, although it is widely acknowledged to be effective as an antidepressant. At the time of this writing it is expected that citalopram, an SSRI available in 51 countries, will soon be approved for use in the United States.

Other so-called atypical antidepressants with mechanisms of action that differ from the SSRIs have also been recently approved . Bupropion (Wellbutrin), a unicyclic aminoketone, was first marketed in 1989. However, to date the pharmacological action underlying its therapeutic efficacy is not completely clear. Venlafaxine (Effexor) is a dual neurotransmitter (serotonin/norepinephrine) reuptake inhibitor and therefore is similar to the TCAs in its mechanism of action, but without the unfavorable side effect burden or cardiac toxicity associated with the TCAs. Nefazodone (Serzone) is chemically related to trazodone and is a weak dual reuptake inhibitor of norepinephrine and serotonin, and a potent $5HT_2$ receptor antagonist. The most recently approved antidepressant is mirtazepine (Remeron), a potent $5HT_2$ and $5HT_3$ receptor antagonist and an α_2-adrenergic receptor agonist. Reversible monoamine oxidase inhibitors, such as moclobemide, which do not require the dietary restrictions of the traditional irreversible MAOIs, are available in many countries but not in the United States.

Issues in the selection of an antidepressant. While major depression is a recurrent disorder for slightly over half of all individuals who suffer an initial episode, at the time of initial presentation the future course of the illness is not known.

Factors to consider in the selection of a medication that may be prescribed for a number of years include efficacy, side effects, potential adverse interactions with other medications, expense, and mechanism of action. The goal of treatment should be returning the patient to a state of complete euthymia, as opposed to simply improving symptoms somewhat, that is, a partial response. Although the initial antidepressant selected, or subsequent monotherapy, may not be sufficient to achieve this goal over the long term, every effort must be made to identify a single agent that will attain this objective.

Potential side effects are a source of concern for both the patient and physician alike. Many side effects of antidepressants are predictable based on knowledge of neurotransmitter receptor interactions. Common side effects and drug mechanisms of action responsible for these responses are presented in Table 4-8.

Occasionally, side effects can be exploited for therapeutic benefit. For example, a patient with major depression and co-morbid irritable bowel syndrome might benefit from a drug with more muscarinic cholinergic receptor antagonism, whereas an older patient with dementia would likely do worse on such a drug because the anticholinergic effects could impair cognitive functioning. Orthostatic hypotension is more problematic for the older female patient with osteoporosis since a fall might fracture a hip, than it would be for a younger patient. Weight gain, which can be significant with the TCAs, is a problem with long-term treatment. Although it may be tempting to utilize a very sedating antidepressant for a patient having difficulty sleeping, it is helpful to remember that the symptoms of depression are just that, symptoms of a disease state. Thus, the underlying syndrome should be treated, not individual symptoms. Thus, the patient with insomnia, although benefiting initially, might subsequently have difficulty awakening in the morning once the depression has improved.

Table 4-8
Predictable Side Effects of Receptor Antagonist Activity

	Receptor type	
Muscarinic cholinergic	*α_1-Adrenergic*	*H_1-Histaminergic*
Dry mouth	Orthostatic	Sedation
Constipation	hypotension	Weight gain
Memory effects		
Blurred vision		
Urinary hesitancy		
Tachycardia		

SOURCE From Schatzberg (1992).

A number of drug-drug interactions occur between antidepressants and other types of medications. These typically involve inhibition of a cytochrome P450 enzyme responsible for degrading other drugs and/or involve displacement of a second drug from protein binding sites. Drug-drug interactions are discussed in greater detail later.

Cost of treatment is a concern, not only for patients but also for physicians and the health care system. Generic TCAs are clearly much less expensive in terms of cost per pill than are the newer generation of antidepressants. Bear in mind that the expense of medication acquisition is typically 4 to 6% of the overall cost of treatment in the outpatient setting, and that newer drugs, because of greater compliance and safety, are generally less expensive when the overall cost of treatment is considered.

There are different stages of treatment for major depression. One approach (Kupfer, 1991) is to divide them into acute, continuation, and maintenance. Acute treatment is the initiation of therapy during a symptomatic phase of the illness and consists of diagnosis, initiation of drug therapy and dose titration, if necessary. This phase is typically measured in weeks. When the symptoms have markedly improved, or remission is achieved, the patient is now in the continuation phase of treatment that has a duration of 4 to 9 months. An episode of depression occurring during this phase is considered a relapse and is conceptualized by many to be a continuation of the same episode that was treated in the acute stage. At the end of the continuation phase, the patient is considered to have recovered from this particular episode of depression. Maintenance treatment is reserved for patients requiring ongoing therapy. The duration of maintenance therapy is indeterminate, with the goal to prevent another episode from occurring. Individuals with recurrent major depression, especially those who have experienced three or more episodes, or two or more particularly severe episodes, are candidates for maintenance treatment. Should another depressive episode occur during this stage it is considered a recurrence, or a new episode, rather than a relapse.

Antidepressant agents. Antidepressants are named on the basis of either their mechanism of action (e.g., MAOIs or SSRIs), or chemical structure (e.g., TCAs or heterocyclic antidepressants). Most antidepressants are believed to exert their therapeutic effect by interacting with noradrenergic, serotonergic, and/or dopaminergic systems. There are orders of magnitude differences in the effects of neurotransmitter uptake inhibitors on individual monoamines. The log ratio of *in vitro* serotonin:norepinephrine reuptake inhibition is shown in Fig. 4-3.

Tricyclic antidepressants. The efficacy of TCAs has been repeatedly demonstrated in placebo-controlled trials over the last three decades. Until the introduction of the newer generation antidepressants, TCAs were the treatment of choice and agents such as imipramine and amitriptyline continue to be a "gold standard" of treatment in many trials. Reuptake inhibition of norepinephrine into presynaptic nerve terminals in brain is the predominant activity thought to be responsible for the therapeutic activity of these drugs, although they also inhibit 5HT reuptake. Clomipramine (Anafranil) is an exception in that it is a more potent and selective serotonin reuptake inhibitor than the other TCAs. Clomipramine is approved for the treatment of OCD in the United States, and has been used as an antidepressant in Europe for many years. The secondary TCAs are more selective as inhibitors of norepinephrine uptake than are their tertiary parent compounds. Noradrenergic reuptake inhibition most likely mediates behavioral activation as well as the increase in blood pressure seen with some patients on TCAs.

The TCAs are the one class of antidepressants for which there is a relationship between serum levels and antidepressant efficacy. The therapeutic plasma level for imipramine is >200 ng/mL of imipramine + desipramine. In contrast, nortriptyline possesses a therapeutic window of between 50 and 150 ng/mL, with lower or higher concentrations associated with less efficacy.

The side effects of TCAs can be a limiting problem in some patients (see Table 4-8). Initial prescribing at a low dose, followed by gradual titration upward, minimizes some side effects. Sedation usually disappears with prolonged exposure to the drug, whereas orthostatic hypotension does not usually

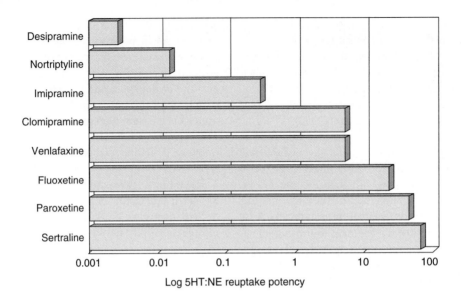

Figure 4–3. *The ratio of 5HT:NE reuptake inhibition selectivity* in vitro *expressed as the log transform. Longer bars are more serotonergic, and shorter bars more noradrenergic in selectivity. Adapted from Richelson (1994).*

diminish over time. Rapid discontinuation of TCAs should be avoided because of the likelihood of anti-cholinergic rebound characterized by insomnia and diarrhea. A more troublesome characteristic of TCAs, however, is their relatively low therapeutic index and untoward effects on the heart as compared to many newer antidepressants. An overdose consisting of a 7- to 10-day supply of many TCAs can be fatal. The toxicity of these drugs in overdose is owing to their fast sodium channel blockade, which confers Type 1a antiarrhythmic properties and cardiac toxicity.

Typical dosing ranges for TCAs and heterocyclic antidepressants are shown in Table 4-9. The usual starting doses range from 25 to 50 mg/day of amitriptyline, desipramine, or imipramine, or 10 to 25 mg of nortriptyline. Patients with comorbid panic disorder should be started at the lower end of the dosing scale because of their extreme sensitivity to side effects. The doses of the TCAs are gradually increased over 7 to 14 days to those on the lower

end of the dosing table (see Table 4-9). After 2 to 3 weeks, the dose may be increased further. Recommendations regarding baseline evaluation of patients for treatment with TCAs usually include an electrocardiogram (ECG) for children and those over 40. However, many clinicians perform a baseline ECG on all patients who are to be treated with TCAs.

There is considerable information about the appropriate dosing of TCAs for maintenance therapy and their efficacy in treating recurrent depression. In contrast to the practice of using one dose for acute treatment and then decreasing the dose for maintenance therapy, studies with TCAs have demonstrated that the dose effective in acute treatment is also the appropriate dose for maintenance or continuation treatment. The effectiveness of continuation TCA therapy in those with recurrent depression has also been demonstrated. In a population of patients with an average of 4.2 episodes of major depression, and 2 within the last 4 years, all were treated with therapeutic doses of imipramine. Those that responded were eligible for randomization to ongoing treatment. Those who continued to receive imipramine, at the original therapeutic dose, had an

Table 4-9

Typical Starting and Therapeutic Dosing Ranges of Tricyclic and Heterocyclic Antidepressants

Generic (Trade)	Starting dose (mg/day)	Usual therapeutic range (mg/day)
Amitriptyline (Elavil, Endep)	25–50	100–300
Amoxapine (Asendin)	50–100	150–400
Clomipamine (Anafranil)	25–50	100–250
Desipramine* (Norpramine)	25–50	100–300
Doxepin (Sinequan Adapin)	25–50	100–300
Imipramine* (Tofranil)	25–50	100–300
Maprotiline (Ludiomil)	25–50	100–225
Nortriptyline* (Aventyl Pamelor)	10–25	50–150
Protriptyline (Vivactil)	10	15–60
Trimipramine (Surmontil)	25–50	100–300
Bupropion (Wellbutrin)	100	300–450
Trazodone (Desyrel)	50	150–500

* Indicates the presence of therapeutic ranges or windows (nortriptyline).

approximately 80% chance of not having a recurrence during the first 3 years. In contrast, those randomized to placebo demonstrated the nature of recurrent depression in that approximately 90% experienced a relapse or recurrence in the first 3 years (Frank et al., 1990).

Although amoxapine (Asendin) and maprotiline (Ludiomil) are tetracyclic antidepressants, they resemble TCAs in many respects. Maprotiline is a norepinephrine reuptake inhibitor. Amoxapine is metabolized to loxapine, an antipsychotic, and therefore is effective as a single agent in the treatment of depression with psychotic features. Because amoxapine is in essence a fixed combination of both an antidepressant and antipsychotic, it is usually not a drug of choice since the doses of the antipsychotic metabolite cannot be individually titrated.

There is also a possibility of tardive dyskinesia with long-term amoxapine treatment.

Clomipramine is a TCA that is unique in its reuptake inhibition profile. In contrast to other TCAs, clomipramine is more selective for serotonin reuptake inhibition, being about 5 times more active in inhibiting serotonin than norepinephrine. Clomipramine is considered by some to be a "mixed reuptake inhibitor" which may confer some advantage in the treatment of the more severely depressed patient. However, this opinion is not a universally shared. The Danish University Antidepressant Group (DUAG) in two separate studies compared clomipramine to either paroxetine (Fig. 4-4) (Danish University Antidepressant Group, 1990) or citalopram (Danish University Antidepressant Group, 1986), an SSRI that is currently avail-

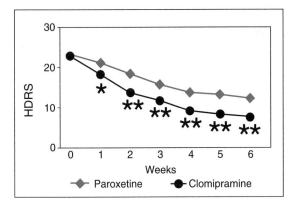

Figure 4–4. *Comparison of the efficacy of paroxetine, a selective serotonin reuptake inhibitor, to clomipramine, a mixed reuptake inhibitor, in inpatients using the HDRS as an outcome measure. The median doses of paroxetine and clomipramine were 30 and 150 mg/day, respectively. There was a significant difference in HDRS scores between the two groups, *p < 0.05, **p < 0.01. From the Danish University Antidepressant Group (1990).*

able only in Europe. These investigators found the mixed reuptake inhibitor clomipramine has greater efficacy than either of the SSRIs. In contrast to these results, a comparison of imipramine and paroxetine (Arminen et al., 1994) revealed no difference in clinical outcome, although the median dose of imipramine (150 mg/day) may have been unacceptably low. An inpatient trial comparing fluoxetine and imipramine revealed no difference in efficacy between the two drugs (Beasely et al., 1993).

The TCAs have some advantages over newer agents including demonstrable efficacy, over 35 years of clinical experience, lower per pill cost, and once daily dosing. Their major drawbacks relate to side effects and safety. Tricyclic antidepressants continue to have a role in the treatment of major depression, although not as first-line medications.

Monoamine oxidase inhibitors. The MAOIs available in the United States are irreversible, nonselective inhibitors of both MAO-A and MAO-B. In other countries, reversible and more selective agents, such as moclobemide, are available, and because of their selectivity for one form of this enzyme, they do not require the dietary restrictions necessary with the older MAOIs. The three MAOIs marketed in the United States are phenelzine (Nardil), tranylcypromine (Parnate), and isocarboxizide (Marplan). All

inhibit MAO-A, which is responsible for the metabolism of norepinephrine, serotonin, and epinephrine, and MAO-B, which metabolizes phenylethylamine, phenylethanolamine, tyramine, and benzylamine. Dopamine is a substrate for both the A and B isoforms, although in the central nervous system (CNS), dopamine is metabolized predominantly by MAO-B.

The therapeutic efficacy of MAOIs corresponds with their inhibition of platelet MAO activity. Typical therapeutic dosing of phenelzine is 45 to 90 mg/day, tranylcypromine 10 to 30 mg/day, and isocarboxizide 30 to 50 mg/day. Phenelzine is often initiated at a dose of 15 mg/day for 2 to 4 days and then increased to 30 mg/day with subsequent 15-mg increases per week. Tranylcypromine is typically started at 10 mg/day for 2 to 4 days and then increased to 20 mg with a further increase 7 days later. Isocarboxizide is usually initiated at 10 mg/day, with increases to 30 to 50 mg/day.

Side effects of MAOIs include orthostatic hypotension, sedation, insomnia, edema, tachycardia, palpitations, sexual dysfunction, and weight gain. Both weight gain and edema appear to be more problematic with the hydrazine MAOI phenelzine than with tranylcypromine. Orthostatic hypotension can be managed by ensuring sufficient hydration, by increasing dietary salt, the use of support stockings, administration of flurohydrocortisol (Florinef), or consumption of small amounts of caffeine.

The untoward interaction of MAOIs with tyramine-containing foods and over-the-counter cold medications prevents them from being drugs of choice in the treatment of depression. Strict adherence to a diet that avoids foods high in tyramine content is a requirement of treatment with MAOIs. Aged or fermented foods such as many cheeses, aged meats, pickled foods, yeast extracts, and many wines and beers are contraindicated, as are most over-the-counter cold remedies, dextromethorphan, meperidine (Demerol), and the epinephrine commonly used in local anesthetics. Although some patients may "cheat" on their diet and not suffer untoward effects, they should be vigorously reminded that tyramine content may vary widely even in a single wheel of cheese and that the potential consequences include the risk of stroke or myocardial infarction. A number of clinicians provide 10-mg doses of nifedipine or

100-mg doses of chlorpromazine for patients to use in the event they experience a severe headache, to be followed by immediate medical attention.

Monoamine oxidase inhibitors are effective antidepressants. They have demonstrated efficacy in major depression, depression with atypical features, depression in bipolar disorder, and in two anxiety disorders, social phobia and panic disorder.

Trazodone. Trazodone is a triazolopyridine compound that is chemically and mechanistically distinct from other antidepressants. In contrast to the TCAs, trazodone is essentially free of anticholinergic or antiarrhythmic properties, characteristics that made it an attractive choice for the treatment of depression. The doses typically required to treat depression are 400 to 600 mg/day, doses at which sedation, and orthostatic hypotension become problematic for many. Starting doses are 50 to 150 mg/day, with divided doses used at a daily dose of 400 to 600 mg.

A rare, but serious, side effect of trazodone is priapism, with the incidence of abnormal erectile function estimated at 1 in 6,000 males. Any abnormal erectile function, such as prolonged or inappropriate erections, should prompt rapid evaluation. Currently, trazodone is often used in combination with SSRIs when patients have persistent insomnia to take advantage of its sedating properties. Most commonly, doses of 25 to100 mg are prescribed to be taken 30 to 60 minutes before bedtime.

Bupropion. Bupropion is an aminoketone compound that is a weak inhibitor of dopamine and norepinephrine, but not serotonin, reuptake. Bupropion is usually taken three-times-a-day, or twice a day in a newly available sustained-release preparation. A major advantage of bupropion compared with other antidepressants, particularly the SSRIs, is its lack of effect on sexual function. Additionally, bupropion has no anticholinergic side effects, and weight gain is very rare. There is some evidence that bupropion is less likely to trigger a switch from depression to mania in patients with bipolar disorder.

The release of buproprion onto the U.S. market was delayed following the emergence of seizures in a population of bulimic patients taking this medication.

The seizure risk at ≤450 mg/day of immediate release bupropion is 0.33 to 0.44% compared to a rate of 0.1% for 100 mg/day of TCAs, or 0.6 to 0.9% for 200 mg/day of TCAs. Starting daily doses of immediate release bupropion are 75 to 100 mg, escalating to a final dose of 150 to 450 mg/day. Dosing of the immediate-release form should be scheduled at a maximum of 150 mg/dose, with at least 4 hours separating doses to minimize the risk of seizures. The sustained-release version, which is often given at 150 mg twice a day, has a reduced seizure risk presumably because of lower peak serum levels. Bupropion has recently received additional FDA approval as a smoking cessation aid and is marketed for this use under the trade name Zyban.

Serotonin Selective Reuptake Inhibitors

The SSRIs currently available in the United States are fluoxetine, sertraline, paroxetine, and fluvoxamine. It is likely that soon this list will include citalopram. All are effective in the treatment of major depression. There is evidence for the efficacy of one or another SSRI in the treatment of dysthymic disorder, bipolar depression, late luteal phase dysphoric disorder, panic disorder, posttraumatic stress disorder, obsessive-compulsive disorder, and social phobia. All members of this class are believed to exert their therapeutic effect by inhibiting the reuptake of serotonin into the presynaptic neuron. Although the SSRIs are more alike than different, and are thought to act by the same mechanism, there are differences in side effects, pharmacokinetics, and potential drug-drug interactions among members of this class. Although a patient may fail to respond to one SSRI, that does not rule out the possibility of responding to another. Nevertheless, many treatment guidelines recommend prescribing an antidepressant that is pharmacologically distinct from one used in a failed trial. The chemical structures of the SSRIs are shown in Fig. 4-5.

Fluoxetine. Fluoxetine is currently the most widely prescribed antidepressant in the world. Since its introduction in 1988, fluoxetine has markedly

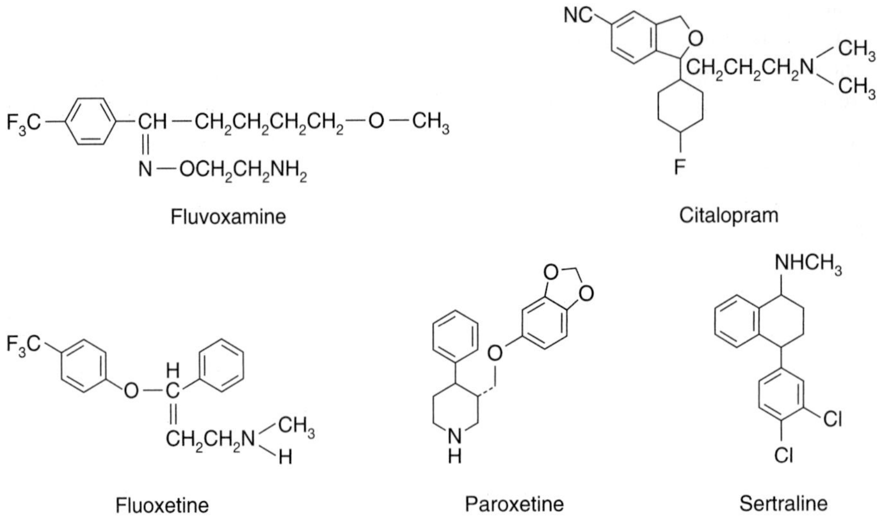

Figure 4–5. *Chemical structures of the SSRIs.*

changed the therapeutic management of depression. Currently, fluoxetine is approved for the treatment of major depression, obsessive-compulsive disorder, and bulimia, with controlled clinical trials having demonstrated its efficacy in a number of other affective and anxiety disorders as well, including late luteal phase dysphoric disorder (premenstrual syndrome) and panic disorder.

In contrast to TCAs, which display a rather steep dose-response curve in depression, fluoxetine is characterized by a flat curve at dosages ranging from 5 to 80 mg/day (Wernicke et al., 1987, 1988). One difficulty in interpreting dose-response data is the long elimination half-life of fluoxetine and norfluoxetine, its primary metabolite, which is also an inhibitor of serotonin reuptake. The elimination half-life of fluoxetine is 1 to 3 days with acute administration, and 4 to 6 days during chronic treatment. Norfluoxetine, however, has an elimination half-life of 4 to 16 days independent of the duration of administration.

Placebo-controlled trials of fluoxetine, and comparator trials with other antidepressants, have consistently demonstrated its efficacy in thousands of depressed patients.

Fluoxetine is free of any significant cardiovascular side effects, a safety profile that represents an important advance over the TCAs. Fluoxetine has no clinically significant affinity for muscarinic cholinergic, H_1-histamine, α_1-adrenergic, or $5HT_1$ or $5HT_2$ seroton receptors, which helps explain its superior side effect profile in comparison to the TCAs. The most prevalent central nervous system side effects of fluoxetine are headache, nervousness, insomnia, drowsiness, anxiety, and tremor. Akathisia, described as a sense of restlessness, and dystonia, a side effect often seen with antipsychotics, is rarely experienced. Common gastrointestinal system side effects include nausea, diarrhea, dry mouth, anorexia, and dyspepsia. In clinical practice, nausea is often less than reported in the premarketing trials and can be minimized by ingestion of the drug during or after meals, and by reducing the initial dose in sensitive individuals. Nausea, when present, tends to be transient.

The incidence of sexual dysfunction in the premarketing trials of fluoxetine was reported to be much lower than that subsequently observed in clinical practice, possibly because patients were not specifically asked about sexual dysfunction during the early trials. Sexual dysfunction with the SSRIs include delayed orgasm or anorgasmia, as well as decreased libido. A number of strategies have been proposed to deal with this side effect, such as a decrease in dosage, drug holidays for shorter half-life SSRIs, or co-administration of buspirone, yohimbine, amantidine, cyproheptadine, or bupropion.

Dosing. The recommended starting dose of fluoxetine is 20 mg per day, although individuals who are sensitive to side effects may be started on a lower initial dose. Many patients with depression or dysthymia are returned to complete euthymia with a dose of 20 mg per day, although others may require a higher dose. Adjustment of the dose of fluoxetine should be accomplished very gradually because the drug may require 40 to 80 days to attain a new steady state. For those individuals who experience a "fading" of the antidepressant effect during SSRI treatment either a dose increase or decrease is frequently helpful. The dose of fluoxetine is often higher for the treatment of OCD than major depression.

Sertraline. Sertraline was the second SSRI to receive approval in the United States for the treatment of depression. It has also been approved for the treatment of OCD and panic disorder. Sertraline has no therapeutically active metabolites.

The efficacy of sertraline in major depression has been demonstrated in a number of clinical trials. It has been shown effective in the prevention of recurrent episodes of depression in a small study in comparison to fluvoxamine. A larger scale study involving the treatment of dysthymia found an average daily dose of sertraline of 139.6 ± 58.5 mg per day was of equal efficacy to an imipramine dose of 198.8 ± 91.2 mg per day (Thase et al., 1996).

The most common side effects associated with sertraline are gastrointestinal complaints such as nausea, diarrhea/loose stools, and dyspepsia. Other common side effects include tremor, dizziness, insomnia, somnolence, increased sweating, dry mouth, and sexual dysfunction.

The recommended starting dose of sertraline is 50 mg per day, although many patients benefit from a lower initial dose such as 25 mg per day for 4 days, followed by 50 mg per day for 5 days, and then 100 mg/day. The average dose of sertraline in flexible dosing blinded controlled trials for depression was over 100 mg per day, with many patients requiring a dose between 100 to 200 mg per day.

Paroxetine. Paroxetine was approved in the United States in 1993, making it the third SSRI marketed in this country. Since then paroxetine has also been approved for the treatment of OCD and panic disorder. Placebo-controlled, double-blind trials of paroxetine in major depression have clearly demonstrated its efficacy in treating this condition. In dose-finding studies, paroxetine exhibited a flat dose-response curve between 20 and 50 mg per day for the treatment of major depression. However, the individual patient may benefit from a dose increase. Outpatient comparison trials of paroxetine with imipramine, clomipramine, nefazodone, and fluoxetine demonstrated comparable efficacy. Two inpatient comparator trials, one with imipramine (Arminen et al., 1994) and the other with amitriptyline (Stuppaeck et al., 1994), showed paroxetine to possess antidepressant efficacy equal to these TCAs. In contrast, one inpatient study with clomipramine and paroxetine found greater efficacy for the former (Danish University Antidepressant Group, 1990). Throughout the comparator trials, paroxetine displayed fewer side effects than the TCAs. A 12-month study demonstrated sustained improvement with paroxetine that was comparable to imipramine, but the TCA group had twice the dropout rate because of intolerable side effects.

The most common side effects of paroxetine are nausea, dry mouth, headache, asthenia, constipation, dizziness, insomnia, diarrhea, and sexual dysfunction. Headache, it should be noted, is a very common side effect in the placebo-treated groups as well. As with the other SSRIs, nausea can be reduced by administering the drug during or after meals. Nausea is transient for most patients. The recommended starting dose for paroxetine is 20 mg per day. Those who are sensitive to side effects often benefit from a starting dose of 10 mg per day for 4 days, increasing to 20 mg per day. In controlled clinical trials, 20 mg/day was found to be the lowest effective dose. If higher doses are needed, the suggested interval is 1 week between increases.

Fluvoxamine. Fluvoxamine is approved in the United States for the treatment of OCD. Like the other SSRIs, fluvoxamine displays efficacy in the treatment of major depression, usually at doses of 100 to 250 mg/day.

Venlafaxine.   Venlafaxine inhibits both serotonin and norepinephrine reuptake. There is evidence to suggest that alterations in both NE and 5HT systems are involved in the pathophysiology of depression. By interacting with both of these systems, but without the side effects of TCAs, or the dietary and medication restrictions of the MAOIs, venlafaxine displays some unique properties in comparison with these other agents. In contrast to the SSRIs, but similar to the TCAs, venlafaxine shows a linear dose-response curve in the treatment of depression (Fig. 4-6).

Venlafaxine has been found to possess similar efficacy to imipramine and trazodone in outpatient trials. In an inpatient trial, venlafaxine (median dose of 200 mg per day) displayed a greater efficacy than fluoxetine (median dose 40 mg per day) after 4 and 6 weeks of therapy (Clerc et al., 1994). Venlafaxine has also been found to be of some benefit in treatment-resistant depression (Nierenberg et al., 1994).

In this study treatment-resistance was defined as a failure to respond to either: three different antidepressants plus augmentation or ECT plus two antidepressant trials plus augmentation. By week 12 of venlafaxine treatment, approximately 20% of these patients were considered either full responders (Hamilton depression scale <9) or partial responders (Hamilton depression scale reduced by ≥50).

The side effect profile of venlafaxine is similar to that of the SSRIs, with the most common being asthenia, sweating, nausea, constipation, anorexia, vomiting, somnolence, dry mouth, dizziness, nervousness, anxiety, tremor, and blurred vision as well as abnormal ejaculation/orgasm and impotence in men. Clinical experience suggests that sexual dysfunction also occurs in women taking this drug. Many of these side effects, especially nausea, can be minimized by starting at a lower dose than is recommended in the package insert. A number of patients do well with a starting dose of 18.75 mg (1/2 of a 37.5-mg pill) twice a day for 6 days before increasing to 37.5 mg twice a day. The effective dose range is 75 to 375 mg/day.

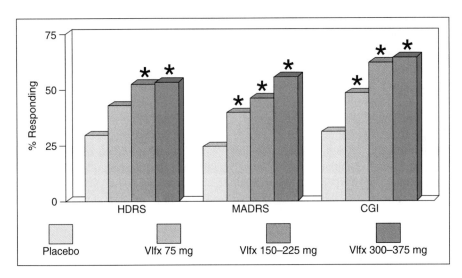

Figure 4–6.   *Venlafaxine dose-response curve. Percent of patients responding in this placebo-controlled trial of venlafaxine (Vlfx) at low dose, 75 mg/day; medium dose, 150 to 225 mg/day; or high dose, 300 to 375 mg/day. Outcome measures were the Hamilton Depression Rating Scale (HDRS), Montgomery Asburg Depression Rating Scale (MADRS), or the Clinical Global Impression (CGI). *p < 0.05 vs. placebo. Adapted from Schweizer et al. (1991).*

An extended-release preparation of venlafaxine (Effexor XR) is now available, and is packaged as 37.5-, 75-, and 150-mg capsules. The suggested starting dose is 37.5 mg/day for 1 week followed by an increase to 75 mg/day. The final dosing range appears to be similar to the immediate release preparation, although clinical trial data are available only with doses up to 225 mg/day. The side effect profile of the extended release is more favorable than the immediate release preparation.

Nefazodone. Nefazodone (Serzone) is an antidepressant chemically related to trazodone. It is thought to be a weak inhibitor of serotonin and norepinephrine uptake into the presynaptic nerve terminal and an antagonist at $5HT_2$ receptors. Nefazodone inhibits α_1-adrenergic receptors, causing orthostatic hypotension. Nefazodone does not appear to possess any clinically significant affinity for α_2- or β-adrenergic, muscarinic cholinergic, $5HT_{1A}$, dopaminergic, or GABAergic receptors. Nefazodone metabolism yields a number of biologically active compounds including hydroxynefazodone, which is pharmacologically similar to the parent compound, meta-chlorophenylpiperazine (mCPP), a serotonin agonist at $5HT_{1B}$ and $5HT_{1D}$ receptors, but an antagonist at $5HT_2$ and $5HT_3$ receptors, and a triazole-dione metabolite that is not well characterized. Steady-state levels of nefazodone are achieved in 4 to 5 days, with an accumulation of nefazodone and hydroxynefazodone two- to fourfold higher than predicted following a single dose. Administration of nefazodone with food delays absorption, causing a 20% decrease in peak serum concentrations.

Nefazodone is approved in the United States for the treatment of major depression. Placebo-controlled trials in patients with DSM III or DSM IIIR major depression have demonstrated the superiority of nefazodone over placebo. The typical effective dose for major depression is usually 400 to 600 mg/day, administered twice a day. In outpatient settings, an initial dose of 50 mg twice a day, with dose increases every 4 to 7 days, is an effective strategy.

The most commonly observed side effects with nefazodone in depressed patients are somnolence, dry mouth, nausea, dizziness, constipation, asthenia, lightheadedness, blurred vision, confusion, and abnormal vision.

Drug-drug interactions with nefazodone are seen with agents that are substrates for cytochrome P450 3A, an enzyme that is potently inhibited by nefazodone, and with any drug that binds extensively to plasma proteins. Because of these interactions the manufacturer warns against combining nefazodone with terfenadine (Seldane), astemizole (Hismanal), or cisapride (Propulsid). The combination of nefazodone and digoxin in young males increases the Cmax, Cmin, and AUC of digoxin 29, 27, and 15%, respectively. Caution should also be exercised when coadministering nefazodone with triazolam (Halcion) or alprazolam (Xanax) since it inhibits benzodiazepine metabolism. Monoamine oxidase inhibitors should not be combined with nefazodone, and a sufficient washout period should be allowed when switching to, or from, nefazodone and an MAOI. Nefazodone tablets are supplied in strengths of 100, 150, 200, and 250 mg.

Mirtazepine. Mirtazepine (Remeron) is a tetracyclic antidepressant with a piperazino-azepine structure. The therapeutic effect of mirtazepine is thought to be due to enhancement of central noradrenergic and serotonergic activity. *In vitro* studies suggest that mirtazepine is an α_2-adrenergic receptor antagonist. By inhibiting this site mirtazepine increases the release of norepinephrine and serotonin from nerve terminals. Mirtazepine is also an antagonist at $5HT_2$ and $5HT_3$, but not $5HT_{1A}$ or $5HT_{1B}$, receptors. Blockade of histamine (H_1) receptors, is thought to be responsible for the marked sedation observed with lower doses of this drug. Orthostatic hypotension, an occasional side effect, is most likely caused by moderate antagonism of peripheral a_1 adrenergic receptors.

Peak plasma levels of mirtazepine are achieved 2 to 4 hours after administration and are not affected by food. The half-life is 20 to 40 hours. Mirtazepine is demethylated and hydroxylated followed by glucuronide conjugation. It is a substrate at the 1A2 and 2D6 isoenzymes of the cytochrome P450 system for hydroxylation, whereas the 3A isoenzyme catalyzes the formation of the N-desmethyl and N-oxide metabolites. There is a linear relationship between plasma levels and dose over the range of 15 to 80 mg/day. The mean elimination half-life for mirtazepine is longer in females (37 hours) than males (26 hours), although the clinical significance of this is unknown.

Mirtazepine was approved for the treatment of major depression based on its efficacy shown in four placebo-controlled trials of adult outpatients with major depression. The mean effective dose in these trials was 21 to 32 mg/day. The most common side effects of mirtazepine are somnolence, increased appetite, weight gain, and dizziness. Increases in nonfasting cholesterol of $\geq 20\%$ above normal limits was observed in 15% of the patients receiving mirtazepine. Agranulocytosis was observed in 2/2,796 patients in premarketing trials, and a third developed neutropenia. Because MAOI should not be combined with mirtazepine, a sufficient washout period should be allowed when switching to, or from, mirtazepine and an MAOI. There are no data suggesting clinically significant drug-drug interactions with mirtazepine and the cytochrome P450 system, although this has not been fully characterized.

Mirtazepine is available in 15- and 30-mg scored tablets. The usual starting dose is 15 mg/day, with subsequent increases after 7 to 14 days. When somnolence is observed as a side effect at 7.5- or 15-mg/day doses, an increase to 30 to 45 mg/day will often reduce this. The dosage of mirtazepine should be lower in elderly patients and those with renal or hepatic disease.

Initiating Treatment

Accurate diagnosis of a major depressive episode, with due attention to other conditions that might present as depression, especially bipolar affective disorder, is the initial step in effective treatment. It is often helpful to establish a baseline measure of severity using rating scales such as the Beck Depression Inventory (Beck et al., 1961), Carroll Rating Scale for Depression (Carroll et al., 1981), or Zung Self-Rating Depression Scale (Zung, 1965), all of which are patient rated, or a clinician rating scale like the Hamilton Depression Rating Scale (Hamilton, 1960) or the Montgomery-Asberg Depression Rating Scale (Montgomery and Asberg, 1979). An accurate baseline assessment aids in quantifying the response to treatment, and assists in attaining full euthymia, the ultimate goal of treatment.

Drug treatment, either alone or in combination with psychotherapy, of major depression is an appropriate choice of therapy. The use of antidepressants must be considered when the intensity of depression is moderate to severe. Currently, the wide array of drugs, and their favorable side effect profiles, ease the initiation of treatment. Newer generation antidepressants are usually the best initial treatment, with MAOIs and TCAs reserved for patients who fail to respond adequately to the newer drugs.

The general approach to initiating treatment for major depression is to establish the diagnosis, rule out any underlying medical reasons for the depression, discuss the diagnosis and treatment options with the patient alone, or with the family or other support group, and then begin therapy. The assessment of suicidal ideation must be a part of the evaluation for any patient with an affective disorder and can often be addressed as follows: "Do things ever get so bad for you that you think about hurting yourself or taking your own life?" The frequency of follow-up visits depends on the severity of the depressive episode and the patient's response to treatment.

Factors that influence the initial choice of antidepressant include:

1. History of prior response in the patient or family history of response to a medication or class of medications. A patient who has been successfully treated in the past with a particular drug, or who has a family member that has, should be started on that medication. Depending on the number or severity of the episodes, consideration should be given to ongoing maintenance therapy.
2. Safety of the drug. Although the newer antidepressants are much safer in overdose than the TCAs or MAOIs, consideration must be given to potential drug-drug interactions or other medical conditions that may be important in selecting a particular antidepressant.
3. Side effect profile. Most newer antidepressant have a favorable side effect profile from a risk-

benefit perspective. Discussion with the patient about side effects and treatment strategies is helpful.

4. Compliance. All of the newer antidepressants need to be taken no more than twice a day, and the majority once a day. This, together with the more favorable side effect profile, significantly enhances compliance with respect to older medications.

5. Expense of medication. Although the cost of a prescription (often $60 to $90 per month, depending on dose), may seem expensive, treatment is always less expensive than no treatment or the poor compliance associated with less expensive, generic TCAs that have a less favorable side effect profile.

6. Availability and necessity of therapeutic drug monitoring. This applies only to a few of the older TCAs since therapeutic blood levels have yet to be established for the newer generation antidepressants.

7. Mechanism of action. The pharmacological effect of the antidepressant is important to consider, not only in selecting an initial drug treatment, but also in deciding on a course of action if the first antidepressant is not effective.

Many patients, and especially those with comorbid anxiety or the elderly, respond better by beginning at a dose slightly less than that recommended in the package insert. Suggested starting dosages are shown on Table 4-10 for the newer generation antidepressants. Drugs that inhibit the reuptake of 5HT are usually better tolerated initially if they are administered with meals.

A gradual dosing initiation usually can be achieved using sample "starter" packages of medications that are supplied by pharmaceutical companies. This saves the patient the expense of purchasing unnecessary medication when starting treatment should the side effects prove intolerable, necessitating a switch to another antidepressant. The dose of antidepressant should be increased to the upper range, as shown on Table 4-10, if the patient is not displaying a full response but experiences no significant side effects.

In general, for many patients with major depression treated in an outpatient setting, 4 to 6 weeks of continuous drug treatment is the appropriate time to begin determining whether the response to the drug selected will be positive. There is a wide range of individual responses to antidepressants and, unfortunately, there is no method to determine who will respond quickly and who will respond more slowly. Quitkin et al. (1996), in a meta-analysis of premarketing trials for the treatment of major depression, asked the question, if patients have not responded at all from baseline by a given week, what are their chances of responding by week 6, a fairly standard treatment duration in clinical trials. Fig. 4-7 shows the rates of response by week 6 if there was no response at earlier weeks. In this group of studies, if a patient had shown no response by week 5, the chances of responding by week 6 was no greater for those in the placebo-treated group.

Others have found similar results. An open-label trial of fluoxetine treatment in major depression addressed the question of predicting outcome after 8 weeks of fluoxetine treatment based on responses at 2, 4, or 6 weeks. In this open label study, 143 outpatients with DSM III-R major depression were administered a fixed dose of 20 mg per day of fluoxetine. Survival analysis was used to calculate the proportion of patients that failed to show a 20% decrease in their Hamilton Depression scale scores by 2, 4, or 6, weeks, but went on to have a 50% or greater decrease at week 8. The proportion of those who did not demonstrate improvement by weeks 2, 4, or 6, but did respond by week 8 were 36.4, 18.9, and 6.5%, respectively, suggesting that in this group the longer time on fluoxetine did not improve the chance for a subsequent recovery (Nierenberg et al., 1995). A study of earlier time points found that 70% of patients that improved after 10 days of fluoxetine could be classified as responders (≥50% decrease in HDRS from baseline) after 4 to 6 weeks of treatment, in contrast to the 39% of patients who did not improve by day 10, but did respond following 4 to 6 weeks of treatment.

An open-label study in 108 patients with major depression treated with fluoxetine at 20 mg/day also addressed the question of nonresponding. Those who did not respond after 3 weeks of treatment were randomized to either a dose increase to 60 mg per day or to continue receiving 20 mg per day for an additional 5 weeks. After 8 weeks of treatment both groups demonstrated improvement, with no statistically significant differences between the two (Fava et al., 1992). Thus, the response rate in this group did not appear to be dose-dependent above 20 mg per day.

The physician must consider a number of factors when a patient fails to respond to treatment. Included is the accuracy of diagnosis, especially unrecognized comorbid substance abuse or anxiety disorders, bipolar affective disorder, or an unrecognized medical condition. The American Psychiatric Association practice guidelines state:

If a patient is considered medication resistant on the basis of an unsatisfactory response to an antidepressant agent for 6–8 weeks, the preferred treatment is:

Table 4-10

Optional Starting Doses and Dose Titration for Patients Sensitive to Side Effects, or Who Have a Comorbid Anxiety Disorder

Newer generation antidepressant medications		
Generic (Trade)	*Starting dose (mg/day)*	*Usual therapeutic range (mg/day)*
Fluoxetine (Prozac)	10 mg × 4 days then 20 mg/day	10–80
Fluvoxamine (Luvox)	50 mg × 4 days, then 100 mg × 4 days, then ↑ by 50 mg each 4–7 days	100–300
Mirtazepine (Remeron)	7.5 mg × 4 days, then 15 mg × 4 days, then 30 mg	30–45
Nefazodone (Serzone)	50 mg bid × 4 days, then 100 mg bid × 7 days, then 150 mg bid × 7 days	150–300 bid
Paroxetine (Paxil)	10 mg × 4 days, then 20 mg. ↑ by 10 mg every 7 days as needed	20–50 mg (depression) 30–60 mg (Panic Disorder, Social Phobia, OCD)
Sertraline (Zoloft)	25 mg × 4 days, then 50 mg × 5 days	100–200
Venlafaxine (Effexor)	18.75 mg × 6 days, then 37.5 mg × 3 days ↑ by 75 mg every 4–7 days as needed	75–375
Venlafaxine XR (Effexor XR)	37.5 mg × 7 days, then 75 mg ↑ by 75 mg every 4–7 days as needed	75–375

These dosing regimens are frequently used by one of the authors (JEK) with good success.

(i)   A trial of an alternative non-MAO inhibitor antidepressant with a different biochemical profile

(ii) Coadministration of the original antidepressant
      plus lithium
      plus thyroid hormone

(iii) Coadministration of a second antidepressant

Other guidelines for the treatment of depression make similar recommendations, with the common suggestion being that failure to respond to treatment should prompt a change in treatment. In the APA guidelines, the change in treatment is to a drug with a different pharmacological profile from that used in the initial trial by either switching to a different chemical class of antidepressant or adding another drug. The decision to augment the current medication or switch to a new one depends on the individual patient and practitioner, as well as the patient's history of prior treatments. The treatment algorithm displayed on Fig. 4-8 lists the different classes of antidepressants that can be considered.

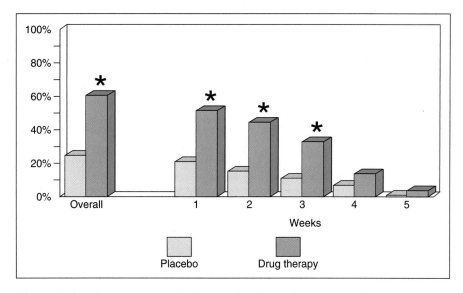

Figure 4–7. *The percentage of subjects who ultimately responded by week 6, if they showed no improvement from baseline at each week. The overall response rate for active antidepressant treatment was just over 60%. For example, if a subject had shown no improvement from baseline by week 3, the chances of responding by week 6 were about 30%. *p < 0.05 versus placebo. Adapted from Quitkin et al., 1996.*

Duration of Treatment

Patients with a first episode of major depression should, in general, be treated for 6 to 12 months after which the antidepressant medication is slowly tapered. This taper can last from 4 to 12+ weeks, depending on the antidepressant and the dose utilized. The continuation phase of treatment should be at the same dose of antidepressant that initially produced the therapeutic effect. Patients with ≥3 episodes of major depression, or those with two severe episodes, are candidates for ongoing maintenance therapy on the dose of antidepressant that produced a beneficial response.

When the patient does not respond to an antidepressant it must be established that the treatment was adequate. This consists of ensuring the accuracy of the diagnosis, especially looking for comorbid anxiety or substance abuse, unrecognized bipolar affective disorder, or an underlying medical condition. In an older patient with a first episode of major depression, medical illness and/or iatrogenic etiologies, such as prescribed medications, must be thoroughly ruled out. Other considerations include noncompliance with the prescribed regimen or an inadequate trial of the antidepressant with either too low a dose or too short a duration of treatment.

As recommended above, patients who do not respond to initial therapy can be switched to a new therapy or can receive augmentation with their present treatment. Switching is changing either from one antidepressant to another in the same or a different class, or to the use of electroconvulsive therapy. Augmentation allows for the broadening of the therapeutic approach by adding a drug with a different mechanism of action from that used initially.

Switching Strategies

An important decision in switching antidepressants is whether the new antidepressant should be of the same class or family as the previous drug. Switching from one TCA to a second TCA has a response rate of 10 to 30%. In contrast, switching from a TCA to

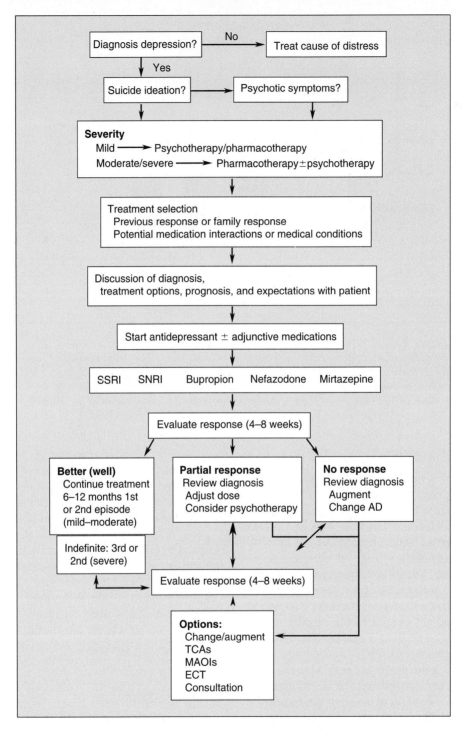

Figure 4–8. *Algorithm for the treatment of a major depressive episode in the outpatient setting. (Abbreviations: SSRI, serotonin selective reuptake inhibitor; SNRI, serotonin-norepinephrine reuptake inhibitor; AD, antidepressant; TCAs, tricyclic antidepressants; MAOIs, monoamine oxidase inhibitors; ECT, electroconvulsive therapy).*

a heterocyclic antidepressant (mostly high dose trazodone or bupropion) has a response rate of 20 to 50%. Administering an MAOI after a TCA nonresponse was successful approximately 65% of the time. When switching to or from a drug with serotonin reuptake inhibition and an MAOI, an adequate washout period must be allowed based on the half-life of the antidepressant. Switching from a TCA to ECT, or from an SSRI to a TCA have response rates of about 50 to 70%. There are no placebo-controlled trials on the effectiveness of switching from one SSRI to another. Open label trials of switching from one SSRI to a second suggests a response rate of 26 to 88%.

When administration of a serotonin reuptake inhibitor is stopped there is a possibility that the patient may develop the serotonin discontinuation syndrome. This is characterized by feelings of malaise, gastrointestinal discomfort, anxiety, irritability and, occasionally, feelings of electric shocks in the arms and legs. The serotonin discontinuation syndrome may occur if a medication is stopped too abruptly or if one or more doses are inadvertently missed. The incidence of this syndrome appears to be inversely related to the half-life of the drug. Thus, short half-life agents, such as paroxetine or venlafaxine, are more problematic than longer half-life drugs, such as fluoxetine. The switch from one serotonin reuptake inhibitor to another can usually be accomplished over the course of 3 to 4 days unless there is evidence of the serotonin discontinuation syndrome in which case it should be done more slowly. When a serotonin reuptake inhibitor is stopped in favor of a drug with a different mechanism of action, the switch must always be more gradual because the new agent will not prevent development of the serotonin discontinuation syndrome.

Augmentation Strategies

Numerous medications are useful as augmentation agents for treatment-resistant depression or for those who only partially respond to an antidepressant. Studies have shown an enhanced antidepressant response with the use of lithium, T_3, TCAs added to SSRIs, buspirone, stimulants, and pindolol. The two most studied strategies are the addition of lithium or T_3 to antidepressants.

The addition of lithium to TCAs appears to be successful in about 40 to 60% of the cases. The response is typically seen from 2 to 42 days, although most patients require a 3- to 4-week trial to determine efficacy. A recent, medium sized, placebo-controlled, double-blind trial examining the efficacy of lithium augmentation included 62 patients who had <50% reduction in the HDRS after 6 weeks of treatment with fluoxetine (20 mg/day) or lofepramine (70–210 mg/day) (Katona et al., 1995). Lithium was given to these subjects in doses to achieve steady-state serum concentrations of 0.6 to 1.0 mEq/L. The response rates after 10 weeks of lithium augmentation were 15/29 (52%) for the group receiving lithium and an antidepressant, and 8/32 (25%) for the placebo and antidepressant group.

Lithium does not appear to be as effective as an augmenting agent in older, as compared to younger, individuals. Zimmer et al. (1991) assessed the response to lithium augmentation in 15 patients 59 to 89 years of age who had experienced no response ($n = 14$) or only a partial response ($n = 2$) to 4 weeks of treatment with nortriptyline. In this case a complete response was noted in only 20% of patients and a partial response in 47%.

Predictors of a positive response to lithium augmentation include bipolar disorder, less severe depression, probably younger age, and a rapid response to lithium. Responders appear to be less likely to have recurrent depression than nonresponders (Nierenberg et al., 1990).

Lithium augmentation is typically initiated at 300 to 600 mg/day and titrated to serum levels of 0.6 to 1.0 mEq/L. Extended-release lithium preparations can be helpful in minimizing the side effects associated with lithium treatment. A baseline laboratory evaluation should be performed as discussed in the context of bipolar disorder.

Thyroid augmentation has been studied most extensively with TCAs, but has also been reported useful in patients receiving SSRIs and MAOIs. Both open-label and double-blind controlled trials suggest that T_3 augmentation is effective. The overall response rate of T_3 augmentation to TCAs is about 50 to 60%. It is important that T_3 and not T_4 be used as an augmentation strategy since studies have shown that T_3 is much more efficacious than T_4 as an augmentation in major depression. Treatment with T_4 for hypothyroidism does not preclude the addition of T_3. Cooke et al. (1992) reported that 5/7 patients with depression who had not responded to 5 weeks of antidepressant treatment had more than a 50% decrease in HDRS after the addition of T_3 in a dose ranging from 15 to 50 μg/day. In general, T_3 augmentation is well tolerated. Starting doses of T_3 are usually from 12.5 to 25 μg/day, with the lower doses being used for those with significant anxiety. The target dose of T_3 is typically 25 to 50 μg/day. Thyroid function should be monitored and the dose of T_3 adjusted to avoid suppression of TSH release.

A number of other drugs have been utilized as augmenting agents in treatment-resistant depressed patients. Most of these agents have been evaluated only in small, open-label trials.

Buspirone is a partial 5-HT1$_A$ receptor agonist that is approved for use in generalized anxiety disorder. Joffe and Schuller (1993) reported on an open trial of buspirone augmentation in 25 patients with major depression who had failed to respond to 5 weeks of treatment with an SSRI (fluvoxamine or fluoxetine) and had also failed two or more previous antidepressant treatment regimens. Complete or partial improvement was observed on the CGI scale in 32 and 36% of these patients, respectively, following the addition of buspirone at 20 to 50 mg/day.

Pindolol is a β-adrenergic receptor antagonist used in the treatment of hypertension. It is also a potent antagonist at 5-HT1$_A$ receptors. Artigas et al. (1994) administered pindolol (2.5 mg three times a day) to eight patients who had not responded (HDRS $\geq$14) after 6 weeks of antidepressant treatment. Rapid improvement within 1 week was noted in five of the eight subjects with HDRS of <7. The preparation of pindolol used may be important. For example, Viskin, a brand of pindolol, may be a different racemic mixture than other preparations.

Other drugs used as augmenting agents include stimulants such as methylphenidate, dexedrine, or amphetamines added to SSRIs, TCAs, and MAOIs. The addition of stimulants to MAOIs should be done cautiously to minimize a potentially dramatic increase in blood pressure. While TCAs were added to SSRIs, the potential interaction between paroxetine, sertraline, and fluoxetine with TCAs must be noted, with TCA blood levels increasing significantly in many patients taking this drug combination. Bupropion has also been added to SSRIs as an augmentation. In patients for whom there is a question of bipolar affective disorder type II (BPAD II) during an episode of major depression the addition of a mood stabilizer may be beneficial.

Treatment of Dysthymic Disorder

Dysthymia is a chronic mood disorder that affects 3 to 6% of the population in the United States. Among patients in psychiatric clinics, dysthymia comprises about one-third of the population. In addition to the deleterious effects of a chronic mood disorder, patients with dysthymic disorder also experience high rates of comorbid anxiety disorders, substance abuse, and major depression. While a limited number of drug trials in dysthymic disorder have been completed, antidepressants that are effective in major depression appear to be effective in this condition as well. The time course of response for patients treated for dysthymic disorder may be slower than for major depression. Vanelle and colleagues (1997) reported on a double-blind, placebo-controlled trial of fluoxetine in the treatment of dysthymic disorder. After 3 months of treatment the group receiving fluoxetine (20 mg/day) had a response rate of 58% (42/72) compared to a rate of 36% (14/39) for the placebo-treated group. Half of the nonresponders in the fluoxetine-treated group responded after the dose was increased to 40 mg/day for an additional 3 months. Sertraline and imipramine were found to be effective in a large, double-blind, placebo-controlled trial of 416 patients with early-onset, primary dysthymia without concurrent major depression (Thase et al., 1996). Response rates, defined by a CGI of 1 or 2 (very much or much improved) were 64, 59, and 44% for imipramine, sertraline, and placebo, respectively. The patients treated with the SSRI experienced fewer side effects than those receiving the TCA.

Pharmacokinetics and Medication Interactions

The newer generation antidepressants have vastly different half-lives, ranging from hours to days, and highly variable degrees of binding to plasma proteins. The pharmacokinetic profiles of many of the newer generation antidepressants are listed on Table 4-11. These characteristics determine frequency of dosing and the potential for inducing serotonin discontinuation syndrome and some drug-drug interactions.

Drug-drug interactions between newer generation antidepressants and other therapeutics is an area that has recently received increased attention. Despite this, there is a relative lack of information on

Table 4-11

Pharmacokinetic Profiles of Newer Generation Antidepressants

Compound	Parent drug ($t_{1/2}$)	Active metabolite ($t_{1/2}$)	Plasma protein binding (%)
Fluvoxamine	16 h		80
Fluoxetine	4–6 days	4–16 days	95
Mirtazepine	20–40 h		85
Nefazodone	2–4 h	4+ hr	>95
Paroxetine	21 h		95
Sertraline	26 h		95
Venlafaxine	5 h	10 hr	27

The half-life of the parent compound, and metabolites if equivalent in activity to the parent compound in the presumed mechanism of therapeutic action, are shown. Plasma protein binding is taken from *in vitro* assays.

the clinical importance and prevalence of drug-drug interactions with these agents. Plasma protein binding with potential displacement of other tightly bound drugs and inhibition of cytochrome P450 enzymes are the two main types of drug-drug interactions that are encountered. Drug-induced induction of cytochrome P450 enzymes is less commonly observed with these substances. Drugs bind in a nonspecific manner primarily to plasma albumin and α_1-acid glycoproteins. When drugs are displaced from those binding sites the amount of available active agent increases, enhancing the response to a given dose. There exists much more evidence regarding the occurrence of drug-drug interactions as a result of cytochrome P450 enzyme inhibition. Clues that a drug-drug interaction is occurring include: increased side effects at a lower than expected dose or therapeutic efficacy at a lower than expected dose. Some drug-drug interactions, however, have only "silent" side effects that may go unnoticed until there is a serious outcome. Ultimately, the pharmacokinetic interactions of various drugs must be considered in terms of the pharmacodynamic results.

A summary of these interactions based on *in vivo* and *in vitro* studies is shown on Table 4-12. Substrates of the different cytochrome P450 isoenzymes are shown on Table 4-13. Medications such as the tertiary TCAs have multiple pathways

of metabolism. A number of clinically relevant medication interactions have been described in the literature, such as fluvoxamine and theophylline via the 1A2 isoenzyme, clozapine and fluvoxamine (1A2), sertraline (2D6), fluoxetine (2D6), or paroxetine (2D6). Paroxetine, fluoxetine, and sertraline all inhibit the metabolism of TCAs through the 2D6 isoenzyme.

The clinical relevance of potential cytochrome P450 inhibition depends on a number of variables. Risk factors for drug-drug interactions include multiple medications, clinically significant renal or hepatic disease, and age. Highly potent cytochrome P450 enzyme inhibitors, such as quinidine and ketoconazole, are also risk factors. An informed awareness of, and monitoring for, potential drug-drug interactions is the best way to maximize clinical care and minimize avoidable risks.

Treatment Algorithms

There are a number of approaches for treating the patient with depression. Some of the variables that need to be considered are the presence or absence of prior major depressive episodes, the severity of the current episode, the amount of support in the home environment, comorbid psychiatric or medical conditions, and whether or not the patient is suicidal. A general approach to the treatment of outpatient depression is shown in Fig. 4-8. The interested reader is also referred to other published treatment algorithms for major depression (American Psychiatric Association, 1993; Nelson et al., 1995).

Table 4-12

Potential Inhibition of the Cytochrome P450 Isoenzyme Pathways by Antidepressants

| Relative rank | Isoenzyme | | | |
	CYP1A2	CYP2C	CYP2D6	CYP3A
Higher	Fluvoxamine	Fluoxetine Fluvoxamine	Fluoxetine Paroxetine	Fluvoxamine Nefazodone TCAs
Moderate	Tertiary TCAs Fluoxetine	Sertraline	Secondary TCAs Sertraline	Fluoxetine Sertraline
Low/ minimal	Bupropion Mirtazapine Nefazodone Paroxetine Sertraline Venlafaxine	Paroxetine Venlafaxine	Bupropion Fluvoxamine Mirtazapine Nefazodone Venlafaxine	Mirtazapine Paroxetine Venlafaxine

Inhibition is characterized as high, moderate, or low/minimal. Within each category of inhibition the compounds are listed alphabetically. Observations based on a combination of *in vitro* and *in vivo* studies.

BIPOLAR AFFECTIVE DISORDER

Bipolar affective disorder (BPAD) is a mood disorder in which episodes of depression and mania or hypomania can be present. The previous term for this disease was manic depression which may convey more of a descriptive sense of the disorder. The distinction is made between BPAD and major depression, which has also been termed unipolar depression, to contrast the mood elevation that can be seen in BPAD. There is no specific sequence for the appearance of depression and mania, and failure to recognize the cyclical nature of the disorder greatly hampers treatment. The key determinates of selecting the most appropriate treatment are accurate diagnosis, whether the condition is rapid or nonrapid cycling, and assessment of the presence or absence of a mixed or dysphoric mania.

Differential Diagnosis

There are many conditions that produce the signs and symptoms of bipolar disorder. Being aware of these is a necessary step in making the correct diagnosis and instituting the most appropriate treatment. The differential diagnosis of BPAD includes mood disorders caused by a general medical condition or substance abuse, major depression, dysthymic disorder, cyclothymic disorder, and psychotic disorders. Additionally, obsessive-compulsive disorder with numerous compulsions can appear to be similar to the increased goal-directed behavior of BPAD. Moreover, a patient with borderline personality disorder who is doing poorly may also share some characteristics of BPAD as a result of the labile affect seen in the personality disorder. In the younger patient, a presentation of depression may be the first affective episode of what will turn out to be BPAD. The DSM-IV defines criteria for mania in terms of duration, symptoms, impairment, and lack of a recognizable drug abuse problem or medication or medical condition that can explain the behavior. The diagnostic criteria for a manic episode are shown on Table 4-14.

Bipolar affective disorder is differentiated from unipolar affective disorder by the presence of differ-

Table 4-13

A Partial List of Commonly Prescribed Medications That Are Substrates for the Cytochrome P450 1A2, 2C, 2D6, or 3A Isoenzymes

1A2 *Antidepressants:* Tertiary TCAs, Fluvoxamine *Antipsychotics:* Clozapine, Haloperidol, Olanzapine, Thioxanthenes, Phenothiazines *Others:* Caffeine, Theophylline, Tacrine, Verapamil, Acetominophen **2C** *Antidepressants:* Amitriptyline, Citalopram, Clomipramine, Imipramine, Moclobemide *Others:* Diazepam, Hexobarbital, Phenytoin, Tolbutamide **2D6** *Antidepressants:* Amitriptyline, Clomipramine, Imipramine, Desipramine, Nortriptyline, Trazodone, Sertraline, Fluoxetine, Paroxetine, Venlafaxine *Antipsychotics:* Chlorpromazine, Clozapine, Perphenazine, Haloperidol, Risperidone, Thioridizine, Olanzapine *Antiarrythmics:* Encainide, Flecainide, Propafenone, Mexiletine β-*Blockers:* Labetalol, Metropolol, Propranolol, Timolol *Opioids:* Codeine, Hydrocodone, Oxycocone *Protease Inhibitors:* Ritonavir *Others:* Dextromethorphan, Amphetamine, Diphenhydramine, Loratadine	**3A** *Benzodiazepines:* Alprazolam, Clonazepam, Midazolam, Triazolam, Diazepam *Antihistamines:* Astemizole, Terfenadine, Loratadine *Calcium Channel Blockers:* Diltiazem, Felodipine, Nifedipine, Verapamil *Antidepressants:* Tertiary TCAs, Nefazodone, Sertraline, Venlafaxine *Antiarrythmics:* Amiodarone, Disopyramide Lidocaine, Quinidine *Protease Inhibitors:* Ritonavir, Indinavir, Saquinavir *Others:* Clozapine, Carbamazepine, Cisapride, Dexamethasone, Cyclosporine, Cocaine, Tamoxifen, Estradiol, Macrolide Antibiotics

Some medications, such as tertiary TCAs and clozapine, have more than one metabolic pathway.

ent phases, including mania, hypomania, and depression. The clinical description of the manic phase (adapted from Goodwin and Jamison, 1990) includes heightened mood, more and faster speech, quicker thought, brisker physical and mental activity levels, more energy (with decreased need for sleep), irritability, perceptual acuity, paranoia, heightened sexuality, and impulsivity. There are a variety of DSM-IV specifiers used to describe bipolar disorder. These are: Bipolar I disorder, single manic episode or most recent episode, hypomanic, mixed, depressed, or unspecified; Bipolar II disorder, most recent episode hypomanic or depressed; or cyclothymic disorder. Additionally, DSM-IV proposes two longitudinal course specifiers with either full interepisode recovery or without it, as well as the presence of a seasonal pattern in the depressive episodes or rapid cycling.

Table 4-14
Diagnostic Criteria for a Manic Episode

A distinct period of abnormally and persistently elevated, expansive, or irritable mood, lasting at least 1 week (or any duration if hospitalization is necessary)

During the period of mood disturbance, three (or more) of the following symptoms have persisted (four if the mood is only irritable) and have been present to a significant degree:

  Inflated self-esteem or grandiosity

  Decreased need for sleep (e.g., feels rested after only 3 hours of sleep.

  More talkative than usual or pressure to keep talking

  Flight of ideas or subjective experience that thoughts are racing

  Distractibility (i.e., attention too easily drawn to unimportant or irrelevant external stimuli)

  Increase in goal-directed activity (either socially, at work or school, or sexually) or psychomotor agitation

Excessive involvement in pleasurable activities that have a high potential for painful consequences (e.g., engaging in unrestrained buying sprees, sexual indiscretions, or foolish business investments)

The symptoms do not meet criteria for a mixed episode.

The mood disturbance is sufficiently severe to cause marked impairment in occupational functioning or in usual social activities or relationships with others, or to necessitate hospitalization to prevent harm to self or others, or there are psychotic features.

The symptoms are not owing to the direct physiologic effects of a substance (e.g., a drug of abuse, a medication, or other treatment) or a general medical condition (e.g., hyperthyroidism).

SOURCE American Psychiatric Association: *Diagnostic and Statistical Manual of Mental Disorders*, 4th ed (DSM-IV). Washington, DC: American Psychiatric Association, 1994.

Mania, as described by the DSM-IV, may have a broad range of severity. Carlson and Goodwin (1973) have described the stages of mania as follows.

Stage I: Increased psychomotor activity, labile affect, expansiveness, grandiosity, overconfidence, sexually preoccupied, still in control

Stage II: More pressured speech, psychomotor activation, increased depression/dysphoria, open hostility, flight of ideas, paranoid and grandiose delusions

Stage III: Desperate, panic stricken, hopeless, frenzied and bizarre psychomotor activity, incoherent, looseness of associations, hallucinations

Different terminologies equate hypomania with stage I, acute mania with stage II, and delirious mania with

stage III. Particularly in stage III, the cross-sectional diagnosis of bipolar disorder as opposed to a schizophrenia is often difficult without the presence of a collateral source of information.

Mixed or dysphoric mania.   Dysphoric or mixed mania is a relatively common presentation yet remains less well-characterized than some other forms of bipolar disorder. It is estimated that 40 to 50% of hospitalized bipolar patients have mixed mania. Mixed mania is characterized by a labile mood and a combination of symptoms that meet the criteria for both a manic episode and an episode of major depression nearly every day during a 1-week period (DSM-IV). There is often a close temporal relationship to a depressive episode. Because mixed mania often has a poorer outcome than "pure" mania, recognition of the mixed state has important treatment implications because anticonvulsants appear to be more effective than lithium in this subtype of bipolar disorder.

Rapid cycling BPAD.   Each episode of mania, depression, or hypomania is counted as a single episode. Rapid cycling occurs in 13 to 20% of all bipolar patients, with an initial onset in 20% and a later onset in 80%. Females predominantly experience rapid cycling, with the majority beginning with a depressive episode. Moreover, patients can alternate between rapid and nonrapid cycling. Similar to mixed mania, the recognition of rapid cycling has important treatment implications since some medications are more effective in this condition than other psychotropic drugs.

Bipolar II.   Bipolar II is characterized by episodes of hypomania and depression. Diagnosis is often complicated by the overlay of personality traits and the fact that the individual is experiencing feelings of being upbeat, energetic, and optimistic during a hypomanic episode. For this reason, it is rare for a person to present for treatment during an hypomanic episode as opposed to depression. Additionally, the patient with bipolar II who comes for treatment during an episode of depression may have difficulty accurately recalling or reporting a more jubilant mood.

A difference between mania and hypomania is the degree of impairment. Indeed, with bipolar II minimal impairment may be difficult for the patient to recognize, underscoring the importance of a collateral history. Still, many patients with episodes of hypomania will find changes in their judgment during the episode that could have significant consequences. The age of onset for bipolar II is about 32 years of age, which is between that of bipolar I and unipolar depression. The number of affective episodes is greater for bipolar II than unipolar depression and the cycle length, or time from the start of one episode to the start of the next, is longer for bipolar II than for bipolar I.

Helpful clues to the diagnosis of bipolar II during a depressed phase when there may not be a clear history of depression include: early age of onset, strong family history of bipolar disorder, previous response to lithium, high frequency of episodes, and pharmacologic hypomania (Weiss et al., 1994). The DSM-IV diagnostic criteria for hypomania are shown on Table 4-15.

Cyclothymia.   Cyclothymia is a bipolar spectrum disorder that is of a markedly lower intensity than is observed in the mood swings and impairment associated with bipolar type I. Similar to dysthymic disorder, however, there is the potential for significant disability and impairment in cyclothymia. The DSM-IV criteria for cyclothymia are shown on Table 4-16.

Features Influencing Treatment and Comorbid Disorders

There are a number of factors and comorbid disorders that influence the course of the disorder, compliance, and selection of medications.

Substance Abuse

Data from the epidemiologic catchment area (ECA) study suggest that patients with bipolar disorder are the most likely of all axis I disorders to experience comorbid substance abuse or dependence. The odds ratio of having substance abuse or dependence in different mood disorders is shown on Table 4-17 (Regier et al., 1988). Bipolar disorder is found in patients in alcohol abuse treatment programs at a rate of 2 to 4% and estimates for bipolar disorder spectrum range from 4 to 30% in cocaine treatment programs. In general, bipolar disorder and cyclothymia are more common in stimulant abusers than in those addicted to opioids or sedative/hypnotics. In patients hospitalized for treatment of bipolar spectrum disorders the rates of substance abuse range from 21 to 58% (Brady and Lydiard, 1992). Patients with comorbid bipolar disorder and substance abuse have lower rates of compliance with therapy, longer hospital stays, and are more difficult to diagnose since stimulant abuse can easily mimic hypomania or mania, and drug withdrawal may have many features of depression.

Table 4-15
Diagnostic Criteria for a Hypomanic Episode

A distinct period of persistently elevated, expansive, or irritable, mood lasting throughout at least 4 days, that is clearly different from the usual nondepressed mood.

During the period of mood disturbance, three (or more) of the following symptoms have persisted (four if the mood is only irritable) and have been present to a significant degree:

  Inflated self-esteem or grandiosity

  Decreased need for sleep (e.g., feels rested after only 3 hours of sleep)

  More talkative than usual or pressure to keep talking

  Flight of ideas or subjective experience that thoughts are racing

  Distractibility (i.e., attention too easily drawn to unimportant or irrelevant external stimuli)

  Increase in goal-directed activity (either socially, at work or school, or sexually) or psychomotor agitation

Excessive involvement in pleasurable activities that have a high potential for painful consequences (e.g., engaging in unrestrained buying sprees, sexual indiscretions, or foolish business investments)

The episode is associated with an unequivocal change in functioning that is uncharacteristic of the person when not symptomatic.

The disturbance in mood and the change in functioning are observable by others.

The episode is not severe enough to cause marked impairment in social or occupational functioning or to necessitate hospitalization, and there are no psychotic features.

The symptoms are not owing to the direct physiologic effects of a substance (e.g., a drug of abuse, a medication, or other treatment) or a general medication condition (e.g., hyperthyroidism)

SOURCE American Psychiatric Association: *Diagnostic and Statistical Manual of Mental Disorders,*
  4th ed (DSM-IV). Washington, DC: American Psychiatric Association, 1994.

Other Disorders

Data from the ECA (Strakowski et al., 1994) show comorbid rates of OCD at 8 to 13%, panic disorder at 7 to 16%, and bulimia at 2 to 15% in patients with bipolar disorder.

Treatment of all three of these conditions with antidepressants is complicated by the presence of the bipolar disorder. For panic disorder comorbid with bipolar disorder, the high rates of substance abuse should be recalled when considering the use of benzodiazepines. Migraine headaches appear at higher rates in individuals with bipolar disorder than in the general population. One study (Merikangas et al., 1990) found migraine sufferers to have a rate of bipolar disorder 2.9 times that of a control population. Interestingly, valproic acid is approved

for the treatment of both bipolar disorder and migraine.

Secondary Mania

Secondary mania is a manic episode produced by an underlying concurrent medical condition, medication, or drug of abuse. Individuals with secondary mania tend to be older and lack a family history of psychiatric disorders. Brain trauma can produce secondary mania with the available data (Strakowski et al., 1994) suggesting it occurs more often with right-sided subcortical lesions (thalamus, caudate) or with cortical lesions with close limbic system connectivity (basotemporal or orbitofrontal cortex).

Secondary mania has been reported in association with multiple sclerosis, hemodialysis, calcium

Table 4-16
Diagnostic Criteria for Cyclothymic Disorder

For at least 2 years, the presence of numerous periods with hypomanic symptoms and numerous periods with depressive symptoms that do not meet criteria for a major depressive episode. (*Note:* In children and adolescents, the duration must be at least 1 year.)

During the above 2-year period (1 year in children and adolescents) the person has not been without the symptoms in criterion above for more than 2 months at a time.

No Major Depressive Episode, Manic Episode, or Mixed Episode has been present during the first 2 years of the disturbance. [*Note:* After the initial 2 years (1 year in children and adolescents) of Cyclothymic Disorder, there may be superimposed Manic or Mixed Episodes (in which case both Bipolar I Disorder and Cyclothymic Disorder may be diagnosed) or Major Depressive Episodes (in which case both Bipolar II Disorder and Cyclothymic Disorder may be diagnosed).]

The symptoms in the first criterion are not better accounted for by Schizoaffective Disorder and are not superimposed on Schizophrenia, Schizophreniform Disorder, Delusional Disorder, or Psychotic Disorder Not Otherwise Specified.

The symptoms are not owing to the direct physiologic effects of a substance (e.g., a drug of abuse, a medication, or other treatment) or a general medical condition (e.g., hyperthyroidism).

The symptoms cause clinically significant distress or impairment in social, occupational, or other important areas of functioning.

SOURCE American Psychiatric Association: *Diagnostic and Statistical Manual of Mental Disorders,* 4th ed (DSM-IV). Washington, DC: American Psychiatric Association, 1994.

replacement, anoxia, head trauma, lyme borreliosis, polycythemia, cerebrovascular disease, cerebral sarcoidosis, tumors, AIDs, neurosyphilis, and as a result of treatment with corticosteroids, amphetamines, baclofen, bromide, bromocriptine, captopril, cimetidine, cocaine, cyclosporine, disulfiram, hallucinogens, hydralazine, isoniazid, levodopa, methylphenidate, metrizamide, opioids, procarbazine, procyclidine, and yohimbine. Keys to a correct diagnosis of secondary mania include an onset late in life, negative family history of mental disorders, new medication, or physiologic insult.

Pharmacotherapy of BPAD. Mood stabilizers such as lithium, carbamazepine, or valproate are the major drugs used to treat BPAD, although newer agents, such as olanzapine, risperidone, lamotrigine, gabapentin, and calcium channel blockers are sometimes employed. Treatment stages are divided between acute stabilization of the manic episode, with polypharmacy sometimes necessary, stabilization, and long-term prophylaxis to prevent future episodes.

Lithium

Lithium has a long history in the treatment of a number of disorders with varying degrees of success and safety. During the early 1900s lithium was a popular component of many "cure-all" patent remedies. Products containing lithium were recommended for the treatment of conditions ranging from malaise to all manner of "nervous system dysfunction." Lithium has also been used as a treatment for gout and was used as a salt substitute in the 1940s. In 1949, Cade described the efficacy of lithium for what he termed psychotic excitement. This discovery would later revolutionize the treatment of bipolar disorder,

Table 4-17

The Adjusted Odds Ratio of Developing Substance Abuse or Dependence (dep) in Different Affective Disorders

	BPAD I	BPAD II	Dysthymia	Unipolar depression
Any substance abuse/dep	7.9	4.7	2.4	1.9
Alcohol dep	5.5	3.1	2.3	1.6
Alcohol abuse	3.0	3.9	0.8	0.9
Drug dep	11.1	3.7	3.6	3.7
Drug abuse	5.9	3.9	3.3	3.6

SOURCE From Regier et al., 1990.

which to that time went virtually untreated. It was not, however, until 1970, that the FDA approved lithium for the treatment for acute mania. Numerous double-blind, placebo-controlled studies have demonstrated the efficacy of lithium in acute mania, with a response rate typically of 70 to 80%. While more recent studies have demonstrated a somewhat lower response rate, this may be due to the presence of more treatment-resistant patients in the trials, or a higher number of those with mixed mania, for which lithium alone is not as effective. Still, of all the mood stabilizers available, clinical experience is greatest for lithium.

Lithium has also been shown to be efficacious as a prophylactic treatment for BPAD. Placebo-controlled trials reveal that about 70% of patients can expect to gain long-term benefit from lithium treatment as reflected by a decrease in the number and the intensity of affective episodes. When patients on prophylactic lithium therapy abruptly terminate treatment approximately 50% relapse within 5 months (Suppes et al., 1991). More gradual discontinuation of lithium treatment appears to decrease the rate of relapse from a 5-year rate of 94% following discontinuation to 53% (Faedda et al., 1993).

Certain features of the patient's illness are predictive of a positive response to lithium. Patients with classic or pure mania, in contrast to the mixed or dysphoric subtype, are good candidates for lithium treatment, as are those who do not have rapid-cycling BPAD. The response rate to lithium in rapid cycling BPAD is about 18 to 25% (Dunner and Fieve, 1974;

Okuma, 1993), as compared to a response rate of about 60% of patients without rapid cycling BPAD (Fig. 4-9). Comorbid substance abuse predicts a poor response to lithium, whereas previous failure to respond to the drug has been shown to predict nothing about the future response to this agent (Bowden et al., 1994).

Even though lithium has one of the lowest therapeutic indices of psychotropic medications, it is used successfully by many BPAD patients. The therapeutic serum level of lithium is generally considered

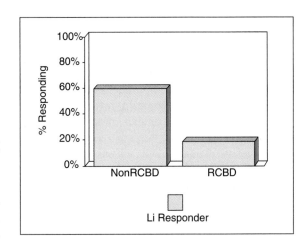

Figure 4–9. *Different response rates among patients with bipolar affective disorder treated with lithium who were rapid cycling (RCBD) or non-rapid cycling (NonRCBD). From Dunner and Fievel, 1974.*

to be between about 0.6 and 1.2 mEq/L, although younger patients may require more, and geriatric patients less. The most common side effects reported with lithium therapy (Goodwin and Jamison, 1990) are excessive thirst, polyuria, memory problems, tremor, weight gain, drowsiness/tiredness, and diarrhea. Those that appear to contribute most to noncompliance are, in descending order, memory problems, weight gain, tremor/incoordination, polyuria, and drowsiness/tiredness. The tremor associated with lithium treatment is worsened by caffeine, which should be discussed with patients who experience it. Tremor is often responsive to treatment with low doses of β-adrenergic receptor blockers. Lithium may produce gastrointestinal side effects such as nausea and loose stools and psoriasis or acne is sometimes precipitated or worsened during the course of treatment. Lithium will also, in many patients, produce a benign granulocytosis. Lithium may affect thyroid function, with the rate of clinical hypothyroidism while on lithium therapy being about 5% (Jefferson, 1990), with about 30% of patients having elevated levels of TSH. There is also an increase (15 to 30%) in thyroid autoantibodies (Deniker et al., 1978; Lazarus, 1986) during lithium therapy. Hyperparathyroidism may also occur during lithium treatment, but is much less common than hypothyroidism (Nordenstrom et al., 1992).

Lithium reduces water reabsorption in the distal tubules and collecting ducts of the kidney, decreasing the ability to concentrate urine, with subsequent polyuria. This action can also lead to polydipsia, and, if patients drink nondiet sodas or fruit juice, can contribute to weight gain over time. There is no convincing evidence that lithium produces irreversible renal dysfunction when administered within the therapeutic dose range.

The cardiac effects of lithium include T-wave flattening and inversion, bradycardia, and increased sinus node recovery time. Since other mood stabilizers, with a more benign cardiac profile, are available, patients with sinus bradycardia or sinus node dysfunction should not be treated with lithium, or be given the drug with extreme caution.

Lithium is available as regular-release (Eskalith, Lithonate, and Lithotabs), controlled-release (Eskal-ith CR), and slow-release (Lithobid) forms, all of which contain lithium carbonate. Lithium citrate is available in a syrup (Cibalith-S), and there are 8 mEq of lithium in both 300 mg of lithium carbonate or 5 mL of lithium citrate. Lithium is completely absorbed following oral administration with peak serum levels achieved within 1 to 1.5 hours with regular-release and 4 to 4.5 hours with controlled- and slow-release formulations. Renal excretion is the primary route of elimination. The half-life of lithium is 18 to 24 h.

Coadministration with nonsteroidal antiinflammatory agents may produce an increase in serum lithium levels, although aspirin and sulindac (Clinoril) do not. Diuretics and angiotensin converting enzyme inhibitors can also increase serum lithium levels by promoting sodium loss and a consequent decrease in lithium excretion.

Lithium in Acute Mania

Lithium is still widely used in the treatment of mania, although the 5- to 10-day lag before attaining clinical benefit often necessitates the use of adjunctive agents. Prior to initiating lithium therapy, renal and thyroid function should be evaluated and an ECG performed. Females of child-bearing potential should also have a serum or urine pregnancy test because of the teratogenic effects of lithium. Treatment is often begun at 600 to 1200 mg/day in divided doses. Most patients achieve a therapeutic serum level between 0.8 and 1.2 mEq/L with the administration of 1200 to 1800 mg/day. Lithium levels should be determined approximately every 4 to 5 days during acute dose adjustment. A number of protocols have been devised to estimate the dose of lithium necessary to achieve therapeutic serum levels. These entail either measuring serum levels 24 h after an initial dose (Cooper et al., 1973), determining 12-, 24-, and 36-h levels (Perry et al., 1982), two blood samples, or a 4-h urine and creatinine clearance (Norman et al., 1982). Despite the variety of methods, many clinicians still dose with a combination of experience-guided strategies taking into consideration clinical efficacy and side effects. Lithium serum levels are obtained 12 h after the last dose when determining therapeutic serum concentrations. Lithium serum levels, as well as renal and thyroid functioning, are typically monitored every 6 to 12 months for the patient stabilized on long-term lithium therapy. Eskalith, Lithonate, Lithotabs, and Lithobid each are available at 300-mg dose strengths. Eskalith CR is a 450-mg dose strength formulation. Five milliliters of the liquid preparation, Cibalith-S, is equivalent to 300 mg of lithium carbonate.

Lithium toxicity may occur at serum levels that would normally be considered therapeutic, especially in the geriatric patient. Early signs of lithium toxicity or intoxication include ataxia, course tremor, and dysarthria. Increased levels of lithium may produce more serious signs such as impaired or decreased consciousness, fasciculations, myoclonus, coma, or even death. Risk factors for lithium toxicity include conditions that produce increase serum levels of the ion such as an excessive intake of lithium, decreased clearance (renal impairment, drug-interactions, low-sodium diets), reduced volume of distribution (dehydration), and factors that increase susceptibility to deleterious side effects such as organicity or older age. Mild toxicity is treated by withholding lithium and ensuring adequate hydration. Increasing severity is treated with forced diuresis or, in life-threatening cases, hemodialysis to clear the lithium. In a suspected overdose at least two lithium serum levels must be established with a period of at least 4 h between them, with the second level being lower than the first. Lithium overdose in combination with an anticholinergic agent may slow absorption of the lithium because of the decreased gastrointestinal mobility, producing a delayed peak serum level.

At one time lithium was believed to produce a markedly increased risk of Ebstein's anomaly in the fetus with maternal exposure. A recent reanalysis of the data suggests that the risk is much lower than was originally believed (Cohen et al., 1994). The use of any psychotropic agent during pregnancy necessitates a careful comparison of risks to benefits. Lithium, however, is probably safer to use during pregnancy, in terms of the developing fetus, than either carbamazepine or valproate. Lithium dosages during pregnancy are usually higher than before pregnancy because of the larger volume of distribution. Because

delivery is accompanied by large changes in fluid volumes the dose of lithium must be adjusted accordingly. Many physicians institute prophylactic treatment of a pregnant bipolar patient shortly before anticipated delivery (Cohen et al., 1995) because of the high risk of relapse in the postpartum period.

Valproate. A number of antiepileptic drugs are useful in the treatment of bipolar affective disorder including valproate (Depakote), carbamazepine (Tegretol and others), lamotrigine (Lamictal), gabapentin (Neurontin), and clonazepam (Klonopin). Valproate is currently approved for the acute treatment of bipolar disorder. Valproic acid was initially used as a drug solvent when Meunier discovered that it possessed antiepileptic properties. Three years later, in 1966, Lambert first reported its beneficial effects in bipolar disorder. The formulation most commonly used in the United States for the treatment of BPAD is an enteric-coated preparation of divalproex sodium (Depakote) that contains sodium valproate and valproic acid in a 1:1 ratio. A valproic acid formulation (Depakene) is available, although it generally produces more gastrointestinal side effects than divalproex sodium.

Valproate is almost completely absorbed following oral administration. Peak serum levels occur about 1 to 4 hours after ingestion of valproic acid and about 3 to 4 hours after ingestion of divalproex sodium. The use of the sprinkle formulation of sodium divalproex delays peak serum concentrations by about 1.5 hours. Food also delays valproate absorption. Valproate is about 90% bound to plasma proteins at serum concentrations of 40 μg/mL, though only about 82% is protein bound at serum concentrations of 130 μg/mL. Protein binding of valproate is reduced in the elderly, patients with chronic hepatic disease or renal disease. Other drugs which bind to plasma proteins, such as aspirin, may displace valproate from its binding site. Because valproate is metabolized primarily in the liver, hepatic disease impairs its clearance and requires a dose reduction. The plasma half-life of valproate is 6 to 16 hours. Numerous mechanisms of action have been proposed to explain the therapeutic efficacy of valproate, including enhancing GABAergic activity, altering sodium or potassium flow at the neuronal membrane, decreasing dopamine turnover, and decreasing glutamic acid N-methyl-D-aspartate receptor-mediated currents.

Valproate has demonstrated an efficacy superior to placebo and equivalent to lithium in the treatment of acute mania. A double-blind, placebo-controlled 3-week trial in inpatients with acute mania who had failed to either respond, or tolerate, a previous trial of lithium revealed that valproate was more efficacious than placebo. Another placebo-controlled, double-blind study with lithium as a comparator had similar results (Bowden et al., 1994). In this case inpatients with manic disorder (Research Diagnostic Criteria) received placebo, valproate at initial dosing of 250 mg tid and adjusted up to 2500 mg/day, or lithium carbonate. The mean doses of valproate among study completers were 1116, 1683, and 2006 mg/day at days 7, 14, and 21, respectively. The mean doses of lithium among study completers were 1312, 1869, and 1984 mg/day at days 7, 14, and 21, respectively. The results indicated valproate had superior efficacy as compared to placebo, and was equivalent to lithium in this regard.

A loading dose strategy for valproate has been developed for use in treating acute mania in an attempt to decrease the response time. Valproate is given at a dose of 20 mg/kg, and in a small open-label study (Keck et al., 1993), 53% of patients had a significant improvement in symptoms with generally good tolerability. Valproate loading using this same strategy (McElroy, 1996) has demonstrated equal times to respond for both valproate and haloperidol, an antipsychotic (Fig. 4-10). The advantage to the rapid response is the ability to use the same agent for both acute and prophylactic treatment.

There are no prospective placebo-controlled studies examining the efficacy of valproate in the prophylactic treatment of BPAD. Open-label studies suggest it is effective in long-term treatment and produces a decrease in the number and intensity of affective episodes. An open-label prospective study of 101 rapid cycling patients with BPAD I or II demonstrated an 87% response or higher in acute or prophylactic antimanic or antimixed state efficacy of valproate (Calabrese et al., 1993). Valproate, like many mood stabilizers, may be more effective in preventing manic or mixed episodes than in preventing episodes of depression. Across four open-label trials, only 58/195 (30%) of acutely depressed patients showed a significant improvement following treatment with valproate (McElroy et al., 1992). Patients with rapid-cycling, mixed or dysphoric mania, or secondary mania, are better candidates for valproate than for lithium. It is not clear if in pure mania or nonrapid cycling whether valproate would possess efficacy different than that observed with lithium.

Valproate is usually well tolerated. The most commonly observed side effects are gastrointestinal complaints, benign hepatic transaminase elevations, and neurological complaints such as tremor or sedation. Gastrointestinal symptoms include

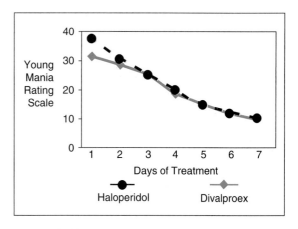

Figure 4–10. *Comparison of the response to valproate vs. haloperidol in inpatients with acute mania. From McElroy et al., 1996.*

nausea, vomiting, dyspepsia, indigestion, anorexia, or diarrhea. These tend to be more prevalent with initiation of treatment and diminish over time. Use of the divalproex sprinkles can further decrease gastrointestinal complaints as can the transient use of histamine H_2 receptor blockers or cisapride (propulsid). Most physicians will allow hepatic transaminase elevations up to two or three times the upper limits of normal without intervention other than perhaps to reduce the dose if clinically indicated. Decreased platelet counts, which are transient, are also occasionally observed with valproate treatment as is a prolongation of bleeding time, petechia or bruising. Patients may also note an increase in appetite and weight gain. There have been reports of hepatic failure in patients receiving valproate, although the population at risk appears to be primarily epileptic children under 2 years of age. The use of valproate during pregnancy has been associated with neural tube defects at a rate of 1 to 1.5% with first-trimester fetal exposure. Congenital heart disease may also be observed in the offspring of mothers treated with valproate. Most of these data are derived, however, from women with epilepsy, a group with a higher rate of offspring with birth defects than the general population.

Valproate may demonstrate drug-drug interactions with other medications that are highly bound to plasma proteins. Additionally, there may be an interaction between valproate and drugs that affect coagulation. In contrast to many other anticonvulsants, valproate does not induce hepatic microsomal enzymes, although it may inhibit the metabolism of other agents.

Valproate is available in a variety of formulations and dosages. The divalproex sodium coated particles in capsules (Depakote sprinkles) are available in a 125-mg size. Divalproex sodium delayed-release capsules (Depakote) are available as 125-, 250-, and 500-mg tablets. Valproic acid (Depakene) is formulated as 250 mg capsules, or as a liquid preparation, containing 250 mg/5 mL.

Prior to initiating valproate treatment the patient's physical health, including liver function and hematology, including platelets, should be assessed. Females of child-bearing potential should also have a pregnancy test because of the teratogenic effects of valproate. Starting doses are typically between 500 and 1000 mg/day in divided doses, although a loading strategy of 20 mg/kg can be utilized. Serum levels of valproate should be frequently monitored during dose titration, with reference ranges drawn at a 12-h trough level. The minimal therapeutic serum concentration is generally considered ≥ 50 μg/mL, with a therapeutic range between 50 to 120 μg/mL. Prophylactic administration of a multivitamin with zinc and selenium is recommended by many to prevent hair loss that may occur with this drug. Weekly to biweekly monitoring of hematological indices, including platelets, and liver function testing is suggested initially. After the patient is stabilized, these tests can be performed less often, with 6-month intervals being appropriate for patients on long-term valproate therapy. Transient increases in transaminases may occur during valproate treatment. These are usually not clinically significant and return to normal if the drug is stopped. Transaminase levels should be followed until a stable level is achieved. A similar approach is used if hematologic indices decrease. The patient should be strongly advised to report abnormal bruising or easy bleeding.

Carbamazepine

Carbamazepine (Tegretol and others) has been used in Europe since the 1960s for the treatment of epilepsy and paroxysmal pain syndromes such as trigeminal neuralgia. It was first reported to have efficacy in BPAD in 1971. Carbamazepine has been available in the United States since 1974 as a treatment of epilepsy, and later with an indication for trigeminal neuralgia. Carbamazepine treatment of bipolar disorder is not an FDA-approved indication, although the drug is often used for this purpose.

Chemically, carbamazepine is a member of the iminostilbene family with structural characteristics similar to the TCAs. Numerous studies have shown it is effective in the treatment of psychomotor and grand mal seizures. The anticonvulsant properties appear to be due to its ability to reduce polysynaptic responses and blockade post-tetanic potentiation. The mechanism of action in the treatment of BPAD is unclear, although actions on potassium channels, and effects on acetylcholine, adenosine, aspartate,

dopamine, GABA, glutamate, norepinephrine, serotonin, and substance P have been postulated to contribute to its antimanic activity (Macdonald, 1990; Post et al., 1991). Carbamazepine also exerts an effect on second messenger systems, decreasing both adenylate and guanylate cyclase activity and slowing the turnover of phosphoinositide (Post et al., 1992).

The oral absorption of carbamazepine is variable, with estimates of 75 to 85% bioavailability. Peak absorption following chronic administration is typically observed at 1.5 h with the suspension formulation, 4 to 5 h with conventional tablets, and 3 to 12 h following ingestion of the extended-release preparation. Approximately 75% of absorbed drug is bound to plasma proteins. Cerebrospinal fluid concentrations of carbamazepine are roughly equivalent to the systemic concentration of free drug. The hepatic cytochrome P450 system is primarily responsible for the metabolism of carbamazepine. A primary metabolite is the 10,11 epoxide that is formed by the cytochrome P450 3A4, has activity similar to the parent compound and is present at about 50% of the concentration of carbamazepine. Coadministration of valproate and carbamazepine produces an accumulation of the 10,11 epoxide metabolite. Like many other anticonvulsants, carbamazepine induces hepatic microsomal enzyme activity. The induction of its own metabolism diminishes its half-life from 25 to 65 h, to 12 to 17 h after 3 to 5 weeks of treatment. The induction of cytochrome P450 3A4 activity by carbamazepine has the potential to produce a number of clinically significant drug interactions. This necessitates a gradual increase in dose to maintain the same serum levels achieved early in treatment. The rate of carbamazepine metabolism returns quickly to normal such that after 7 days off of the drug over 65% of the autoinduction is lost (Schaffler et al., 1994). This suggests that with the noncompliant patient for whom carbamazepine is restarted, the initial dosing levels should be reduced over what may have been therapeutic during earlier treatment, with subsequent gradual upward titration as autoinduction reoccurs.

The efficacy of carbamazepine in bipolar disorder has been demonstrated in a number of studies, mostly with small sample sizes, and in comparisons to placebo, lithium, or neuroleptics. Pooled data from studies in which concurrent lithium or neuroleptics were not administered show a 50% efficacy rate for carbamazepine in acute mania compared to 56 and 61% for lithium or antipsychotic treatment, respectively; none of these differences was statistically significant from one another (Keck et al., 1992). The onset of action for carbamazepine is similar to neuroleptics and may be slightly faster than for lithium. Like other mood stabilizers, carbamazepine appears to be less efficacious in the treatment of depression, with only a 30 to 35% response rate generally observed. Carbamazepine has been demonstrated to have more efficacy in the treatment of patients with rapid cycling (Okuma, 1993). Predictors of response to carbamazepine include rapid cycling and mixed or dysphoric mania. Failure to respond to another anticonvulsant does not predict a poor outcome with carbamazepine (Post et al., 1984).

The most commonly encountered CNS side effects associated with carbamazepine are dizziness, drowsiness, disturbances of coordination, confusion, headache and fatigue. Gradual upward titration of the dose helps minimize responses. Carbamazepine toxicity can produce ataxia, dizziness, diplopia or sedation. Higher serum concentrations of carbamazepine lead to nystagmus, ophthalmoplegia, cerebellar signs, impairment of consciousness, convulsions, and respiratory dysfunction. Nausea, vomiting, and gastrointestinal distress, if it occurs, is more common early in treatment. Carbamazepine produces a decrease in white blood cell count in a number of patients, but values usually remain above 4000. Thrombocytopenia is also occasionally observed during treatment with this drug. Idiosyncratic blood dyscrasias occur at a rate between 1/10,000 and 1/125,000 patients. Carbamazepine can produce a rash which prompts discontinuation of the drug by many physicians. Hyponatremia will sometimes occur with carbamazepine treatment and is thought to be owing to its antidiuretic effect. The incidence of hyponatremia is between 6 and 31%, with the elderly at higher risk.

Carbamazepine is teratogenic, with first-trimester exposure being associated with an increased incidence of neural tube defects, fingernail hypoplasia, craniofacial defects, and developmental delay.

Carbamazepine interacts with a number of other drugs since the cytochrome P450 3A4 enzyme is induced during carbamazepine therapy. The reader is referred to the list of substrates for this enzyme for more details (Table 4-13). Oral contraceptives are of particular importance because they may be less effective during carbamazepine treatment.

Prior to initiating carbamazepine therapy the physical health of the patient, including liver function and hematology, including platelets, should be assessed. Females of childbearing potential should also have a pregnancy test performed. Starting doses of carbamazepine are typically between 200 to 400 mg/day in divided doses, although a loading dose strategy of 20 mg/kg has been described. Serum levels of carbamazepine should be checked during dose titration, with reference ranges drawn at a 12-h trough level. The therapeutic range is generally considered to lie between 4 and 12 μg/mL, although this is extrapolated from data obtained while treating epileptic patients. The usual dose range for carbamazepine is between 1000 to 2000 mg/day. Because there is no clear relationship between clinical outcome and serum concentrations of carbamazepine, dosing should be guided by clinical response rather than by aiming for a predetermined serum level. Autoinduction of its metabolism will often require a dose increase after 3 to 5 weeks of treatment, which can sometimes amount to as much as a doubling of the dose. Carbamazepine is available as 100-mg chewable tablets, 200-mg standard release tablets, and 100-, 200-, and 400-mg extended release tablets. It is also available as a liquid suspension at a concentration of 100 mg/5 mL.

Other Agents

Clozapine (Clozaril) and olanzapine (Zyprexa) are atypical antipsychotics for which there is evidence of efficacy in the treatment of acute mania. The necessity of weekly white blood cell counts and the side effect profile of clozapine usually limits its use to treatment resistant BPAD patients. Olanzapine, in contrast, does not require hematologic monitoring, and has a favorable side effect profile. There are ongoing placebo-controlled studies of olanzapine as monotherapy in acute mania. The usual therapeutic dose of olanzapine in the treatment of acute mania is between 10 and 20 mg, often given at bedtime as a single dose.

Lamotrigine (Lamictal) and gabapentin (Neurontin) are two newer generation anticonvulsants that may possess efficacy in mania, although no controlled studies have been conducted. Neither drug requires that serum levels be followed. Gabapentin was approved in 1993 for the treatment of epilepsy. While it is structurally similar to γ-aminobutyric acid (GABA), its precise mechanism of action remains undefined. Gabapentin has about 60% bioavailability, though this decreases with larger doses. It exhibits negligible (<3%) binding to serum proteins, has a serum half-life of 5 to 7 h and is excreted unchanged in the urine. The most common side effects associated with gabapentin are sleepiness, dizziness, unsteadiness, nystagmus, tremor, and double vision. The initial dose of gabapentin is 300 mg/day, with increases of 300 mg every 3 to 5 days. The usual dosing range in BPAD is 900 to 3200 mg/day. There does not appear to be a drug-drug interaction between Gabapentin, valproate, or carbamazepine.

Lamotrigine was approved in 1994 as a treatment for epilepsy and, like gabapentin, has found some utility as a mood stabilizer. Similar to gabapentin, lamotrigine has favorable side effect profile, but little data demonstrating its efficacy in BPAD. Lamotrigine may exert its anticonvulsant effects by inhibiting voltage-gated sodium channels. It is also a weak antagonist at 5HT3 receptors. The bioavailability of lamotrigine is 98% and is not affected by food. Peak serum concentrations occur 1.4 to 4.8 h after ingestion. The most common side effects reported for lamotrigine are dizziness, headache, double vision, unsteadiness, nausea, blurred vision, sleepiness, rash, and vomiting. The presence of a rash deserves special attention because they may progress to Stevens-Johnson syndrome and, rarely, toxic epidermal necrolysis which may be fatal.

Lamotrigine therapy is complicated by concurrent treatment with valproate or carbamazepine. Without concurrent carbamazepine or valproate, the initial dosing of lamotrigine is 25 to 50 mg per day with increases of 25 to 50 mg every 1 to 2 weeks. The therapeutic dose, though this is determined on the basis of clinical effect, appears to be 100 to 400 mg/day. Doses of 50 mg/day and above are often administered as divided doses. With concurrent valproate, the initial dose of lamotrigine is 12.5 mg/day, with a gradual increase. Because valproate inhibits the metabolism of lamotrigine a rapid dose escalation in the presence of valproate is associated with a higher incidence of rash. When carbamazepine, which induces drug metabolism, is coadministered, the dose of lamotrigine can be increased at a faster rate.

Calcium channel blockers have been used in the treatment of BPAD, although their role is not completely clear. Verapamil is the most widely studied of this class for the treatment of BPAD. Nimodipine may have efficacy in patients with ultrarapid cycling.

Clonazepam, (Klonopin) a high-potency benzodiazepine, has been used as monotherapy in acute mania, and as adjunctive medication in early treatment. While clonazepam has been reported to be superior to placebo (Edwards et al., 1991), lithium (Chouinard et al., 1983) and comparable to haloperidol (Chouinard, 1987), but less effective than lorazepam (Bradwejn et al., 1990), the total number of patients included in these trials is remarkably small. With the variety of mood stabilizers available today, most clinicians utilize benzodiazepines as an adjunct to other antimanic drugs, rather than as monotherapy.

Bipolar Depression

There is much less information on the treatment of depression in the patient with BPAD than on the treatment of mania. This is despite the often severe level of impairment observed in the depressed or mixed phases of BPAD. It is also difficult to assess treatment response in bipolar patients owing to the relatively high rate of spontaneous remission, the switch into mania, and the presence of multiple medications that is now more the rule than the exception. The treatment approach for the patient with BPAD-depression depends on the severity of the depression and their current treatment. Reinstitution of a mood stabilizer, if the patient is not currently taking one, is the first step. For those on mood stabilizers, the dose should be increased to the upper end of the therapeutic range if it can be tolerated.

Lithium treated patients who develop an episode of depression should have their serum lithium levels and thyroid function assessed to rule out lithium-induced hypothyroidism. The response rate to lithium as an antidepressant in BPAD is about 30% (Zornberg and Pope, 1993) as is the overall response rate to valproate or carbamazepine. Antidepressants are clearly effective in the treatment of the depressive component of BPAD. Double-blind, placebo-controlled trials of antidepressants for the treatment of depression in BPAD yield a response rate of 48 to 86% (Kalin, 1997). Imipramine (Baumhackl et al., 1989; Cohn et al., 1989); (Himmelhoch et al., 1991), desipramine (Sachs et al., 1994), moclobemide (Baumhackl et al., 1989), bupropion (Sachs et al., 1994), tranylcypromine (Himmelhoch et al., 1991), and fluoxetine (Cohn et al., 1989) have all demonstrated efficacy in the treatment of BPAD depression.

The question of antidepressant-induced mania in these patients is important. A retrospective review of clinical trials suggests a switch rate of 3.7% for both sertraline and paroxetine, compared to 4.2% with placebo, and 11.2% with TCAs (Peet, 1994). Premarketing trials of SSRIs have shown a switch rate of about 1% for these drugs in the treatment of major depression, obsessive-compulsive disorder-or panic disorder.

The cycle length in BPAD may be shortened in some patients treated with antidepressants. Wehr et al. (1988) compared 51 rapid cycling patients to 19 nonrapid cycling patients, the vast majority female. In 73% of the rapid cyclers, but only 26% of the nonrapid cyclers, the initial episode of hypomania or mania occurred during antidepressant therapy. Just over half (51%) of the rapid cycling group demonstrated cycle acceleration with antidepressant use, and a slowing down when antidepressants were discontinued. The TCAs cause a greater switch rate into mania and are less effective than either SSRIs or

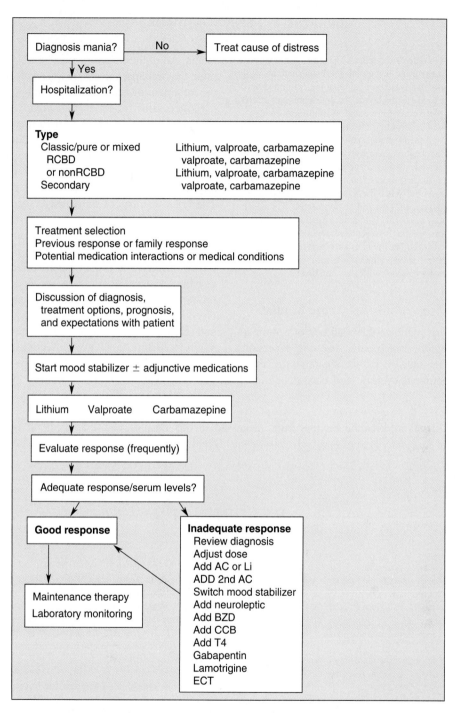

Figure 4–11. *Algorithm for the treatment of acute mania. (Abbreviations: RCBD, rapid cycling bipolar affective disorder; nonRCBD, nonrapid cycling bipolar affective disorder; AC, anticonvulsant, such as carbamazepine, valproate, gabapentin, or lamotrigine; Li, lithium; BZD, benzodiazepine; CCB, calcium channel blocker; ECT, electroconvulsive therapy).*

MAOIs. A recent controlled double-blind study demonstrated the efficacy of paroxetine in bipolar depressed patients with lithium levels that were suboptimal. For the lithium treated patients with optimal plasma levels, the antidepressant effects of lithium and paroxetine were equal to lithium alone.

The decisions confronting the clinician treating a BPAD patient who is depressed include a consideration of the risks of antidepressant-induced mania or hypomania, and the potential acceleration of episode cycling. In general, optimization of the mood stabilizer is the first order of business. Thyroid axis function should be assessed. When these measures are not successful, antidepressants or ECT should be considered. The SSRIs and bupropion may be less likely to induce mania or hypomania and, by extension, less likely to accelerate mood cycling, than either TCAs or MAOIs. The use of mood charts to track cycling frequency and response to treatments is helpful in the treatment of what is, for many patients, a lifelong condition.

Treatment Algorithms for Acute Mania

The factors that optimize the treatment of acute mania are; recognition of bipolar disorder, especially problematic in stage III mania, awareness of rapid cycling or nonrapid cycling, and classic or mixed mania. All of these factors must be weighed to determine the best approach to treatment. A flowchart for the treatment of acute mania is shown in Fig. 4-11.

Successful treatment can greatly enhance the quality of life for the patient with major depression or bipolar affective disorder. This chapter has focused on pharmacotherapy for these conditions, although combined pharmacotherapy and psychotherapy represents optimal treatment for most patients. The consequences of untreated or partially treated affective disorders on relationships and issues of compliance are just two of the areas that often require intervention. Although the available pharmacotherapy for affective disorders is quite effective, modern psychopharmacology is a very recent addition to the physician's armanentarium. For thousands of years, physicians have relied on empathy, communication, and caring as the primary therapeutic modality. While medications to treat affective disorders are truly life-saving advances, they represent only one component of our overall treatment approach.

For additional information on the drugs discussed in this chapter, see chapter 19 in *Goodman and Gilman's The Pharmacological Basis of Therapeutics* (Ninth Edition), McGraw-Hill, New York, 1996.

REFERENCES

American Psychiatric Association: Practice guideline for major depressive disorder in adults. *Am J Psychiatry* 1993;150(4)(Suppl):1–26.

Arminen SL, Ikonen U, Pulkkinen P, et al.: A 12-week double-blind multi-centre study of paroxetine and imipramine in hospitalized depressed patients. *Acta Psychiatr Scand* 1994;89:382–389.

Artigas F: Pindolol induces a rapid improvement of depressed patients treated with serotonin reuptake inhibitors. *Arch Gen Psychiatry* 1994;51:248–251.

Baker M, Dorzab J, Winokur G, Cadoret R: Depressive disease: Classification and clinical characteristics. *Comp Psychiatry* 1971;12:354–365.

Baumhackl U, Biziere K, Fischbach R, et al.: Efficacy and tolerability of moclobemide compared with imipramine in depressive disorder (DSM-III): An Austrian double-blind, multicentre study. *Br J Psychiatry* 1989;155(Suppl 6):78–83.

Beasely CM Jr, Holman SL, Potvin JH: Fluoxetine compared with imipramine in the treatment of depression. A multicenter trial. *Ann Clin Psychiatry* 1993;5:199–207.

Beck AT, Ward CH, Mendelson M, et al.: An inventory for measuring depression. *Arch Gen Psychiatry* 1961;4:53–63.

Bowden CL, Brugger AM, Swann AC, et al.: Efficacy of divalproex vs. lithium and placebo in the treatment of mania. *JAMA* 1994;271(12):918–924.

Bradwejn J, Shriqui C, Koszycki D, et al.: Double-blind comparison of the effects of clonazepam and lorazepam in mania. *J Clin Psychopharmacol* 1990;10:403–408.

Brady KT, Lydiard RB: Bipolar affective disorder and substance abuse. *J Clin Psychopharmacol* 1992;12:17S–22S.

Calabrese JR, Woyshville MJ, Kimmel SE, Rapport DJ: Predictors of valproate response in bipolar rapid cycling. *J Clin Psychopharmacol* 1993;13(4):280–283.

Carlson GS, Goodwin FK: The stages of mania: A longitudinal

analysis of the manic episode. *Arch Gen Psychiatry* 1973;28:221–228.

Carroll BJ, Feinberg M, Smouse PE, et al.: The Carroll rating scale. *Br J Psychiatry* 1981;138:194–200.

Chouinard G: Clonazepam in acute and maintenance treatment of bipolar disorder. *J Clin Psychiatry* 1987;48:29S–36S.

Chouinard G, Young SN, Annable L: Antimanic effect of clonazepam. *Biol Psychiatry* 1983;18:451–486.

Clerc GE, Ruimy P, Verdeau-Pauilles J, French Inpatient Study Group: A double-blind comparison of venlafaxine and fluoxetine in patients hospitalized for major depression and melancholia. *Int Clin Psychopharmacol* 1994;9:139–143.

Cohen LS, Friedman JM, Jefferson JW, et al.: A reevaluation of risk of in utero exposure to lithium. *JAMA* 1994;271(2):146–150.

Cohen LS, Sichel DA, Robertson LM, et al.: Postpartum prophylaxis for women with bipolar disorder. *Am J Psychiatry* 1995;152:1641–1645.

Cohn JB, Collins G, Ashbrook E, Wenicke JF: A comparison of fluoxetine, imipramine, and placebo in patients with bipolar depressive disorder. *Int Clin Psychopharmacol* 1989;4:313–322.

Cooke RG, Joffe RT, Levitt AJ: T_3 augmentation of antidepressant treatment in T_4-replaced thyroid patients. *J Clin Psychiatry* 1992;53:16–18.

Cooper TB, Berner PE, Simpson GM: The 24-hour serum lithium level as a prognosticator of dosage requirements. *Am J Psychiatry* 1973;130:601–603.

Danish University Antidepressant Group: Citalopram: Clinical effect profile in comparison with clomipramine. A controlled multicenter study. *Psychopharmacology* 1986;90:131–138.

Danish University Antidepressant Group: Paroxetine: A selective serotonin reuptake inhibitor showing better tolerance, but weaker antidepressant effect than clomipramine in a controlled multicenter study. *J Affect Disord* 1990;18:289–299.

Deniker P, Eygiem A, Bernheim R, et al.: Thyroid antibody levels during lithium therapy. *Neuropsychobiology* 1978;4:270–275.

Depression Guideline Panel: Depression in Primary Care: Volume 2. Treatment of Major Depression. Clinical Practice Guideline, Number 5, Rockville, MD, U.S. Department of Health and Human Services, Public Health Service, Agency for Health Care Policy and Research, 1993.

Dunner DL, Fieve RR: Clinical factors in lithium carbonate prophylaxis failure. *Arch Gen Psychiatry* 1974;30:229–233.

Edwards R, Stephenson U, Flewett T: Clonazepam in acute mania: a double-blind trial. *Aust NZ J Psychiatry* 1991;25:238–242.

Faedda GL, Tondo L, Baldessarini RJ, et al.: Outcome after rapid versus gradual discontinuation of lithium treatment in bipolar disorders. *Arch Gen Psychiatry* 1993;50:448–455.

Fava M, Rosenbaum JF, Cohen L, et al.: High-dose fluoxetine in the treatment of depressed patients not responsive to a standard dose of fluoxetine. *J Affect Disord* 1992;25:229–234.

Frank E, Kupfer DJ, Perel JM, et al.: Three-year outcomes for maintenance therapies in recurrent depression. *Arch Gen Psychiatry* 1990;47:1093–1099.

Goodwin FK, Jamison KR: *Manic-Depressive Illness*. New York, Oxford University Press, 1990.

Hamilton M: A rating scale for depression. *J Neurol Neurosurg Psychiatry* 1960;23:56–62.

Himmelhoch JM, Thase ME, Mallinger AG, Houck P: Tranylcypromine versus imipramine in anergic bipolar depression. *Am J Psychiatry* 1991;148:910–916.

Jefferson JW: Lithium: The present and the future. *J Clin Psychiatry* 1990;51(Suppl 8):4–19.

Joffe RT, Schuller DR: An open study of buspirone augmentation of serotonin reuptake inhibitors in refractory depression. *J Clin Psychiatry* 1993;54:269–271.

Kalin N: Management of the depressive component of bipolar disorder. *Depression and Anxiety* 1997;4:190–198.

Katona CLE, Abou-Saleh MT, Harrison DA, et al.: Placebo-controlled trial of lithium augmentation of fluoxetine and lofepramine. *Br J Psychiatry* 1995;166:80–86.

Keck PE Jr, McElroy SL, Nemeroff CB: Anticonvulsants in the treatment of bipolar disorder. *J Neuropsychiatry Clin Neurosci* 1992;4:395–405.

Keck PE Jr, McElroy SL, Tugrul KC, et al.: Valproate oral loading in the treatment of mania. *J Clin Psychiatry* 1993;54:305–308.

Kupfer DJ: Long-term treatment of depression. *J Clin Psychiatry* 1991;52 (Suppl 5):28–34.

Lazarus JH: *Endocrine and Metabolic Effects of Lithium*. New York, Plenum, 1986.

Macdonald RL: Carbamazepine: mechanisms of action, in Levy RH, Dreifuss FH, Mattson RH, et al. (eds): *Antiepileptic Drugs*. New York, Raven, 1990, pp. 447–455.

McElroy SL, Keck PE, Pope HG, Hudson JI: Valproate in the treatment of bipolar disorder: Literature review and clinical guide lines. *J Clin Psychopharmacol* 1992;12:42S–52S.

McElroy SL, Keck PE, Stanton SP, et al: A randomized comparison of divalproex oral loading versus haloperidol in the initial treatment of acute psychotic mania. *J Clin Psychiat* 1996;57:142–146.

Merikangas KR, Angst J, Isler H: Migraine and psychopathology. Results of the Zurich cohort study of young adults. *Arch Gen Psychiatry* 1990;147:573–578.

Montgomery SA, Asberg M: A new depression scale designed to be sensitive to change. *Br J Psychiatry* 1979;134:382–389.

Nelson JC, Docherty JP, Henschen GM, et al.: Algorithms for the treatment of subtypes of unipolar major depression. *Psychopharmacol Bull* 1995;31(3):475–482.

Nemeroff CB, DeVane CL, Pollock BG: Newer antidepressants and the cytochrome P450 system. *Am J Psychiatry* 1996;153:311–320.

Nierenberg AA, McLean NE, Alpert JE, Worthington JJ: Early nonresponse to fluoxetine as a predictor of poor 8-week outcome. *Am J Psychiatry* 1995;154:426–428.

Nierenberg AA, Feighenr JP, Rudolph R, et al.: Venlafaxine for treatment-resistant unipolar depression. *J Clin Psychopharmacol* 1994;14:419–423.

Nierenberg AA, Price LH, Charney DS, Heninger GR: After lithium augmentation: A retrospective follow-up of patients with antidepressant-refractory depression. *J Affect Dis* 1990;18:167-175.

Nordenstrom J, Strigard K, Perbeck L, et al.: Hyperparathyroidism associated with treatment of manic-depressive disorders with lithium. *Eur J Surg* 1992;158:207–211.

Norman KP, Cerrone KL, Reus VI: Renal lithium clearance as a rapid and accurate predictor of maintenance dose. *Am J Psychiatry* 1982;139:1625–1626.

Okuma T: Effects of carbamazepine and lithium on affective disorders. *Neuropsychobiology* 1993;27:138–145.

Peet M: Induction of mania with selective serotonin re-uptake inhibitors and tricyclic antidepressants. *Br J Psychiatry* 1994;164:549–550.

Perry PJ, Alexander B, Dunner FJ, et al: Pharmacokinetic protocol for predicting serum lithium levels. *J Clin Psychopharmacol* 1982;2:114–118.

Post RM, Altshuler LL, Ketter TA, et al.: Antiepileptic drugs in affective illness: clinical and theoretical implications, in Smith D, Treiman D, Trimble M (eds): *Advances in Neurology*, vol 55. New York, Raven, 1991, pp. 239–277.

Post RM, Berettine W, Uhde TW, et al.: Selective response to the anticonvulsant carbamazepine in manic depressive illness: A case study. *J Clin Psychopharmacol* 1984;4:178–185.

Post RM, Weiss RB, Chuang DM: Mechanisms of action of anticonvulsants in affective disorders: Comparison with lithium. *J Clin Psychopharmacol* 1992;12:23S–35S.

Quitkin FM, McGrath PJ, Stewart JW, et al.: Chronological milestones to guide drug change. When should clinicians switch antidepressants? *Arch Gen Psychiatry* 1996;53:785–792.

Richelson, E: Pharmacology of antidepressants: characteristics of the ideal drug. *MAYO Clinic Proc.* 1994;69:1069–1081.

Regier DA, Boyd JH, Burke JD Jr, et al.: One-month prevalence of mental disorders in the United States; based on five epidemiologic catchment area sites. *Arch Gen Psychiatry* 1988;45:977–986.

Sachs GS, Lafer B, Stoll AL, et al.: A double-blind trial of bupropion versus desipramine for bipolar depression. *J Clin Psychiatry* 1994;55:391–393.

Schaffler L, Bourgeois BF, Luders HO: Rapid reversibility of autoinduction of carbamazepine metabolism after temporary discontinuation. *Epilepsia* 1994;35:195–198.

Schweizer E, Weise C, Clary C, et al: Placebo-controlled trial of venlaflaxine for the treatment of major depression. *J Clin Psychopharmacol* 1991;11:233–236.

Strakowski SM, McElroy SL, Keck PW Jr, West SA: The co-occurrence of mania with medical and other psychiatric disorders. *Intl J Psychiatry Med* 1994;24:305–328.

Stuppaeck CH, Geretsegger C, Whitworth AB, et al.: A multicenter double-blind trial of paroxetine versus amitriptyline in depressed inpatients. *J Clin Psychopharmacol* 1994;14:241–246.

Suppes T, Baldessarini RJ, Faedda GL, Tohen M: Risk of recurrence following discontinuation of lithium treatment in bipolar disorder. *Arch Gen Psychiatry* 1991;48:1082–1088.

Thase ME, Fava M, Halbreich U, et al.: A placebo-controlled, randomized clinical trial comparing sertraline and imipramine for the treatment of dysthymia. *Arch Gen Psychiatry* 1996;53:777–784.

Van Der Meyden CH, Kruger AJ, Muller FO, et al.: Acute oral loading of carbamazepine-CR and phenytoin in a double-blind randomized study of patients at risk for seizures. *Epilepsia* 1994;35:189–194.

Vanelle JM, Attar-Levy D, Poirier MF, et al.: Controlled efficacy study of fluoxetine in dysthymia. *Br J Psychiatry* 1997;170:345–350.

Wehr TA, Sack DA, Rosenthal NE, Cowdry RW: Rapid cycling affective disorder: Contributing factors and treatment responses in 51 patients. *Am J Psychiatry* 1988;145:179–184.

Weiss MK, Tohen M, Zarate C Jr, Iversen A: Diagnosis and management of bipolar II disorder. *Comp Ther* 1994;20:121–124.

Wells KB, Stewart A, Hays RD, et al.: The functioning and well-being of depressed patients: Results from the Medical Outcomes Study. *JAMA* 1989;262:914–919.

Wernicke JF, Dunlop SR, Dornseif BE, et al.: Low-dose fluoxetine therapy for depression. *Psychopharmacol Bull* 1988;24:183–188.

Wernicke JF, Dunlop SR, Dornseif BE, Zerbe RL: Fixed-dose fluoxetine therapy for depression. *Psychopharmacol Bull* 1987;23:164–168.

Zimmer B, Rosen J, Thornton JE, et al.: Adjunctive lithium carbonate in nortriptyline-resistant elderly depressed patients. *J Clin Psychopharmacol* 1991;11:254–256.

Zornberg GL, Pope HG Jr: Treatment of depression in bipolar disorder: New directions for research. *J Clin Psychopharmacol* 1993;13:397–408.

Zung WW: A self-rating depression scale. *Arch Gen Psychiatry* 1965;12:63.

ATTENTION DEFICIT AND DEVELOPMENTAL DISORDERS

D.M. Kaplan, M.A. Grados, and A.L. Reiss

The terms attention-deficit/hyperactivity disorder _(ADHD) and_ developmental disorders _are based on descriptions of clinical phenomena rather than diseases, although there has been much effort to demarcate these entities in terms of a medical model; that is, with specific etiologies and pathophysiologies. Fragile X syndrome, with its comorbid mental retardation and hyperactivity, and increased incidence of autism, is one such example. This chapter is divided into four sections: ADHD, and three categories of developmental disabilities: learning disorders, focusing on developmental reading disorder, mental retardation, and autistic disorder._

Attention deficit hyperactivity disorder (ADHD) is a commonly diagnosed condition and is often the "bread and butter" of clinical practice for child and adolescent psychiatrists and pediatric neurologists. It also is treated by many pediatricians, who usually defer to the previous two specialists when treatment with psychostimulants fail. The condition may be lifelong and therefore can be well conceptualized as a developmental disorder. Adult ADHD, for example, has recently received much attention, although there is still much to learn about its pathophysiology, clinical features, and management. Although autistic disorder has been viewed as a fascinating "other-worldly" anomaly, studied, for example, by many of the best minds in child and adolescent psychiatry, authorities in mental retardation have suffered from low professional status, reflecting the position in society of this group of patients.

Psychopharmacology is only one of the modalities, albeit an important one, for the management of ADHD and the other developmental disorders. Just as there is importance in managing these disorders with a number of simultaneous interventions based on a "biopsychosocial-educational" perspective, so is there enormous value in a multidisciplinary ap-

proach. Psychopharmacology in this area still suffers from a paucity of new agents. Apart from the psycho-stimulants, few drugs have been adequately tested in these conditions, although the new generation of atypical antipsychotic drugs holds promise. Clinical psychopharmacologic trials for the pediatric age group lag behind their adult counterparts, necessitating the cautious use of drugs not formally approved for this purpose.

Psychopharmacologic management can be very effective when practiced by individuals who remain current with regard to the last information on brain–behavior interactions, and to approaches used to improve the feelings and functioning of patients. The practice of psychopharmacology for ADHD and the other developmental disorders is maximized by physicians able to truly empathize with their patients, challenging themselves with the question, "Is this how I'd want a member of _my_ family treated?"

PSYCHOPHARMACOLOGY OF ADHD

Attention-deficit/hyperactivity disorder (ADHD) is a description of a behavioral syndrome with a number of possible biopsychosocial etiologies. Its essential feature is a persistent pattern of inattention and/or hyperactivity-impulsivity that is more frequent and severe than is typically observed in individuals of the same age. ADHD is one of the most prevalent childhood and adolescent psychiatric disorders, making up as much as 50% of clinic populations (Cantwell, 1996).

Diagnosis

The diagnosis of ADHD has been modified continuously as described in the various editions of the *Diagnostic and Statistic Manual* (DSM) of the American Psychiatric Association (APA), with changing relative emphasis of the core symptoms. According to the DSM-IV, ADHD is subdivided into ADHD-Combined Type (both inattention and hyperactivity-impulsivity), ADHD-Predominantly Inattentive Type, and ADHD-Predominantly Hyperactive-Impulsive Type. Significant symptoms must be present for 6 months or more and be apparent in more than one setting (home, school, work, or social situations). The symptoms must cause significant impairment and be apparent before the age of 7.

Epidemiology

Community-based studies confirm that ADHD is the most prevalent psychiatric disorder in childhood and adolescence, with estimates of 5 to 10% in the elementary school population. Up to 7% of American school-aged children are treated with stimulants, 90% of the time with methylphenidate. Approximately 25% of children in special education programs are placed on a psychostimulant. ADHD is found more commonly in males, 9:1 in clinical samples and 4:1 in epidemiologic samples. This ratio may be owing, in part, to referral bias and differential patterns of symptom expression between genders.

Etiology

The etiology of ADHD is unknown. Fragile X syndrome, fetal alcohol syndrome, very low birth weight children, and a very rare genetic thyroid disorder can present behaviorally with ADHD but these cases comprise only a small percentage of the total. The search for an etiology has led to studies in the fields of genetics, neurochemistry, and structural and functional neuroimaging, among others. For example, reduced size in the rostrum and rostral body of the corpus callosum has been reported. Single photon emission computerized tomography (SPECT) studies have revealed focal cerebral hypoperfusion of striatum and hyperperfusion in sensory and sensorimotor areas of the cortex. Family genetic factors have been implicated in the etiology of ADHD for the past 25 years, with heritability estimated between 0.55 and 0.92. Family aggregation studies have indicated that ADHD and its comorbid problems run in families. Reduced levels of brain dopamine and norepinephrine turnover have been suggested by many studies, however brain neurochemistry is complex and single neurotransmitter theories are probably overly simplistic. Psychosocial and environmental factors, such as food additives or sugar intoxication, are not thought to play a primary etiologic role in ADHD (Cantwell, 1996).

Natural History

The normally exuberant preschool child can pose a diagnostic problem, although the preschooler with ADHD will often have additional symptoms such as temper tantrums, and argumentative, aggressive, and fearless behavior. Elementary school children often have difficulties with the cognitive demands of school as well as peer group problems. Through adolescence, symptoms of ADHD may change in quality or severity; a lower number of symptoms has been suggested as a cutoff point for the diagnosis in adolescence and possibly adulthood as well. For example, the core symptoms of ADHD might manifest as an internal sense of restlessness in older persons rather than gross motor activity. Difficulty in completing independent academic work might characterize adolescent ADHD and risk-taking behaviors such as frequent car or bike accidents might be additional manifestations of the disorder.

Three potential outcomes of ADHD have been described: "Developmental delay" (30% of subjects) where the individual outgrows the symptoms in early adulthood, "continual display" (40% of subjects) where impairment continues into adult life, and "developmental decay" (30% of subjects), where more serious psychopathology, such as substance abuse or antisocial personality disorders, develops alongside the ADHD symptoms. ADHD is thought to be a lifelong disability although, at present, adult ADHD has uncertain construct validity (Wilens and Biederman, 1992; Shaffer, 1994), with a varying response to psychostimulants. The disorganized adult with ADHD might require the use of written lists as reminders and might be plagued by shifting activities, unfinished projects, procrastination, and explosive outbursts. Probably only a minority of children proceed to adult ADHD, and the diagnosis is complicated by frequent comorbidity with, for example, depression and antisocial personality disorder.

Comorbidity

Up to two-thirds of elementary school age children with ADHD have at least one other diagnosable psychiatric disorder. There is an increased incidence of conduct disorder, oppositional defiant disorder, learning disorders, communication disorders, anxiety and mood disorders, Tourette syndrome, or chronic tics. Also described is an inability to appreciate social cues or a lack of social "savoir-faire."

Assessment and Diagnosis

At present the diagnosis of ADHD is purely clinical since there are no laboratory tests or biologic markers that can be used to confirm the diagnosis. Diagnostic tools that are used include parent, child, and teacher interviews, observations of the parent and child, behavioral rating scales, physical and neurologic examinations, and cognitive testing. Audiology and vision testing might also be required. At the initial visit, a detailed developmental and symptomatic history should be taken, including medical, neurological, family, and psychosocial histories. Symptoms should only be considered meaningful if they exceed those expected of a child at the same age and cognitive level.

A variety of general or specific rating scales may be employed to gather information. A widely used

example of the former is Achenbach's Child Behavior Checklist (CBCL) with parent and teacher versions that can be used as a broad-based screen. More specific scales developed for ADHD include those devised by Connors, which include the Connors Parent Rating Scale (CPRS), the Connors Teachers Rating Scale (CTRS), the Connors Teacher's Questionnaire (CTQ), and the Abbreviated Rating Scale (ARS) (Conners and Barkley, 1985). Other specific scales for ADHD are Swanson's SNAP and Pelham's Disruptive Behavior Disorder Scale. Specialized tests such as the Continuous Performance Task (CPT) or the Paired Associate Learning (PAL) should not be used alone to provide a definitive diagnosis of ADHD.

The following approach has been found to obviate false positives and negatives in the diagnosis of ADHD.

1. A comprehensive interview of all parenting figures and relevant school personnel focusing on essential symptoms complemented by a developmental, academic, family, social, medical, and mental health history.
2. A developmentally appropriate interview with the child assessing symptoms pertaining to ADHD as well as anxiety, depression, suicidality, and psychosis.
3. A medical evaluation screening for sensory deficits and neurological problems.
4. Cognitive assessment of strengths and weaknesses in this area.
5. The use of general and more specific rating scales for ADHD.
6. Assessments of speech and language and fine and gross motor function when necessary.

ADHD is diagnosed in the United States using the criteria of the *Diagnostic and Statistic Manual* of the American Psychiatric Association (Table 5-1). Although DSM-III, DSM-III-R, and DSM-IV differ on the arrangement of the core symptoms, there is general global consistency among them (Cantwell, 1996). DSM-IV divides the symptoms into an inattention domain and a hyperactivity/impulsivity domain, with each dimension having nine symptoms.

Table 5-1
DSM-IV Criteria for Attention Deficit/Hyperactivity Disorder

A. Either 1 or 2:

1. Six (or more) of the following symptoms of **inattention** have persisted for at least 6 months to a degree that is maladaptive and inconsistent with developmental level.

Inattention
   a. Often fails to give close attention to details or makes careless mistakes in schoolwork, work, or other activities
   b. Often has difficulty sustaining attention in tasks or play activities
   c. Often does not seem to listen when spoken to directly
   d. Often does not follow through on instructions and fails to finish schoolwork, chores, or duties in the workplace (not because of oppositional behavior or failure to understand instructions)
   e. Often has difficulties organizing tasks and activities
   f. Often avoids, dislikes, or is reluctant to engage in tasks that require sustained mental effort (such as schoolwork or homework)
   g. Often loses things necessary for tasks or activities (e.g., toys, school assignments, pencils, books, or tools)
   h. Is often easily distracted by extraneous stimuli
   i. Is often forgetful in daily activities

2. Six (or more) of the following symptoms of **hyperactivity-impulsivity** have persisted for at least 6 months to a degree that is maladaptive and inconsistent with developmental level.

Hyperactivity
   a. Often fidgets with hands or feet or squirms in seat
   b. Often leaves seat in classroom or in other situations in which remaining seated is expected
   c. Often runs about or climbs excessively in situations where it is inappropriate (in adolescents or adults, may be limited to selective feelings of restlessness)
   d. Often has difficulty playing or engaging in leisure activities quietly
   e. Is often "on the go" or often acts as if "driven by a motor"
   f. Often talks excessively

Impulsivity
   g. Often blurts out answers before questions have been completed
   h. Often has difficulty awaiting turn
   i. Often interrupts or intrudes on others (e.g., butts into conversations or games)

B. Some hyperactive-impulsive or inattentive symptoms that caused impairment were present before the age of 7 years.
C. Some impairment from the symptoms is present in two or more settings (e.g., at school [or work] and at home).
D. There must be clear evidence of clinically significant impairment in social, academic, or occupational functioning.
E. The symptoms do not occur exclusively during the course of a Pervasive Developmental Disorder, Schizophrenia, or other Psychotic Disorder, and are not better accounted for by another mental disorder (e.g., Mood Disorder, Anxiety Disorder, Dissociative Disorder, or a Personality Disorder).

Code based on type:
Attention-Deficit/Hyperactivity Disorder, Combined Type: If both Criteria A1 and A2 are met for the past 6 months
Attention-Deficit/Hyperactivity Disorder, Predominantly Inattentive Type: If Criterion A1 is met but Criterion A2 is not met for the past 6 months
Attention-Deficit/Hyperactivity Disorder, Predominantly Hyperactive-Impulsive Type: If Criterion A2 is met but Criterion A1 is not met for the past 6 months

For individuals (especially adolescents and adults) who currently have symptoms but no longer meet full criteria, "In Partial Remission" should be specified.
SOURCE From American Psychiatric Association, 1994.

The combined type requires that the individual has six or more symptoms of the nine symptoms from both the inattention and the hyperactivity/impulsivity domains. The predominantly inattentive type consists of six or more inattention symptoms and five or fewer hyperactive/impulsive symptoms. The predominantly hyperactive/impulsive type consists of six or more symptoms of the hyperactive/impulsive dimension and five or fewer of the inattention dimension. In all cases, the symptoms must be more frequent and severe than those of children of comparable developmental level and must cause significant functional impairments.

Clinical Description

Typically, individuals with ADHD have trouble staying on task, are distractible, and appear as if their mind is elsewhere. They may avoid situations in which close attention to details or organizational skills are needed. A pattern of losing necessary objects or general forgetfulness is often observed. Hyperactivity may be manifested by fidgetiness, excessive running or climbing, by constantly appearing to be "on the go," or by excessive talking. Hyperactivity may improve with age, manifesting in adolescence or adulthood only as a subjective sense of restlessness. Impulsivity may be manifested by impatience, difficulty in delaying responses, blurting out answers, and trouble waiting one's turn. Associated with the disorder are low self-esteem, low frustration tolerance, noncompliance, aggression, poor social functioning, and learning disorders. These deficits lead to impairments in academic, peer, and family functioning. Symptoms can be found as early as age 3, where clinical observations might include pronounced motor activity, excessive climbing, aggressiveness, and destructiveness (Greenhill, 1995).

Nonpharmacologic Treatment of ADHD

The decision to employ medication is based on the severity of the symptoms and the preferences of the child, parents, caretaker, and school. It also depends on the ability of the environment to mitigate and cope with the child's problem behaviors and the success or failure of previous treatments. At present, a multiple-modality approach combining medical and psychosocial therapies is regarded as preferable. Medical and psychosocial treatment have complimentary effects and psychosocial interventions may improve symptoms during the period when the effect of the medication has diminished.

A number of home- and school-based nonpharmacologic strategies (including behavioral modification) as well as parent management training, such as contingency management techniques, and a daily school-home report card or a point-token response system are utilized. Cantwell (1996), reports that parent management training helps to reduce disruptive behavior at home, increase confidence in the parenting role, and decrease family stress. Other possible techniques mentioned by Cantwell are: parent counseling; modification of the school milieu; social skills group therapy; and individual counseling or therapy to treat low self-esteem, depression, or anxiety, and improve impulse control and social skills. The most appropriate educational environment is a structured classroom with the child placed in front of the room, close to the teacher, where he or she may be less easily distracted and more able to focus. Children with ADHD respond to predictable well-organized schedules and rules. Tangible rewards, reprimands, and time-outs can be used in both school and home settings. School placement is very important, varying from a regular classroom with or without individual tutoring, a resource program, a self-contained special class, or a special school. The clinician can play an important role in assessing the need for specialized educational interventions and in facilitating school placement.

A number of summer treatment programs have been developed that address not only academic performance but also behavioral management and social skills. Information about support groups, such as Children and Adults with Attention Deficit Disorders (CHADD), might prove useful for parents, providing group support and knowledge about working with school systems and resources in the community. Older siblings can also serve as positive reinforcement for their affected brother or sister. Additionally, literature is now available for parents, teachers, and the children themselves describing ADHD in nontechnical language. Assessment and treatment of parental, marital, and family psychopathology and dysfunction will usually enhance all other therapeutic endeavors.

Pharmacologic Treatment of ADHD

Central nervous system stimulants is the major class of drugs indicated for ADHD. Among these the most commonly used are methylphenidate (Ritalin), dextroamphetamine sulfate (Dexedrine), and pemoline (Cylert). In addition to dextroamphetamine sulfate, there is a mixed amphetamine salt, recently marketed as Adderall, which combines racemic amphetamine with dextroamphetamine. The popularity of methylphenidate and dextroamphetamine has been reinforced by their rapid, dramatic, and normalizing effects and low cost. They are relatively safe medications with a wide range of tolerated doses and wide therapeutic margins. Symptoms most likely to improve with these medications are restlessness, hyperactivity, impulsivity, disruptive, and aggressive behaviors.

Stimulants decrease activity in structured settings such as the classroom, reducing oppositionality, aggression, and conduct symptoms, thereby improving behavior, academic performance, and productivity. In less restricted situations, however, they have yielded inconsistent results. Drug treatment has also shown positive changes in mother-child, sibling, family, teacher-child, and peer interactions. In addition, participation in leisure time activities such as sports or games may be improved by these medications.

Comorbidity

Comorbidity is generally high among children with ADHD. This calls into question the validity of ADHD as a distinct clinical entity. British clinicians have a higher threshold for a diagnosis of ADHD, even when using the same diagnostic criteria, and some British psychiatrists even doubt the existence of the disorder as a discrete clinical entity. Children with comorbid diagnoses might react differently to certain medications. For example, comorbid anxiety has been reported to predict a reduced response to stimulants or to increase their untoward effects. Although, in general, psychostimulants are probably more effective than behavioral interventions, and possibly almost as effective as stimulants and behavioral therapy together, this depends to a large extent on comorbidity.

Decision Tree for Medication in ADHD

Methylphenidate is usually the first choice for ADHD, but dextroamphetamine is often equally effective, having similar effects on hyperactivity, inattention, distractibility, and impulsivity. Although dextroamphetamine and methylphenidate seem to be equally effective, not all children respond equally well, and about one-quarter respond favorably to one or the other but not both. However, methylphenidate might be slightly more effective than dextroamphetamine in reducing motor activity. A more variable effect has been found among preschoolers and adults. Notably, an 18% placebo effect for children with ADHD demonstrate the remarkable efficacy of stimulants.

Magnesium pemoline is probably less effective than the other two stimulants. Until recently it was considered the third choice of psychostimulant after methylphenidate and dextroamphetamine; however, recent reports of increasingly severe liver toxicity, including liver failure, have decreased enthusiasm for pemoline. A reasonable third choice after methylphenidate and dextroamphetamine is the atypical antidepressant bupropion (Wellbutrin), which, in spite of its known risk for lowering the seizure threshold, has been found effective for ADHD (Conners et al., 1996).

The next option would be either a tricyclic thought to have acceptable cardiac risk, that is, nortriptyline or imipramine, or one of the α-adrenergic agonists (first choice if the patient has tics or there is a family history of tics or Tourette syndrome). The two available α-adrenergic agonists are clonidine (available both in tablet and skin patch forms) and guanfacine (available in tablet form alone), which is less sedating than clonidine. Mood stabilizers, such as sodium valproate, lithium, and carbamazepine, should be considered next, particularly if there is a suspected comorbid or family history of mood disorder. Desipramine might also be considered if there is no evidence of cardiac problems on history or ECG. Even so, caution must be exercised with desipramine since it has been associated with four sudden deaths. Indeed, in three of these cases desipramine was prescribed for ADHD. It should be noted that dietary management and vitamin therapies have not proven their usefulness in the treatment of ADHD and might even be harmful (Aman and Singh, 1988).

Mechanisms of Action of the Psychostimulants

The psychostimulants are amine (noncatecholamine) sympathomimetics and function as indirect aminergic agonists. Their primary effect is to increase the levels of dopamine and norepinephrine in the synaptic cleft by blocking their reuptake into the presynaptic neuron (Greenhill, 1995). Dextroamphetamine (Dexedrine) releases cytoplasmic dopamine and blocks dopamine, norepinephrine, and serotonin reuptake. Methylphenidate (Ritalin) has structural and pharmacologic properties similar to amphetamine, although its mode of action is somewhat different. Thus, methylphenidate does not release dopamine although it blocks catecholamine reuptake, with greater effects on dopamine than on norepinephrine. The chemical structures of dextroamphetamine and methylphenidate are shown in Figure 5-1. The psychostimulants are well absorbed when taken orally and readily cross the blood-brain barrier. Food enhances their absorption. In children, stimulants achieve peak plasma levels in 2 to 3 hours with a half-life of 4 to 6 h, although there is a large interindividual variation. Subjective clinical effects seem to peak earlier than plasma levels, at approximately 1 to 3 h. Methylphenidate reaches peak plasma levels in 1 to 2 h (more rapidly than dextroamphetamine), begins taking effect within 30 min, and has a half-life of 2.5 h. Some studies suggest that behavioral benefits occur mainly during the absorption phase. Pemoline, which is structurally different from other stimulants, also blocks dopamine reuptake, although it has minimal sympathomimetic effects. In children, its onset of action appears to be about as rapid as other stimulants, it reaches peak serum level in 2 to 4 h, and has a half-life of 12 h, potentially enabling once per day dosing.

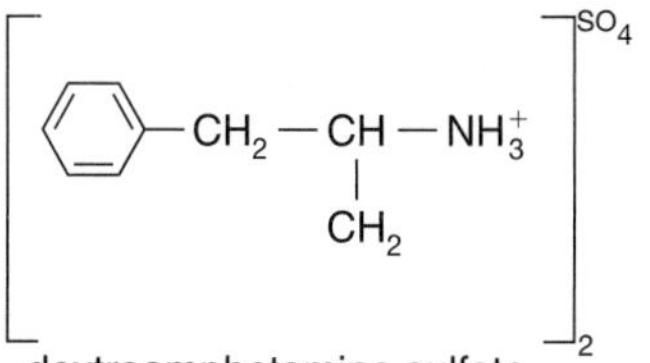

Dextroamphetamine and methylphenidate improve performance on tests of attention, vigilance, reaction time, short-term memory, and visual and verbal learning. This may be due to an improved executive function "signal-to-noise" ratio, manifesting as more focused attention and less distraction by extraneous stimuli. These stimulant actions are not specific for individuals with ADHD, with nonaffected children and adults showing similar cognitive and behavioral effects. Despite improved performance on various measures, children's overall academic performance and achievement have not conclusively shown long-term improvement when treated with psychostimulants. Also, long-term social gains, such as better life adjustment, or better jobs have not been demonstrated with these medications.

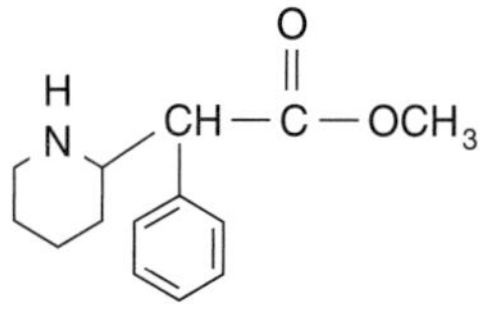

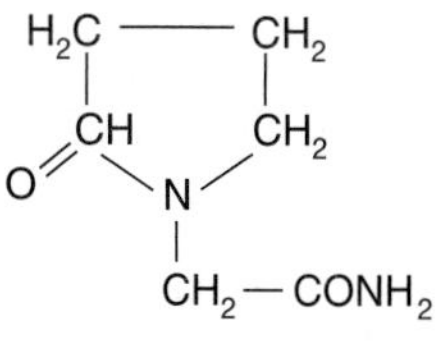

There is a suggestion that the stimulants have a dissociation of dose-response curves with improvements in one domain (e.g., hyperactivity) occurring while decrements are seen in others (e.g., attention). Known as the "Sprague effect" (Sprague and Sleator, 1977), this might be owing to a type of cognitive constriction interfering with cognitive flexibility in a subgroup of patients at doses where the behavioral effects of the medication are maximized. In these cases, the dose should be lowered. This impairment in cognitive functioning might be particularly disadvantageous for developmentally disabled children who may already be overfocused and perseverative (Harris, 1995).

Physiologic and Psychophysiologic Effects of the Psychostimulants

Stimulants excite the medullary respiratory center, without any significant effects on respiratory rate. They also stimulate the reticular activating system, sometimes resulting in insomnia, which may account for some of their effects on attention and task performance. Direct actions on the cardiovascular system mildly elevate systolic and diastolic blood pressure (Greenhill, 1995), although this is rarely of clinical significance. Stimulants also relax the bronchial smooth muscle, cause some contraction of the urinary bladder sphincter, and have unpredictable gastrointestinal effects. Dextroamphetamine has been reported to suppress mean-sleep-related prolactin.

Adverse Effects of the Psychostimulants

The most common short-term adverse effects of the stimulants are insomnia, anorexia, and weight loss. Appetite suppression is probably owing to an effect on the lateral hypothalamic nucleus that mediates

Figure 5–1. *The chemical structures of dextroamphetamine, methylphenidate, and piracetam.*

satiety. This sometimes results in rebound hunger, necessitating a late evening meal.

Although growth suppression is generally thought to be temporary, there are reports of statistically significant decreases in height and weight velocity during chronic treatment with dextroamphetamine and methylphenidate. This might prove important for those individuals who do not seem able to adjust to the growth suppression. Generally, dextroamphetamine's longer half-life, and its effect on prolactin suppression, might lead to more pronounced weight and height suppression. Less common adverse effects are dizziness, headache, nausea, abdominal pain, and drowsiness; however, these are generally short-lived and rarely require drug treatment be terminated. Stomachache, nausea, and loss of appetite can be managed by reducing the dosage or changing the dosing schedule by, for example, giving stimulants in the middle of the meal, using sustained-release preparations, or adding antacids. As a rule, relatively few adverse effects occur with dosages below 1 mg/kg of methylphenidate or 0.5 mg/kg of dextroamphetamine per day.

An important concern with stimulant therapy is the possible triggering, unmasking, or exacerbation of tics or irreversible Tourette syndrome, although cases have been reported where both the tics and the ADHD improved with this treatment. Other common untoward effects of stimulants are dysphoria, flattening of affect, and irritability, particularly among developmentally disabled children. Behavioral rebound on withdrawal, or wearing off of the psychostimulants, can also be a problem. In this case, behavior becomes worse than baseline, with over-talkativeness, irritability, noncompliance, and insomnia beginning 5 to 15 h after the last dose and lasting half an hour or more. Sometimes behavioral signs are confused with an exaggeration of presenting complaints (Greenhill, 1995). Behavioral rebound most often occurs in preschoolers, and slow-release preparations, or a small afternoon dose of methylphenidate, might help.

Rare untoward effects of stimulants are leukocytosis, toxic psychosis with tactile and visual hallucinations, mania, paranoia, choreoathetosis (pemoline), cardiac arrhythmias (particularly rare with pemoline), hypersensitivity, and angina. A possible lowered seizure threshold with methylphenidate and increased seizure threshold with dextroamphetamine has been suggested although, overall, it is believed that at therapeutic doses there is no significant effect on seizure activity, particularly if the patient's seizures are already controlled with antiepileptics.

Of great public concern is the possible abuse potential of psychostimulants. Although euphoria is noted with these agents in normal young adults, none is reported among normal or hyperactive prepubertal children. Although there is some abuse potential, it has been mostly limited to adult drug abusers and individuals with antisocial personality disorders who are using methylphenidate or dextroamphetamine intravenously. Recently, however, there have been news reports of abuse of methylphenidate by children and adolescents. As a result, methylphenidate and dextroamphetamine are DEA class II substances, with a number of states requiring prescriptions in triplicate. Pemoline, on the other hand, is a noncontrolled class IV substance. Concerns have also been raised that psychostimulants have been inappropriately prescribed to children not conforming to acceptable classroom behavior, leading to public skepticism about the use of the psychostimulants in general.

Contraindications to the Psychostimulants

Contraindications are few and include psychosis and tics or Tourette's syndrome (a relative contraindication). Tourette's should be distinguished from mild transient tics that are common in children. According to a recent study, tics subsided in a substantial majority of children in spite of continued treatment with stimulants. If this does not occur, adjunct treatment of the tics with clonidine, guanfacine, haloperidol, or pimozide is usually effective. Other contraindications are a medical condition precluding the use of sympathomimetics, or drug abuse among family members of a child with ADHD or in an adult being treated for ADHD. If the latter is a problem, pemoline, the least euphorigenic of the stimulants, bupropion, or a tricyclic antidepressant should be considered. Borderline personality disorder is another relative contraindication for psychostimulants since they might increase mood lability.

CLINICAL PHARMACOLOGY OF ADHD

Dosing Strategy

Medication therapy can be divided into baseline, titration, and maintenance phases. Baseline data required include height, weight, blood pressure, heart rate, and blood count. The use of rating scales is important to record the extent and severity of core and associated symptoms, the most popular being the Connors Teachers Rating Scale (CTRS) and the Connors Parents Rating Scale (CPRS). Standardized scoring methods for the CTRS can be used to generate a hyperactivity factor scale (Greenhill, 1995).

Monitoring Response

A 25% decline in global teacher rating on the hyperactivity factor of the Connors Teacher Questionnaire (CTQ) is generally considered a moderately satisfactory response to therapy. Another method of monitoring response is the use of a computerized Continuous Performance Test that assesses impulsivity (errors of commission) and inattention (errors of omission). The Abbreviated Rating Scale (ARS) is popular as a monitoring instrument. Completed by the parent or teachers, this test has demonstrated validity, and its 10-point scale, yielding a maximum severity rating of 30, is uncomplicated and it can be rapidly completed.

Routine Blood Work

Risk of hepatitis and hepatic failure with pemoline mandates monitoring of liver function tests at initiation and every 6 months thereafter. Regarding the other stimulants, a baseline full blood count and blood chemistry is sometimes performed and, if normal and in the absence of symptoms, there is usually no need to repeat these studies during titration and maintenance phases.

Dosing

It is recommended that either methylphenidate or dextroamphetamine be attempted with the individual who has never received stimulants before since few naive patients fail to respond to these agents (Elia and Rapaport, 1991). There are various dosing strategies for these drugs (Figure 5-2). The first is a stepwise titration method. Preschoolers can start on a single 7:30 or 8:00 A.M. dose of 2.5 to 5.0 mg of methylphenidate, given after breakfast, checking carefully for intensity and duration of response. It is recommended that this morning dose be titrated upward by 2.5 to 5.0 mg increments until a satisfactory response is obtained. The second dose, if needed, should be given 30 min before the effect of the first dose appears to wear off. The second dose should be initiated at one-half the maximum of the first dose and, again, titrated upward in incremental fashion until desired results are obtained. In this way the patient will have smooth coverage with less risk of rebound. The dose can be increased to a maximum of 10 to 15 mg bid, with dose changes every 3 to 7 days until the therapeutic effect or adverse events occur. An afternoon (third) dose of 2.5 to 10 mg, again 30 min before the response to the previous dose has terminated, or just before homework, might be added. For school-aged children the titration might begin with 5 mg in place of 2.5 mg.

The second strategy is to dose by weight using 0.3 to 1.2 mg/kg, with most preferring 0.3 to 0.6 mg/kg. The maximal recommended dose is 60 mg/day.

A third strategy entails the use of empiric starting doses, where the usual beginning dose of dextroamphetamine is 5 mg bid (for ages 6 or older), of methylphenidate is 5 mg bid, and of pemoline is 18.75 mg, increasing by 18.75 mg weekly to 75 mg/day or until desired clinical response is seen. Manufacturers recommend a maximum daily dose of methylphenidate of 112.5 mg. Pemoline's 12-h half-life allows for once or twice daily dosing, which can serve to overcome the stigma of the child being medicated at school and the reluctance of some school authorities to administer medication. If the patient has never taken stimulants before, half the usual starting dose can be considered initially. Adderall, a new mixed salt amphetamine, is increasingly being prescribed because of its possibly improved pharmacokinetics and longer duration of action. It can be given once or twice a day at doses similar to dextroamphetamine. Lack of improvement after 2 wk at a maximum dosage of dextroamphetamine or methylphenidate, or 5 weeks of pemoline, is an indication to terminate the medication and reevaluate the patient.

Because psychostimulants cause anorexia and gastric discomfort, and their absorption is enhanced with meals, it is advisable to administer them with or immediately after meals. Different dosages may be optimum for different behaviors; for example, lower for cognitive improvement versus higher for overall clinical improvement. Dosages must be reevaluated as the child grows, with increases corresponding to increases in lean body weight and decreases sometimes necessary after

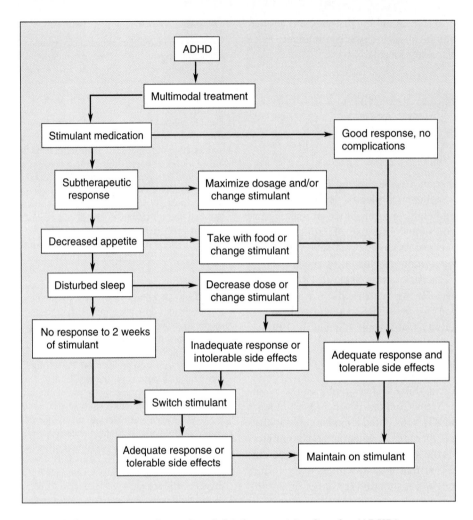

Figure 5–2. *Treatment of attention deficit/hyperactivity disorder (ADHD).*

puberty. Upon commencing a medication trial, a written record should be made of possible risks and benefits as well as plans for future trials if this should fail. Obviously, signed informed consent, as well as assent by the child or adolescent, should be clearly recorded in the chart.

Detailed dosing instructions should be written by the caretaker and checked by the service provider with a copy kept for the chart. A separate running list of new medications started and stopped, as well as changes in dosage, provides a convenient way of tracking medication trials, helps plan future trials, and provides a logical therapeutic plan for insurance companies, should it be required. At the outset of the maintenance phase, a regimen should be established for a pattern of regular revisits, the frequency of ratings, and off-drug periods.

Wherever possible, tentative duration of treatment should be stated, alleviating some of the parents/caretakers misgivings about medication. Planning in single school-year units is convenient, with a possible drug-free trial period during a non-stressed portion of the school year (Greenhill, 1995). Sometime after the initiation period, doses can be set slightly lower. Regular visits enable observation, assessment of beneficial and untoward effects, and a review of academic and social progress. Counseling and educational guidance can also be given at this time. Medication compliance should be assessed, with parents/caretakers encouraged to bring the child's medication bottle for a pill count. At each monthly visit height, weight (preferably plotted on growth charts), blood pressure, and heart rate should be monitored. An annual complete physical examination, including full blood count and liver function studies (biannually for pemoline) is advisable.

Stimulant medication usually can be halted abruptly without adverse consequences. It is uncertain whether tolerance develops to the benefits of these drugs. Often, "pseudotolerance" is noted, which is usually related to poor compliance (Greenhill, 1995), although it might be owing to attenuation of a placebo response or lower efficacy of a generic preparation. During the maintenance phase, both written and verbal contact, if possible, should be maintained with the teacher and/or principal in addition to the regular completion of rating scales, such as the CTPS and the Abbreviated Rating Scale (ARS). The rating scales should be obtained at least every 4 months and particularly during medication or dosage changes or during exacerbation of symptoms. Methylphenidate is approved only for those 6 years of age and upward, although many clinicians use it as a first choice for preschoolers. There has been limited experience with methylphenidate in adults. In this case the dose can be administered at 1 mg/kg per day or more, up to a maximum of 60 mg/day.

Drug Holidays

In the past, drug holidays were recommended to compensate for growth suppression. Today it is appreciated that learning occurs both in and outside the classroom and that stimulants have the potential to improve peer and family relationships. Therefore, drug holidays are not routinely recommended and should be individualized. For example, some parents will elect not to dose over weekends if the child is relatively manageable. This decision is often influenced by the exaggerated public concern about the dangers of the psychostimulants, particularly their abuse potential. The drug can be discontinued once a year to assess whether there is a continued need for treatment.

Drug Combinations

Clonidine is frequently combined with the psychostimulants, particularly methylphenidate. This combination is used particularly for sleep disturbance owing to ADHD or insomnia caused by the psychostimulants themselves. There have been concerns regarding the use of clonidine with methylphenidate, with four recently reported sudden deaths of children receiving this combination. The exact role, if any, of these medications in the deaths is unclear. A conservative approach might be to refrain from simultaneous dosing with these medications, particularly when treating children with cardiovascular disease, using the clonidine only for sedation before bed. Open studies of tricyclic antidepressants and α-adrenergic agonists administered to children and adolescents with ADHD and comorbid tic disorder have yielded positive results. Clonazepam has also been used successfully with methylphenidate for tics. Other combinations used occasionally include the addition of a tricyclic antidepressant to a stimulant. A serotonergic agent, such as fluoxetine or sertraline, has also been combined with a stimulant, particularly in cases of a comorbid mood disorder. However, this combination may enhance agitation.

Toxicity

The use of a monoamine oxidase inhibitor together with a stimulant is contraindicated owing to the risk of a potentially fatal hypertensive crisis. Systemic agents used for asthma, such as theophyline, can produce palpitations, tachycardia, dizziness, and agitation, making it preferable to use inhaled bronchodilators or steroids. Dextroamphetamine blocks the action of propranolol and slows absorption of phenytoin and phenobarbital. Methylphenidate can elevate blood levels of some antidepressants, coumarin anticoagulants, and phenylbutazone.

Dose forms of the psychostimulants. Methylphenidate is available in 5-, 10-, and slow-release 20-mg tablet forms. Both regular and slow-release forms are efficacious, although 20-mg sustained-release MPH is probably not equivalent to 10 mg bid. Sustained-release preparations of methylphenidate have not been widely accepted by clinicians despite their greater ease of use. Those prescribing the sustained-release form generally increase the total daily dose by 30 to 50%.

Dextroamphetamine is available as 5-mg tabs and as long-acting dextroamphetamine spansules in 5-, 10-, and 15-mg forms. The sustained-release form of dextroamphetamine does not vary in dosage from the regular form. Pemoline is available in 18.75-, 37.5-, and 75-mg tablets as well as 37.5-mg chewable tablets. The mixed amphetamine salt preparation (Adderall) is available in 10- and 20-mg tablets. The recommended starting dose for preschoolers 3 to 5 years of age is 2.5 mg daily, and for children 6 years and older 5 mg one to two times per day.

NONSTIMULANT MEDICATIONS FOR ADHD

Approximately 25 to 30% of patients diagnosed with ADHD do not respond satisfactorily to stimulant drugs (Green, 1995). The use of nonstimulants, alone or in combination with stimulants to achieve a synergistic effect, is often helpful in these patients. Currently there is insufficient information about etiologically distinct subgroups of ADHD that might respond differentially to medication, be they stimulants, nonstimulants or both. Nonstimulant medications utilized occasionally for ADHD include the atypical antidepressant bupropion, the α-agonists clonidine and guanfacine, the tricyclic antidepressants such as nortriptyline, mood stabilizers such as valproic acid, and newer antipsychotics such as risperidone.

The use of nonstimulant medications for an off-label indication is acceptable to the American Medical Association "if the proposed use is based on rational scientific theory, expert medical opinion, or controlled clinical studies." It states further that "experience states that the official label lags behind scientific knowledge and publications." Green (1995) notes that "clinicians who prescribe nonstimulant drugs are usually on solid ground if a trial of stimulant medication has failed or if they document scientifically valid reasons for preferring a nonstimulant drug."

Bupropion

Bupropion is an antidepressant of the aminoketone class (Green, 1995). Limited experience indicates that buproprion is effective for the treatment of children and adolescents with ADHD. In one study there was evidence that it improved their cognitive performance as well. In addition, children with prominent symptoms of conduct disorder as well as ADHD appear to respond particularly well to bupropion (Conners et al., 1996). Relatively common side effects of bupropion include allergic rashes and edema, agitation, dry mouth, insomnia, headache, nausea, vomiting, constipation, and tremor. A rarer side effect is induction of hypomania.

The most serious side effect of bupropion is seizures, with an incidence of 0.4% of adult patients receiving up to 450 mg/day, increasing as the dose increases. There seems to be increased risk of seizures in patients with comorbid eating disorders. Divided doses are recommended to reduce the risk of seizures. The risk for children and the developmentally disabled, although probably greater, has not been clearly documented. Bupropion has also been found to exacerbate tics in children with ADHD and Tourette syndrome and is therefore relatively contra-indicated in this situation. Bupropion is administered in two or three daily doses beginning at 37.5 to 50 mg bid with a titration over 2 weeks to a usual maximum of 250 mg/day (300 to 400 mg/day in adolescents) (Conners et al., 1996).

TRICYCLIC ANTIDEPRESSANTS

There is a great deal of research experience on the use of tricyclic antidepressants (TCAs) in the treatment of ADHD, with some studies suggesting that approximately 70% of these patients respond to desipramine. Until recently the antidepressants have been the most frequently prescribed second-line drugs for treating ADHD (Green, 1995). Many clinicians have been prescribing the tricyclics less in recent years because of the growing appreciation for the risk of cardiotoxicity, especially in prepubertal children, and the problems associated with overdosing. Many of the TCAs are thought to reduce hyperactivity and impulsivity and improve mood in patients with ADHD. Those with comorbid anxiety disorder or depression may respond better to the TCAs than to stimulants. The effects of these drugs on concentration and learning is uncertain, however, and sedation can be a problem.

Generally, the TCAs have relatively long half-lives, obviating the need for school dosing. Behavior after school and in the evenings is typically rated better than with stimulants. The mechanism of action of the TCAs in ADHD appears to be different from that thought to be important in depression. Thus, optimal doses are usually considerably lower and onset of clinical response is usually more rapid with ADHD patients than with depressed patients. There is evidence that although some ADHD patients may not respond to one TCA they may respond to another (Green, 1995).

CARDIOTOXICITY OF THE TRICYCLICS

Children display different pharmacokinetics than adolescents or adults. Moreover, a smaller fat-to-muscle ratio in children leads to a decreased volume of distribution and a lack of protection from overdose by fat stores. Children also metabolize these drugs more readily than adolescents or adults, and therefore display greater swings in blood levels. Because TCAs lower the seizure threshold, they must be used with caution in epileptic patients.

Large interindividual differences in plasma levels occur for the same dose of TCAs in children. Because between 3 and 10% of the population has a genetic variation characterized by a decreased activity in cytochrome P-450 2D6, they metabolize TCAs more slowly and therefore may develop toxic serum levels even at doses lower than 5 mg/kg (Green, 1995). This may lead to cardiovascular and central nervous system toxicity and may be confused with exacerbation of symptoms. Because there is a minimal correlation between dose and serum levels of TCAs (Wilens, 1993), and serum levels correlate with potentially serious untoward effects, monitoring of drug and metabolite serum levels should be considered mandatory in ADHD (Green, 1991). It is recommended that TCAs be administered to children in two or three divided doses if more than 1 mg/kg per day is given, to minimize the untoward effects of peak plasma levels. For this reason long-acting preparations, such as imipramine pamoate capsules, are not recommended (Green, 1995).

Toxic responses to the TCAs are a concern for all age groups, but particularly children and adolescents. Particularly troubling is the slowing of cardiac conduction which, as demonstrated on the ECG, results in an increase in P-R and QRS intervals, cardiac arrhythmias, tachycardia, and heart block (Green, 1995). At least five sudden deaths have been reported in children 12 years of age and younger taking desipramine with tachyarrhythmias, such as torsade de pointes, being the suspected cause. Three of these deaths occurred after exercise. Four of the deaths were children 9 years old or younger, with the fifth being a 12-year-old. Because of this it is recommended that an ECG be obtained at baseline, during titration, and at maintenance levels, with emphasis on the measurement of the QTc interval. Thus, guidelines for administering TCAs for the treatment of ADHD include an ECG at baseline, at 3 mg/kg per day and at a final dose of not greater than 5 mg/kg per day. The following parameters are advised: PR interval equal to 210 ms, QRS interval widening not greater than 30% over baseline, QTc interval less than 450 ms, maximum HR equal to 130/min, maximum systolic BP equal to 130, and maximum diastolic BP equal to 85. Once steady state plasma levels are obtained, ECGs can be assessed semiannually. One report indicated that 10% of children and adolescents treated with desipramine for ADHD had an incomplete right bundle branch block, which is considered normal for children up to age 10, with a QRS interval of 120 ms or greater, and 18% had sinus tachycardia with a ventricular rate of 100 beats per minute or greater. It is unknown if these findings increase the risk of complications with desipramine.

On 24-h ECG recordings of children receiving long-term desipramine, a significantly higher rate of single or paired premature atrial contractions and runs of supraventricular tachycardia were found with decreased rates of sinus pauses and junctional rhythm. However, desipramine levels correlated only with paired premature atrial contractions. Because parasympathetic input to the heart decreases substantially with age, and desipramine may increase the ratio of sympathetic to parasympathetic drive more in younger patients, reductions in heart period variability would be associated with increased vulnerability for serious arrhythmias.

In 1992, the American Academy of Child and Adolescents Psychiatry reported that the risk of sudden death for children 5 to 14 years old treated with desipramine at therapeutic doses is approximately the same as the risk for similarly aged children in the general population, between 1.5 and 4.2 million/year. The issue, however, remains controversial. Some experts have proposed severe restrictions on the use of desipramine whereas others disagree, noting there is as yet no established cause of the deaths nor any scientific evidence that they were related to the drug. Green (1995) believes that because the number of sudden deaths is so small, the reason for death unknown, and because no specific cardiac finding has any known predictive value, it is mandatory that both ECG changes and serum drug and metabolite levels be monitored to ensure they are maintained within recommended parameters whenever TCAs are prescribed. Until further data are gathered it is advisable to follow these conservative guidelines and to favor nortriptyline and imipramine as first-choice TCAs for the treatment of prepubertal children. Moreover, a patient or family history of cardiac disease should be a relative contraindication to TCAs use in general.

Tricyclic Antidepressants Most Frequently Used for ADHD

Owing to the previously detailed risk of cardiotoxicity, the TCAs are utilized less frequently for treating ADHD than before, with nortriptyline being favored by many. Wilens (1993), in a chart review of 58 treatment-resistant ADHD patients found that nortriptyline at a mean daily dose of 73.6 mg induced a moderate response in 48% of the subjects whether or not there was a comorbidity. Significantly, more of the "markedly improved" subjects had serum nortryptiline levels between 50 and 150 ng/mL. Untoward effects were mild in these patients and no significant conduction abnormalities were noted. Nortriptyline has also been found effective in ADHD and comorbid tic disorder/Tourette syndrome.

Desipramine and imipramine are the most studied and, until fairly recently, were the most frequently used TCAs for ADHD. At present, desipramine is still widely used, with data suggesting both efficacy and relative safety from cardiotoxicity if it is used in the recommended dose ranges (i.e., <3 mg/kg per day). Because imipramine is used to treat nocturnal enuresis, it is probably the most widely prescribed TCA for children. Imipramine has been found effective for both ADHD and Tourette syndrome in some studies, although high rates of untoward effects and tolerance have been problematic. In a controlled study, although amitriptyline proved effective for some children, reducing hyperactivity and aggression in the home and school environments, untoward effects, particularly sedation, made it difficult to tolerate the required dosages. Another TCA used with children and adolescents is clomipramine. Its side effects include sedation, dry mouth, blood dyscrasias, and an increased risk of seizures.

OTHER PHARMACOTHERAPEUTIC AGENTS USED FOR ADHD

Selective Serotonin Reuptake Inhibitors

The selective serotonin reuptake inhibitors (SSRIs), which include fluoxetine, sertraline, paroxetine, fluvoxamine, are now being prescribed more frequently than the TCAs because of their significantly safer side effect profile, especially with regard to cardiotoxicity and lethality of overdose (Green, 1995).

Although there has been limited experience with these agents, positive findings have been reported for ADHD children and adolescents treated with fluoxetine, with and without comorbid disorders. Further studies are needed to compare the efficacy of the SSRIs to the TCAs or bupropion in treating this condition (Green, 1995). Possible side effects with the SSRIs include restlessness, hyperactivity, behavioral activation, insomnia, impulsivity, and suicidal ideation.

α-Adrenergic Agonists

Clonidine and guanfacine are α_2-adrenergic receptor agonists used for the treatment of ADHD. Although there is limited evidence of their efficacy when given alone, in conjunction with stimulants they may help in the treatment of associated hyperactive/hyperarousal behavior and they may be beneficial for children with tics.

Clonidine.   Clonidine, an antihypertensive agent, is an α_2-noradrenergic receptor agonist that acts at presynaptic sites in the brain to inhibit endogenous release of norepinephrine (Hunt et al., 1991). Clonidine increases frustration tolerance and task orientation and decreases hyperarousal in ADHD, with the best responders being those whose onset of symptoms was at an early age and who are hyperaroused, hyperactive, energetic, impulsive and uninhibited with frequent comorbid conduct or oppositional disorders (Hunt et al., 1990). It is thought that clonidine may not be of value in treating distractibility in

ADHD without hyperactivity. It is recommended that the dose of clonidine should be increased gradually, beginning initially with one-half tablet (0.05 mg) per day, increasing by half a tablet every 3 days until a total daily dosage between 3 and 5 μm/kg in 3 or 4 divided doses is achieved (Hunt et al., 1990).

Clonidine may also be administered by transdermal patch. In one study it was found that the daily dosage had to be increased in about one-third of patients when they switched from oral administration to a transdermal patch. In approximately half of these patients the efficacy of the patch diminished after 5 days. This may be owing to a 12- to 16-h half-life for adults versus an 8- to 12-h half-life for adolescents and 4 to 6 h for prepubertal children. It usually takes about 1 month of treatment for significant clinical improvement to occur with clonidine. Children with ADHD have benefited from clonidine for up to 5 years. When discontinued, the clonidine dose should be reduced gradually over a period of 2 to 4 days to avoid hypertensive crises and withdrawal symptoms, such as nervousness, agitation, and headache (Green, 1995).

The untoward effect most frequently reported with clonidine is sedation. Typically, this occurs about 1 h after taking the medication and lasts about 30 to 60 min. Tolerance to sedation is normally seen after 3 weeks of treatment. The mean blood pressure decreases by about 10% on this dose of clonidine. About 5% of children and adolescents develop clinical depression while taking the drug, particularly those with a family history of mood disorders (Hunt et al., 1990). The drug should probably be avoided with these patients. Because ADHD is a comorbid diagnosis in approximately 50% of children with Tourette disorder, and 20 to 50% of such patients develop worsening of their tics if treated with stimulants, clonidine may be considered an alternative treatment for these patients as well as those unable to tolerate the side effects of stimulants.

Clonidine and methylphenidate in comorbid ADHD and conduct/ODD.   Hunt et al. (1990) reported on the use of clonidine together with methylphenidate for children with ADHD and coexisting conduct or oppositional defiant disorder who suffered from high arousability and distractibility. The combined use of these drugs might enable a reduction in the dosage of methylphenidate. This can be valuable when there are significant untoward effects with methylphenidate such as rebound insomnia or significant height or weight suppression.

Guanfacine Hydrochloride (Tenex)

Gaunfacine hydrochloride has also been used as a treatment for children and adolescents with ADHD, particularly those with comorbid tics. An antihypertensive agent, guanfacine is a selective α_2-adrenergic receptor agonist. It differs from clonidine in being a more selective α_2-agonist (Green, 1995). In an open study on 10 subjects with ADHD and Tourette's syndrome, daily doses of guanfacine ranged from 0.75 to 3.0 mg, with the optimal dose found to be 1.5 mg for most subjects. Group analysis did not reveal significant improvement of ADHD symptoms, although three subjects had moderate improvement and one showed marked improvement. Group means of tics, however, were significantly reduced. The most commonly reported side effects were lethargy, headache, insomnia, and dizziness, all of which remitted over 3 to 4 days. Guanfacine may be particularly useful for children and adolescents who have comorbid ADHD and chronic tics.

ANTIPSYCHOTIC DRUGS

The majority of the studies comparing antipsychotics with stimulants in the treatment of ADHD were performed over 20 years ago, with most reporting that stimulants were more effective (Green, 1991). Although antipsychotics were found to display some efficacy, most clinicians are reluctant to use them because of the risk of irreversible tardive dyskinesia, neuroleptic malignant syndrome, and a decrease in cognition and learning due to their sedative effects (Green, 1995). It is now believed that antipsychotics used to treat ADHD have minimal effects on cognition if used at appropriate dosages. There also is some evidence that thioridazine may be superior to stimulants in treating subgroups of developmentally disabled children with ADHD (Aman et al., 1991).

Overall however, primarily because of the risks of tardive dyskinesia, the older generation of anti-psychotics are rarely justified for the treatment of ADHD. Newer agents, such as risperidone, which have a lower incidence of parkinsonism and tardive dyskinesia, might occasionally be indicated for particularly disruptive ADHD. Olanzepine, one of the newest atypical antipsychotics, may have a superior side effect profile than risperidone, although it is yet to be tested as a treatment for disruptive ADHD.

Monoamine Oxidase Inhibitors

The nonselective monoamine oxidase inhibitors phenelzine (Nardil) and tranylcypromine (Parnate) have been used primarily as antidepressants. Their potentially serious side effects, particularly hypertensive crises, and the difficulty of adhering to a tyramine-free diet, as well as numerous drug restrictions, limit their use in children and adolescents. Accordingly, neither of these preparations is recommended for children or adolescents (Green, 1995), although tranylcypromine has been reported to be effective in ADHD. Because selegiline (Deprenyl) is a selective MAO-B inhibitor, hypertensive crisis usually only occurs at higher doses, making it somewhat safer to use for ADHD with comorbid Tourette. Selegiline is available in 5-mg tablets and can be prescribed up to a maximum daily dose of 15 mg divided into morning and noon doses.

MISCELLANEOUS DRUGS FOR ADHD

The mood stabilizers lithium, carbamazepine, and valproic acid do not seem to have a positive effect on core ADHD symptoms, although symptoms of episodic discontrol, or a diagnosed or undiagnosed cyclical mood disorder, may be positively affected with these agents (Cantwell, 1996). Other drugs that do not appear useful for idiopathic ADHD not associ-

ated with a comorbid disorder are the benzodiazepines and mianserin (Green, 1995).

PSYCHOPHARMACOLOGY OF DEVELOPMENTAL LEARNING DISORDERS

Adequate learning depends on a number of factors, including innate cognitive capacities, motivation, familiarity with the language spoken at school, matching of academic expectations, and quality of classroom instruction. Academic failure can have devastating effects on the self-image, leading to social isolation and exclusion from full cultural and economic participation in society (King, 1991).

Historical Background

Prior to the 1940s, children who had academic difficulties in the United States were considered mentally retarded, emotionally disturbed, or socioculturally deprived. Later academic difficulties were thought to be neurologically based and unfortunate terms such as "minimal brain damage" (reflecting hypothesized neuroanatomic damage) and "minimal brain dysfunction" or MBD (reflecting hypothesized neurophysiologic dysfunction) were popularized. Following this, the terms "dyslexia" for reading disorder, "dysgraphia" for writing disorder, and "dyscalculia" for mathematics disorder were coined, implying common etiology and treatment strategies. Today it is believed that the etiologies are probably different for each with the terms reading, writing, and mathematics disorder now being preferred.

Definition of Learning Disorders

The developmental learning disorders are defined in the DSM-IV as inadequate development of academic, language, speech, and motor skills that are not owing to a demonstrable neurologic disorder, mental retardation, a pervasive developmental disorder, or deficient educational opportunities (American Psychiatric Association, 1994). A learning disorder is diagnosed if an individual's ability is substantially below what would be expected given the person's chronologic age, measured intelligence, and age-appropriate education. "Substantial" is usually taken to mean two standard deviations below that expected from chronologic age and IQ.

In the United States, the term often used by educators is "learning disability" (Silver, 1996). The definition of learning disorders has importance as it defines levels of funding and access to federally mandated special education classes. There are a number of differences between the definition of a learning disability and that of a learning disorder. A learning disorder, as defined by the Education for all Handicapped Children Act, excludes those whose learning problems are a result of visual, hearing, or motor handicaps or of mental retardation, emotional disturbance, or environmental, cultural, or economic disadvantage. Therefore, many dual-diagnosed children, with mental retardation and reading disabilities beyond that predicted by their IQ might arbitrarily be denied needed remedial services. These exclusionary criteria have led to the proposal of a new definition of a learning disorder by the federal interagency Committee on Learning Disabilities, which would not exclude individuals with mental retardation, ADHD, or social and emotional disturbance from being diagnosed additionally with a learning disorder.

Classification of Learning Disorders

The DSM-IV lists the following learning disorders:

1. Reading disorder
2. Mathematics disorder
3. Disorder of written expression
4. Communication disorders
5. Developmental expressive language disorder
6. Mixed receptive/expressive language disorder
7. Phonologic disorder (articulation disorder)
8. Motor skills disorder

These are placed on its axis II, so as not to be overlooked, as they occur frequently in conjunction with other disorders (Table 5-2).

Table 5-2
DSM-IV Diagnostic Criteria for Reading Disorder

A. Reading achievement, as measured by individually administered standardized tests of reading accuracy or comprehension, is substantially below that expected given the person's chronologic age, measured intelligence, and age-appropriate education.
B. The disturbance in Criterion A significantly interferes with academic achievement or activities of daily living that require reading skills.
C. If a sensory deficit is present, the reading difficulties are in excess of those usually associated with it.

If a general medical (e.g., neurologic) condition or sensory deficit is present, code the condition on Axis III.
SOURCE From the American Psychiatric Association, 1994.

Prevalence and Epidemiology of Learning Disorders

The prevalence of learning disabilities is unknown, primarily because of different case definitions. In the interim, the Centers for Disease Control and Prevention has estimated that 5 to 10% of school-aged children are affected by learning disabilities. Males outnumber females by 2:1 to 5:1, although this might be the result of a referral bias related to the increased incidence of disruptive behavior among males with learning disorders. The incidence of reading disorder in American inner cities can be gauged by a study of Baltimore public school sixth graders that found that 28% of the children were 2 or more years below grade level.

Comorbidity

Those with learning disorders might suffer comorbid social, emotional, behavioral, psychiatric, or neurologic disorders. Indeed, it has been suggested that learning disorders are part of a continuum of neurologic dysfunction (Silver, 1996). For example, learning disorders are common after serious head injury and in cerebral palsy, as are reading disorders in individuals with seizures and neurofibromatosis. Twenty to twenty-five percent of individuals with learning disabilities have ADHD and 30 to 70% of individuals with ADHD have a learning disorder. It should be noted that children with comorbid ADHD are far more likely to be referred for special education. The incidence of Tourette's syndrome is also significantly greater among the learning disordered, whereas approximately one-third of the reading disordered suffer from conduct disorder and vice versa.

Peers frequently ostracize, ridicule, and tease the learning disabled child which results in passivity, depression, or somatic complaints. The child with a learning disorder might act the class clown. Some with nonlanguage-related disability may also have difficulty learning social skills, missing social cues such as facial expression, tone of voice, or body language. This profile has been termed nonverbal learning disability, and appears to be associated with depression.

Diagnostic Criteria for Learning Disorders

The diagnosis of a learning disorder is one of exclusion. Because individuals with learning disorders are often first referred for professional help because of behavior problems, it is important to ascertain whether these problems are the cause or the consequence of the academic failure. Although this differentiation is not always simple to make, there are some guidelines. For example, a child with primary emotional problems will not usually demonstrate an uneven profile of cognitive strengths and weaknesses. The clinician should inquire about school performance for each academic area and, if a particular difficulty is noted, further investigations, including cognitive and achievement tests, should be initiated.

The tests used to evaluate learning disorders utilize an information processing, or cybernetics model (Silver, 1996). This is based on the different stages required for processing of information. Thus, information is first perceived and recorded, then in-terpreted, integrated, and stored for later retrieval. Finally, an individual must be able to retrieve and communicate this information. A psychoeducational assessment determines intellectual ability and cognitive style, looking with particular emphasis on discrepancies between intellectual potential and academic performance. Thus, discrepancies within each test are noted and the current level of academic skills measured with standardized achievement tests, bearing in mind that, by definition, half of all children will automatically score below average on these tests.

A neurologic examination is an important part of the initial to check for both soft neurologic signs and to exclude gross central nervous system pathology. As an example, headaches should always be investigated so as not to miss rare progressive lesions, such as recurrent bleeds from a vascular malformation involving the temporal lobe speech areas. Other professionals, including a speech and language pathologist, might be enlisted to clarify areas of language disability, and an occupational therapist utilized to test gross, fine motor, or sensory-motor functioning.

It is best to diagnose learning disorders as early as possible, as timely intervention is effective and avoids the trauma of later failure. Characteristics seen in preschoolers that are suggestive of learning disabilities are delayed motor development, language delays, speech disorders, poor concept development, and poor cognitive abilities as reflected in play (Harris, 1995).

Pathophysiology of Learning Disorders

The pathophysiology of learning disorders has not been clearly elucidated and is probably multifactorial. School difficulties might stem from attention deficits, memory impairment, receptive and expressive language disorders, problems with reasoning and abstraction, and organizational difficulties. Visual or auditory perceptual disabilities might also be the cause of the disorder. Visual perceptual disabilities might relate to difficulty in distinguishing subtle differences in shapes, such as differentiating d from b, or 6 from 9. There might be difficulty with figure-ground discrimination, or in estimating depth, resulting in motor clumsiness (Silver, 1996). Other difficulties include problems distinguishing subtle differences in sounds, separating sounds from background noise, or processing sound inputs quickly (Silver, 1996).

Even if learning disorders are biologically determined, sociocultural variables influence their development and expression. Environmental factors, such as the inner city's "culture of poverty" (King, 1991), and emotional factors, often cause performance below academic potential. Emotional factors might include oppositional and narcissistic personality traits and the need to thwart parental expectations. There also is an increased incidence of learning disorders in later children of large families. Cigarette use and light alcohol consumption by pregnant women has been associated with academic difficulties in their children, with the long-term impact on the fetus of medications taken during pregnancy still being investigated. Moreover, autoimmune etiologies have also been proposed.

Clinical Description of Learning Disorders

Reading is a complex motor, perceptual, cognitive, and linguistic process. It requires the ability to distinguish lexical (letter) representations and transform them into phonetic (sound) representations (Shepherd and Uhry, 1993), the ability to discern the syntax of phrases and sentences, an understanding of the semantic meaning of words and sentences, and an adequate short-term memory. A reading disorder may be part of a general developmental language disorder or may be specific, with little evidence of a language disorder. There is a high correlation between reading skills, mathematics, and spelling skills, and children with reading disorders seem to have higher rates of articulation difficulties (with the reverse also true). Poor readers may suffer from difficulties with the pragmatics of conversation.

Reading disorders should be viewed as lifelong disabilities, as affected adults, particularly males, continue to have reading difficulties. Individuals with a reading disorder will continue to read and spell at a slower rate than their peers, they complete fewer years of education, and fewer become professionals. With early recognition, however, and appropriate special education intervention, individuals can learn to compensate. In fact there is a striking number of successful artists and craftsmen who have suffered from reading disorders, among them the writers Hans Christian Andersen and Gustave Flaubert.

Pathophysiology of Reading Disorders

Processing deficits.   It is now believed that a reading disorder reflects deficits in basic language capabilities rather than deficits in cognitive-perceptual processes. Reading is thought to involve the acquisition of two systems; first, a lexical or sight reading system, and second, a phonologic system for unfamiliar words. Children with a reading disorder have difficulty transitioning from the first to the second system. As a result, there might be disjointed reading or guessing. The usual processing problems in a reading disorder may occur in one of three ways.

1. The ability to decode is impaired but comprehension is intact
2. Intact decoding with impaired comprehension (hyperlexia)
3. Both decoding and comprehension might be impaired

Most students with a reading disorder have problems with rapid automatic decoding, although it should be noted that silent reading may be strong in spite of weak oral reading. Because spelling is based on word recognition, it also is often impaired. Visual-evoked potential studies suggest perceptual anomalies in the reading disordered with, for example, a failure of visual circuits to provide temporal resolution (Harris, 1995). It is suggested that the magnocellular system involving the retina, the lateral geniculate nucleus, and the primary visual cortex process visual stimuli at a slower rate, explaining why words might seem to blur, fuse, or jump off the page. Visual tracking problems might lead to the skipping of words and comprehension difficulties might necessitate repeated reading of the same material. Visual perception anomalies might also affect social functioning, forcing the individual to rely on context, repetition, and facial expression to comprehend stimuli from the environment.

Genetics

Studies have shown strong familial aggregation for reading disorders, with a high concordance rate for identical twins. Although a single gene model of inheritance with environmental modification has been proposed, it would seem that reading disorders are genetically heterogeneous.

Neuroanatomic Findings

Reading disorders are possibly linked to abnormal cerebral organization and lateralization. A lack of normal asymmetry of the superior surface of the temporal lobe (planum temporale), affecting the processing of both spoken and written language, has been noted in some affected individuals. This has been supported by findings of a loss of the normal asymmetry of this area when visualized with MRI. This lack of normal asymmetry has also been noted for the posterior brain. In other studies, congenital abnormalities of the corpus callosum were associated with phonologic aspects of reading disorders. Functional imaging studies of children with reading disorders have also proven useful in unraveling the pathophysiology of this disability. For example, there appears to be a relative reduction in the frontal activation normally seen during attention-demanding tasks, whereas PET scan evaluations of males with a reading disorder have demonstrated abnormalities in cerebral blood flow in the left temporoparietal region.

Minor cortical malformations have also been described with, for example, multiple foci of glial scarring in the perisylvian cortex and ectopic neurons thought to be owing to disordered cortical neuronal migration. These malformations are believed to occur during gestation or the early postnatal period.

Treatment of Reading Disorders

Nonpharmacologic treatment.   The treatment of reading disorders is essentially nonpharmacologic. All reading disorders require highly individualized special education based on an ongoing assessment of the individual's strengths and weaknesses. Conceptual and cognitive strengths are targeted to utilize more than one sensory modality (Silver, 1996). Both the reading difficulties and the language disorder, which is frequently present, should be considered. Remedial teaching, spelling, and writing might also be required. There are numerous reading techniques, although no particular method has been found to be significantly superior to the others.

One of the most frequently used treatment methods is a synthetic, alphabetic, and multisensory approach called the Orton-Gillingham method. The individual is taught letter-sound associations involving auditory, visual, and motor aspects of speech and written language. Once the reading and writing of basic words has been mastered, attempts are made at constructing sentences. The teaching of reading, spelling, and writing occurs simultaneously with instruction involving extended practice and the linking of weak skills to stronger ones. Speech and learning skills are also taught. A new microcomputer program which shows promise for a sub-group of language disordered children has been developed to improve word recognition and decoding skills (Merzenich et al., 1996).

School setting can significantly alleviate difficulties associated with this disability. First, the correct level of academic intervention should be ascertained, with a number of possible options depending on the severity of the disorder. The student might require tutoring in a regular class, daily remedial instruction, a self-contained class, or a school for the learning disabled. If in a regular class, extra time should be allocated for written tests, spelling errors should be noted (without affecting grades), foreign languages should not be mandatory, and oral examinations should be offered (Harris, 1995). Compensatory skills such as computer-based programs can be developed, and talents, hobbies, and leisure activities should be encouraged to develop competency and camaraderie. Adolescents might need help in vocational planning and independence skills.

The school should protect the student from negative labeling (Harris, 1995) and teachers and parents should be alert for secondary depression, anxiety, or a sense of inferiority requiring individual, group, or family psychotherapy. Disorganization, low self-esteem, emotional lability, and poor interpersonal skills make the management of children with learning disabilities challenging. Within the family setting the learning disabled tend to suffer from intense sibling rivalry as well as the humiliation of being surpassed by younger siblings.

Since parents need help in dealing with disappointment, anger, and guilt, the clinician must provide ongoing support and counseling and must serve as an advocate for the child in dealing with the school system. For the older student there are helpful remedial services in many higher education or training programs. Parent and advocacy groups also are useful as are a number of lay books on the subject.

Pharmacologic Treatment

The nootropics.   A new class of pharmacologic agents, the nootropics or "knowledge-enhancing" drugs, is thought to have potential for treating cognitive disorders such as learning and attentional disorders, organic brain syndromes, and mental retardation (Conners, 1993). It should be noted, however, that proponents of new nootropics frequently make exaggerated claims for these agents (Conners, 1993), making it necessary for the physican to protect patients and their families from being seduced by scientifically unsubstantiated claims. One drug that seems to display some efficacy is piracetam. Although various analogues of piracetam, such as primeracetam, have been studied there is no clear evidence of their therapeutic efficacy and none have yet been approved for human use. Drugs such as hydergine, while having been used in adults with memory disorders, they have not been shown to have any significant effect on cognition in children. Moreover, there is at present no evidence to suggest that any particular dietary manipulation, including megavitamins, mineral supplements, or additive-free diets are effective in treating learning disorders or in enhancing cognitive functioning.

Pharmacotherapy for Comorbid Disorders

Pharmacotherapy has been attempted for both the primary learning disorder and comorbid disorders. Although stimulants have proved effective in the short-term of children with a reading disorder and ADHD, they are ineffective for treating a reading disorder alone. Stimulants can also sometimes improve the handwriting of children with a learning disorder and comorbid ADHD. Anxiolytics have been prescribed for comorbid anxiety or anxiety secondary to learning disorders, although no significant benefits have been found.

Piracetam. Piracetam, a 2-oxo-1-pyrrolidine acetamide (Figure 5-1), has been targeted for the primary deficits associated with a reading disorder. It was originally developed as an analog of the neurotransmitter γ-aminobutyric acid (GABA) for the treatment of motion sickness, although it is not thought to be either a GABA receptor agonist or antagonist (Conners, 1993). Rather, piracetam appears to decrease hippocampal acetylcholine levels, to modify norepinephrine content in brain, and to alter metabolism by increasing the concentration of ATP (Conners, 1993). The significance of these effects in its mechanism of action is unknown. Piracetam blocks the effects of hypoxic amnesia suggesting that its effects on memory may relate to oxygen consumption (Conners, 1993). There are also data suggesting piracetam might facilitate transfer of information between the cerebral hemispheres through the corpus callosum. Studies with reading disordered adults indicate that piracetam enhances verbal learning. For example, EEG studies of visual evoked potentials suggested that piracetam facilitates processing of visual linguistic stimuli in the left parietal cortex. In a multisite year-long study using event-related potentials, piracetam was shown to significantly increase reading age in reading disordered individuals. Verbal, but not nonverbal, functioning also showed improvement in this study. In a separate study involving 257 reading disordered boys, improved reading speed was noted with piracetam without any significant improvements in reading accuracy or comprehension. Yet another, lengthier, multisite study demonstrated a small improvement in oral passage reading without any improvement in reading speed or on information processing, language, or memory. Moreover, a European study suggested that piracetam has an advantageous effect on kindling-induced learning deficits. Piracetam appears to be quite safe, displaying no significant adverse effects.

Piracetam appears to hold some promise for treating reading disorders, particularly on word and syllable identification. However, it cannot be recommended at this time as a sole agent for developmental reading disorder (Harris, 1995). Further studies to assess its effectiveness, when given alone or in combination with therapies such as remedial reading instruction and training in phonologic awareness, are required. Trials with piracetam should, for example, focus on visual and auditory processing speed (Harris, 1995). Currently, there are no data suggesting that it has a role in treating those nonreading deficits associated with reading disorder. Although piracetam has been approved in Mexico, Canada, and Europe, it is not yet available in the United States (Conners, 1993).

PSYCHOPHARMACOLOGY OF MENTAL RETARDATION

The psychopharmacologic treatment of mental retardation is entering a new era characterized by improved diagnoses, an enhanced understanding of underlying neuropsychiatric pathogenic mechanisms, and the availability of therapeutic agents.

The assessment and treatment of children and adults with mental retardation should be multimodal, taking into account the individual's functioning in school, work, and the community. Treatment possibilities encompass a wide spectrum of interventions, including individual, group, family, behavioral, vocational, physical and occupational therapies, among others. Psychopharmacologic management is also an option.

The use of psychotropic drugs in mentally retarded individuals requires attention to legal and ethical considerations. In the 1970s, the international community acknowledged the rights of the mentally retarded regarding proper medical care. These rights were specified in the "Declaration on the Rights of Disabled Persons." This declaration advocated "a right to proper medical care" and "the same civil rights as other human beings. Disabled persons shall be able to avail themselves of qualified legal aid when such aid proves indispensable for the protection of their persons."

The declaration of the right of mentally retarded individuals to proper medical care was followed by close supervision of possible excesses in overly restrictive care and, in particular, by concern over the use of psychotropics as a method of restraint. The courts have generally upheld the notion that an individual should be placed under physical or chemical restraints only in "the occurrence of, or serious threat of, extreme violence, personal injury, or attempted suicide." Furthermore, the courts usually demand that "an individualized estimation of the possibility and type of violence, the likely effects of drugs on a particular individual, and an appraisal of alternative, less restrictive courses of action" must be made to provide the "least restrictive alternative" (Aman and Singh, 1988). Thus, in making treatment decisions concerning the use of psychotropics in mentally retarded individuals, risks and benefits need to be weighed carefully. The best interests of the mentally retarded patient are considered through alternate judgment when there is a historical lack of judgment, with "substituted judgment" advisable when there is some knowledge of the individual's current or past preferences (Aman and Singh, 1988).

In the last two decades the doctrine of the "least restrictive alternative" has prompted a review of the use of psychotropics in the mentally retarded. Prevalence figures for the use of psychotropics were found to be 30 to 50% of individuals in institutional settings, 25 to 35% of mentally retarded adults in the community, and 2 to 7% of mentally retarded children in the community. Psychotropics were found to be used most frequently with older patients, those with higher restriction placements, and those with higher rates of social, behavioral, and sleep problems. Gender, IQ, and the type of behavioral problem did not seem to correlate with the use of psychotropics in the mentally retarded. It should be noted that although 90% of mentally retarded individuals live in nonresidential settings, there have been few systematic studies conducted outside of institutions.

Clinical Description: Psychiatric Disorders in Mental Retardation

Children and adults with mental retardation have high rates of psychiatric disorders. Overall, 50% of individuals with mental retardation manifest a psychiatric disorder that warrants intervention. The high proportion of mental illness in this population is the multidetermined product of neuropsychiatric disor-

ders, medical vulnerabilities, genetic syndromes, social disadvantage, and high-stress family environments. It is postulated that individuals with mild mental retardation display psychiatric manifestations similar to those without mental retardation, whereas moderate to severely retarded individuals display more externalizing disorders, pervasive developmental disorders, and behaviors that are idiosyncratic to this population (Bregman, 1996). The identification of specific behavioral patterns is crucial to implementing effective therapy. In this context, information should be obtained from parents, teachers, employers, and relatives to reliably identify particular behavioral syndromes. The use of standardized rating scales is highly recommended to establish baseline and follow-up data.

Diagnostic Criteria: Rating Scales in Mental Retardation

Although psychiatric disorders accompanying mental retardation are often difficult to characterize, effective treatment requires that behavioral syndromes be accurately identified (Feinstein and Reiss, 1996). The use of observationally based rating scales are highly recommended in assessing the effectiveness of pharmacologic trials (Table 5-3). Thus, response to medication may be followed with the Aberrant Behavior Checklist-Community Version (ABC-CV), an informant-based instrument that is sensitive to "state symptoms." For hyperactivity and attentional difficulties, the Conners rating scale has proven to be highly reliable. For example, this scale was used to establish the efficacy of methylphenidate in attention-deficit hyperactivity disorder accompanying mental retardation (Handen et al., 1992). Because internalizing disorders, such as anxiety and depression, are more difficult to assess in individuals with mental retardation, instruments specific for this population are recommended, such as the Psychopathology Inventory for Mentally Retarded Adults (PIMRA), the Reiss Screen for Maladaptive Behavior, and the Emotional Disorders Rating Scale-DD (Feinstein et al., 1988). The Diagnostic Assessment for the Severely Handicapped (DASH), another

Table 5-3

Examples of Instruments Used to Assess Psychopathology in Mental Retardation

Instrument	Informant	Use
Aberrant Behavior Checklist-Community Version (Aman, 1985)	Primary caregiver	State symptoms (drug-sensitive)
Conners Rating Scales (Goyette, 1985)	Parent and teacher	Hyperactivity, Inattention
Psychopathology Inventory for Mentally Retarded Adults (PIMRA) (Senatore, 1985)	Primary caregiver and self-report	General diagnostic
Emotional Disorders Rating Scales-DD (Feinstein, 1988)	Primary caregiver	General affective and behavioral syndromes

instrument for assessing psychopathology, applies algorithms that result in DSM criteria.

When considering treatment for the mentally retarded it is crucial to identify specific syndromes such as major depressive disorder, bipolar disorder, anxiety disorder, or a pervasive developmental disorder when they are present. Frequently, however, default treatments for specific behaviors, such as self-injurious behavior (SIB), aggression, and behavioral outbursts are necessary.

Diagnostic Criteria: Mental Retardation and Psychiatric Syndromes

Mental retardation is a nonspecific diagnosis that adheres to criteria stipulated in DSM-IV (Table 5-3). Both heritable and nonheritable causes of mental retardation often have characteristic neuropsychiatric manifestations, a clinical phenomenon that has led to the description of "behavioral phenotypes." Among genetic disorders with accompanying mental retardation and characteristic behavioral expressions are fragile X syndrome, Turner syndrome, Rett syndrome, Down syndrome, Williams syndrome, Prader-Willi syndrome, Lesch-Nyhan syndrome, and Lowe syndrome, among others. While autism has marked behavioral singularities there are no current identifiable genetic markers, although the condition is suspected to be highly familial.

Fragile X syndrome. Fragile X syndrome is an X-linked condition caused by mutations, usually characterized by an excessive number of CGG trinucleotide repeats within the promoter site, of the FMR1 gene located at Xq27.3. Carrier males pass the premutation to their daughters but not their sons. The CGG repeat can expand to the full mutation (disease-associated) status when passed through a female meiotic cycle. The full mutation is characterized by hypermethylation of the FMR1 promoter region and a CGG repeat sequence ranging from approximately 200 to many thousands. Each child of a carrier female has a 50% chance of inheriting the fragile X mutation, which can be passed silently down through generations before a child is affected by the syndrome. The phenotype associated with the full mutation is characterized by mental retardation, long narrow face, prominent ears, jaw, and forehead, high arched palate, strabismus, poor muscle tone, flat feet, and macroorchidism. Also common in males are hand-flapping or hand-biting, as well as an unusual speech pattern characterized by a fast and fluctuating rate of speech with sound, word, or phrase repetition. Affected males also commonly manifest attention span problems, hyperactivity, motor delays, and socially avoidant behavior toward peers or strangers in the presence of a normal attachment patterns to caregivers.

Gaze aversion is a frequent and striking feature of affected males. Affected females have a milder form of impairment which is characterized by avoidant symptoms or social phobia (Freund, 1993), as well as learning disabilities, including math deficits and attentional deficits, even though their IQ may be within the normal range. Thus, the fragile X full mutation is typically associated with anxiety symptoms, attentional deficits, hyperactivity, stereotypies, and occasional mood disorders.

Turner syndrome.   Turner syndrome is a chromosomal condition causing short stature and infertility in females that results from a complete or partial absence of one X chromosome. Psychological testing of these individuals reveals relative deficiencies in visuospatial and nonverbal task execution. Behaviorally, females with Turner syndrome are described as more immature, hyperactive, and "nervous." They also have poor peer relations, difficulty in schooling, and problems in concentrating.

Estrogen replacement therapy has been used for decades to treat Turner syndrome to promote development of secondary sexual characteristics and to maintain tissue and bone integrity. Estrogen treatment has also been reported to have a positive effect on self-esteem in females with this condition. Growth hormone was recently approved to facilitate growth in Turner syndrome.

Down syndrome.   John Langdon Down first identified this condition which, in 95% of the cases, is caused by trisomy 21. The condition is characterized by epicanthal folds over the eyes, flattened bridge of the nose, a single palmar crease, decreased muscle tone, and cardiac abnormalities. Individuals with Down syndrome usually show adequate sociability although the condition is characterized by early dementia, dyskinesias, and mood disorders.

A clinical diagnosis of dementia predicts behavioral maladaption in Down syndrome. Studies of adaptation in Down syndrome also show significant deficits in communication relative to daily living and socialization skills, with expressive language being significantly weaker than receptive skills.

Williams syndrome.   Williams syndrome is a genetic disorder caused by deletion of one or more genes at, or surrounding, the elastin locus (7q11.23). This condition is characterized by a typical "elfin" facies, cardiovascular malformations, high blood pressure, elevated blood calcium levels, and behavioral abnormalities. Unique pixie-like facial features—almond shaped eyes, oval ears, full lips, small chins, narrow faces, and broad mouths—are common components of the phenotype.

High, superficial sociability with adults has been frequently described in children with Williams syndrome. Other abnormalities include concentration difficulties, excessive anxiety, poor peer relationships, and poor visuospatial and motor skills. In addition, autistic features, developmental and language delays, problems in gross motor skills, hypersensitivity to sounds, abnormal eating habits, and perseverative behaviors have been noted with Williams syndrome.

Prader-Willi syndrome.   Prader-Willi syndrome is caused by a microdeletion in chromosome 15, with breakpoints at sites 15q11 and 15q13 that are inherited from the father. This condition was first described in 1956 by Prader as a syndrome characterized by obesity, short stature, cryptorchidism, and mental retardation. Other features of this disorder are obsessional thinking about food, compulsive eating habits, compact body build, underdeveloped sexual characteristics, and poor muscle tone.

Individuals with Prader-Willi syndrome have delays in language and motor development as well as learning disabilities. Food-related behaviors are prominent, including food stealing, gorging, hoarding, and indiscriminate eating of various foods. Associated behavioral problems include sleep disturbances, irritability, temper tantrums, and a high pain threshold. A range of compulsive behaviors, including skin picking, nail biting, nose picking, lip biting, and hair pulling, are also observed with this condition.

Lesch-Nyhan syndrome. Lesch-Nyhan syndrome is inherited as an X-linked recessive disorder that affects only males. It is caused by an inborn error of purine metabolism characterized by the absence of hypoxanthine-guanine phosphoribosyltransferase. The condition is characterized by hyperuricemia, impaired kidney function, joint pain, choreoathetosis, spasticity, compulsive self-mutilation, and mental retardation.

Individuals with Lesch-Nyhan disease manifest characteristic behaviors, of which the most prominent is persistent and severe self-injurious behavior (SIB). A considerable variability in self-injury is present, which appears related to perceived internal stress rather than to environmental influences. Even though patients often cannot inhibit self-injury they can predict its onset and request restraints. Aggression against others can be as prevalent as SIB in these patients. A study of these patients revealed stress reduction, teeth extraction, and physical restraint were the most commonly used management techniques, with behavior modification having limited efficacy. The severity of self-injury does not appear to change over time, with age of onset being a predictor of outcome.

The development of animal models of Lesh-Nyhan disease have provided insights into the pathogenesis of SIB. Transgenic mice deficient in hypoxanthine-guanine phosphoribosyltransferase do not display any neurological dysfunction. However, after administration of 9-ethyladenine, a neuroactive compound that acts in the basal ganglia, these animals displayed SIB. A recent positron emission tomography (PET) study of Lesch-Nyhan patients found a significant reduction of dopaminergic nerve terminals and cell bodies throughout the brain. These dopaminergic deficits appear to be pervasive and developmental in origin, suggesting they contribute to the characteristic neuropsychiatric manifestations of the disorder. When an inhibitor of dopamine neuronal uptake is administered repeatedly to normal adult rats, SIB is elicited that is temporally associated with a 30% reduction on the concentration of striatal dopamine, an increased turnover of serotonin, and a robust induction of substance P and neurokinin A synthesis. In this case, SIB can be blocked by lesions of the dopaminergic system or by D1 or D2 dopamine receptor antagonists. Not surprisingly, therefore, risperidone, an antipsychotic, has been reported to provide benefit in Lesch-Nyhan syndrome.

Cornelia de Lange syndrome. In 1933, Cornelia de Lange, a Dutch pediatrician, described two children with similar features, including low birthweight, delayed growth and small stature, microcephaly, thin eyebrows that meet at midline (synophrys), long eyelashes, short upturned nose, and thin, downturned lips. Other findings with this syndrome included hirsutism, small hands and feet, partial joining of the second and third toes, incurved fifth fingers, gastroesophageal reflux, seizures, heart defects, cleft palate, bowel abnormalities, and feeding difficulties.

Most individuals with Cornelia de Lange syndrome have moderate to severe mental retardation. Although the transmission of this disorder has not yet been fully characterized, the offspring of some mildly affected individuals display the full disorder. Behavioral characteristics include autistic spectrum manifestations such as infrequent facial expressions of emotion, self-injurious behaviors, stereotypic movements, and comfort associated with vestibular stimulation or vigorous movement.

Lowe syndrome. The oculocerebrorenal syndrome of Lowe is an X-linked disorder characterized by congenital cataracts, cognitive impairment, and renal tubular dysfunction. Maladaptive behaviors, particularly stubbornness, hyperactivity, temper tantrums, and stereotypic behaviors are frequently associated with this condition.

Pharmacotherapeutics: Psychotropics and Mental Retardation

Because individuals with both mental retardation and psychiatric disorders are often multiply and chronically medicated for behavioral control (Baumeister et al., 1993), it is vital to recognize the short- and long-term effects of these agents so as to employ

Table 5-4
Mental Retardation

A. Significantly subaverage intellectual functioning: an IQ of approximately 70 or below on an individually administered IQ test (for infants, a clinical judgment of significantly subaverage intellectual functioning).
B. Concurrent deficits or impairments in present adaptive functioning (i.e., the person's effectiveness in meeting the standards expected for his or her age by his or her cultural group) in at least two of the following areas: communication, self-care, home living, social/interpersonal skills, use of community resources, self-direction, functional academic skills, work, leisure, health, and safety.
C. The onset is before the age of 18 years.

Code based on degree of severity reflecting level of intellectual impairment:
Mild Mental Retardation
IQ level 50–55 to approxmately 70
Moderate Mental Retardation
IQ level 35–40 to 50–55
Severe Mental Retardation
IQ level 20–25 to 30–35
Profound Mental Retardation
IQ level below 20 or 25
Mental Retardation, Severity Unspecified: When there is strong presumption of mental retardation but the person's intelligence is untestable by standard tests (e.g., for individuals too impaired or uncooperative, or with infants)

This condition is coded on Axis II.

only those with the least potential for causing adverse effects. Thus, monitoring of medication use in long-term treatment settings can sometimes lead to a decline in the amount of psychotropic use without adversely affecting outcome. In particular, the antipsychotics which are the most widely used psychotropic agents in this population, carry a high risk for side effects, including irreversible tardive syndromes, such as tardive dyskinesia and tardive dystonia. Although antipsychotics can control aberrant behavior by suppressing behavior generally, they also specifically reduce stereotyped and self-injurious behavior. In addition, opioid antagonists and serotonin reuptake inhibitors have been used in controlling self-injurious and stereotyped behaviors. Mood stabi-

lizers, such as lithium (Lithobid), valproic acid (Depakote), and carbamazepine (Tegretol), are helpful in managing cyclical mood changes and behavioral outbursts. β-Adrenergic receptor blocking agents, such as propranolol (Inderal), have been shown to be useful in treating aggression and disruptive behaviors. Stimulants, such as methylphenidate (Ritalin), dextroamphetamine (Dexedrine), pemoline (Cylert), and α_2-adrenergic receptor agonists such as clonidine (Catapres) and guanfacine (Tenex), are of benefit in the treatment of hyperactive and inattentive syndromes in individuals with mental retardation (Table 5-4).

Combined treatment with antipsychotics, anticonvulsants and mood-enhancing or stabilizing agents is fraught with problems associated with pharmacokinetic and pharmacodynamic interactions. Physicians should refer to authoritative and updated sources of information to predict such possible interactions before initiating multiple medication regimens.

Mental Retardation and Self-Injurious/Aggressive Behavior

Self-injurious behavior in individuals with mental retardation commonly consists of inappropriate and persistent head banging, self-biting, and self-hitting. Other topographies are also possible, such as inflicting self-injury by scratching, pinching, and falling to the ground. Approximately 5 to 15% of mentally handicapped individuals are reported to engage in SIB and SIB is the major reason for failure of community placement for persons with mental retardation. Because these behaviors are commonly multidetermined, a thorough evaluation of SIB should include an assessment of environmental, medical, and psychological factors. The initial evaluation should consist of a functional analysis of behavioral determinants using abbreviated forms for this purpose. Medical conditions often precipitate bursts of SIB because of a lack of the capacity to communicate physical complaints. In addition, because psychiatric conditions may underlie SIB and therefore, careful attention must be paid to accompanying symptoms.

Aggressive behavior is often a concomitant of SIB, or it may present independently. On occasion, there are oscillations between the manifestations of SIB and aggressive behavior in a given individual, with a worsening of one being accompanied by an improvement in the other.

Antipsychotics.   Given the importance of curbing destructive behaviors, many psychotropics have been examined to treat these conditions, with none being found as effective as antipsychotics. Antipsychotics efficacy may be due to the apparent hyperactivity of brain dopaminergic systems in SIB. Trials of chlorpromazine (Thorazine), thioridazine (Mellaril), and risperidone (Risperdal) have all shown efficacy in curbing destructive behaviors. Open trials of flu-phenazine (Prolixin) and haloperidol (Haldol) yielded positive data in the management of self-injurious and aggressive behaviors. Aggressive behaviors may not respond as consistently as SIB to antipsychotic treatment. It is possible that neurobiologic factors are more important in SIB, whereas environmental factors have a greater influence in aggressive behaviors.

The major drawback in the use of antipsychotics is the relatively high frequency of drug-induced movement disorders. Surveys of individuals with mental retardation show that between one-third and two-thirds show signs of tardive dyskinesia (TD), a chronic, sometimes irreversible, form of orofacial dyskinesia that can be induced by some antipsychotics. However, it has been suggested that a sizable proportion of mentally retarded individuals, up to one-third in some studies, may have a TD-like movement disorder in the absence of antipsychotic use. This indicates that susceptibility to TD may be disproportionately high in this patient population. Risk factors for TD during treatment with antipsychotics include length of treatment, dosage, and the age of the patient. The importance of this is highlighted by the fact that up to 33% of children and adults with mental retardation who receive antipsychotics develop TD. Parkinsonism and other types of extrapyramidal side effects, including tremors, muscular rigidity and acute dystonias, affect up to one-third of patients taking these drugs. Akathisia, a syndrome of motor restlessness with an impulse to be in constant motion, occurs in up to 15% of patients on antipsychotics. Use of these drugs is also associated with a risk of neuroleptic malignant syndrome (NMS), an infrequent, but potentially fatal, complication. Risk factors for NMS include male gender and high-potency antipsychotics. A recent study found 21% mortality among those mentally retarded individuals who experienced NMS. Baseline and follow-up measures of movement disorders with the Abnormal Involuntary Movement Scale (AIMS), Dyskinesia Identification System Condensed User Scale (DISCUS), and/or Akathisia Scale (AS) are mandatory when prescribing antipsychotic medications to mentally retarded individuals. While the new, atypical antipsychotics, such as clozapine (Clozaril) and olanzapine

(Zyprexa) may pose less risk for antipsychotic-induced movement disorders, they have yet to be tested in controlled clinical trials involving mentally retarded individuals. It should be noted that although clozapine is an effective antipsychotic, it is associated with a significant risk of agranulocytosis and seizures. Olanzapine, sertindole, quetiapine, and ziprasidone are newer atypical antipsychotics that will undoubtedly be used in the future for treating the mentally retarded because their lower side effect profiles are superior to those of conventional antipsychotics.

Nevertheless, the recent development of alternatives to antipsychotics such as the serotonin selective reuptake inhibitors and mood stabilizers, coupled with more refined diagnostic tools for identifying specific psychiatric abnormalities in mentally retarded individuals, may reduce the need for using antipsychotics routinely in treating SIB and aggression.

Mood-stabilizers. Lithium (Lithobid, Eskalith), carbamazepine (Tegretol), and valproic acid (Depakote) are mood-stabilizing agents. Both severe aggression and SIB, even in the absence of mood disturbance, have been treated successfully with lithium, with clinical impression and rating scales showing significant improvement of aggression in virtually all studies. Although less data are available regarding the effectiveness of carbamazepine and valproic acid in the treatment of SIB and aggression in persons with mental retardation, the results with lithium suggest they may be useful as well.

β-Adrenergic receptor blockers. Propranolol (Inderal) is a β-adrenergic receptor blocking agent that may be beneficial in managing aggressive behavior associated with increased adrenergic tone. By blocking some receptor responses to norepinephrine, propranolol decreases the chronotropic, inotropic, and vasodilator responses to this neurotransmitter. Inhibition of these physiologic manifestations of stress may, in itself, help reduce aggressive behavior. Because high serum propranolol levels have been noted in patients with Down syndrome, its bioavailability may be increased for some reason in these patients. Although it has been reported that impulsive

outbursts of rage have been successfully managed with propranolol in some mentally retarded individuals, controlled trials are necessary to establish this therapeutic benefit.

Opioid receptor antagonists. Naltrexone (Trexan) and Naloxone (Narcan), opioid receptor antagonists, have been used in the treatment of SIB. Both naltrexone and naloxone are opioid receptor antagonists that block the effects of endogenous opioids. Naloxone is only available in injectable form, and has a shorter half-life than naltrexone. Although initial open trials of opioid receptor antagonists showed promise in the treatment of SIB, more recent controlled trials have not revealed any difference from placebo. The induction of dysphoric mood and the lack of replication in controlled studies, suggests this class should not be considered a primary treatment for SIB, although such drugs may be useful in select cases.

Serotonin reuptake inhibitors. The similarity of SIB to stereotypical behaviors may explain the positive response of some patients to serotonin reuptake inhibitors such as clomipramine (Anafranil), fluoxetine (Prozac), fluvoxamine (Luvox), sertraline (Zoloft), and paroxetine (Paxil). SIB, aggression, stereotypy, and ritualistic behaviors have been shown to respond to fluoxetine, especially if comorbid compulsive behaviors are present (Bodfish and Madison, 1993). Similar results were obtained with clomipramine, including reductions in SIB and ritualistic and perseverative behaviors. Double-blind studies are needed to determine whether these drugs are useful in all patients with SIB or whether they target a select group with comorbid compulsive/perseverative behaviors. Because these drugs have a tendency to cause behavioral activation their use may be limited in the treatment of this condition.

Mental Retardation and Mood Disorders

Recent advances in the diagnosis of depression and dysthymic disorder in mentally retarded patients may facilitate the use of more specific treatments for these conditions. However, the response to antidepressants is not uniform in mentally retarded individuals, with dysphoria, hyperactivity, and problem behaviors often occurring with antidepressant use. In a retrospective review of the response to TCAs in mentally retarded adults, only 30% were found to benefit significantly, with symptoms of agitation, aggression, SIB, hyperactivity, and temper outbursts being mostly unabated.

Greater response predictability is associated with mood stabilizers in the treatment of cyclic mood disorders in mental retardation. Although lithium is known to alter sodium transport in nerve and muscle cells, and to alter the metabolism of catecholamines, its precise mechanism of action as a mood stabilizer is unknown. Lithium blood levels must be monitored when using this ion, as well as baseline thyroid and hematological parameters. One double-blind and several open trials of lithium in treating bipolar disorder in mental retardation have yielded encouraging results. Side effects of lithium therapy include gastrointestinal distress, eczema, and tremors.

Valproic acid (Depakene) and divalproex sodium (Depakote) are anticonvulsants and mood-stabilizing agents that may act by modifying the brain levels of GABA. Although significant liver toxicity has been reported with valproic acid, this is typically seen in infants during the first six months of treatment. Nonetheless, initial and periodic monitoring of liver function is mandatory when prescribing this medication. Valproic acid has been reported to produce up to an 80% positive response rate in mood symptoms, SIB and aggression in mentally retarded patients. Carbamazepine (Tegretol), another anticonvulsant that is efficacious as a mood-stabilizing agent, may also be of benefit in treating abnormalities in mood in mentally retarded patients. Because both aplastic anemia and agranulocytosis have been reported in association with carbamazepine use, baseline and follow-up hematologic testing are mandatory when prescribing this agent. Patients should be made aware of the early toxic signs and symptoms of a hematologic problem, such as fever, sore throat, rash, mouth ulcers, easy bruising, and petechial or purpuric hemorrhage. Despite its anticonvulsant properties, carbamazepine should be used with cau-

tion in patients with a mixed seizure disorder that includes atypical absence seizures, because it may precipitate generalized tonic-clonic convulsions in these patients. The response to carbamazepine has not been as predictable as to lithium and valproic acid in the treatment of affective syndromes in persons with mental retardation.

Mental Retardation and Anxiety Disorders

Buspirone. Buspirone (Buspar) is an antianxiety agent unrelated to the benzodiazepines, barbiturates, or other sedative/hypnotics. Preclinical studies indicate that buspirone has a high affinity for serotonin (5-HT1A) receptors, and moderate affinity for D2-dopamine receptors in brain. The latter effect may be responsible for a syndrome of restlessness that sometimes appears shortly after initiation of treatment with buspirone. Other side effects of buspirone include dizziness, nausea, headache, nervousness, lightheadedness, and excitement. Although buspirone has not been used in controlled studies for the management of anxiety in mentally retarded individuals, it has been found to be helpful in reducing SIB.

Mental Retardation and Stereotypical Behavior

Fluoxetine (Prozac) is a selective serotonin reuptake inhibitor that is effective in treating depression and obsessive-compulsive behavior. Because the metabolism of fluoxetine involves the CYP2D6 system, concomitant therapy with drugs metabolized by this enzyme, such as TCAs, may lead to drug interactions with adverse consequences. Studies have shown that previously stable plasma levels of imipramine and desipramine increased by two- to ten-fold when fluoxetine was used as an add-on therapy. Moreover, because of its long half-life, such an effect may linger for 3 weeks or longer after fluoxetine therapy is discontinued. Possible side effects of fluoxetine include anxiety (10–15%), insomnia (10–15%), altered appetite and weight (9%), activation of mania/

hypomania (1%), and seizures (0.2%). Also seen are asthenia, tremor, sweating, gastrointestinal complaints, including anorexia, nausea, and diarrhea, and dizziness or lightheadedness.

Other selective serotonin reuptake inhibitors, such as sertraline, fluvoxamine, paroxetine, and the nonselective agent clomipramine, may prove useful in managing stereotypical behaviors, especially if a compulsive component is present. Clomipramine is a dibenzazepine TCAs with specific antiobsessional properties. In a recent study, clomipramine was found to be effective in the management of anger, and compulsive, ritualized behaviors in adults with autism. While the other serotonin reuptake inhibitors are likely to demonstrate beneficial effects in the treatment of stereotypical behaviors in mentally retarded patients, controlled studies have yet to be performed with these agents.

Mental Retardation and Hyperactivity/Inattention

Despite the long-standing observation that up to 20% of children with mental retardation have an accompanying syndrome of hyperactivity/inattention, it has only been in the last two decades that specific treatments for these syndromes have been attempted.

Stimulants. Methylphenidate (Ritalin) is a mild central nervous system stimulant that differentially reduces ADHD symptoms in individuals with mental retardation (Aman et al., 1991). Methylphenidate is a short-acting stimulant with a peak effect in children at 4.7 hours (1.3–8.2 hours) for the slow-release preparation (Ritalin-SR) and 1.9 hours (0.3–4.4 hours) for the tablets. The beneficial effects of stimulants are more marked in individuals with mild to moderate mental retardation, with favorable response predicted by the presence of impulsivity, attentional deficits, conduct problems, motor incoordination, and perinatal complications. Because of its stimulant properties, methylphenidate is contraindicated in the presence of marked anxiety, tension, and agitation. It also is relatively contraindicated in patients with glaucoma, motor tics, or with those who have

a family history or diagnosis of Tourette's syndrome. Methylphenidate may inhibit the metabolism of coumarin anticoagulants, anticonvulsants, such as phenobarbital, diphenylhydantoin, or primidone, as well as drugs such as phenylbutazone and TCAs. Given this possibility, it may be necessary to decrease the dose of these drugs when they are given concomitantly with methylphenidate. The most common adverse reactions to methylphenidate are anxiety and insomnia, both of which are usually dose-dependent. Other adverse effects include allergic reactions, anorexia, nausea, dizziness, palpitations, headache, dyskinesia, drowsiness, tachycardia, angina, cardiac arrhythmia, abdominal pain, and weight loss with prolonged use.

Dextroamphetamine sulfate (*d*-amphetamine, Dexedrine) is the dextro isomer of *d,l*-amphetamine sulfate. Peripheral actions of amphetamines include elevations of systolic and diastolic blood pressures and weak bronchodilator and respiratory stimulant actions. Ingestion produces, on average, a peak dextroamphetamine blood level in 2 hours. The half-life of dextroamphetamine is approximately 10 hours. Acidifying agents decrease, and alkalinizing agents increase, the absorption of dextroamphetamine. Dextroamphetamine has been shown to be effective in the treatment of ADHD in children with mental retardation.

α-Adrenergic receptor agonists. Clonidine (Catapres) and guanfacine (Tenex) are α-adrenergic receptor agonists that have been used successfully in managing hyperactivity. Clonidine, an imidazoline derivative, stimulates α-adrenergic receptors in the brain stem, thereby reducing sympathetic outflow, decreasing peripheral resistance, renal vascular resistance, heart rate, and blood pressure. Clonidine acts rapidly, decreasing blood pressure within 30 to 60 min after an oral dose, and peaking within 2 to 4 h. Tolerance to its effects develops on continued use. Sudden cessation of clonidine administration can result in nervousness, agitation, headache, and tremor accompanied, or followed, by a rapid increase in blood pressure and elevated levels of plasma catecholamines. Because clonidine may potentiate bradycardia and AV block, caution must be exercised in patients taking agents such as digitalis, calcium channel blockers or β-adrenergic receptor antagonists which affect sinus node function or AV nodal conduction. The most frequent dose-related side effects associated with clonidine are dry mouth (40%), drowsiness (33%), dizziness (16%), constipation (10%), weakness (10%), and sedation (10%). Guanfacine (Tenex), another α_2-adrenergic receptor agonist, also decreases peripheral vascular resistance and reduces heart rate. Guanfacine has been used successfully in the treatment of ADHD in children and may have a specific effect in enhancing prefrontal brain function. As with clonidine, the use of guanfacine in combination with phenothiazines, barbiturates, or benzodiazepines may enhance the sedative response to these agents. Most of the side effects associated with guanfacine are mild. They include dry mouth, sedation, asthenia, dizziness, constipation, and impotence. The use of clonidine or guanfacine in the mentally retarded is not usually influenced by the presence of tics, as these tend to be more difficult to ascertain than in nonmentally retarded individuals. However, if a tic disorder or a family history of Tourette's syndrome is present, they may be first-line drugs in the treatment of ADHD in persons with mental retardation.

PSYCHOPHARMACOLOGY OF AUTISM AND PERVASIVE DEVELOPMENTAL DISORDERS

Because there are no drugs specifically approved for the treatment of autism or associated pervasive developmental disorders, the pharmacologic management of these conditions is adjunctive to educational, behavioral, and psychosocial interventions. Inasmuch as autistic children are highly susceptible to the emergence of neuropsychiatric disorders, these conditions merit specific treatment when they occur.

In considering pharmacotherapy for autistic disorder it is not always appropriate to extrapolate from related psychiatric conditions because of possible differences in the pathophysiology and the response

to medications in this patient population. Thus, it is common to find problems such as short attention span, hyperactivity, tics, obsessive-compulsive traits, mood, and anxiety in autistic children. These should be differentiated from the autistic child's inherent lack of joint attention, paucity of social reciprocity, propensity for stereotypies/need for sameness, and difficulty in regulating basic affective exchanges. The treatment of symptoms in autistic disorder and pervasive developmental disorder should therefore be based on an understanding of the specificity of autism.

Clinical Description: Psychiatric Disorders in Autism

Autistic disorder. Autistic disorder was first identified by Leo Kanner in 1943 who described a group of children with a sense of aloneness that was not a retreat into fantasy but rather an absence of social awareness. Other aspects of deviant functioning, such as delay in language development, restricted interests, and stereotypies were also described by Kanner. Today autism is recognized as a developmental and neurobiologically based disorder that manifests in children early in life, usually before 3 years of age. Although autism is now clearly differentiated from childhood schizophrenia, a very rare disorder, the core deficit in autism has not yet been identified. Explanations based on theory of mind, symbolic deficits, or executive deficits have been only partially supported over time.

In 1961 it was noted that patients with autism had elevated serotonin (5-hydroxytryptamine) levels in the blood. Subsequently it was found this is due to an increase in the platelet content of serotonin. More recent data indicate that treatment with specific serotonin reuptake inhibitors produces a reduction in ritualistic behavior and aggression in some autistic individuals and that a reduction in brain serotonin causes a worsening of stereotyped behavior. Thus, abnormalities in the regulation of serotonin may explain some of the features of autism.

Autism is conceptualized as a spectrum of disorders, with more severe cases showing a classical presentation which includes language delays, social deficits, and stereotypical behaviors beginning at an early age. Autism is accompanied by mental retardation in 75% of the patients, whereas the opposite end of the spectrum is represented by Asperger syndrome, high functioning autism and atypical autism.

Asperger disorder.   Asperger syndrome is characterized by social isolation in combination with odd and eccentric behavior, labeled "autistic psychopathy." This is characterized by a deficit in understanding others' emotional expression and an inability to engage in social reciprocity with peers. It has been proposed these children have a personality disorder compensated for by overachievement in restricted domains, such as intellectual pursuits. Up to 35% of individuals with Asperger syndrome have a high frequency of co-occurring psychiatric conditions, including mood disorders, obsessive-compulsive disorder, and schizophrenia.

High-functioning autism is not clearly differentiated from Asperger syndrome. The neuropsychological profile of individuals with Asperger syndrome coincides with a group of neuropsychological strengths and deficits described by the term nonverbal learning disabilities, suggesting an empirical distinction from high functioning autism. Projective testing has shown that individuals with Asperger syndrome may have richer inner lives, more elaborate fantasies, and be more focused on their inner experiences than individuals with high functioning autism. Pedantic speech was recently studied in both groups and found to be more frequent in Asperger syndrome, suggesting it may aid in empirically differentiating the two conditions.

"Atypical autism" describes a syndrome that fails to meet the age of onset criteria and/or does not fulfill the three required diagnostic criteria for autism (APA, 1994). The term pervasive developmental disorder (PDD) has been adopted in the official nomenclature but carries an imprecise meaning, and can be viewed as an umbrella concept that embraces all of these conditions. Pervasive developmental disorder not otherwise specified (PDD-NOS) is a descriptive term that attempts to describe children with atypical autism (Table 5-5).

Rett syndrome.   Related to, but probably different pathogenically from, autistic disorder are Rett syndrome and childhood disintegrative disorder. Rett syndrome was first recognized by Andreas Rett in 1966 as a neurological disorder primarily affecting females. This genetic condition is characterized by normal development until 6 to 18 months of age with ensuing severe to profound mental retardation, microcephaly, loss of purposeful hand movements, hand-wringing stereotypies, shakiness of the torso and, possibly, the limbs, unsteady stiff-legged gait, hyperventilation, apnea, aerophagia, seizures (in 80% of cases), teeth grinding, difficulty chewing, and hypoactivity. As opposed to autistic disorder, a patient with Rett disorder typically has normal social development with adequate social reciprocity and cuddling in the first few months of life. Brain imaging studies show a diffuse cortical atrophy and/or hypoplasia with particular volume loss of the caudate nucleus.

Childhood disintegrative disorder.   Childhood disintegrative disorder (CDD), or Heller syndrome, is a rare condition with poor prognosis. In 1908 Heller described a group of children with "dementia infantilis." These children had apparent normal development until 3 to 4 years of age at which time there was an onset of behavior problems, language loss, and mental retardation. Current criteria require an apparently normal development up to 2 years of age, with significant loss of previously acquired skills such as language, social skills, bowel and bladder control, play, and motor skills to diagnose CDD. Further, impairment of at least two of the three areas impaired in autistic disorder, language, social skills, and stereotypical behaviors, are required for the diagnosis of CDD. In general, CDD remains a diagnosis of exclusion.

Diagnostic Criteria: Diagnostic Instruments in Autism

Several standardized and reliable instruments are available to assess and diagnose autistic disorder. While current research protocols rely heavily on the Autism Diagnostic Interview-Revised (ADI-R), this

Table 5-5
Autistic Disorder

A. A total of six (or more) items from 1, 2, and 3 with at least two from 1, and one each from 2 and 3:

1. Qualitative impairment in social interaction, as manifested by at least two of the following:
    a. Marked impairment in the use of multiple nonverbal behaviors such as eye to eye gaze, facial expression, body postures, and gestures to regulate social interaction
    b. Failure to develop peer relationships appropriate to developmental level
    c. A lack of spontaneous seeking to share enjoyment, interests, or achievements with other people (e.g., by a lack of showing, bringing, or pointing out objects of interest)
    d. Lack of social or emotional reciprocity

2. Qualitative impairments in communication as manifested by at least one of the following:
    a. Delay in, or total lack of the development of spoken language (not accompanied by an attempt to compensate through alternative modes of communication such as gesture or mime)
    b. In individuals with adequate speech, marked impairment in the ability to initiate or sustain a conversation with others
    c. Stereotyped and repetitive use of language or idiosyncratic language
    d. Lack of varied, spontaneous make-believe play or social imitative play appropriate to developmental level

3. Restricted repetitive and stereotypic patterns of behavior, interests, and activities, as manifested by at least one of the following:
    a. Encompassing preoccupation with one or more stereotyped and restricted patterns of interest that is abnormal either in intensity or focus
    b. Apparently inflexible adherence to specific, nonfunctional routines or rituals
    c. Stereotyped and repetitive motor mannerisms (e.g., hand or finger flapping or twisting, or complex whole-body movements)
    d. Persistent preoccupation with parts of objects

B. Delays or abnormal functioning in at least one of the following areas, with onset prior to age 3 years: (1) social interaction, (2) language as used in social communication, or (3) symbolic or imaginative play.

C. The disturbance is not better accounted for by Rett Disorder or Childhood Disintegrative Disorder.

instrument is too cumbersome for routine clinical use. In this regard the Childhood Autism Rating Scale (CARS) is favored. Diagnostic instruments used to assess maladaptive behaviors in mental retardation are also applicable to autistic children, with the Aberrant Behavior Checklist-Community Version (ABC-CV) and the Conners Scales for Hyperactivity/Inattention being preferred.

Pharmacologic Treatment of Autism and Associated Behavioral Syndromes

As in mental retardation, the treatment of autism requires a host of interventions to treat multiple domains of functioning, including social, educational, psychiatric, and behavioral. Some have advocated a behavioral treatment approach as the main component in the management of maladaptive behaviors in autism. Indeed, over 250 studies have been conducted utilizing behavioral techniques. Target behaviors are divided into categories, such as aberrant behaviors, social skills, language, daily living skills, and academic skills, with specific treatments delineated for each. For example, aberrant behaviors can undergo a functional analysis to identify predisposing environmental factors which may be subject to interventions. Behavioral techniques can use positive or negative reinforcers with an extinction component. Other therapeutic approaches, especially functional communication and occupational therapy, can ameliorate symptoms and enhance the quality of life of the autistic child. However, often there are symptoms that do not seem to be environmentally determined or, even if they are environmentally exacerbated, are intense enough or independent enough of the environment that they warrant pharmacotherapeutic intervention. Thus, the use of psychotropics in autism entails a careful assessment of the clinical condition in conjunction with other facets of the multimodal approach to treatment.

Once the need for psychotropic treatment is established, consideration must be given to the multiple psychological and family issues that arise from the presence of a family member with a developmental disorder. The use of medication in this context requires a thoughtful strategy to minimize problems associated with possible unexpressed anger toward the child, the wish for a magical cure, unresolved parental guilt, and unrealistic expectations for the response to pharmacotherapy. Further, it is important to remember that few psychotropic medications have completed controlled trials in the treatment of autistic children. When prescribing psychotherapeutics to autistic patients it is important to recognize that these individuals commonly have difficulty in communicating discomfort or distress from side effects, except perhaps by a worsening of target behaviors. The use of medication to control behaviors of autistic children therefore relies on establishing baseline and follow-up target symptoms and behaviors, using quantitative or semiquantitative measures of symptoms and careful monitoring of side effects. Since mental retardation and autistic disorder often coexist, most of the scales employed in the former retain their validity for the latter.

Autism and Self-Injurious Behavior/Aggression

Antipsychotics. Although effective for hyperactivity, fidgetiness, and stereotypical behaviors, antipsychotic use in autistic disorder should be reserved for the most severe cases of uncontrollable behaviors such as severe self-injury or refractory aggression (Figure 5-3). This is because there is a high risk for long-term side effects with antipsychotics. Trifluoperazine (Stelazine), pimozide (Orap), and haloperidol (Haldol) have been used in double-blind controlled trials in children with autism, and all have displayed a potential for extrapyramidal symptoms and tardive dyskinesia in this population. Risperidone (Risperdal), an atypical antipsychotic, and sulpiride, a benzamide derivative, have also been used with limited success in children with autism and SIB.

Autism and Mood Disorders

Significant mood symptoms are common in children with autism. The presentation of affective disorders in autism and autistic-like disorders appears to be most common in patients with IQs in the mentally

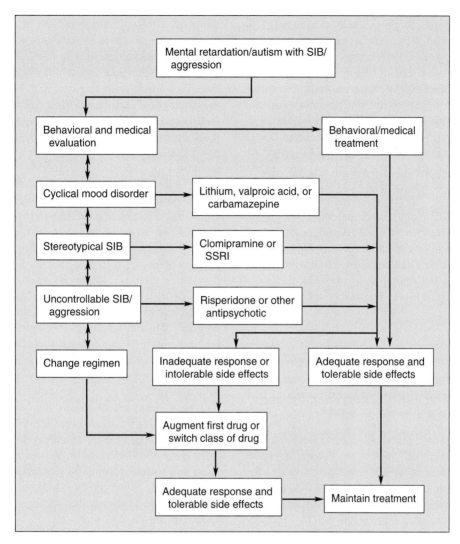

Figure 5–3. *Treatment of mental retardation/autism with SIB/aggression.*

retarded range, with 35% experiencing a childhood-onset of affective illness (Lainhart and Folstein, 1994). Some 50% of these patients have a family history of affective disorder or suicide. This tendency is supported by a recent family study of psychiatric disorders in autistic probands that found high rates of affective disorder and social phobia in relatives. It has been suggested that limbic abnormalities found in autopsy cases of autism may be related to mood dysregulation.

Mood-stabilizing agents. Lithium has been used in the treatment of cyclic manic-like symptoms in autism, such as decreased need for sleep, hypersexuality, increased locomotor activity, and irritability. Although an early controlled trial of lithium in autistic disorder was inconclusive, there are multiple case reports suggesting that lithium is useful in controlling these symptoms in autistic individuals, especially if there is a family history of mood disorders.

Anticonvulsants. Valproic acid (Depakene), divalproex sodium (Depakote), and carbamazepine (Tegretol) may also be efficacious when cyclical irritability, insomnia, and hyperactivity are present in autism. An open trial of valproate indicated that it may be effective in controlling behavioral symptoms in children with autism and EEG abnormalities. Target blood levels for both drugs are in the upper range of those used for seizure control, 8 to 12 μg/mL for carbamazepine and 80 to 100 μg/mL for valproic acid. Baseline hematologic and liver function tests should be obtained for both drugs and monitored regularly. Lamotrigine (Lamictal), a new anticonvulsant, is currently being tested in a controlled trial for behavioral symptoms in autistic children. Because up to 33% of autistic individuals have seizures, a trial with an anticonvulsant in the setting of an abnormal EEG and seizure-like episodes is a reasonable option.

Autism and Anxiety

Individuals with autism commonly manifest anxiety in the form of psychomotor agitation, self-stimulating behaviors, and signs of distress. Moreover, family studies suggest high rates of social phobia in first-degree relatives of autistic probands.

Benzodiazepines. Benzodiazepines have not been studied systematically in autistic disorder, probably owing to concerns with oversedation, paradoxical excitement, tolerance, and addiction. Clonazepam (Klonopin), which is unique among the benzodiazepines for upregulating serotonin 5-HT1 receptors, has been used as an anxiolytic, antimanic, or antistereotypic agent in autism. Lorazepam (Ativan) is usually reserved for the management of acute agitation and is available in oral or injectable form.

Buspirone. Buspirone (Buspar), a partial serotonin receptor agonist (5-HT-1A), is a useful anxiolytic. However, there is only limited information on its use in autistic disorder (Realmuto et al., 1989).

Autism and Stereotypical Behavior

Selective serotonin reuptake inhibitors. Selective serotonin reuptake inhibitors (SSRIs) such as

fluoxetine (Prozac), sertraline (Zoloft), fluvoxamine (Luvox), and paroxetine (Paxil), and the nonselective inhibitor clomipramine may be of benefit in treating some of the behavioral problems associated with autism. Fluoxetine has been reported to be effective in the treatment of autism. In a group of autistic adults, fluvoxamine was effective in a controlled trial in reducing repetitive thoughts and behavior, maladaptive behavior, aggression, and in improving some aspects of social relatedness, especially language usage. The treatment response to fluvoxamine was not correlated with age level of autistic behavior or IQ. Other than mild sedation and nausea in a few patients, fluvoxamine was well tolerated. The use of clomipramine is discouraged in children because of its potential to cause potentially fatal cardiotoxicity. Antipsychotics such as haloperidol appear to decrease levels of hyperactivity, stereotypies, and emotional lability, and to normalize object relations and social withdrawal in autistic patients. Potential side effects, however, limit the widespread use of these agents. The dopamine receptor antagonist amisulpride, that has been shown to improve negative symptoms in schizophrenia, may have some utility in treating stereotypical behaviors in autism, although controlled studies are needed to demonstrate this advantage. While clozapine, an atypical antipsychotic, has been effective and well-tolerated in the treatment of childhood-onset schizophrenia, this group was carefully differentiated from autistic children, leaving the question open as to whether the agent may be of benefit in this condition as well.

Autism and Hyperactivity/Inattention

Stimulants. Stimulants often do not produce predictable results in treating hyperactivity in autistic children (Figure 5-4) as compared to nonautistic patients. Typically, stimulants produce a decrease in the level of disruptive activity in autism, with a possible concomitant increase in stereotypic and ritualistic behaviors. In some cases a stimulant may produce behavioral toxicity and worsening of disruptive behaviors. This may occur when lack of joint attention in autistic children is confused with, and treated as,

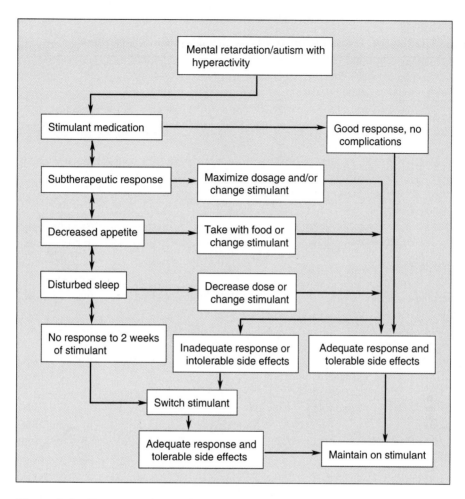

Figure 5–4.   *Treatment of mental retardation/autism with hyperactivity.*

the short attention span characteristic of attention-deficit hyperactivity disorder (ADHD).

α-Adrenergic receptor agonists.   α-Adrenergic receptor agonists such as clonidine (Catapres) and guanfacine (Tenex) downregulate noradrenergic locus ceruleus neurons, thereby reducing anxiety and hyperactivity. Transdermal and oral clonidine have been successfully used in managing hyperactivity and impulsivity in controlled trials with autistic children, although excessive sedation and tolerance to the beneficial effect limits this approach.

β-Adrenergic receptor antagonists.   Propranolol (Inderal) may be useful in managing impulsivity and aggression in autistic disorder. Cardiac parameters, such as pulse and blood pressure should be monitored carefully, with the dose titrated to the antihypertensive range.

Opioid receptor antagonists.   Naltrexone (Trexan) is of some benefit in managing hyperactivity in autistic children, but is without affect on social/cognitive deficits.

Table 5-6

Psychotropics Used in the Treatment of ADHD and Developmental Disorders

Drug	Main indications	Total daily dose	Schedule	Adverse effects
Antipsychotics				EPS
Haloperidol (Haldol)	Severe, uncontrollable	1–10 mg (variable)	bid-tid	Tardive Dyskinesia
Risperidone (Risperdal)	aggression or SIB	3–6 mg/day (variable)	bid	Acute Dystonia NMS
Mood-Stabilizers				
Lithium (Lithobid)	Cyclical Mood Symptoms	150–1200 mg	bid-tid	Polyuria, hypothyroidism, tremors, acne
Valproic Acid (Depakote)		250–1500 mg	bid-tip	Hepatic toxicity, thrombocytopenia
Carbamazepine (Tegretol)		200–1500 mg	bid-tid	Bone marrow suppression
Anti-Obsessional Agents				
Clomipramine (Anafranil)	Repetitive, ritualistic, and stereotypical behaviors	150–600 mg up to 5 mg/kg per day	bid-tid	Anticholinergic effects, overdose fatal
Fluoxetine (Prozac)		10–80 mg	qd	Insomnia, headaches, anxiety, GI symptoms
Sertraline (Zoloft)		25–200 mg	qd-bid	Anxiety, insomnia, GI symptoms
Fluvoxamine (Luvox)		25–150 mg	bid-tid	Fatigue, anxiety, GI symptoms
Paroxetine (Paxil)		10–40 mg	qd-bid	Fatigue, sweating, GI symptoms
Stimulants				
Methylphenidate (Ritalin)	Hyperactivity, impulsivity, and inattention	0.3–1.0 mg/kg per day	bid-qid	Anorexia, insomnia, depression, psychosis with high doses,
Dextroamphetamine (Dexedrine)		approx. 50–75% of MPH dosage	bid-qid	increased heart rate, induction of tics
Pemoline (Cylert)		56.25–75 mg	qd	

(*Continued*)

Table 5-6

Psychotropics Used in the Treatment of ADHD and Developmental Disorders (*Continued*)

Drug	Main indications	Total daily dose	Schedule	Adverse effects
Anxiolytics				
Buspirone (Buspar)	Anxiety	15–60 mg	bid-tid	Dizziness, nausea, headache
Clonazepam (Klonopin)	Anxiety, cyclical mood symptoms	0.1–0.2 mg/kg	qd-bid	Sedation, behavior changes
Lorazepam (Ativan)	Acute agitation	2–6 mg	bid-tid	Sedation, dizziness, weakness
Other Agents				
Propranolol (Inderal)	Aggression	120–500 mg	bid-qid	Lightheadedness, insomnia, lassitude, bronchospasm
Naltrexone (Trexan)	SIB	25–50 mg	qd	Nausea, depression, withdrawal effects, hepatotoxicity
Clonidine (Catapres)	Hyperactivity	0.2–0.6 mg	tid-qid	Dry mouth, sedation, dizziness
Guanfacine (Tenex)	Hyperactivity	1–2 mg	qd	Dry mouth, sedation, dizziness

EPS = Extrapyramidal Syndrome
NMS = Neuroleptic Malignant Syndrome
MPH = Methylphenidate

For additional information on the drugs discussed in this chapter see chapters 10, 17, 18, 19, and 23 in *Goodman and Gilman's The Pharmacological Basis of Therapeutics* (Ninth Edition), McGraw-Hill, New York, 1996.

REFERENCES

Aman MG, Singh NN (eds): *Psychopharmacology of the Developmental Disabilities*. New York: Springer Verlag, 1988.

Aman MG, Marks RE, Turbott SH, Wilsher CP, et al.: Methylphenidate and thioridazine in the treatment of intellectually subaverage children: Effects on cognitive-motor performance. *J Am Acad Child Adolesc Psychiatry* 1991;30:816–824.

American Psychiatric Association: *Diagnostic and Statistical Manual of Mental Disorders*, 4th ed. Washington, DC: American Psychiatric Association, 1994.

Baumeister AA, Todd ME, Sevin JA: Efficacy and specificity of pharmacological therapies for behavioral disorders in persons with mental retardation. *Clin Neuropharmacol* 1993;16(4):271–294.

Bodfish JW, Madison JT: Diagnosis and fluoxetine treatment of compulsive behavior disorder in adults with mental retardation. *Am J Ment Retard* 1993;98:360–367.

Bregman JD: Pharmacologic interventions. *Child Adolesc Clin North Am Ment Retard* 1996;5(4):853–880.

Cantwell DP: Attention deficit disorder: a review of the past 10 years. *J Am Acad Child Adolesc Psychiatry*1996;35:978–987.

Conners CK, Barkley R: Rating scales and checklists for child psychopharmacology. *Psychopharmacol Bull* 1985;21:816–832.

Conners CK: Nootropics and foods, in Werry JS, Aman MG (eds): *Practitioner's Guide to Psychoactive Drugs for Children and Adolescents*. New York, Plenum Medical, 1993.

Conners CK, Casat CD, Gualtieri CT, Weller E, et al.: Bupropion hydrochloride in attention deficit disorder with hyperactivity. *J Am Acad Child Adolesc Psychiatry* 1996;5:1314–1321.

Elia J, Rapaport J: Methylphenidate versus dextroamphetamine: Why both should be tried, in Osman B, Greenhill LL (eds): *Ritalin: Theory and Patient Management*. New York, Mary Ann Liebert, 1991, pp 243–265.

Feinstein C, Kaminer Y, Barrett R, Tylenda B: The assessment of mood and affect in developmentally disabled children and adolescents: The emotional disorders rating scales. *Res Dev Disabil* 1988;9:109–121.

Feinstein C, Reiss AL: Psychiatric disorder in mentally retarded children and adolescents. *Child Adolesc Clin North Am* 1996;5(4):827–852.

Freund LS, Reiss AL: Psychiatric disorders associated with fragile X in the young female. *Pediatrics* 1993;91:321–329.

Green WH: *Child and Adolescent Clinical Psychopharmacology*. Baltimore, Williams & Wilkins, 1991.

Green HW: The treatment of attention-deficit disorder with nonstimulant medications, in Riddle M (ed): *Pediatric Psychopharmacology*. Philadelphia, W.B. Saunders, 1995; *Child Adolesc Clin North Am* 1995;4(1):169–195.

Greenhill LL: Attention-deficit hyperactivity disorder, in Riddle M (ed): *Pediatric Psychopharmacology*. Philadelphia, W.B. Saunders, 1995; *Child Adolesc Clin North Am* 1995;4(1):123–168.

Handen BL, Breaux AM, Janosky J, et al.: Effects and noneffects of methylphenidate in children with mental retardation and ADHD. *J Am Acad Child Adol Psychiatry* 1992;31(3):455–461.

Harris JC: Learning disorders, in *Developmental Neuropsychiatry*. New York, Oxford University Press, 1995, pp. 142–180.

Hunt RD, Capper L, O'Connell P: Clonidine in child and adolescent psychiatry. *J Child Adol Psychopharmacol* 1990;1:87–102.

Hunt RD, Lau S, Ryu J: Alternative therapies for ADHD, in Greenhill LL, Osman BB (eds): *Ritalin: Theory and Patient Management*. New York, Mary Ann Liebert, 1991, pp 75–95.

King RA: Learning disorders, in Noshpitz JD, King RA (eds): *Pathways of Growth: Essentials of Child Psychiatry*. New York, John Wiley & Sons, 1991, pp 377–397.

Lainhart JE, Folstein SE: Affective disorders in people with autism: a review of published cases. *J Autism Dev Dis* 1994;24(5):587–601.

Merzenich MM, Jenkins WM, Johnston P, et al.: Temporal processing deficits of language-learning impaired children ameliorated by training. *Science* 1996;271:77u–81.

Realmuto GM, August GJ, Garfinkel B: Clinical effect of buspirone in autistic children. *J Clin Psychopharmacol* 1989;9:122–125.

Shaffer D: Attention deficit hyperactivity disorder in adults. *Am J Psychiatry* 1994;151: 633–638.

Shepherd MJ, Uhry JK: Reading disorder, in Silver LB (ed): *Child Adolesc Clin North Am Pediatric Learning Disabil* 1993;2:193–208.

Silver LB: Developmental learning disorders, in Lewis M (ed): *Child and Adolescent Psychiatry: A Comprehensive Textbook*, 2nd ed. Baltimore, Williams & Wilkins, 1996.

Sprague RL, Sleator EK: Methylphenidate in hyperkinetic children: differences in dose effects on learning and social behavior. *Science* 1977;198:1274–1276.

Wilens TE, Biederman J: The stimulants, *Psychiatric Clin North Am* 1992;15:191–222.

Wilens TE, Biederman J, Geist DE, et al.: Nortriptyline in the treatment of ADHD: A chart review of 58 cases. *J Amer Acad Child Adolesec Psychiat* 1993;32:343–349.

OBSESSIVE-COMPULSIVE DISORDER AND TOURETTE'S SYNDROME

Wayne K. Goodman and Tanya Murphy

Detailed in this chapter are the diagnosis and pharmacological management of obsessive-compulsive disorder (OCD) and Tourette's syndrome (TS). Other topics include the recognition and treatment of body dysmorphic disorder and trichotillomania, which are sometimes referred to as obsessive-compulsive (OC) spectrum disorders. Although OCD is classified as an anxiety disorder in DSM-IV, its distinct presentation, pathobiology, and pharmacotherapy warrant separate consideration from the other anxiety disorders described in this volume. The pairing of OCD and TS in this chapter is based on a growing literature indicating that TS and some forms of childhood-onset OCD may be biologically related. In fact, some have suggested that childhood-onset OCD and TS may represent different phenotypic expressions of the same underlying diathesis. The lines of evidence supporting a clinically meaningful relationship between OCD and TS are summarized in this chapter. As an example, OC symptoms and tics—the cardinal features of OCD and TS, respectively—are comorbid at higher than expected rates, with more than 50% of TS patients exhibiting OC symptoms (Fig. 6-1). Although only about 20% of cases with a principal diagnosis of OCD appear to have a personal or family history of chronic tics, their presence may have implications for pharmacological management.

OBSESSIVE-COMPULSIVE DISORDER

Presenting Symptoms

As defined in DSM-IV, obsessive-compulsive disorder (OCD) is an anxiety disorder characterized by recurrent, unwanted, and distressing thoughts, images, or impulses (obsessions) and/or repetitive, rule-governed behaviors that the person feels driven to perform (compulsions) (Table 6-1). Both obsessions and compulsions need not be present to satisfy diagnostic criteria. The majority of patients have both obsessions and compulsions, with a minority experiencing either alone. The patient usually tries to actively dismiss or neutralize the obsessions by seeking reassurance, avoiding situational triggers (if present), or engaging in compulsions. In most cases, compulsions serve to alleviate anxiety. It is not uncommon, however, for the compulsions themselves to engender anxiety, such as when they become very arduous or time-consuming.

Common types of obsessions include concerns with contamination (e.g., fear of dirt, germs, or innocuous residues), safety and harm (e.g., being responsible for a fire), unwanted acts of aggression (e.g., impulsively harming a beloved grandchild), unacceptable sexual or religious thoughts (e.g., sacrilegious images of Christ in a devout Catholic), or the need for symmetry or exactness (Table 6-2).

Common compulsions include excessive cleaning (e.g., ritualized hand washing), checking behav-

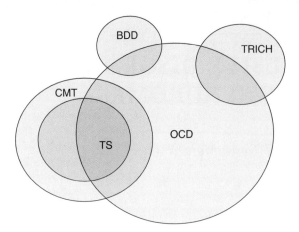

Figure 6–1. *Venn diagram of clinical overlap between obsessive-compulsive disorder (OCD) and related disorders. Abbreviations: BDD, body dysmorphic disorder; CMT, chronic multiple (motor or vocal) tics; TRICH, trichotillomania; TS, Tourette's syndrome.*

iors, ordering and arranging rituals, counting, repeating routine activities (e.g., going in or out of a doorway), and hoarding (e.g., collecting useless scraps of paper). Although most compulsions are observable behaviors, some are performed as mental rituals (e.g., silent recitation of nonsense words to vanquish a horrific image) (Table 6-2).

Most OCD patients have multiple types of obsessions and compulsions. For example, a patient may complain primarily of obsessive-compulsive symptoms involving asbestos contamination, but a detailed interview may disclose that the patient silently counts floor tiles and hoards junk mail, other bona-fide symptoms of OCD. For this reason, the administration of a comprehensive symptom inventory, such as the symptom checklist of the Yale-Brown Obsessive-Compulsive Scale (Y-BOCS) (Goodman et al., 1989), is often helpful in the initial evaluation.

A hallmark of the disorder is that at some point during the course of the illness the person recognizes the senselessness, or at least excessiveness, of his or her thoughts or behaviors (Fig. 6-2). Indeed, it is the presence of insight that distinguishes OCD from a psychotic process. The symptoms may be bizarre, but the patient recognizes their absurdity. For example, one patient feared he would accidentally discard his 5-year-old daughter so he rechecked envelopes before mailing to make sure that she was not inside. He readily acknowledged this was an impossibility, but was so tormented by pathological doubt that his anxiety would escalate uncontrollably unless he checked. The degree of insight varies considerably among patients and may even fluctuate within a particular individual over time and according to the situation. To accommodate this, DSM-IV permits inclusion of patients who currently exhibit little insight into their behaviors (specified as "poor insight") as long as they possessed insight at some point during the course of the illness.

When does normal checking behavior end and pathological checking begin? A diagnosis of OCD is warranted when the symptoms cause marked distress, are time-consuming, taking more than 1 h a day, or significantly interfere with functioning. Someone who needs to check the door exactly six times before leaving the house but is otherwise free of obsessive-compulsive symptoms may have a compulsive symptom, but does not have OCD. The impairment associated with OCD ranges from mild, with little interference in functioning, to extreme, when the person is incapacitated.

There are few modifications needed for making the diagnosis of childhood OCD, with the clinical presentation in children and in adults being remarkably similar. Although most children recognize that the symptoms are unwanted, it may be more difficult to evaluate insight in younger patients with OCD. Not all rituals in childhood should be considered pathological (Evans et al., 1997), since a need for sameness and consistency may promote a sense of security at times of transition. For example, many normal children engage in bedtime rituals such as arranging their bedding in a particular way, ensuring that their toes are covered, or checking for "monsters" under the bed. Childhood rituals should be suspected as signs of OCD when they become maladaptive (i.e., time-consuming or distressing) and persistent.

Abuse of stimulants such as amphetamine and cocaine may induce repetitive behaviors that resemble the rituals of OCD. Punding is a Swedish slang

Table 6-1

Diagnostic Criteria for Obsessive-Compulsive Disorder

A. Either obsessions or compulsions:

Obsessions are recurrent and persistent thoughts, impulses, or images that are experienced at some time during the disturbance as intrusive and inappropriate and cause marked anxiety or distress. These thoughts, impulses, or images are not simply excessive worries about real problems. The person attempts to ignore or suppress such thoughts, impulses, or images, or to neutralize them with some other thought or action. The person recognizes that the obsessional thoughts, impulses, or images are a product of his or her own mind (not imposed from without as in thought insertion).

Compulsions are repetitive behaviors or mental acts that the person feels driven to perform in response to an obsession, or according to rules that must be applied rigidly. These behaviors or mental acts are aimed at preventing or reducing distress or preventing some dreaded event or situation; however, these behaviors or mental acts either are not connected in a realistic way with what they are designed to neutralize or prevent or are clearly excessive.

B. At some point during the course of the disorder, the person has recognized that the obsessions or compulsions are excessive or unreasonable.

C. The obsessions or compulsions cause marked distress, are time consuming (take > 1 h a day), or significantly interfere with functioning.

D. If another Axis I disorder is present, the content of the obsessions or compulsions is not restricted to it, for example:

Preoccupation with food (eating disorder)
Hair pulling (trichotillomania)
Concern with appearance (body dysmorphic disorder)
Preoccupation with drugs (substance use disorder)
Preoccupation with having a serious illness (hypochondriasis)
Preoccupation with sexual urges or fantasies (paraphilia)

E. The disturbance is not due to the direct physiological effects of a substance or a general medical condition.

---

term that describes individuals who compulsively perform meaningless activities (e.g., assembling and disassembling household products) during intoxication with stimulants (Goodman et al., 1990). Stereotyped behaviors can be produced in laboratory animals by administration of stimulants and dopamine agonists (Goodman et al., 1990).

One explanation for why OCD may go undetected is that patients are often secretive about their obsessive-compulsive symptoms out of concern that they will be perceived as "crazy." In fact, many become experts at camouflaging their symptoms by either performing them in private, avoiding situations likely to trigger them, or, in the case of compulsions

Table 6-2
Common Types of Obsessions and Compulsions

Obsessions

- Fear of contamination by dirt or germs
- Fear of a terrible event such as fire, illness, or death
- Fear of harming oneself or others
- Excessive need for order or symmetry
- Personally unacceptable sexual or religious thoughts
- Superstitious fears

Compulsions

- Excessive cleaning or washing
- Excessive checking (for example, of locks or appliances)
- Excessive ordering or arranging of objects
- Ritualized counting
- Repeating routine activities (such as going through a doorway)
- Hoarding or collecting useless objects
- Mental rituals (for example, reciting nonsense words to banish an unwanted image)

that must be performed in public, inconspicuously incorporating them into ordinary activities. Patients with OCD are often reluctant to divulge their embarrassing or unacceptable thoughts unless they are specifically questioned about them. It behooves the physician to inquire about OC symptoms in patients who present with depression or anxiety, two common comorbid states that may mask OCD. These and other possible indicators of OCD and related disorders are listed in Table 6-3. OCD may be suspected in patients who have no known risk factors for AIDS but repeatedly request HIV testing. Recurrent, unfounded concerns about toxins and other environmental exposures may also signal a case with contamination fears. Physical signs of OCD are not common, but can include an unexplained dermatitis that may be secondary to excessive hand washing or use of caustic agents or alopecia of unknown origin that may sug-

gest compulsive hair pulling. Individuals who make frequent visits to the plastic surgeon but are never satisfied with the results may have body dysmorphic disorder and OCD. Depression in the immediate postpartum period is a well-recognized and serious clinical event. Postpartum OCD can occur together with depression, and its recognition is critical to appropriate therapeutic management.

Course

The onset of OCD is typically in adolescence or early adulthood, with less than 10% of patients first developing clinically significant symptoms after age 35 years. Onset has been reported as early as age 2 years, with nearly 15% of cases occuring before puberty. Boys are more often affected than girls, and their average age of onset is earlier. In adults with OCD, the overall sex ratio is close to 1:1. This contrasts with both depression and panic disorder, where there is a clear preponderance of women. The lifetime prevalence of OCD has been estimated as between 2 and 3% of the U.S. population.

The course of the illness is usually chronic, with either waxing and waning of symptoms in about 85% of patients or a progressive deterioration in about 5 to 10%. Only 5% of patients follow a true episodic course with periods in which they are totally free of symptoms, and even a smaller percentage experience

Table 6-3
Clues to an Underlying Diagnosis of OCD and Related Disorders

- Anxiety
- Depression
- Illness concerns (e.g., AIDS, cancer, poisoning)
- Tics
- Signs of unexplained dermatitis or alopecia of unknown origin (trichotillomania)
- Excessive concerns with appearance (body dysmorphic disorder)
- Postpartum depression

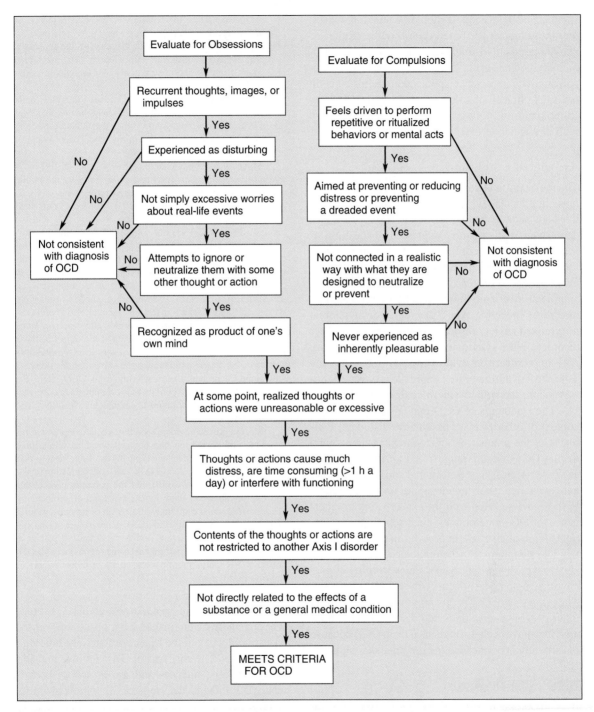

Figure 6–2. Steps required in making a diagnosis of obsessive-compulsive disorder (OCD).

spontaneous remission. It should be noted, however, that these figures are based on follow-up studies of clinical populations that may be biased toward chronicity (Goodman et al., 1994). It is possible that many patients who experience spontaneous remissions do not seek clinical attention or are lost to follow-up. In the majority of cases, the onset is not associated with any apparent external precipitant.

Associated Conditions

The most common comorbid major psychiatric diagnosis in patients with OCD is depression, with two-thirds of patients having a lifetime history of major depression, and one-third depressed at the time of first evaluation (Goodman et al., 1994). In fact, it is the development of depression that may prompt the OCD patient to present for treatment. There is also significant overlap between OCD and other anxiety disorders, including panic disorder, social phobia, generalized anxiety disorder, and separation anxiety disorder. Other syndromes with excess comorbidity risk in comparison with expected rates include Tourette's syndrome (TS), anorexia nervosa, trichotillomania, and body dysmorphic disorder (Fig. 6-1).

The symptoms of OCD may also appear in the context of other primary psychiatric disorders. Estimates of the number of schizophrenic patients who display OC symptoms range from 1 to 20% (Goodman et al., 1994). It is noteworthy that some of the novel antipsychotics, such as clozapine and risperidone, have been associated with the exacerbation or emergence of OC symptoms in some schizophrenic patients (Goodman et al., in press). Literature suggests that OC symptoms of schizophrenics respond favorably to typical anti-OC agents, but worsening of psychotic symptoms can occur with anti-OC treatment. The symptoms of OCD occur commonly in autism and other pervasive developmental disorders. Traditionally, they have been distinguished from OCD because of difficulty in confirming the presence of insight.

Differential Diagnosis

It is important to differentiate OCD from several other commonly encountered conditions before making a final diagnosis (Fig. 6-2).

As noted earlier, the presence or previous evidence of insight distinguishes OCD from a primary psychotic process. Obsessions may involve unrealistic fears but, unlike delusions, they are not fixed, unshakable convictions. To distinguish obsessions from psychotic symptoms like thought insertion (e.g., "aliens are transmitting telepathic messages to me"), a patient with OCD must attribute the intrusive thoughts to his or her own mind. An obsession can sometimes be misdiagnosed as an auditory hallucination when the patient, especially a child, refers to it as "the voice in my head" even though it is recognized as his or her own thoughts.

Much miscommunication exists because of the loose usage of the words *obsession* and *compulsion* by the public and professionals alike. To be bona-fide symptoms of OCD, obsessions and compulsions are strictly defined as described earlier in this chapter. A key point to remember is that the compulsions of OCD are not considered inherently pleasurable: at best, they relieve anxiety. As a contrasting clinical example, although patients seeking treatment for "compulsive" eating, gambling, or masturbating may feel unable to control behaviors that are acknowledged as deleterious, at some time in the past these acts were experienced as gratifying. By the same token, sexual obsessions are relabeled as preoccupations when it is evident that the person either derives some sexual satisfaction from these thoughts or the object of these thoughts is coveted. A woman who says she is "obsessed" with an ex-boyfriend, even though she knows she should leave him alone, is probably not suffering from OCD. Here the diagnostic possibilities would include erotomania (as depicted in the movie *Fatal Attraction*), pathological jealousy, and unrequited love.

Morbid preoccupations, sometimes called depressive ruminations, of depression can be mislabeled as obsessional thinking. The depressed patient typically dwells on matters that are meaningful to most people (e.g., one's accomplishments or other measures of self-worth), but the patient's perceptions and interpretations of these events or issues are colored by the depressed mood state. In contrast with obsessions, morbid preoccupations are usually defended by the patient as realistic concerns. Another difference is that the depressed patient is often preoccupied with past mistakes and regrets, whereas the person with OCD is more concerned about recent events or averting future harm.

The worries of generalized anxiety disorder (GAD) can be distinguished from obsessions on the basis of content and the absence of anxiety-relieving compulsions. The concerns of GAD involve real-life situations (e.g., finances and job or school performance), although the degree of apprehension is clearly excessive. In contrast, true obsessions usually reflect unrealistic fears such as inadvertently poisoning dinner guests.

The differential diagnosis between certain complex motor tics and certain compulsions (e.g., repetitive touching) can be problematic. By convention, tics are distinguished from tic-like compulsions based on whether the patient attaches a purpose or meaning to the behavior. For example, if a patient feels an urge to repeatedly touch an object this would be classified as a compulsion only if it was preceded by a need to neutralize an unwanted thought or image; otherwise it would be labeled a complex motor tic.

The distinction between the somatic obsessions of OCD and the somatic preoccupations of hypochondriasis is not always clear. One difference between the two syndromes, as defined in DSM-IV, is that patients with hypochondriasis are afraid they have a serious medical problem, whereas patients with OCD are more afraid they will acquire an illness. There are exceptions to these rules, however, as some of those who fear they have an illness (e.g., AIDS) exhibit an overall clinical picture more consistent with OCD. Consequently, an added requirement has been adopted that the patient perform multiple compulsions, such as ritualized checking for enlarged lymph nodes or excessive hand washing, to qualify for OCD. Doctor shopping or making repeat office visits are not considered true compulsions. The presence, or past history, of other OC symptoms not associated with somatic concerns increases confidence that the clinician is dealing with a case of OCD. The unfounded fear of spreading an illness is also a characteristic of OCD. Finally, the course of hypochondriasis tends to fluctuate more than that of OCD.

Panic attacks can be present in OCD, but an additional diagnosis of panic disorder should not be considered unless the attacks occur spontaneously. Some patients with OCD report the occurrence of panic attacks following exposure to a fearful stimulus such as a trace of blood encountered by someone with an AIDS obsession. In contrast with panic disorder, the individual is not afraid of the panic attack; rather, he or she is fearful of the consequences of contamination.

There continues to be debate regarding the relationship of "compulsive" self-injurious behaviors to compulsions vis-à-vis OCD. At present, self-mutilation behaviors (e.g., self-enucleation, severe nail biting) should not be considered as compulsions when diagnosing OCD. Likewise, behaviors that actually result in physical harm to others are outside the bounds of OCD. While patients with OCD may have unfounded fears about acting on violent and irrational impulses, they do not act on them. In evaluating a patient with violent or horrific thoughts, the physician must decide, based on clinical judgment and the patient's history, whether these symptoms are obsessions or part of the fantasy life of a potentially violent person. If the thoughts appear to be voluntarily produced, then they should not be viewed as obsessions.

The relationship between OCD and compulsive traits or personality is the subject of many diagnostic questions. Historically, the distinction between OCD and obsessive-compulsive personality disorder (OCPD) has been blurred in the psychiatric literature. DSM-IV has perpetuated the nosological confusion between the Axis I anxiety disorder and the Axis II personality disorder by selecting very similar diagnostic labels. Although some patients with OCD may have traits listed as criteria for OCPD, particularly perfectionism, preoccupation with details, and indecisiveness, most OCD patients do not meet the full criteria for OCPD, which also includes restricted expression of feelings, stinginess, and excessive devotion to productivity. Studies of comorbidity suggest that no more than 15% of patients with OCD meet the full criteria for OCPD (Goodman et al., 1994). The quintessential OCPD patient is a workaholic, draconian supervisor who, at home, shows contempt for displays of tender emotions and insists that the family submit to his will. Moreover, this individual does not have insight into his behavior and is not likely to seek psychiatric help on his own. Strictly defined, obsessions and compulsions are not present in OCPD. Hoarding behavior is generally regarded as a symptom of OCD although it is listed as a criterion for OCPD. Being detail oriented, hardworking, and productive is not the same as having OCPD; in fact, these traits are considered advantageous and adaptive in many settings, including medical school.

For purposes of the present discussion, a conservative approach to the phenomenology of OCD was adopted. Because OCD is at the crossroads of affective, psychotic, and movement disorders, it is not surprising that some real-life cases challenge a clinician's ability to define and categorize them. While standardized diagnostic criteria for psychiatric conditions are designed to be reliable, their validity must withstand empirical testing.

Pathogenesis

A condition resembling OCD has been recognized for more than 300 years. Each stage in the history of OCD has been influenced by the intellectual and scientific climate of the time. Early theories regarding the cause of a malady similar to OCD stressed the role of distorted religious experience, with English writers from the eighteenth and late seventeenth centuries attributing intrusive blasphemous images to the work of Satan. Even today, some patients with obsessions of "scrupulosity" still wonder about demonic possession and may seek exorcism. The French nineteenth-century accounts of obsessions emphasized the central role of doubt and indecisiveness. In 1837, the French clinician Esquirol used the term *folie du doute,* or the doubting madness, to refer to this cluster of symptoms (Pitman, 1994). Later French writers, including Pierre Janet in 1902, stressed loss of will and low mental energy as underlying the formation of OC symptoms (Pitman, 1994).

The greater part of the twentieth century was dominated by psychoanalytic theories of OCD. According to psychoanalytic theory, OC symptoms are defense mechanisms (e.g., doing-undoing and reaction formation) that represent maladaptive attempts to deal with unresolved unconscious conflicts from early stages of psychosexual development. Psychoanalysis offers an elaborate metaphor for the mind, but it is not grounded in evidence based on studies of the brain. These theories have lost favor because they have not led to effective and reproducible treatments. The psychoanalytic focus on the symbolic meaning of obsessions and compulsions has given way to an emphasis on the form of the symptoms: recurrent, distressing, and senseless forced thoughts and actions. The content of symptoms may reveal more about what is most important to or feared by the patient than why that particular individual developed OCD in the first place. Alternatively, the content, such as grooming and hoarding, may be related to the activation of fixed action patterns (i.e., innate complex behavioral subroutines) mediated by the brain areas involved in OCD (Swedo, 1989).

In contrast with psychoanalysis, learning theory models of OCD have gained momentum as a result of the success of behavior therapy. Behavior therapy does not concern itself with the psychological origins or meaning of OC symptoms. Rather, it is theorized that obsessions and compulsions are acquired sequentially as the result of classical, then instrumental conditioning (Meyer, 1996). Learning theory does not account for all aspects of OCD. For example, it does not adequately explain why some compulsions persist even when they produce, rather than reduce, anxiety. Because compulsions are viewed as a response to obsessions, learning theory does not account for cases in which only compulsions are present. It is also incompatible with OC symptoms that develop directly as the result of brain injury. These limitations notwithstanding, the effectiveness of a behavior therapy technique referred to as exposure and response prevention has been confirmed in numerous studies (van Balkom et al., 1994).

For the last 30 years, the neurotransmitter serotonin [5-hydroxytryptamine(5-HT)] has remained the leading target for investigations of the neurochemical underpinnings of OCD. The bulk of the evidence implicating brain serotonin systems is derived from drug response data, namely, the preferential efficacy of potent selective serotonin reuptake inhibitors (SSRIs) in OCD (see discussion of treatment later in this chapter). Theories of pathogenesis that rely heavily on the presumed mechanism of action of an effective therapy can, however, be misleading. It is conceivable that SSRIs may exert their therapeutic effect in OCD by enhancing the functioning of intact compensatory systems rather than correcting a primary disturbance. More direct measures of neurochemical challenges, or functional neuroimaging, are needed to confirm a pathophysiological role for serotonin. Though tending to support a derangement in serotonin function, such studies have failed to elucidate the precise nature of the suspected disturbance (Barr et al., 1992). An example of this are studies of the behavioral and biochemical effects of the mixed serotonin agonist/antagonist *meta*-chlorophenylpiperazine in OCD, which have yielded inconsistent findings, not only between, but also within, individual laboratories (Barr et al., 1992). In contrast with panic disorder, there is little support for a role of noradrenergic pathways in the neurobiology of OCD.

Recent studies on the origins of OC behavior and OCD have been influenced by the following developments: (1) evidence for possible involvement of neurotransmitters other than serotonin and neuromodulators; (2) advances in the understanding of brain neurocircuitry; (3) identification of putative subtypes; and (4) the role of autoimmune factors. Some modern theories of pathobiology incorporate many or all of these elements.

A growing body of evidence, including data from functional neuroimaging studies, implicates circuitry of the basal ganglia and orbitofrontal cortex in the pathophysiology of OCD. Increased metabolic activity in the orbitofrontal cortex and anterior cingulate gyrus has been the most consistent finding in positron emission tomography (PET) and functional magnetic resonance imaging (fMR) studies of OCD (Schwartz, 1997). Some investigators have proposed that increased activity in these areas is secondary to impaired modulation by the interconnected caudate nucleus. Baxter and colleagues (1996) have proposed that an imbalance between the direct and indirect pathways of the basal ganglia thalamocortical circuitry is responsible for inappropriately activating the orbitofrontal cortex and cingulate cortex (Baxter et al., 1996). This provokes faulty error detection signals, alerting the organism that something is wrong (when it is not) and that corrective action needs to be taken. In the patient with OCD, this process is manifested as intrusive disturbing thoughts and the emergence of self-protective behaviors such as checking and cleaning.

The working assumption of the scientific community is that OCD is heterogeneous with respect to etiology. Direct evidence for this is furnished by accidents of nature. Numerous case reports document that von Economo's encephalitis, head trauma, carbon monoxide poisoning, stroke, Sydenham's chorea, Huntington's disease, and other bilateral insults to structures of the basal ganglia can be associated with the development of OC symptoms (Goodman et al., 1990). The wide variations seen in treatment response, course, and comorbidity of OCD are consistent with multiple pathogenic forms of the illness. Underlying heterogeneity may also explain why it has been so difficult to discover a consistent biologic abnormality. TS-related OCD, or OCD with comorbid chronic tics, is the putative subtype that has received the most empirical support. As discussed later, a dysregulation in dopamine function has been implicated in TS. Based on preclinical and clinical data, Goodman and colleagues proposed that OC symptoms may be mediated or controlled by an interplay of serotonin and dopamine neuronal systems in TS-related OCD (Goodman et al., 1990).

It has been proposed that some cases of childhood-onset OCD may be related to an infection-triggered autoimmune process similar to that of Sydenham's chorea, a late manifestation of rheumatic fever (Swedo et al., 1994). Indeed, over 70% of cases of Sydenham's chorea have OC symptoms (Swedo et al., 1994). The etiology of Sydenham's chorea is thought to involve the development of antibodies to group A β-hemolytic streptococcal infection that cross-react with basal ganglia and other brain areas (Murphy et al., 1997). Swedo has coined the term PANDAS (pediatric autoimmune neuropsychiatric disorders associated with strep) to describe cases of childhood-onset OCD that resemble Sydenham's chorea with respect to acute onset following a GABHS infection, accompanying neurological signs, and an episodic course (Swedo, 1994). This exciting new avenue of research will undoubtedly be the subject of intense investigation in the coming years.

There has been a recent trend to look beyond the monoamine neurotransmitter systems and explore the role of other neurochemicals in this disorder, including neuropeptides. Leckman and coworkers (1994) have proposed that abnormalities in oxytocin-mediated neuronal function may be present in some patients with OCD. In one study, cerebrospinal fluid levels of oxytocin were elevated in a subgroup of "pure" OCD patients compared with either healthy control subjects or patients with tics, with or without OCD (Leckman et al., 1994). Additional studies are needed to examine the contribution of neuropeptides to the pathophysiology and treatment of OCD.

Pharmacotherapeutics

In the past, OCD was generally viewed as unresponsive to a range of conventional therapies. Traditional talk therapy based on psychoanalytic principles was rarely successful in reducing the severity of obsessions or compulsions, and the success rate with a range of different medications was just as disappointing. The 1980s witnessed renewed optimism about the prognosis of OCD as new, more effective forms of behavior therapy and pharmacotherapy were introduced and subjected to large-scale testing. The form of behavior therapy that has been most effective in OCD is referred to as exposure and response prevention. Exposure consists of confronting the patient with situations that evoke obsessional distress; response prevention involves instruction on how to resist performing compulsive rituals (Foa et al., 1985).

At present, the mainstay of the phamacotherapy of OCD is a trial with either clomipramine or an SSRI. The pharmacology of SSRIs is reviewed in detail in Chap. 4. Only those properties of SSRIs specific to their use in OCD are discussed here. Clomipramine is both a tricyclic and an inhibitor of serotonin reuptake. Although tricyclics are discussed in Chap. 4, this chapter addresses those features of clomipramine that distinguish it from other members of its class.

The modern era in the pharmacotherapy of OCD began in the late 1960s with the observation that clomipramine, but not other tricyclic antidepressants such as imipramine, was effective in OCD. Clomipramine, the 3-chloro analogue of the tricyclic imipramine, is 100-fold more potent as an inhibitor of serotonin uptake than the parent compound. These distinctive clinical and pharmacological properties of clomipramine led to the hypothesis that serotonin might be involved in the pathophysiology of OCD (Goodman et al., 1990). The superiority of clomipramine over placebo and nonserotonergic antidepressants has been confirmed in numerous double-blind trials (DeVeaugh-Geiss et al., 1991). Clomipramine is the most thoroughly studied drug in OCD and was the first to receive U.S. Food and Drug Administration (FDA) approval for this indication. Desmethylclomipramine, a major metabolite of clomipramine, potently blocks reuptake of both sero-tonin and norepinephrine. During chronic treatment, desmethylclomipramine attains higher plasma levels than the parent compound. Most side effects of clom-ipramine can be predicted from its receptor binding profile. Thus, as with other tricyclic antidepressants, side effects typical of anticholinergic blockade (e.g., dry mouth and constipation) are common. Likewise, nausea and tremor are common with clom-ipramine as is the case with SSRIs. Impotence and anorgasmia occur with clomipramine. Many patients complain of sedation and weight gain. Safety con-cerns with clomipramine include prolongation of the QT interval and seizures. The risk of seizures in-creases significantly at doses above 250 mg daily. Intentional overdose with clomipramine can be lethal.

In recent years, trials have been conducted in OCD patients with a newer generation of antidepres-sant drugs that are both potent and selective inhibitors of serotonin reuptake. Included in this group are fluvoxamine, paroxetine, sertraline, and fluoxetine. Unlike clomipramine, none of these medications loses its selectivity for blocking serotonin reuptake in vivo. Also, in contrast with clomipramine and other tricyclics, these drugs lack significant affinity for histaminic, cholinergic, and α-adrenergic recep-tors. All potent SSRIs tested to date have proved efficacious in controlling the symptoms of OCD. As was previously demonstrated for clomipramine,

fluvoxamine was shown more effective than desipra-mine in reducing OC symptoms (Goodman et al., 1990). An FDA indication for OCD in adults has been granted for fluvoxamine, fluoxetine, paroxetine, and sertraline. The anti-OC efficacy of fluvoxamine has also been confirmed in children. The SSRIs are generally well tolerated, with the most common side effects being nausea, somnolence, insomnia, tremor, and sexual dysfunction, in particular anorgasmia. There are few significant safety concerns, and the risk associated with overdose is small.

Antidepressants that do not significantly block serotonin reuptake (e.g., desipramine) are generally ineffective in treat-ing OCD. In this respect, OCD contrasts sharply with depres-sion and panic disorder, two psychiatric illnesses that, in most studies, respond equally well to antidepressants regardless of their selectivity in inhibiting monoamine reuptake. This and other differences in the comparative efficacy of medications and electroconvulsive therapy (ECT) in the treatment of OCD, depression, and panic disorder are summarized in Table 6-4. As noted, potent SSRIs and clomipramine are generally less effective in OCD than in depression or panic disorder. Indeed, the response of depression or panic disorder to treatment is often all-or-none, whereas OCD is more likely to show a graded and incomplete response to treatment. Based on conser-vative outcome criteria, approximately 40 to 60% of patients with OCD experience a clinically meaningful response to a trial with an SSRI or clomipramine.

Acute blockade of serotonin reuptake appears to be the critical first step in a chain of neural events leading to anti-OC efficacy. Based on electrophysiological studies in laboratory animals, Blier and coworkers (1996) proposed that enhance-ment of serotonin neurotransmission in the orbitofrontal cortex

Table 6-4

Comparative Efficacy of Somatic Treatments for OCD, Depression, and Panic Disorder

	SSRIs (e.g., fluvoxamine)	TCAs (e.g., clomipramine)	(e.g., imipramine)	MAOIs (e.g., phenelzine)	ECT	Benzos (e.g., alprazolam)
OCD	XXX	XXX	X	X	X	X
Depression	XXX	XXX	XXX	XXX	XXX	—
Panic disorder	XXX	XXX	XXX	XXX	—	XXX

NOTE Efficacy range = X (minimal evidence/weak effect) to XXX (much evidence/strong effect).

KEYS SSRIs, Selective serotonin reuptake inhibitors; TCAs, tricyclic antidepressants;

    MAOIs, monoamine oxidase inhibitors; ECT, electroconvulsive therapy;

    benzos, benzodiazepines.

during chronic SSRI administration is related to the mechanism of action of these agents in OCD.

Now that there are several potent SSRIs to choose from, an important clinical question is whether there are significant differences in the anti-OC efficacy of these drugs. A meta-analysis comparing published multicenter trials found that clomipramine is significantly superior to the SSRIs fluoxetine, sertraline, and fluvoxamine (Griest et al., 1995). Meta-analyses are subject to a number of limitations, however, including the possibility that the apparent differences in drug efficacy actually reflect underlying differences in patient characteristics. The early multicenter clomipramine trials were conducted at a time when there were no effective alternatives, whereas in subsequent studies many cases resistant to other medications (including clomipramine) were included. The best way to determine the comparative efficacy of treatments is a randomized, head-to-head, double-blind comparison. The results of several such studies comparing clomipramine with SSRIs have been published recently (Koran et al., 1996; Bisserbe et al., 1997). By and large, these studies failed to find evidence for the superiority of clomipramine over the SSRIs tested thus far. With regard to side effects, the outcome is different. There are fewer serious side effects with the SSRIs, and they are generally better tolerated than clomipramine.

Clinical Pharmacology

Practical guidelines to the pharmacologic management of OCD are discussed in this section, and key decision points are summarized as an algorithm in Fig. 6-3.

Acute pharmacological treatment. The recognition and accurate diagnosis of OCD are the first steps in the proper treatment of this condition. If the diagnosis of OCD is overlooked, then inappropriate treatment may be prescribed. For example, patients with OCD often present with symptoms of depression or anxiety, but not all antidepressants and few, if any, anxiolytic medications are effective antiobsessional agents. Likewise, treatments that have proved effective for OCD may be of little value in treating the symptoms of other disorders, such as the delusions of schizophrenia or the character traits of obsessive-compulsive personality disorder.

The treatment of choice for OCD is a 10- to 12-week trial with an SSRI at adequate doses. It is hard to justify beginning with clomipramine given the superior tolerability and safety of SSRIs and their comparable efficacy. Which SSRI to prescribe initially is based on expected side effect profile and pharmacokinetic considerations. In the individual patient, however, it is quite difficult to predict the best fit with a particular agent. In the early stages of treatment the primary objective is to promote compliance. Although patients may be experiencing marked distress and functional impairment, most have had symptoms for years before presenting for treatment. The dose of SSRI can be increased incrementally every 3 to 4 days in outpatients (even faster in inpatients), but this dose escalation should be reduced if the patient is troubled by side effects, particularly nausea. Fluoxetine, paroxetine, and sertraline can be given as a single daily dose. The package insert recommends initiating clomipramine and fluvoxamine therapy on a twice-daily regimen, but in most cases these drugs can be given as a single daily dose, usually at night because they tend to be sedating. In contrast, fluoxetine tends to be activating and is best administered in the morning so that sleep is not disrupted. If the patient reports insomnia while taking fluvoxamine, then the schedule should be reversed such that the bulk (or all) of the dose is taken in the morning.

Although there is consensus among experts that the duration of an adequate medication trial must be between 10 and 12 weeks, there is less uniformity of opinion with regard to what constitutes an adequate dose. Some, but not all, fixed-dose trials of SSRIs and clomipramine indicate that higher doses are significantly superior to lower doses in the treatment of OCD. In the case of paroxetine in OCD, 20 mg per day did not separate from placebo; the lowest effective dose was 40 mg per day (Wheadon et al., 1993). By and large, studies of fluoxetine in OCD suggest that 60 mg per day is more effective than 20 mg per day, but that 20 and 40 mg per day are still more effective than placebo (Tollefson et al., 1994). As the 60-mg-per-day dose of fluoxetine is associated with more side effects than lower doses, the preferred clinical practice is to give patients with OCD 40 mg for about 8 weeks before increasing the dose further. In the final analysis, the criteria for an adequate trial must be defined in relation to the medication(s) in question. Adequate trials in OCD of clomipramine, fluvoxamine, fluoxetine, sertraline,

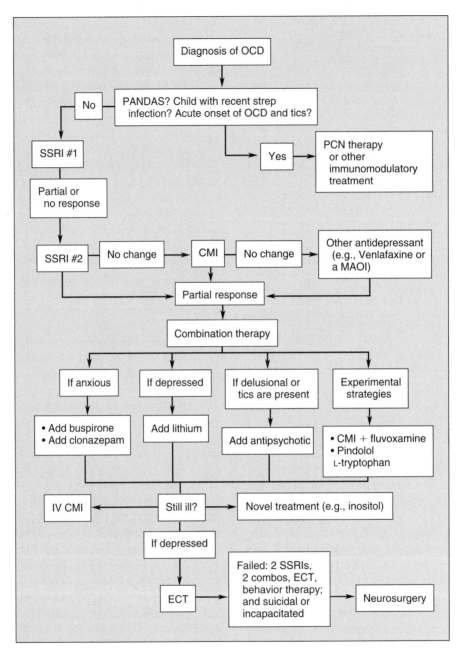

Figure 6–3. *Algorithm for medical management of obsessive-compulsive disorder (OCD). Abbreviations: CMI, clomipramine; ECT, electroconvulsive therapy; MAOI, monoamine oxidase inhibitor; PANDAS, pediatric autoimmune neuropsychiatric disorders associated with strep; PCN, penicillin; SSRI, selective serotonin reuptake inhibitor.*

and paroxetine would be 10 to 12 weeks of treatment with a minimum mean daily dose of 150, 150, 40, 150, and 40 mg, respectively, for at least the final 8 weeks. Although a trial of fluoxetine with 40 mg per day for 8 of 12 weeks might be deemed adequate, a nonresponder to such a trial should probably not be labeled as fluoxetine-resistant until the dose is increased to 80 mg per day as tolerated.

Based on the multicenter trial of fluvoxamine in children 8 years or older and adolescents with OCD (Riddle et al., 1994), it is advisable to start patients in this age range on fluvoxamine 25 mg at bedtime. This dose should be continued for approximately 3 days and then increased by 25-mg increments every 3 to 4 days until a maximum daily dose of 200 mg is achieved. Fluvoxamine should be given twice per day for daily doses of 75 mg or greater, with the larger dose given at bedtime. In general, lower maximal dosages of SSRIs and clomipramine should be used in the elderly and in patients with hepatic insufficiency.

Long-term treatment. Important clinical questions remain unanswered regarding the long-term management of OCD patients who have responded to an acute drug trial. Compared with an ample database on long-term treatment of depression, there is currently little known about how long medication should be continued in OCD. In clinical practice, most patients are given medications for at least 1 year; some seem to require indefinite treatment. The relapse rate with abrupt discontinuation of medication is high in OCD—as much as 90% in some studies (Pato et al., 1990). It is yet to be established in a controlled study whether a gradual taper of medication over a longer period of time (e.g., 6 months or more), as is usually done in clinical practice, produces a lower relapse rate. An alternative to outright discontinuation is a dose reduction to a new stable level. Both clinical experience and a recent report (Ravizza et al., 1996) suggest that patients with OCD can be maintained successfully at lower doses than those required to produce an initial treatment response.

Adverse events have been associated with abrupt discontinuation of clomipramine and the SSRIs, paroxetine, fluvoxamine, and sertraline. Relatively fewer reports of withdrawal syndromes following abrupt cessation of fluoxetine may reflect the long half-lives of the parent drug and its metabolite nor-fluoxetine. The constellation of symptoms reported with the SSRIs is somewhat variable, but has most frequently included flulike symptoms, vertigo or dizziness, insomnia, vivid dreams, irritability, and headaches lasting from several days to more than 1 week. No medically significant events have been documented, but patients often describe marked discomfort. To reduce the risk of a discontinuation syndrome, a gradual taper is recommended for clomipramine and all SSRIs except fluoxetine.

Management of side effects. Because of the chronic nature of the illness, management of even mild drug-induced side effects may have a bearing on compliance and quality of life. In clinical experience at this institution, the most significant complaints associated with chronic treatment with clomipramine are weight gain, somnolence, sexual dysfunction (impotence or anorgasmia), dry mouth, urinary hesitancy, constipation, and tremor. Elevations in hepatic transaminase levels can occur with clomipramine, and therefore liver function tests should be assessed at least annually or when symptoms of drug-induced hepatitis appear. The dosage of clomipramine may need to be lowered when it is given with medications known to increase plasma concentrations of tricylic antidepressants. Clinically problematic complaints associated with chronic SSRI administration include daytime drowsiness, disturbed sleep, anorgasmia, weight gain (not as common or marked as with clomipramine), and tremors. Drowsiness seems to be most prominent in the afternoon, especially during monotonous activities such as driving a motor vehicle. Because side effects are often dose-related, dosage reduction is always the first consideration. The addition of a second medication, however, may be indicated to counteract the side effects of insomnia or sexual dysfunction.

In evaluating insomnia in a patient receiving an SSRI, it is important to rule out the possibility it is secondary to an inadequately treated comorbid depression or persistent obsessional thoughts. Once this is done, the clinician is often faced with choosing a medication for symptomatic treatment of this side effect. The triazolopyridine antidepressant, trazodone (50 to 100 mg at bedtime), has been a popular choice because of its nonaddictive sedative properties (Nierenberg et al., 1994). An alternative to trazodone may be a hypnotic benzodiazepine. It should be remembered that fluvoxamine may increase plasma concentrations of triazolobenzodiazapines such as alprazolam by inhibiting their hepatic metabolism; lorazepam metabolism is unaffected by fluvoxamine. Zolpidem is structurally distinct from benzodiazepines, yet acts as an agonist at benzodiazepine receptors; some evidence suggests that its abuse potential is less and its amnesic effects are fewer compared with benzodiazepines.

Sexual dysfunction in patients receiving psychotropic medications is best approached through a systematic evaluation to determine causality. For cases in which the medication seems responsible, the literature offers several different approaches to consider. Cyproheptadine is an antihistamine and $5\text{-}HT_2$ receptor antagonist that has been reported to reverse anorgasmia and ejaculatory delay secondary to serotonergic medications such as fluoxetine (Arnott and Nunn, 1991). Sedation is common with cyproheptadine and may present a dose-limiting side effect. An open trial of the α_2-adrenergic receptor antagonist yohimbine has also been reported to counter the sexual side effects of clomipramine and fluoxetine in six patients (Jacobson, 1992). There has been one case report of fluoxetine-induced sexual side effects resolving in a 50-year-old male with the addition of bupropion (Labbate and Pollack, 1994). The mechanism by which bupropion resolved this sexual dysfunction is unknown. The benefit of a drug holiday has been evaluated in an open trial of 30 patients experiencing SSRI-induced sexual dysfunction (Rothschild, 1995). Patients receiving paroxetine and sertraline, but not fluoxetine, reported significant improvement in sexual functioning following a 2-day drug holiday.

Approaches to Treatment of Refractory OCD

Despite progress in the pharmacologic treatment of OCD, approximately 50% of patients fail to respond to an apparently adequate trial with a single drug. Furthermore, even among responders, few become completely asymptomatic. New and better approaches for treating medication-resistant OCD are needed.

Dosage escalation and switching antidepressants. If a patient has had a limited response to, but few side effects with, an SSRI or clomipramine, the next logical step is to increase to the highest recommended dose. Fortunately, the SSRIs are generally safe even at high doses. In contrast, clomipramine should not be administered in doses above 250 mg per day without careful medical monitoring (e.g., serial ECGs) and unless clinically indicated.

Although there is debate in the literature regarding the value of prescribing an SSRI after an OCD patient has not responded to clomipramine, there are numerous anecdotal examples of therapeutic success with one SSRI following failure with a different drug, including clomipramine. These authors advocate changing to a different SSRI if there has been no improvement at all following an adequate trial with another member of this class. With partial gains, a combination treatment approach is generally recommended instead. Naturally, if the patient does not tolerate one SSRI, it is advisable to try a different one, selected on the basis of its expected side effect profile.

Other classes of antidepressants may be considered in patients who have failed to show any response to SSRIs or clomipramine. Preliminary evidence suggests that venlafaxine may benefit some patients with OCD. The monoamine oxidase inhibitor phenelzine may also be useful in some cases of OCD, but it is difficult to predict who will respond on the basis of baseline clinical characteristics.

Combination strategies: Adding another agent to the SSRI or clomipramine. The patient who has had a partial response to SSRI or clomipramine monotherapy or failed to show any improvement following two consecutive trials with different SSRIs is a candidate for combination treatment. To date, the rationale for the majority of drug combination strategies has been to add agents to ongoing SSRI or clomipramine therapy that may modify serotonergic function, such as tryptophan, fenfluramine, lithium, buspirone, pindolol, or another SSRI. Addition of an antipsychotic is also a possibility.

Addition of tryptophan, the amino acid precursor of serotonin, has been reported helpful at a case report level only. At present, oral tryptophan supplements are not available in the United States because of evidence linking some preparations to the eosinophilia myalgia syndrome, a serious and potentially fatal hematologic/connective tissue illness. Blier and Bergeron (1996) in Canada, where tryptophan is readily available, described the benefits of adding tryptophan to a subgroup of patients with OCD taking a combination of an SSRI and pindolol.

In small open-label studies, addition of the serotonin releaser and reuptake blocker d,l-fenfluramine (Pondimen) or dexfenfluramine (Redux) to an SSRI led to improvement in OCD; however, no controlled trials have been conducted. In September 1997, the manufacturer (Wyeth-Ayerst) removed these products from the worldwide market after reports of cardiac complications (Connolly et al., 1997). Other safety concerns with these agents include primary pulmonary hypertension, possible neurotoxicity, and serotonin syndrome when combined with SSRIs.

Coadministration of lithium is a proven method for enhancing the action of antidepressants in patients with depression. Lithium has been hypothesized to potentiate antidepressant-induced increases in serotonin neurotransmission by enhancing presynaptic serotonin release in some brain regions. Despite several earlier encouraging reports, the efficacy of lithium addition in OCD has not been corroborated in controlled trials (Goodman et al., in press). Although the overall yield is low in OCD, individual patients, particularly those with marked depressive symptoms, may benefit from lithium augmentation.

In two open-label studies, addition of the $5HT_{1a}$ partial agonist buspirone to ongoing fluoxetine treatment in patients with OCD led to greater improvement in OC symptoms than did continued treatment with fluoxetine alone (Goodman et al., in press). These initially encouraging findings have not been confirmed in three subsequent double-blind trials (Goodman et al., in press). Adjunctive buspirone may be useful for treatment of OCD with concomitant symptoms of generalized anxiety disorder.

Pindolol is a nonselective β-adrenergic receptor antagonist that binds with high affinity to the $5HT_{1a}$ receptor and blocks the presynaptic actions of $5HT_{1a}$ agonists. Some studies have shown that pindolol may hasten or augment antidepressant action in depressed patients. Similar studies in OCD are inconclusive thus far (Goodman et al., in press), but additional trials are under way.

In clinical practice, a number of SSRI-resistant OCD patients receive simultaneous treatment with two SSRIs. There is scant empirical or theoretical support, however, for this strategy. The advantage of dual SSRI therapy over a higher dose of a single agent is hard to explain based on the current understanding of the pharmacodynamic properties of these drugs. Suitable empirical studies would require a high-dose SSRI monotherapy control group and double-blind conditions.

Antipsychotics alone do not appear effective in OCD, but there is emerging evidence that conjoint SSRI-antipsychotic treatment may be beneficial in a subset of patients with tic-related OCD (McDougle et al., 1994). To date, the putative subgroup that has received the most attention has been OCD with a comorbid chronic tic disorder. Results from a double-blind, placebo-controlled study of haloperidol addition to fluvoxamine-refractory patients with OCD support the efficacy of this combination treatment strategy. Patients who had an unsatisfactory response to 8 weeks of fluvoxamine monotherapy were randomized to either 4 weeks of haloperidol or placebo in addition to a fixed daily dosage of fluvoxamine. The fluvoxamine-haloperidol combination was preferentially effective in reducing OC symptoms in the patients with a comorbid tic disorder. A number of preliminary reports suggest that risperidone, an atypical antipsychotic that blocks both dopamine and $5HT_2$ serotonin receptors, might alleviate OC symptoms when added to ongoing SSRI therapy.

Novel and experimental drug treatments. A variety of alternative drug treatments have been used in OCD. Of those considered here, intravenous clomipramine is the only treatment supported by a reasonable degree of empirical evidence. Recent studies on the therapeutic use of the second messenger precursor inositol have been extended to OCD. Various trials with immunomodulatory treatments (e.g., prednisone, plasmapheresis, IV immunoglobins) or antimicrobial prophylaxis

(e.g., penicillin) are under way at the National Institute of Mental Health and elsewhere.

Nonpharmacologic biological approaches. Nonpharmacologic biologic treatments of OCD have included electroconvulsive therapy (ECT) and neurosurgery. ECT, regarded as the gold standard for treating depression, is generally viewed as having limited benefit in OCD despite sporadic reports of its success in treatment-resistant cases (Rudorfer, 1997). In some instances the favorable response to ECT is short-lived.

Modern stereotactic surgical procedures should not be equated with the relatively crude neurosurgical approaches of the past. Recent evidence suggests that stereotactic lesions of the cingulum bundle (cingulotomy) or anterior limb of the internal capsule (capsulotomy) may produce substantial clinical benefit in some patients with OCD without causing appreciable morbidity (Baer et al., 1995). A number of unanswered questions about neurosurgical treatment of OCD remain: (1) What is the true (placebo-corrected) efficacy of surgery? (2) Which procedure (i.e., cingulotomy, capsulotomy, limbic leucotomy) is best? (3) What is the optimal placement of lesions? and (4) Can the best candidates for surgery be predicted? At present, stereotactic psychosurgery should be viewed as the option of last resort in the gravely ill patient with OCD who has not responded to well-documented adequate trials over a 5-year period with several SSRIs and clomipramine, exposure and response prevention, at least two combination strategies (including combined SSRI and behavior therapy), an MAOI trial, a trial with a novel antidepressant (e.g., venlafaxine), and ECT (if depression is present).

OC-SPECTRUM DISORDERS

Some neuropsychiatric conditions have been referred to as OC-spectrum disorders on the basis of clinical similarities to OCD (i.e., recurrent disturbing ideation and/or irresistible urges), higher than expected comorbidity with OCD, and favorable response to SSRIs. For example, autistic patients may exhibit classic compulsive symptoms such as repeating routine activities, ordering, hoarding, incessant questioning, touching, tapping, and other stereotyped behaviors. Although major depression is the most frequently encountered comorbid major psychiatric disorder—and its ruminations have been likened to obsessions—it is not thought of as belonging to the OC-spectrum because of its distinct clinical features, course, and treatment response. Furthermore, the development of depression is usually presumed secondary to having OC symptoms. Of the OC-spectrum disorders, Tourette's syndrome is the only one to date for which a relationship with some forms of OCD is supported by family and genetic data (Pauls et al., 1986).

Although it is beyond the scope of this chapter to discuss the validity of a particular disorder's inclusion among the OC spectrum, several general caveats warrant mention. Some authors (Hollander and Cohen, 1996) have conceptualized OC-spectrum disorders and OCD itself as falling along a continuum from pure obsessiveness at one end, to compulsivity, and finally to impulsivity at the other end. One problem with this schema is that differentiating compulsive from impulsive behavior can be problematic. In addition, the hypothesis that OC-spectrum cases fall along different points of the compulsive-impulsive continuum needs to explain how both compulsive and impulsive behavior can coexist in the same individuals. For example, some cases of comorbid OCD and TS display both compulsive (e.g., ritualized

Table 6-5
List and DSM-IV Classification of OC-Spectrum Disorders

Childhood-onset disorders
Tourette's syndrome (TS)*
Autism
Prader-Willi syndrome
Somatoform disorders
Body dysmorphic disorder (BDD)*
Hypochondriasis
Eating disorders
Anorexia nervosa
Bulimia nervosa
Binge-eating disorder
Impulse control disorders
Trichotillomania*
Pathological gambling
Compulsive nail biting (onychophagia)
Kleptomania
Compulsive buying
Paraphilias

* Discussed in text.

Table 6-6
Diagnostic Criteria for Body Dysmorphic Disorder

A. Preoccupation with an imagined defect in appearance. If a slight physical anomaly is present, the person's concern is markedly excessive.

B. The preoccupation causes clinically significant distress or impairment in social, occupational, or other important areas of functioning.

C. The preoccupation is not better accounted for by another mental disorder (e.g., dissatisfaction with body shape and size in anorexia nervosa).

grooming) and impulsive (e.g., inappropriate touching) behaviors. The aforementioned limitations of the OC spectrum construct notwithstanding, the conditions listed in Table 6-5 have been frequently classified as such. Of those listed in the table, only the pharmacologic treatment of body dysmorphic disorder (BDD), trichotillomania, and TS are discussed in the following.

Body Dysmorphic Disorder

One of the OC-spectrum disorders to receive the most attention is body dysmorphic disorder, for which the diagnostic criteria are listed in Table 6-6. The central feature of BDD is a preoccupation with an imagined or inconsequential defect in physical appearance. In the DSM-IV Field Trials, 12% of OCD cases also met criteria for BDD (Simeon et al., 1995). The phenomenologies of BDD and OCD are similar in many respects. Both are characterized by recurrent, disturbing, and intrusive thoughts. In the case of OCD, the content may involve a variety of different subjects (e.g., contamination or fear of acting on unwanted impulses). The concerns of BDD, by definition, always involve a minor or imagined physical anomaly. The most frequent concerns relate to the face and head (e.g., nose size, facial shape, skin texture, wrinkles, or blemishes); less frequently, other aspects of the body are the focus of attention (e.g., breast asymmetry and foot size). BDD is often accompanied by repeated checking (e.g., examining the imagined defect in the mirror) or touching, behaviors that are very similar to those found in classic OCD. Instead of engaging in checking rituals, some patients with BDD may endeavor to avoid all reminders of their flawed appearance by removing mirrors and covering all reflective surfaces in their home (Phillips, 1995).

In contrast with OCD, patients with BDD usually are convinced that their irrational preoccupations are justifiable. When presented with contradictory evidence, however (e.g., a nomogram showing that one's measured head size is within normal limits), a BDD patient will acknowledge that there is no objective support for the concern. Thus, the overvalued ideas of BDD fall somewhere between obsessions and delusions with respect to how strongly false beliefs are held to be valid. In clinical practice, the distinction between BDD and a somatic delusion is not always straightforward, nor may it be meaningful (Phillips et al., 1994).

There have been no controlled treatment studies of BDD, but several open-label case series suggest that SSRIs and clomipramine are beneficial for many of these patients, even some with delusional ideation. In a retrospective analysis of 50 patients with BDD, those treated with clomipramine, fluoxetine, or fluvoxamine seemed to do better than those treated with tricyclic antidepressant (Hollander et al., 1993). Phillips and McElroy (1996) conducted an open-label trial of fluvoxamine (up to 300 mg per day) in 20 patients with BDD. Based on stringent outcome criteria, 14 of 20 (70%) responded. The authors note that "delusional patients were as likely to respond as nondelusional subjects, and insight significantly improved." In experience at this institution, BDD tends to be less responsive to pharmacotherapy than is OCD.

Trichotillomania

Among the impulse control disorders, trichotillomania has been examined most closely with respect to its relationship with OCD. The diagnostic criteria for trichotillomania are listed in Table 6-7. As noted, the key features of trichotillomania are (1) recurrent hair pulling, (2) mounting tension preceding the act, and (3) pleasure or relief accompanying the act. The sites most often affected are the scalp, eyebrows, eyelashes, extremities, and pubic hair. Some patients eat their hair (trichotillophagia). The bald spots can be obvious and may require wigs or extensive makeup to camouflage. Rather than feeling gratification following hair pulling, patients are more likely to experience regret over the disfigurement or frustration with their loss of self-control.

Although hair pulling can occur during periods of heightened stress, patients seem most vulnerable during times of idleness as while watching TV, reading, or driving home from work. This observation has led to the suggestion that trichotillomania is better conceptualized as a habit disorder than as an impulse control disorder. Habit reversal is a behavior therapy technique that seems most beneficial for treating trichotillomania and was originally developed for maladative habits (Azrin et al., 1980). Some authors have

Table 6-7
Diagnostic Criteria for Trichotillomania

A. Recurrent pulling out of one's hair resulting in noticeable hair loss.

B. An increasing sense of tension immediately before pulling out the hair or when attempting to resist the behavior.

C. Pleasure, gratification, or relief when pulling out the hair.

D. The disturbance is not better accounted for by another mental condition and is not due to a general medical condition (e.g., a dermatologic condition).

E. The disturbance causes clinically significant distress or impairment in social, occupational, or other important areas of functioning.

posited that pathologic grooming is the common thread running between trichotillomania, onychophagia, and some forms of OCD (Swedo, 1989).

Despite similarities between trichotillomania and OCD, the differences between them are equally noteworthy. While early reports of trichotillomania emphasized its co-occurence with OCD and favorable response to SSRIs (Swedo et al., 1989), later studies indicate that trichotillomania often exists in isolation (Christenson et al., 1992) and that pharmacotherapy often fails (Christenson and Crow, 1996). In contrast with OCD, many more women than men are affected. The hypothesis that OCD and trichotillomania are mediated by shared brain pathways was called into question after functional neuroimaging studies revealed differences between the two disorders (Swedo et al., 1991).

Although there are successful double-blind, controlled trials with clomipramine, SSRI efficacy in trichotillomania has not been supported by most controlled trials of fluoxetine (Christenson et al., 1991). Christenson and Crow (1996) completed an 8-week open trial of fluvoxamine (up to 300 mg per day) in 19 patients with trichotillomania. Subjects improved on four of five outcome measures, with the reduction from baseline ranging from 22 to 43%. Only 4 of 19 subjects (21%), however, qualified as responders based on stringent criteria, and a loss in efficacy appeared by the end of 6 months. Even among responders to an acute trial with an SSRI, spontaneous relapse is common in trichotillomania. Additional studies are needed to investigate the effectiveness of other agents and combinations of agents in the treatment of this perplexing condition.

TOURETTE'S SYNDROME

Definition and Historical Aspects

Tourette's syndrome is a childhood-onset neuropsychiatric disorder characterized by multiple motor and phonic tics and by a constellation of associated behavioral problems that often become the focus of clinical attention. The latter may include symptoms of OCD and attention deficit hyperactivity disorder

(ADHD) (Coffey and Park, 1997). TS is named after George Gilles de la Tourette, a French neurologist and student of Charcot, who reported nine cases in 1885 that resemble the modern definition of the syndrome (Tourette, 1885). The first medical reference to a probable case of TS was Itard's (Itard, 1825) description of a French noblewoman who lived her life as a recluse owing to her socially inappropiate vocalizations. But the earliest historical account of TS may be from a treatise on witchcraft, *Malleus Maleficarum (The Witch Hammer)*, about a fifteenth-century individual:

When he passed any church, and genuflected in honour of the Glorious Virgin, the devil made him thrust his tongue far out of his mouth; and when he was asked whether he could not restrain himself from doing this, he answered: "I cannot help myself at all, for so he uses all my limbs and organs, my neck, my tongue, and my lungs, whenever he pleases, causing me to speak or to cry out; and I hear the words as if they were spoken myself, but I am altogether unable to restrain them; and when I try to engage in prayer he attacks me more violently, thrusting out my tongue" (Kramer and Sprenger, 1971).

According to current terminology, the involuntary tongue thrusting would be categorized as copropraxia, an example of a complex motor tic (see discussion later). Although one might argue that the blasphemous thoughts are obsessions (intrusive, distressing ideas), the resultant actions, unlike compulsions, do not neutralize the discomfort; rather, they engender further distress. Patients with OCD may worry about acting on unwanted impulses, but rarely do so.

The lifetime prevalence of TS and related chronic tic disorders has been estimated as 3.4% in the U.S. population (Zohar et al., 1992) and up to 20% of children in special education (Kurlan et al., 1994). Males are affected much more frequently than females. TS can be a devastating and lifelong condition and, unfortunately, there have been few recent advances in its treatment.

Presenting Symptoms

Tics include a broad range of motor or phonic actions that are experienced as irresistible but may be suppressible for a period of time. The extent to which these actions are suppressible varies according to the severity, type, and timing of the tics. Many simple and rapidly executed tics (such as a bout of eye blinking and head jerks) are uncontrollable, whereas other tics may appear intentional because they occur in response to an urge and can be delayed. Some patients employ camouflage techniques to conceal tics. For example, a teenage boy may substitute a more socially appropriate tic such as touching of the abdomen in place of a less appropriate gesture such as crotch grabbing. Tics vary over time with respect to anatomic location and severity with the tendency to suddenly disappear and be replaced by new ones. This variation may lead to the mistaken impression that the individual can voluntarily drop certain tics and adopt new ones at any time. In approximately 90% of patients surveyed, tics are often preceded by an unpleasant sensation of a need to make a movement or sound called a premonitory urge or experience (Leckman et al., 1993).

Certain conditions may affect the intensity of the tics. During sleep, tics subside but may not disappear entirely. Tics are often more noticeable while a person is relaxed, such as while watching television at home, as well as during times of stress. Tics may be minimal or nonexistent while the patient is highly focused, as in the description of a surgeon by Oliver Sacks (1995): ". . . [before surgery he exhibited] constant sudden dartings and reachings with the hands, almost but never quite touching his unscrubbed, unsterile shoulder, his assistant, the mirror, sudden lungings, and touchings of his colleagues with his feet; and a barrage of vocalizations— Hooty-hooo! Hooty-hooo!"—suggestive of a huge owl.

"The scrubbing over, . . . Bennett took the knife, made a bold, clear incision—there was no hint of any ticcing or distraction—and moved straightaway into the rhythm of the operation. Twenty minutes passed, fifty, seventy, a hundred. The operation was often complex—vessels to be tied, nerves to be found—but the action was confident, smooth, moving forward at its own pace, with never the slightest hint of Tourette's. . . ."

Classification

Motor and phonic tics are further subclassified according to their complexity: simple or complex (Table 6-8). Simple motor tics are rapid or darting movements involving a single muscle group. In contrast with tremors, tics are nonrhythmic. Examples of simple motor tics include eye blinking, head jerks, and shrugging. Complex motor tics are slower and orchestrated, resembling normal movements or gestures, but are unusual in their timing and intensity. Examples include facial grimacing, touching, twirling, copropraxia (obscene gestures), and echopraxia (imitating the movements of others). Motor tics are often clonic in nature but may be dystonic. Clonic tics are abrupt and of short duration and usually repetitious such as

Table 6-8
Classification of Tics

	Motor	Phonic
Simple	Rapid, darting, meaningless (e.g., eye blinking, head jerks, shoulder shrugs, tongue thrusting, nodding, abdominal tensing, toe movements)	Fast, meaningless sounds (e.g., coughing, throat clearing, sniffing, grunting, "uh, uh, uh")
Complex	Slower, seemingly purposeful (e.g., head gestures, dystonic postures, gyrating, copropraxia, repeated touching, grooming hair, knuckle popping, jumping, twirling, spitting)	Linguistically meaningful speech (e.g., coprolalia, echolalia, palalalia, "yeah, yeah," "oh, my")

with eye blinking or tapping. Dystonic tics are also abrupt but are more sustained in posture such as prolonged mouth opening or sustained trunk bending accompanied by jaw clenching. Tics often occur in bouts with several different movements or sounds appearing in rapid sequence.

Simple vocal tics are fast, meaningless sounds such as sniffing, grunting, or throat clearing, and may be attributed to "allergies." Complex vocal tics involve higher-order processing: they are linguistically meaningful, ill-timed utterances such as phrases, echolalia (repetition of other's speech), palilalia (repetition of one's own speech), and coprolalia (use of socially inappropriate language). Some authors have suggested that vocal tics should be considered motor tics that happen to involve contractions of muscles of the respiratory system (Jankovic, 1992).

Many clinicians mistakenly believe that the presence of coprolalia is essential in making the diagnosis of TS when in fact it is present in only a minority of patients. Coprolalia, in fact, is relatively rare, occurring in 2 to 27% of patients with TS, with onset typically during adolescence (Robertson and Yakeley, 1997). The more severe the disorder, the more likely coprolalia will be found (Robertson and Yakeley, 1997). Some researchers label copropraxia and coprolalia as part of the spectrum of socially inappropriate behaviors or vocalizations known as coprophilia (Shapiro et al., 1987). In a large series of patients with Tourette's syndrome, 32% reported coprolalia, 13% reported copropraxia, and 38% reported any type of coprophilia (Shapiro et al., 1987). In another TS study of nonobscene, socially inappropriate comments and actions, 22% reported the habitual insulting of other people, 30% reported having the urge to insult, 40% indicated they tried to suppress the urge, and 24% tried to disguise their insults by trying to say something different that was not insulting (Kurlan, 1996). The insults were generally of the "You're fat, ugly, stupid, etc." type. Insulting behavior and comments were strongly associated with ADHD, conduct disorder, coprolalia, copropraxia, and mental coprolalia and were most often seen in younger males (Kurlan et al., 1994).

Diagnostic Criteria and Assessment

Transient tic disorders (TTD) are common, affecting up to one-fourth of schoolchildren (Kurlan et al., 1994). Criteria include the presence of tics for at least 4 weeks but less than 12 months (Fig. 6-4). A child may have several episodes of transient tic disorder before eventually developing a chronic tic disorder or TS. Chronic tic disorders (CT) are either vocal or motor tics (but not both) lasting longer than 1 year. The criteria for Tourette's syndrome requires that at least one vocal tic and multiple motor tics be present at some point in the illness, although they

Table 6-9
Diagnostic Criteria for Tourette's Syndrome

A. Both multiple motor and one or more vocal tics have been present at some time during the illness, although not necessarily concurrently. (A *tic* is a sudden, rapid, recurrent, nonrhythmic, stereotyped motor movement or vocalization.)

B. The tics occur many times a day (usually in bouts) nearly every day or intermittently throughout a period of more than 1 year, and during this period there is never a tic-free period of more than 3 months.

C. The disturbance causes marked distress or significant impairment in social, occupational, or other important areas of functioning.

D. The onset is before age of 18 years.

E. The disturbance is not due to the direct physiological effect of a substance (e.g., stimulants) or a general medical condition (e.g. Huntington's disease or postviral encephalitis).

SOURCE American Psychiatric Association: *Diagnostic and Statistical Manual of Mental Disorders*, 4th ed. Washington, DC, American Psychiatric Association, 1994.

do not need to occur concurrently (Table 6-9). For example, a 16-year-old boy with multiple motor tics but no phonic tics at the time of examination would still qualify for the diagnosis of TS if he had vocal tics when he was 12. Some view the distinction between TS and chronic multiple motor tics as artificial given that family studies suggest a similar pattern of transmission (Pauls and Leckman, 1986). The symptoms of TS must be present for greater than 1 year with the tic-free interval not exceeding 3 months. Onset must be before age 18, although this criterion has varied in the past. Onset of a tic disorder after the age of 18 would have to be classified as "Tic disorder not otherwise specified" (Table 6-10).

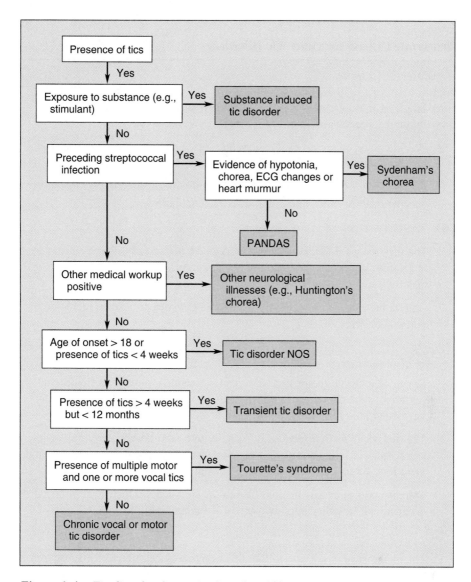

Figure 6–4. *Tic disorder diagnosis algorithm. Abbreviations: NOS, not otherwise specified; PANDAS, pediatric autoimmune neuropsychiatric disorders associated with strep.*

Some concern has arisen on how to classify mild tics. Current DSM-IV criteria for all tic diagnoses require that the tic symptoms cause "marked distress or significant impairment in functioning." Many children with tics never come to clinical attention. Mild to moderate tics, however, may cause some distress, and even when pharmacologic suppression of tics is not necessary the presence of tics may influence the treatment of comorbid disorders such as OCD or ADHD. In this respect, tics may serve as a useful clinical marker to document even when they are not the focus of treatment. Epidemiologic and family-genetic studies are influenced by classification of tic severity: a higher incidence of tic disorders is found if mild tics

Table 6-10

Diagnostic Criteria for Other Tic Disorders

Transient tic disorder

A. Single or multiple motor or vocal tics (i.e., sudden, rapid, recurrent, non-rhythmic, stereotyped motor movements or vocalizations).

B. The tics occur many times a day, nearly every day for at least 4 weeks, but no longer than 12 consecutive months.

C. The disturbance causes marked distress or significant impairment in social, occupational, or other important areas of functioning.

D. The onset is before age of 18 years.

E. The disturbance is not due to the direct physiological effect of a substance (e.g., stimulants) or a general medical condition (e.g., Huntington's disease or postviral encephalitis).

F. Criteria have never been met for Tourette's disorder or chronic motor or vocal tic disorder.

Chronic motor or vocal tic disorder

A. Single or multiple motor or vocal tics (i.e., sudden, rapid, recurrent, non-rhythmic, stereotyped motor movements or vocalizations), but not both, have been present at the time of the illness.

B. The tics occur many times a day (usually in bouts) nearly every day or intermittently throughout a period of more than 1 year, and during this period there is never a tic-free period of more than 3 months.

C. The disturbance causes marked distress or significant impairment in social, occupational, or other important areas of functioning.

D. The onset is before age of 18 years.

E. The disturbance is not due to the direct physiological effect of a substance (e.g., stimulants) or a general medical condition (e.g., Huntington's disease or postviral encephalitis).

F. Criteria have never been met for Tourette's disorder.

Tic disorder not otherwise specified

This category is for disorders characterized by tics that do not meet criteria for a specific tic disorder. Examples include tics lasting less than 4 weeks or tics with an age of onset after 18 years of age.

SOURCE American Psychiatric Association: *Diagnostic and Statistical Manual of Mental Disorders*, 4th ed. Washington, DC, American Psychiatric Association, 1994.

meet the threshold for a case, whereas a lower incidence is found if DSM-IV criteria are followed.

Assessment of the disorder involves a physical examination that includes a careful neurological examination to rule out physical causes of abnormal movements such as hyperthyroidism. Minor nonspecific neurologic abnormalities, or "soft signs," are frequently found in patients with TS. Choreiform movements have been reported with an increased frequency in patients with a tic disorder, OCD, and ADHD (Denckla, 1989). Psychiatric screening for comorbid disorders and a cognitive evaluation for learning disabilities are essential in the evaluative process as these disorders may cause the patient the most disability. Assessment of the tics typically involves clinician ratings of the type, frequency, and severity of each tic. An excellent example of this type of assessment tool is the Yale Global Tic Severity Rating Scale (YGTSS) (Leckman et al., 1996). Self or parent reports, such as the Tourette Syndrome Symptom Checklist (TSSL) (Cohen and Leckman, 1984), are important as well. Asking the patient to reproduce his or her tics often brings out a volley of tics. Because tics may occur at a low level in novel situations such as a doctor's office, however, home videotapes of tics provide an excellent tool for acute evaluation of tics and a means to monitor treatment progress.

Course

The average age of onset of motor tics is 7 years and often progresses in a rostral-caudal fashion. The average age of onset of vocal tics is 11 years. Waxing and waning of symptom type and severity is the general course of the disorder, with progression of symptom severity until midadolescence. Partial remission or stabilization occurs in many cases by late adolescence or early adulthood. The majority of adults with TS, however, report continued significant interference in daily functioning, and one-third report severe interference (Erenberg et al., 1987).

Associated Conditions

Comorbid disorders are reported frequently in patients with TS and are generally a significant source of disability. Many patients, however, still attain high achievement despite many obstacles. Samuel Johnson, a prominent eighteenth-century literary figure, is an excellent example. He suffered from severe TS with marked OC symptoms. He also engaged in self-injurious behaviors and suffered from depressive symptoms (Murray, 1980).

How much the associated disorders are part of TS or comorbid with it is still under debate. It appears through the genetic association of OCD with TS that OC behavior is an integral component of the disorder. Support exists as well for including self-injurious behaviors (Robertson et al., 1996) and some cases of ADHD (Pauls et al., 1990) as integral features of the syndrome. Other disorders commonly seen in TS include personality disorders (Robertson et al., 1997) affective disorders, non-OCD anxiety disorders, personality disorders, sleep disorders, learning disabilities, and phonological disorders (Coffey and Parks, 1997).

Recent studies relying on systematic assessment procedures and specific diagnostic criteria indicate that about 40 to 60% of TS patients display OC symptomatology (Leckman et al., 1995). The available epidemiologic data suggest that the population prevalence of OCD is between 2 and 3% and, thus, it is highly unlikely that this association is due to chance alone. Studies have shown that TS patients with prenatal exposure to maternal stress (Leckman et al., 1990) and male TS patients with childbirth complications were more likely to develop OCD (Santangelo et al., 1994). The appearance of OC symptoms in TS patients appears to be an age-dependent phenomenon, with OC symptoms increasing through adolescence and young adulthood, whereas tic symptoms tend to decrease (Brunn, 1984). Repetitive counting, ordering and arranging, tapping, rubbing, touching, and symmetry ("evening up") compulsions are the most common type of compulsions reported in TS patients (Holzer et al., 1994). Typical contamination obsessions and washing rituals are less common.

As noted earlier, differentiating between certain compulsions and tics can be difficult. By convention, an action is classified as a compulsion if it seems designed to neutralize the discomfort associated with an antecedent thought (obsession). In some cases, however, "obsessions" may represent post-hoc constructs that are invented to explain one's uncontrollable behaviors. Alternatively, what were once tics may later be incorporated in the individual's repertoire of compulsive behavior. For example, consider a 21-year-old patient who had eye-blinking tics at 8 years who now reports he must blink exactly six times to rid himself of horrific images of death. Sometimes a tic is identified by the company it keeps: if the movement is associated with other clear-cut tics, it is probably a tic itself. In all likelihood, tic-like compulsions (e.g., blinking, touching, tapping) and certain complex motor tics are at the crossroads of OCD and TS and will continue to defy attempts to dissect them at a clinical level.

The symptoms of ADHD, hyperactivity, inattentiveness, and impulsivity, are seen in approximately 50% of patients with TS and often appear before the onset of tics. A child with moderate to severe TS will generally look distractible, fidgety, and impulsive; therefore, differentiating ADHD symptoms among a background of tics may be challenging. Whether ADHD is a core feature of TS or simply a comorbid condition has yet to be elucidated. Pauls and colleagues (1990) postulate that there may be two types of TS with comorbid ADHD: one in which the ADHD is independent of the TS and one in which the ADHD is secondary to the occurrence of TS. Some researchers have reported that the presence of ADHD conferred a higher risk for increased tic severity and other comorbid disorders. Children with ADHD and TS often have severe difficulty with impulse control including failure to inhibit aggression (Cohen, 1980; Comings and Comings, 1987). Aggression may coincide with highly unpredictable, affectively charged episodes, compounding the child's frustration with himself or herself and provoking scorn by peers and family. One study reported that the combination of OCD and ADHD in patients with TS correlated highly with the presence of rage attacks (Park et al., 1993).

Differential Diagnosis

Owing to the highly variable and complex nature of TS, the differential diagnoses span a wide array of neurologic and psychiatric disorders that include Sydenham's chorea, Huntington's chorea, dystonia muscularum deformans, blepharospasm, neuroacanthocytosis, postviral encephalitis, drug-induced movement disorders, OC behavior, and stereotypies associated with autism, mental retardation, and psychosis. Laboratory tests should be performed with the differential diagnosis and therapeutic interventions in mind (Table 6-11).

Differentiating between simple tics and other abnormal movements involves assessment of the duration, location, timing, and associations of the movement. For example, typical chorea is of longer duration and occurs randomly in different muscle groups. Sydenham's chorea occurs suddenly as a constellation of behavioral changes and abnormal movements following a streptococcal infection. Some of these abnormal movements may be tic-like. Likewise, TS may have choreiform-like movements upon the back-

Table 6-11
Differential Diagnosis of Tics

Characteristics of tics	Differential diagnosis
Abrupt	Myoclonus Chorea Hyperekplexia Paroxysmal dyskinesia Seizures
Premonitory symptoms (urge—relief)	Stereotypy (akathisia) Restless legs Dystonia
Suppressibility	All hyperkinesias (most typical in tics)
Decrease with distraction *and* concentration	Akathisia Psychogenic hyperkinesias
Decrease during skilled tasks	Chorea
Increase with stress	Most hyperkinesias
Increase with relaxation after a period stress	(parkinsonian tremor)
Multifocal, migratory	Chorea Myoclonus
Fluctuate spontaneously	Paroxysmal dyskinesias Seizures
Present during sleep	Myoclonus (segmental) Periodic movements Painful legs/moving toes Other hyperkinesias Seizures

SOURCE Janovic J: Diagnosis and classification of tics and Tourette syndrome. *Adv Neurol* 1992;58:7–14.

ground of simple and complex motor or vocal tics. Careful attention to the history and course of the illness and examination for other signs of rheumatic fever should aid in the differential between Sydenham's chorea and TS.

Dystonia is distinguished from dystonic tics by its more continuous nature and the usual absence of clonic tics. Myoclonus is typically seen in one location, whereas tics tend to vary in location and occur in "runs." Ocular movements such as jerks or sustained eye deviation are seen in few movement disorders other than tic disorders. The exceptions include (1) eye dystonia, an adverse response to neuroleptic therapy; (2) ocular spasms as a consequence of encephalitis lethargica; (3) ocular myoclonus, which often accompanies palatal myoclonus; and (4) opsoclonus. Idiopathic blepharospasm, in its mild form, may be difficult to differentiate from eye-blinking and eye-closing tics but generally the presence of tics at other sites helps with the diagnosis of a tic disorder. Blepharospasm generally affects the older adult population, whereas TS typically has its onset in early childhood.

Pathogenesis

Genetics. Tourette's syndrome is thought to be inherited as an autosomal single dominant gene with incomplete but high penetrance and variable expression that may include OCD, chronic tics (CT) (Pauls and Leckman, 1986; Eapen et al., 1993), and transient tic disorder (TTD) (Kurlan et al., 1988). From genetic analyses, it appears that CT (and perhaps TTD) is a variant expression of TS. In twin studies, monozygotic twins demonstrate a higher concordance rate (77 to 100% for any tic disorder) than dizygotic twins (23% for any tic disorder) (Price et al., 1986). Strong discordance was observed, however, in monozygotic twins when tics were classified according to severity (Hyde et al., 1992). Genetic linkage studies are under way to identify the chromosomal location of the putative TS gene (Heutnik et al., 1993).

Basal ganglia dysfunction. Basal ganglia dysfunction is implicated as the primary site of pathology in TS. Other movement disorders such as Parkinson's disease and Huntington's chorea have known basal ganglia dysfunction. Accumulating evidence from neuroimaging studies suggest that patients with TS may have abnormalities in basal ganglia structure or function. For example, TS patients were found to have slightly smaller left basal ganglia volumes compared with normal controls, particularly in the lenticular nucleus (a basal ganglia structure thought to be involved in motor control) (Peterson et al., 1993). Also, normal basal ganglia asymmetry is absent or reversed in many TS patients (Singer et al., 1993). In addition, there appears to be a significant mean reduction of blood flow to the left lenticular nucleus (Riddle et al., 1992). Another study showed a significant decrease in right basal ganglia activity in five of six subjects with TS but not in normal controls (Klieger et al., 1997). In a study of 50 TS patients, hypoperfusion of the left caudate, anterior cingulate, and left dorsolateral prefrontal cortices was found (Moriarity et al., 1995).

In a quantitative MRI study of monozygotic twins discordant for tic severity, relative reductions in the right caudate and left lateral ventricular volumes were found in the more severely affected twin. Loss of the normal lateral ventricular asymmetry was also found. Other basal ganglia volumes and asymmetries did not differ within pairs, although there was a loss of the normal asymmetry for the caudate nuclei in all the twins concordant for handedness (Hyde et al., 1995). In a study of monozygotic twins with discordant TS severity, binding of the radioactively tagged D2 dopamine receptor antagonist, iodobezamide, was significantly greater in the caudate nucleus in the more severely affected patients. The differences in tic severity among TS patients has been hypothesized to be due to dopamine D2 receptor supersensitivity (Wolf et al., 1996). These twin studies suggest the importance of environmental factors affecting the phenotype of TS.

Neurochemical hypotheses. Dopamine dysfunction has been implicated in the pathobiology of TS based on symptom suppression by dopamine receptor antagonists and exacerbation with substances that increase central monaminergic activity (L-dopa, stimulants). Postmortem studies suggest either an increase in dopaminergic neurons or increased presynaptic dopamine uptake sites in the caudate and putamen. This finding is supported by a study showing a 37% increase in striatal binding of a ligand specific for presynaptic dopamine transport sites (Singer et al., 1991). Another finding that supports dopaminergic involvement is decreased turnover of central dopamine as reflected in reduced cerebrospinal fluid levels of homovanillic acid (HVA) (Leckman et al., 1995).

Norepinephrine (NE) dysfunction has been implicated by the therapeutic effects of α_2-adrenergic receptor agonists and other neurochemical studies (Leckman et al., 1995). Children and adults with TS have a blunted growth hormone response when challenged with clonidine. Increased levels of CSF NE and its major metabolite MHPG have been reported in TS patients when compared with both normal controls and patients with OCD. Patients with TS have increased plasma adrenocorticotropin (ACTH) before and after lumbar puncture and also have significantly greater excretion of urinary NE than the normal controls. Urinary NE of TS patients significantly correlated with clinician ratings of tic severity (Leckman et al., 1995).

Chappell and colleauges (1996) showed significantly higher CRF (corticotropin-releasing factor) in CSF of patients with TS compared with patients with OCD and healthy controls. The relationship between CRF and NE in mediating the stress response may underlie the association of tic exacerbations with increased anxiety and stress.

Opioid system involvement has been implicated in the pathogenesis of TS via endogenous opioid projections from the striatum to the pallidum and substantia nigra (Leckman et al., 1988). Other support includes findings that the GABAergic projection neurons express dynorphin (an endogenous opioid) and that the prodynorphin gene is positively regulated by D1-like DA receptors. The preproenkephalin gene is under the tonic inhibitory influence of dopamine D1 receptors. Variations in dynorphin have been reported in patients with TS (Haber et al., 1986; Leckman et al., 1988). Other systems implicated in the pathobiology of TS include the serotonergic, cholinergic, and excitatory and inhibitory amino acid pathways (Leckman et al., 1995).

Environmental factors. Monozygotic twin studies, with twin pair discordance for TS symptomatology, reveal that the more severely affected twin tends to have a lower birthweight than the less severely affected sibling (Leckman et al., 1987; Hyde et al., 1992). Other environmental factors possibly involved in the phenotypic expression of TS include prenatal exposure to substances, maternal stress, excessive heat, cocaine, stimulants, or anabolic steroids (Leckman et al., 1995). Infections may also play a role, particularly group A (β-hemolytic) streptococcal infections (Swedo et al., 1997).

Swedo and colleagues (1997) have postulated an autoimmune neuropsychiatric disorder that may be a partial expression of Sydenham's chorea with a presentation of the TS phenotype. The characteristics of this disorder include a dramatic onset of illness characterized by OC symptoms, adventitious movements, and/or hyperactivity, waxing and waning course, and history or clinical evidence of recent strep throat. During the acute phase, an abnormal neurological examination is found with hypotonia, dysarthria, and choreiform movements. Kiessling showed increased antineuronal antibodies to caudate in patients with Tourette's syndrome (Kiessling et al., 1993), which parallels Husby's findings of increased antineuronal antibodies in patients with Sydenham's chorea (Husby et al., 1976). Recent studies have demonstrated the presence of a B-cell marker found in rheumatic fever patients in some patients with childhood-onset OCD and tic disorders (Murphy et al., 1997; Swedo et al., 1997).

Pharmacotherapeutics

The clinician should determine if the severity of the symptoms warrants pharmacotherapy (Fig. 6-5). Drug studies of TS are affected by the natural waxing and waning course of the disorder, with remission and exacerbations not necessarily occurring in response to pharmacotherapy. Short-term symptom fluctuations should be treated conservatively. In general, the treatment goal is intermediate symptom relief: total suppression of tics is unlikely and medication side effects might be excessive. Education of patient, family, and school personnel is essential to promoting understanding and tolerance of the symptoms. Comorbid disorders may be the most significant source of distress and impairment in functioning

and should be addressed as well. It is possible that treatment of comorbid ADHD, OC behavior, anxiety, and depression may lead to reduction of symptoms secondary to the associated reduction in stress.

Neuroleptics and related medications. For nearly three decades, dopamine D2 receptor antagonists such as haloperidol and pimozide have been the backbone of treatment for TS (Table 6-12). Approximately 70% of patients with TS initially exhibit clinically meaningful suppression of tics with these agents. Long-term follow-up studies suggest, however, that a smaller percentage maintain their improvement (Cohen and Leckman, 1984). Haloperidol has generally been considered the first-line treatment of TS, partly because it was the first drug used in the treatment of TS and because it was believed to be safer than pimozide. Comparison studies on the efficacy and tolerability of haloperidol and pimozide have been equivocal. On an individual basis, some patients show a preferential response to one neuroleptic over the another. In a controlled study of haloperidol, pimozide, and placebo, haloperidol was slightly more effective than pimozide, with the dosage ratio of pimozide to haloperidol of 2:1. Adverse effects were essentially the same, with the exception of QTC prolongation with pimozide (Shapiro et al., 1989). A recent study by Sallee and colleagues (1997), however, showed that milligram for milligram, pimozide was

Table 6-12

Selected Medications and Available Dosages for Tourette's Syndrome

Antipsychotics
Haloperidol (Haldol)—tablets of 0.5, 1, 2, 5, 10, 20 mg Pimozide (Orap)—2-mg tablets Fluphenazine (Prolixin)—1-mg tablets
α$_2$-Adrenergic receptor agonists
Clonidine (Catapres)—tablets of 0.1, 0.2 mg; transdermal patches of 0.1, 0.2, 0.3 mg Guanfacine (Tenex)—tablets of 1, 2 mg

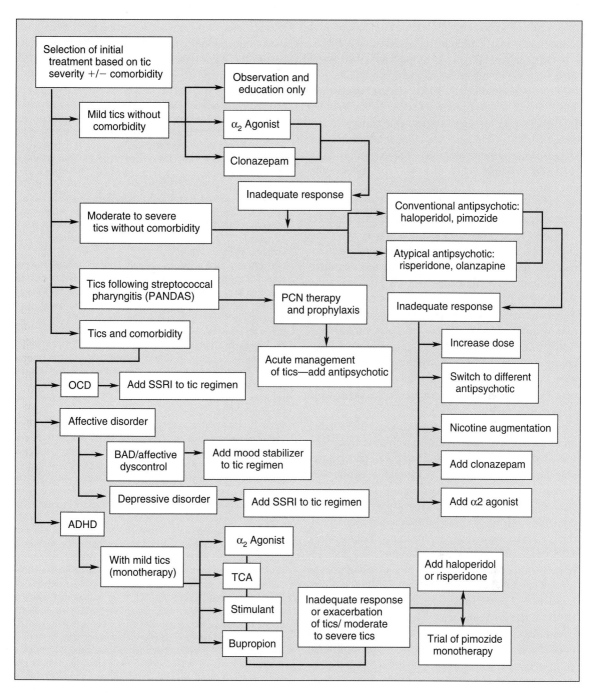

Figure 6–5. *Tic disorder treatment algorithm. Abbreviations: ADHD, attention deficit hyperactivity disorders; BAD, bipolar affective disorder; PCN, penicillin; TCA, tricyclic antidepressant.*

more efficacious and better tolerated than haloperidol in the treatment of children and adolescents with TS.

Other dopaminergic drugs that have had some success in the treatment of TS include fluphenazine, sulpiride (Robertson et al., 1990), risperidone (Brunn and Budman, 1993; Lombroso et al., 1995; Van der Linden et al., 1994), and tetrabenazine (Jankovic and Beach, 1997). Fluphenazine, a phenothiazine, has shown some promise in open studies. Sulpiride, a selective dopamine D2 receptor antagonist with structural similarity to metoclopramide, has been reported to be effective in suppressing tics. Sulpiride is not available in the United States. Side effects stemming from prolactin elevation may be problematic (Robertson et al., 1990). A related medication, tiapride, has shown mixed results in the treatment of children and adolescents with TS but also is not available in the United States (Eggers et al., 1988). Tetrabenazine, which depletes presynaptic stores of monoamine neurotransmitters, has shown modest efficacy in the treatment of TS in an open trial (Jankovic and Beach, 1997). It is associated with bothersome side effects including a 28.5% incidence of parkinsonism and a 15% incidence of depression (Jankovic and Beach, 1997).

A new generation of antipsychotics was recently approved for the treatment of psychiatric disorders. Included in this group are clozapine, risperidone, olanzapine, and quetiapine. Clozapine has not been shown effective in the treatment of TS; however, risperidone shows promise. The affinity of risperidone for dopamine D2 receptors is approximately 50 times greater than that of clozapine (Caine et al., 1979). Recently, encouraging findings have been reported from open-label studies of risperidone in the treatment of TS (Brunn and Budman, 1993; Lombroso et al., 1995; Robertson et al., 1996); double-blind studies are under way. The incidence of extrapyramidal side effects and tardive dyskinesia appears to be less with risperidone compared with traditional antipsychotics. The comparative efficacy of risperidone versus other neuroleptics in TS has not been formally examined. Thus, at present, the main advantage of risperidone may be with regard to tolerability and safety. No studies on the treatment of TS have been reported for quetiapine and olanzapine, although some clinicians are reporting success with the use of olanzapine in the treatment of TS. Obviously, before the use of these medications can be recommended, controlled research is needed.

Mechanism of action. While antipsychotics have many complex interactions through many different neurotransmitter receptor types, the main action for efficacy in the treatment of TS is believed to be blockade of dopamine D2 sites in the brain. Indeed, this property is shared by all antipsychotics with tic-supressing activity. Pimozide and fluphenazine also block calcium channels, which may be responsible for EKG changes associated with these medications. Risperidone has approximately 50% the dopamine D2 receptor affinity and more than 500-fold the 5HT₂ receptor affinity of haloperidol. Tetrabenazine reduces the accumulation of dopamine in presynaptic storage vesicles.

Side effects. Side effects frequently limit the therapeutic potential of antipsychotics and lead to noncompliance or discontinuation of therapy. Side effects such as fatigue, intellectual dulling, and memory problems interfere with success at work and school. Weight gain may lead to the patient's dissatisfaction with his or her appearance in addition to health problems. In a recent case report, liver function abnormalities were found in young males on risperidone therapy following excessive weight gain. Evidence of fatty liver infiltrates were found by hepatic ultrasound. Extrapyramidal side effects are the likely result of dopamine D2 receptor blockade in the caudate and substantia nigra and include akathisia, parkinsonism, and dystonia. In adult studies, extrapyramidal side effects were minimal, although children may have an increased risk for dystonia. Prolactin secretion is under tonic inhibitory control of dopamine and is increased by agents that block dopamine. Increased prolactin levels may result in breast changes, galactorrhea, amenorrhea, and sexual dysfunction. Prolactin levels may be useful in limiting dosage and extrapyramidal symptoms in patients on pimozide therapy (Sallee et al., 1997). With chronic use, tardive dyskinesia develops in 10 to 20% of patients treated with an antipsychotic for more than 1 year. Children, elderly females, African Americans, and patients with mood disorders have a higher risk. Tardive dyskinesia may be difficult to assess on the background of tics. Case reports of children developing school phobia after initiation of antipsychotic therapy have been described. Dysphoria during antipsychotic therapy is a frequent side effect, but actual depression may be particularly problematic with tetrabenazine (Jankovic and Beach, 1997). Electrocardiogram changes (QTC interval prolongation) have been reported with pimozide, which has led experts to recommend ECG monitoring and a maximum daily dose of 10 mg. Additionally, dosages of primozide above 20 mg per day are associated with increased seizure risk.

Contraindications. Parkinson's disease, CNS depression, and known drug hypersensitivity are contraindications to neuroleptics. Use in pregnancy and breast feeding has not been approved; use in these conditions should be used in circumstances only where the severity of TS is such that it outweighs the risk to the child. Pimozide and possibly fluphenazine have potential to cause cardiovascular effects owing to calcium channel blockade. Conditions where use of pimozide is contraindicated include congenital long QT syndrome, cardiac arrhythmias, or concurrent use with macrolide antibiotics (clarithromycin, erythromycin, azithromycin, dirithromycin) or medications that prolong the QT interval.

Toxicities. Antipsychotic overdose can produce seizures, cardiac arrhythmias, and other life-threatening events. Neuroleptic malignant syndrome, although uncommon, is another serious risk even at routine dosages. Hypotension, sedation, and severe extrapyramidal reactions such as acute dystonias and rigidity can occur. Case reports of sudden death with pimozide have been described in schizophrenic patients on high doses of 80 mg daily.

α_2-Adrenergic receptor agonists.

Clonidine and guanfacine are marketed as antihypertensives; however, clonidine has been used for a number of years to treat tic disorders and ADHD. Clonidine has become the first-line treatment by many clinicians because it does not produce adverse neurological effects such as EPS or tardive dyskinesia. Partial or no benefit on tic severity, however, has been seen in placebo-controlled trials with this agent (Goetz, 1992). Motor tics seem to benefit most from clonidine (Leckman et al., 1991). Response to clonidine is often delayed, requiring 3 to 6 weeks of treatment before a clinical response is noted. Perhaps clonidine's greatest utility is improving the associated behavioral symptoms such as overactivity, poor frustration tolerance, sleep difficulties, and aggression that are commonly seen in TS and ADHD patients. Many patients cannot tolerate clonidine-induced sedation and postural hypotension. Of greater concern are patients with poor compliance with subsequent rebound side effects and recent reports of sudden death in children on clonidine therapy.

Recently, guanfacine has been found beneficial in these disorders, with fewer side effects than clonidine. Studies of guanfacine's efficacy have been small, open studies. Before advocating its use for treatment of TS or ADHD, placebo-controlled studies on guanfacine's safety and efficacy for the treatment of these disorders are needed.

Mechanism of action. Clonidine demonstrates presynaptic α_2-adrenergic autoreceptor agonism at low dosages; at higher doses, it may also exert postsynaptic agonism. The mode of action is thought to be related to inhibition of norepinephrine release. In addition to clonidine's effect on the noradrenergic system, it appears to have indirect effects on dopaminergic activity as reflected in studies of homovanillic acid (HVA) levels (Leckman et al., 1995).

Side effects. The most common side effects associated with clondine are sedation, dizziness, bradycardia, constipation, dry mouth, and weight gain. Occasionally children will appear irritable and dysphoric shortly after the initiation of the drug. Onset or exacerbation of depression has been reported. An abrupt withdrawal of clonidine may lead to rebound hypertension, tachycardia, motor restlessness, agitation, muscle aches, sweating, increased salivation, and possibly manic-like symptoms. A marked exacerbation of tics upon clonidine withdrawal has been described that may be long-lasting despite reinitiation of clonidine therapy (Leckman et al., 1986). A few cases of sudden death have been reported in children who are undergoing or have recently undergone clonidine therapy. In most of these cases, other factors were involved and it is uncertain if the use of clonidine was causal (Cantwell et al., 1997).

Contraindications. Clonidine therapy should probably be avoided in patients with preexisting myocardial or valvular disease, especially left ventricular outflow tract obstruction, syncope, and bradycardia. A relative contraindication is renal disease because of the associated risks for cardiovascular disease. Careful monitoring for changes in pulse, blood pressure, and ECGs is recommended in addition to pretreatment screening for risks of cardiovascular disease (Cantwell et al., 1997).

Toxicities. Serious adverse effects can occur with acute withdrawal or overdose. Children may be particularly susceptible to both situations. For example, parents may not be aware of the importance of strict medication compliance and the child has episodes of withdrawal with medication lapses. Overdose may occur secondary to confusing the clonidine with another prescribed medication such as methylphenidate and the child takes three pills instead of one, for example. As little as 0.1 mg has been reported to cause toxicity in children. Symptoms of overdose include bradycardia, CNS depression, initial hypertension then hypotension, respiratory depression, and hypothermia.

Other treatments.

Although tricyclic antidepressants (TCA) may mildly improve tics, their greatest benefit may be in treating patients with mild tic severity but who have comorbid ADHD, depression, or an anxiety disorder (Singer et al., 1995; Sandyk and Bamford, 1988). Tricyclics may also be helpful in those patients with comorbid nocturnal enuresis or sleep disorders. Cardiac effects of increased pulse and ECG changes (increased QRS, PR, and QTC intervals) with potential risk of serious cardiac toxicity necessitate monitoring of ECGs, plasma drug levels, vital signs, and drug interactions. Seven cases of sudden death possibly associated with desipramine and imipramine have been reported (Varley and McClellan, 1997). Selegiline has also been found helpful in patients with tic disorders and comorbid ADHD (Feigin et al., 1996; Jankovic, 1993).

In open studies of antipsychotic nonresponders, nicotine has been reported to potentiate the action of antipsychotics in suppressing motor and vocal tics in TS patients (Dursun and Reveley, 1997; Silver et al., 1996). Silver and colleagues (1996) showed significant reduction in tic severity after a 24-h administration of transdermal nicotine. Symptom improvement lasted on average 11 days if outliers were excluded (Silver et al., 1996). Other open-label studies have shown similar results in addition to the possibility of using transdermal nicotine as monotherapy for the treatment of TS (Dursun and Reveley, 1997). Double-blind, placebo-controlled studies are under way. Nicotine is known to have effects on many neurotransmitter systems and its action on the nicotinic cholinergic receptors stimulates release of β-endorphin, dopamine, serotonin, norepinephrine, acetylcholine, and corticosteroids. The mechanism whereby nicotine potentiates antipsychotic effects on TS patients is unknown. The neuroleptic potentiating effect can be inhibited with the nicotinic receptor antagonist mecamylamine.

The benzodiazepine with the most support for the use in TS is clonazepam. Clonazepam may be useful (1) as a single-agent treatment of tics, particularly for motor tics; (2) with TS and comorbid anxiety disorders such as panic disorder; and (3) as an augmentation agent (Goetz, 1992; Steingard et al., 1994).

Several other medications have been reported to show some success in case reports and open-label studies in the treatment of TS including naloxone, antiandrogens, calcium channel blockers, lithium, and carbamazepine (LeWitt, 1993). Botulinum toxin injections (Scott et al., 1966) have been used to treat a few cases of severe coprolalia.
Treatment of comorbid OCD. Most recent studies indicate that SSRIs produce little tic improvement or, occasionally, an exacerbation (Como and Kurlan, 1991). SSRIs are the drug of choice, however, for OC behavior, and the addition of an antipsychotic may enhance anti-OC efficacy in patients with both OCD and TS.
Treatment of tic disorders and comorbid ADHD. The use of stimulants for therapy of ADHD with comorbid tics continues to be controversial (Robertson and Eapen, 1992). Some observations suggest that stimulants exacerbate and perhaps precipitate tics in a significant number of patients. Stimulant therapy was closely associated with persistent exacerbation of tics in 24% of individuals with TS treated with a stimulant

(Price et al., 1986). The high comorbidity of ADHD with TS may, in some cases, falsely lead the clinician to believing that the treatment of the ADHD caused the tics. Tics generally return to baseline after discontinuation of the stimulant but may decrease in severity with continued use. Two studies of stimulant therapy for children with ADHD and comorbid tic disorder suggest that ADHD can be successfully treated without worsening tics (Castellanos et al., 1997; Gadow and Sverd, 1990). For some children, a mild increase in tics is more acceptable than the hardship of moderate to severe ADHD. Some specialists recommend the use of stimulants to offset the adverse effects of antipsychotics. There is an impression that pemoline may exacerbate tics more than methylphenidate and dextroamphetamine. Treatment with TCAs and α_2-adrenergic receptor agonists may be the most conservative approach regarding the concern over tic exacerbation, although efficacy is modest. Another consideration for the treatment of ADHD is the use of bupropion. A recent study shows comparable efficacy to methylphenidate in the treatment of ADHD (Barrickman et al., 1995), but case studies of tic exacerbation have also been reported with bupropion (Spencer et al., 1993). Two studies support the use of selegiline for treatment of ADHD comorbid with a tic disorder. Improvement in ADHD was reported in both studies, with improvement in the tic disorder in one (Feigin et al., 1996) and no worsening of the tic disorder in the other (Jankovic, 1993).
Treatment of comorbid mood disorders. Treatment of comorbid depression with standard antidepressant therapy should involve considerations of other associated symptoms such as ADHD and OC symptoms and interactions with current tic suppressing therapy. Reports of tic exacerbation or precipitation have been reported with the SSRIs, TCAs, and bupropion. Mood stabilizers should be considered for the treatment of affective instability, unchecked aggression, or mania.

Clinical Pharmacology

Dosing.   Start with 0.25 mg of haloperidol, 0.5 mg of pimozide, 0.5 mg fluphenazine, or 0.25 mg of risperidone; increase doses by the same increment every 5 to 7 days. Dosage range of haloperidol is 0.5 to 10 mg; pimozide, 1.5 to 10 mg; fluphenazine, 2 to 15 mg; risperidone, 0.5 to 8 mg. Dosing may be given in one to three divided doses depending on tolerance to side effects and breakthrough symptoms. Pimozide has a long half-life and may successfully be given as a single bedtime dose. Cardiac monitoring should be done with pimozide therapy with extra precautions if doses exceed 10 mg. The dose should not be increased if there is significant QTC prolongation. The manufacturer recommends discontinuation with the occurrence of T-wave inversion or U waves. Monitoring liver functions should be done with all antipsychotics but particularly with pimozide and risperidone. Monitoring for signs of tardive dyskinisia should be done every 3 months. Some clinicians advocate prophylactic use of anticholinergic agents such as benzotropine and diphenhydramine to prevent the occurrence of extrapyramidal side effects. Many clinicians, however, wait until they are required.

Dosing of α_2-adrenergic receptor agonists. Clonidine has been used extensively by psychiatrists, neurologists, and pediatricians although clonidine has not been approved by the FDA for use in tic disorders or psychiatric disorders. Safety and efficacy studies for these purposes are still very much needed. Guanfacine has only recently begun to be used, and much less support exists in the medical literature for its use. Because profound sedation can occur with a little as 0.05 mg of clonidine, especially in children, very small initial doses are recommended. In general, start with one-fourth to one-half tablet (0.1 mg) of clonidine by mouth at bedtime, increasing by 0.025- to 0.05-mg increments every 3 to 4 days as tolerated in three to four divided doses up to a maximum dose of 0.4 mg per day. Alternatively, a transdermal patch may be used, which comes in 0.1-, 0.2-, and 0.3-mg sizes. Patches should be changed every 4 to 7 days depending on the age of the patient, with younger patients needing more frequent changes. Limitations to the patch include difficulty keeping the patch in place either from swimming, excessive perspiration, or the child's removing it, and allergic reaction at the site of the patch. Some clinicians have success by placing the patch in the center of the back after administering diphenhydramine hydrochloride (Benadryl) cream or spray. Efficacy may not be seen for several weeks with either the transdermal or oral routes. Guanfacine is available in 1- and 2-mg tablets; the dose is started at 0.5 mg and increased every 7 days, with doses given twice daily and a daily dosage range of 0.5 to 4.0 mg. A baseline ECG and vital signs should be done with each dosage increase and after every 3 months of maintenance therapy. Also, ECGs and orthostatic blood pressure and pulse measures should be done if symptoms of dizziness, palpitations, hot flashes, or excessive lethargy are reported.

Initial dosing of clonazepam is approximately 0.5 mg, increasing the dose by 0.5 mg every 5 days as tolerated until maximum therapeutic benefits are seen. The side effects of sedation are likely to limit the rate of increased dosage. The maintenance dosage range is 1.0 to 6.0 mg.

Studies support using 7-mg transdermal nicotine patches for one 24-h application at approximately 2-week intervals for neuroleptic augmentation. Duration of response is highly variable from a few days to several weeks.

For additional information on the drugs discussed in this chapter see chapters 10, 17, 18, 19, and 52 in *Goodman & Gilman's The Pharmacological Basis of Therapeutics* (Ninth Edition), McGraw-Hill, New York, 1996.

REFERENCES

Arnott S, Nutt D: Successful treatment of fluvoxamine-induced anorgasmia by cyprophetadine. *Br J Psychiat* 1991;52:163–164.

Azrin NH, Nunn RG, Frantz SE: Treatment of hairpulling (trichotillomania): A comparison study of habit reversal and negative practice training. *J Behav Ther Exp Psychiat* 1980;11:13–20.

Baer L, Rauch SL, Ballantine T, et al: Cingulotomy for intractable obsessive-compulsive disorder. *Arch Gen Psychiat* 1995;52:384–392.

Barickman LL, Perry PJ, Allen AJ, et al: Bupropion versus methylphenidate in the treatment of attention-deficit hyperactivity disorder. *J Am Acad Child Adolesc Psychiat* 1995;34:649–657.

Barr LC, Goodman WK, Price LH, et al: The serotonin hypothesis of obsessive-compulsive disorder: Implications of pharmacologic challenge studies. *J Clin Psychiat* 1992;53(4,suppl):29–37.

Baxter LR, Saxena S, Brody AL, et al: Brain mediation of obsessive-compulsive disorder symptoms: Evidence from functional brain imaging studies in the human and non-human primate. *Sem Clin Neuropsychiat*, in press.

Bisserbe JC, Lane RM, Flament MF, et al: A double-blind comparison of sertraline and clomipramine in outpatients with obsessive-compulsive disorder. *Eur Psychiat* 1997;12:82–93.

Blier P, Bergeron R: Sequential administration of augmentation strategies in treatment-resistant obsessive-compulsive disorder: Preliminary findings. *Intern Clin Psychopharm* 1996;11:37–44.

Brunn RD, Budman CL: Risperidone as a treatment for Tourette's syndrome. *J Clin Psychiat* 1996;57(1):29–31.

Brunn RD, Budman CL: The natural history of Gilles de la Tourette's syndrome, in Kurlan R (ed): *Handbook of Tourette's Syndrome and Related Tic and Behavior Disorders.* New York, Marcel Dekker, 1993, pp 27–42.

Caine ED, Polinsky RJ, Kartzinel R, et al: The trial use of clozapine for abnormal involuntary movement disorders. *Am J Psychiat* 1979;136:317–320.

Cantwell DP, Swanson J, Connor DF: Case study: Adverse response to clonidine. *J Am Acad Child Adolesc Psychiat* 1997;36:539–544.

Castellanos FX, Giedd JN, Elia J, et al: Controlled stimulant treatment of ADHD and comorbid Tourette's syndrome: Effects of stimulant and dose. *J Am Acad Child Adolesc Psychiat* 1997;36(5):589–596.

Chappell P, Leckman J, Goodman W, et al: Elevated cerebrospinal fluid corticotropin-releasing factor in Tourette's syndrome: Comparison to obsessive-compulsive disorder and normal controls. *Biol Psychiat* 1996;39:776–783.

Chappell PB, Riddle MA, Scahill L, et al: Guanfacine treatment of comorbid attention-deficit hyperactivity disorder and Tourette's syndrome: Preliminary clinical experience. *J Am Acad Child Adolesc Psychiat* 1995;34(9):1140–1146.

Christenson GA, Crow SJ: The characterization and treatment of trichotillomania. *J Clin Psychiat* 1996;57(suppl 8):42–49.

Christenson GA, Mackenzie TB, Mitchell JE, et al: A placebo-controlled double-blind crossover study of fluoxetine in trichotillomania. *Am J Psychiat* 1991;148:1566–1571.

Christenson GA, Mackenzie TB, Mitchell JE: Characteristics of 60 adult chronic hair pullers. *Am J Psychiat* 1992;15:777–790.

Coffey BJ, Park KS: Behavioral and emotional aspects of Tourette syndrome. *Neurol Clin* 1997;15(2):277–289.

Cohen DJ, Leckman JF: Tourette syndrome: Advances in treatment and research. *J Am Acad Child Adolesc Psychiat* 1984;23:123–125.

Cohen DJ: The pathology of the self in primary childhood autism and Gilles de la Tourette syndrome. *Psychiat Clin North Am* 1980;3:383–402.

Comings DE, Comings BG: A controlled study of Tourette syndrome. VII. Summary: A common genetic disorder causing disinhibition of the limbic system. *Am J Hum Genet* 1987;41:839–866.

Como PG, Kurlan R: An open-label trial of fluoxetine for obsessive-compulsive disorder in Gilles de la Tourette's syndrome. *Neurology* 1991;41(6):872–874.

Connolly HM, Crary JL, McGoon MD, et al: Valvular heart disease associated with fenfluramine-phentermine. *N Engl J Med* 1997;337:581–588.

Denckla MB. Neurological examination, in Rapoport J (ed): *Obsessive-Compulsive Disorder in Children and Adolescents.* Washington, DC, American Psychiatric Press, 1989, pp 107–115.

DeVeaugh-Geiss J, Katz R, Landau P, et al: Clomipramine hydrochloride in the treatment of patients with obsessive-compulsive disorder. *Arch Gen Psychiat* 1991;48:730–738.

Dursun SM, Reveley MA: Differential effects of transdermal nicotine on microstructured analyses of tics in Tourette's syndrome: An open study. *Psychol Med* 1997;27(2):483–487.

Eapen V, Pauls DL, Robertson MM: Evidence of autosomal dominant transmission in Tourette's syndrome: United Kingdom cohort study. *B J Psychiat* 1993;162:593–596.

Eggers C, Rothenberger A, Berghaus U: Clinical and neurobiological findings in children suffering from tic disease following treatment with tiapride. *Eur Arch Psychiat Neurol Sci* 1988;237(4):223–229.

Erenberg G, Cruse RP, Rothner AD: The natural history of Tourette syndrome: A follow-up study. *Ann Neurol* 1987;22:383–385.

Evans DW, Leckman JF, Carter A, et al: Ritual, habit, and perfectionism: The prevalence and development of compulsive-like behavior in normal young children. *Child Devel* 1997;68(1):58–68.

Feigin A, Kurlan R, McDermott MP, et al: A controlled trial of deprenyl in children with Tourette's syndrome and attention-deficit disorder. *Neurology* 1996;46(4):965–968.

Foa EB, Steketee GS, Ozarow BJ: Behavior therapy with obsessive-compulsives: From theory to treatment, in Mavissakalian M, Turner SM, Michelson L (eds): *Obsessive-Compulsive Disorder: Psychological and Pharmacological Treatment.* New York, Plenum Press, 1985, pp 49–129.

Gadow KD, Sverd J: Stimulants for ADHD in child patients with Tourette's syndrome: the issue of relative risk. *J Dev Behav Pediatr* 1990;11(5):269–271.

Gilles de la Tourette G: Étude sur une affection nerveuse caractrise par de l'incoordination mortice accompagne d'echolalie et de coprolalie. *Arch Neurologie* 1885;9:19–42.

Goetz CG: Clonidine and clonazepam in Tourette syndrome, in Chase N, Friedhoff A, Cohen D (eds): *Advances in Neurology. Tourette Syndrome: Genetics, Neurobiology, and Treatment.* New York, Raven Press, 1992.

Goodman WK, McDougle CJ, Price LH, et al: Beyond the serotonin hypothesis: A role for dopamine in some forms of obsessive-compulsive disorders: *J Clin Psychiat* 1990;51:36-43.

Goodman WK, Price LH, Delgado PL, et al: Specificity of serotonin reuptake inhibitors in the treatment of obsessive-compulsive disorder: Comparison of fluvoxamine and desipramine. *Arch Gen Psychiat* 1990;47:577–585.

Goodman WK, Price LH, Rasmussen SA, et al: The Yale-Brown Obsessive Compulsive Scale (Y-BOCS): Part I. Development, use and reliability. *Arch Gen Psychiat* 1989;46:1006–1011.

Goodman WK, Rasmussen SA, Foa EB, et al: Obsessive-compulsive disorder, in Prien RF, Robinson DS (eds): *Clinical Evaluation of Psychotrophic Drugs: Principles and Guidance.* New York, Raven Press, 1994, pp 431–466.

Goodman WK, Ward HE, Kablinger AS, et al: Biological approaches to treatment-resistant obsessive compulsive disorder, in Goodman WK, Rudorfer MV, Maser J (eds): *Obsessive-Compulsive Disorder: Contemporary Issues in Treatment.* Hillsdale, NJ, Lawrence Erlbaum, in press.

Griest JH, Jefferson JW, Kozak KA, et al: Efficacy and tolerability of serotonin transport inhibitors in obsessive-compulsive disorder: A meta-analysis. *Arch Gen Psychiat* 1995;52:53–60.

Haber SN, Kowall NW, Vonsattel JP, et al: Gilles de la Tourette's syndrome: A postmortem neuropathological and immunohistochemical study. *J Neurol Sci* 1986;75:225–241.

Heutink P, Sandkuyl LA, van de Wetering BJM, et al: Linkage and Tourette syndrome. *Lancet* 1993;337:122–123.

Hollander E, Cohen LJ, Simeon D: Body dysmorphic disorder. *Psychiat Ann* 1993;23(7):359–364.

Hollander E, Cohen LJ: Psychobiology and psychopharmacology of compulsive spectrum disorders, in Oldham JM, Hollander E, Skodol AE (eds): *Impulsivity and Compulsivity.* Washington DC, American Psychiatric Press, 1996, p 143.

Holzer JC, Goodman WK, McDougle CJ, et al: Obsessive-compulsive disorder with and without a chronic tic disorder: A comparison of symptoms in 70 patients. *Brit J Psychiat* 1994;164:469–473.

Husby G, Van de Rijn I, Zabriskie JB, et al: Antibodies reacting with cytoplasm of subthalmic and caudate nuclei neurons in chorea and acute rheumatic fever. *J Exp Med* 1976;144:1094–1110.

Hyde TM, Aaronson BA, Randolph C, et al: Relationship of birth weight to the phenotypic expression of Gilles de la Tourette's syndrome in monozygotic twins. *Neurology* 1992;42:652–658.

Hyde TM, Stacey ME, Coppola R, et al: Cerebral morphometric abnormalities in Tourette's syndrome: A quantitative MRI study of monozygotic twins. *Neurology* 1995;45(6):1176–1182.

Itard JMG: Memoire sur quelques fonctions involuntaires des appareils de la locomotion de la prehension et de la voix. *Arch Gen Med* 1825;8:385–407.

Jacobson FM: Fluoxetine-induced sexual dysfunction and an open trial of yohimbine. *J Clin Psychiat* 1992;53:119–122.

Jankovic J, Beach J: Long-term effects of tetrabenazine in hyperkinetic movement disorders. *Neurology* 1997;48(2):358–362.

Jankovic J: Deprenyl in attention-deficit associated with Tourette's syndrome. *Arch Neurol* 1993;50(3):286–288.

Jankovic J: Diagnosis and classification of tics and Tourette syndrome, in Chase N, Friedhoff A, Cohen D (eds): *Advances in Neurology.* New York, Raven Press, 1992, pp 7–14.

Kiessling LS, Marcotte AC, Culpepper L: Antineuronal antibodies in movement disorders. *Pediatrics* 1993;92(1):39–43.

Klieger PS, Fett KA, Dimitsopulos T, et al: Asymmetry of basal ganglia perfusion in Tourette's syndrome shown by technetium-99m-HMPAO SPECT. *J Nucl Med* 1997;38(2):188–191.

Koran LM, McElroy SL, Davidson JRT, et al: Fluvoxamine versus clomipramine for obsessive-compulsive disorder: A double-blind comparison. *J Clin Psychopharmacol* 1996;16:121–129.

Kramer H, Sprenger J: *Malleus Maleficarum.* New York, Dover Publications, 1971, pp 131–132.

Kurlan R, Behr J, Medved L, Como P: Transient tic disorder

and the spectrum of Tourette's syndrome. *Arch Neurol* 1988;45:1200–1201.

Kurlan R, Daragjati C, Como P, et al: Non-obscene complex socially inappropriate behavior in Tourette's syndrome. *J Neuropsychiat Clin Neurosci* 1996;8(3):311–317.

Kurlan R, Whitmore BA, Irvine C, et al: Tourette's syndrome in a special education population: A pilot study involving a single school district. *Neurology* 1994;44:699–702.

Labbate LA, Pollack MH: Treatment of fluoxetine-induced sexual dysfunction with bupropion: A case report. *Ann Clin Psychiat* 1994;53:212–213.

Leckman JF, Dolnansky ES, Hardin MT, et al: Perinatal factors in the expression of Tourette's syndrome: An exploratory study. *J Am Acad Child Adolesc Psychiat* 1990;29:220-226.

Leckman JF, Goodman WK, North WG, et al: The role of central oxytocin in obsessive-compulsive disorder and related normal behavior. *Psychoneuroendocrinology* 1994;19(8):723–749.

Leckman JF, Hardin MT, Riddle MA, et al: Clonidine treatment of Gilles de la Tourette's syndrome. *Arch Gen Psychiat* 1991;48(4):324–328.

Leckman JF, Ort S, Caruso KA, et al: Rebound phenomena in Tourette's syndrome after abrupt withdrawal of clonidine: Behavioral, cardiovascular, and neurochemical effects. *Arch Gen Psychiat* 1986;43(12):1168–1176.

Leckman JF, Pauls DL, Cohen DJ: Tic disorders, in Bloom FE, Kupfer DJ (eds): *Psychopharmacology: The Fourth Generation of Progress.* New York, Raven Press, 1995, pp 1665–1674.

Leckman JF, Price RV, Walkup JT, et al: Nongenetic factors in Gilles de la Tourette's syndrome. *Arch Gen Psychiat* 1987;44:100.

Leckman JF, Riddle MA, Berrettini WH, et al: Elevated CSF dynorphin A [1-8] in Tourette's syndrome. *Life Sci* 1988;43:2015–2023.

Leckman JF, Riddle MA, Hardin MT, et al: The Yale global tic severity scale: Initial testing of a clinician-rated scale of tic severity. *J Am Acad Child Adolesc Psychiat* 1989;28:566–573.

Leckman JF, Walker DE, Cohen DJ: Premonitory urges in Tourette's syndrome. *Am J Psychiat* 1993;150:98–102.

Lewitt PA: Pharmacotherapy beyond the catechoaminergic systems, in Kurlan R (ed): *Handbook of Tourette's Syndrome and Related Tic and Behavior Disorders.* New York, Marcel Dekker, 1993, pp 389–400.

Lombroso PJ, Scahill L, King RA, et al: Risperidone treatment of children and adolescents with chronic tic disorders: A preliminary report. *J Am Acad Child Adolesc Psychiat* 1995;34(9):1147–1152.

McDougle CJ, Goodman WK, Leckman JF, et al: Haloperidol addition in fluvoxamine-refractory obsessive-compulsive disorder: A double-blind, placebo-controlled study in patients with and without tics. *Arch Gen Psychiat* 1994;51:302–-308.

Mesulam MM, Petersen RC: Treatment of Gilles de la Tourette's syndrome: Eight-year, practice-based experience in a predominantly adult population. *Neurology* 1987;37:1828–1833.

Meyer V: Modification of expectations in cases with obsessional rituals. *Beh Res Ther* 1996;138:584–592.

Moriarty J, Costa DC, Schmitz B, Trimble MR, et al: Brain perfusion abnormalities in Gilles de la Tourette syndrome. *Br J Psychiat* 1995;167:249–254.

Murphy TK, Goodman WK, Fudge MW, et al: B Lymphocyte antigen D8/17: a peripheral marker for Tourette's syndrome and childhood-onset obsessive-compulsive disorder? *Am J Psychiat* 1997;154:402–407.

Murray TJ: Dr. Samuel Johnson's tics and gesticulations. *Br Med J* 1979;1:1610–1614.

Nierenberg AA, Adler LA, Peselow E, et al: Trazodone for antidepressant-associated insomnia. *Am J Psychiat* 1994;151:1069–1072.

Park S, Como PG, Cui L, Kurlan R: The early course of the Tourette's syndrome clinical spectrum. *Neurology* 1993;43(9):1712–1715.

Pato MT, Hill JL, Murphy DL: A clomipramine dosage reduction study in the course of long-term treatment of obsessive-compulsive disorder patients. *Psychopharmacol Bull* 1990;26:211–214.

Pauls DL, Leckman JF: The inheritance of Gilles de la Tourette syndrome and associated behaviors: Evidence for autosomal dominant transmission. *N Engl J Med* 1986;315:993–997.

Pauls DL, Pakstis AJ, Kurlan R, et al: Segregation and linkage analyses of Tourette's syndrome and related disorders. *J Am Acad Child Adolesc Psychiat* 1990;29:195–203.

Pauls DL, Towbin KE, Leckman JF, et al: Gilles de la Tourette's syndrome and obsessive-compulsive disorder: Evidence supporting a genetic relationship. *Arch Gen Psychiat* 1986;43:1180–1182.

Peterson B, Riddle MA, Cohen DJ, et al: Reduced basal ganglia volumes in Tourette's syndrome using three-dimensional reconstruction techniques from magnetic resonance images. *Neurology* 1993;43(5):941–949.

Phillips KA, McElroy SI: An open-label study of fluvoxamine in body dysmorphic disorder. *Biol Psychiat* 1996;39(7):625.

Phillips KA, McElroy SL, Keck PE Jr, et al: A comparison of delusional and nondelusional body dysmorphic disorder in 100 cases. *Psychopharmacol Bull* 1994;30(2):179–186.

Phillips, KA: Body dysmorphic disorder: Clinical features and drug treatment. *CNS Drugs* 1995;3(1):30–40.

Pitman RK: Obsessive-compulsive disorder in Western history, in Hollander E, Zohar J, Marazzati D, et al (eds): *Current Insights in Obsessive-Compulsive Disorder.* New York, John Wiley & Sons, 1994, pp 3–10.

Price RA, Leckman JF, Pauls DL, et al: Gilles de la Tourette's syndrome: Tics and central nervous system stimulants in twins and nontwins. *Neurology* 1986;36(2):232–237.

Ravizza L, Barzega G, Bellino S, et al: Drug treatment of obsessive-compulsive disorder (OCD): Long-term trial with clomipramine and selective serotonin reuptake inhibitors. *Psychopharmacol Bull* 1996, 32(1): 167–173.

Riddle M, Rasmussen AM, Woods SW, et al: SPECT imaging of cerebral blood flow in Tourette's syndrome. *Adv Neurol* 1992;58:207–212.

Riddle MA, Claghorn J, Gaffney G, et al: A controlled trial of fluvoxamine for OCD in children and adolescents. *Biol Psychiat* 1994;14:78–79.

Robertson MM, Banerjee S, Hiley PJF, et al: Personality disorder and psychopathology in Tourette's syndrome: A controlled study. *Br J Psychiat* 1997;171:283–286.

Robertson MM, Eapen V: Pharmacologic controversy of CNS stimulants in Gilles de la Tourette syndrome. *Clin Neuropharmacol* 1992, 15(5):408–425.

Robertson MM, Schnieden V, Lees AJ: Management of Gilles de la Tourette syndrome using sulpiride. *Clin Neuropharmacol* 1990;13(3):229–235.

Robertson MM, Yakeley J: Gilles de la Tourette syndrome and obsessive-compulsive disorde, in Fogel BS, Schiffer RB, Rao SM (eds): *Neuropsychiatry.* Baltimore, MD, William & Wilkins, 1996, 827–870.

Rothschild AJ: Selective serotonin reuptake inhibitor-induced sexual dysfunction: Efficacy of a drug holiday. *Am J Psychiat* 1995;152:1514–1516.

Rudorfer MV: Electroconvulsive therapy in treatment refractory obsessive-compulsive disorder, in Goodman WK, Rudorfer MV, Maser J (eds): *Obsessive-Compulsive Disorder: Contemporary Issues in Treatment.* Hillsdale, NJ, Lawrence Erlbaum, 1997, in press.

Sacks O: *An Anthropologist on Mars.* New York, Alfred A. Knopf, 1995, p 95.

Sallee FR, Dougherty D, Sethuraman G, et al: Prolactin monitoring of haloperidol and pimozide treatment in children with Tourette's syndrome. *Biol Psychiat* 1996;49(10):1044–1050.

Sallee FR, Nesbitt L, Jackson C, et al: Relative efficacy of haloperidol and pimozide in children and adolescents with Tourette's disorder. *Am J Psychiat* 1997;154(8):1057–1062.

Sallee FR, Sethuraman G, Rock CM: Effects of pimozide on cognition in children with Tourette syndrome: Interaction with comorbid attention-deficit hyperactivity disorder. *Acta Psychiatr Scand* 1994;90(1):4-9.

Sandyk R, Bamford CR: Beneficial effects of imipramine on Tourette's syndrome. *Int J Neurosci* 1988;39(1-2):27–29.

Santangelo SL, Pauls DL, Goldstein JM, et al: Tourette's syndrome: What are the influences of gender and comorbid obsessive-compulsive disorder? *J Am Acad Child Adolesc Psychiat* 1994;33:795-804.

Schwartz JM: Obsessive-compulsive disorder. *Sci Med* 1997;4:14–23.

Scott BL, Jankovic J, Donovan DT: Botulinum toxin injection into vocal cord in the treatment of malignant coprolalia associated with Tourette's syndrome. *Mov Disord* 1966;11(4):431–433.

Shapiro AK, Shapiro E, Young JG, et al (eds): Signs, symptoms and clinical course, in *Gilles de la Tourette Syndrome,* 2d ed. New York, Raven Press, 1987, pp 127–193.

Shapiro E, Shapiro AK, Fulop G, et al: Controlled study of haloperidol, pimozide and placebo for the treatment of Gilles de la Tourette syndrome. *Arch Gen Psychiat* 1989;46:722–730.

Silver AA, Shytle RD, Philipp MK, et al: Case study: long-term potentiation of neuroleptics with transdermal nicotine in Tourette's syndrome. *J Am Acad Child Adolesc Psychiat* 1996;35(12):1631–1636.

Simeon D, Hollander E, Stein D, et al: Body dysmorphic disorder in the DSM-IV field trial for obsessive-compulsive disorder. *Am J Psychiat* 1995;152:1207–1209.

Singer HS, Brown J, Quaskey S, et al: The treatment of attention-deficit hyperactivity disorder in Tourette's syndrome: A double-blind placebo-controlled study with clonidine and desipramine. *Pediatrics* 1995;95(1):74–81.

Singer HS, Hahn IH, Moran TH: Abnormal dopamine uptake sites in postmortem striatum from patients with Tourette's syndrome. *Ann Neurol* 1991;30:558–562.

Singer HS, Reiss AL, Brown JE, et al: Volumetric MRI changes in basal ganglia of children with Tourette's syndrome. *Neurology* 1993;43(5):950–956.

Spencer T, Biederman J, Steingard R, et al: Bupropion exacerbates tics in children with attention-deficit hyperactivity disorder and Tourette's syndrome. *J Acad Child Adolesc Psychiat* 1993;32(1):211–214.

Steingard RJ, Goldberg M, Lee D, et al: Adjunctive clonazepam treatment of tic symptoms in children with comorbid tic disorders and ADHD. *J Am Acad Child Adolesc Psychiat* 1994;33(3):394–399.

Swedo SE, Leonard HL, Kiessling LS: Speculations on antineuronal antibody-mediated neuropsychatric disorders of childhood. *Pediatrics* 1994;93(2):323–326.

Swedo SE, Leonard HL, Mittleman BB, et al: Identification of children with pediatric autoimmune neuropsychiatric disorders associated with streptococcal infections by a marker associated with rheumatic fever. *Am J Psychiat* 1997;154(1):110–112.

Swedo SE, Leonard HL, Rapoport JL, et al: A double-blind comparison of clomipramine and desipramine in the treatment of trichotillomania (hair pulling). *N Engl J Med* 1989;321:497–501.

Swedo SE, Rapoport JL, Leonard HL, et al: Regional cerebral glucose metabolism of women with trichotillomania. *Arch Gen Psychiat* 1991;48:828–833.

Swedo SE: Rituals and releasers: An ethological model of obsessive-compulsive disorder, in Rapoport JL (ed): *Obsessive-Compulsive Disorder in Children and Adolescents.* Washington DC, American Psychiatric Press, 1989, pp 269–288.

Swedo SE: Sydenham's chorea: A model for childhood autoimmune neuropsychiatric disorders. *JAMA* 1994;272(2):1788–1791.

Tollefson GD, Rampey AH Jr, Genduso LA: A multicenter investigation of fixed-dose fluoxetine in the treatment of obsessive-compulsive disorder. *Arch Gen Psychiat* 1994;51:559–567.

van Balkom AJLM, van Oppen P, Vermeulen AWA, et al: A meta-analysis on the treatment of obsessive-compulsive disorder: A comparison of antidepressants, behavior and cognitive therapy. *Clin Psych Rev* 1994;14:359–382.

Van der Linden C, Bruggeman R, van Woerkom TC: Serotonin-dopamine antagonist and Gilles de la Tourette's syndrome: An open pilot dose-titration study with risperidone [letter]. *Mov Disord* 1994;9:687–688.

Varley CK, McClellan J: Case study: Two additional sudden deaths with tricyclic antidepressants. *J Am Acad Child Adolesc Psychiat* 1997;36:390–394.

Wheadon DE, Bushnell WD, Steiner M: A fixed dose comparison of 20, 40, or 60 mg paroxetine to placebo in the treatment of obsessive-compulsive disorder. *Proc Amer Coll Neuropsychopharm* 1993;32:143.

Wolf SS, Jones DW, Knable MB, et al: Tourette sydrome: Prediction of phenotypic variation in monozygotic twins by caudate nucleus D2 receptor binding. *Science* 1996;273:1225–1227.

Zabriskie JB, Lavenchy D, Williams RC Jr, et al: Rheumatic fever-associated B cell alloantigens as identified by monoclonal antibodies. *Arthrit Rheumat* 1985;28(9):1047–1051.

Zohar AH, Ratzoni G, Pauls DL, et al: An epidemiological study of obsessive-compulsive disorder and related disorders in Israeli adolescents. *J Am Acad Child Adolesc Psychiat* 1992;31:1057–1061.

C H A P T E R 7

SLEEP DISORDERS

Andrew Winokur

Several epidemiological surveys have provided data confirming the prevalence of sleep disorders in the general population. These conditions exact a substantial toll in human suffering, impaired quality of life and productivity, and fatalities attributable to sleepiness-related traffic accidents, and they have numerous other health implications. Additionally, the economic cost associated with sleep disorders is thought to be enormous. Studies such as the 1991 and 1995 Gallup surveys indicate that symptoms of sleep disturbances are often not reported by patients, and their diagnoses are often overlooked by physicians. Thus, a substantial percentage of patients with prominent symptoms of disturbed sleep do not receive appropriate treatment.

As detailed in this chapter, effective management of sleep disorders requires recognition of symptoms that may be subtle or hidden on initial presentation. The clinician must develop a sensitive eye and ear to detect such symptoms, including specific questions to elicit responses suggesting sleep problems. Once such symptoms are identified, a systematic and comprehensive evaluation must be performed to arrive at a clearly delineated diagnosis and identify, if possible, an underlying etiology. Treatment plans are developed most rationally on the basis of a sound diagnosis and an understanding of the underlying mechanism of sleep disturbance.

Treatment options for sleep disorders vary as a function of diagnosis and etiology. In many cases, a thoughtful integration of pharmacological and nonpharmacological options provides the most satisfactory and meaningful improvement. Because medications play an important role in the treatment of a number of the sleep disorders, familiarity with pharmacological treatment options is a prerequisite for employing these agents in an optimal manner. In particular, it is crucial to understand both the advantages and disadvantages of the drugs employed in the treatment of these conditions. In some instances, knowledge of subtle differences between drugs can have a significant impact on the efficacy and tolerability of the therapeutic regimen. Although diagnosing and treating sleep disorders present some formidable challenges, they also represent a distinct opportunity to attain a significant degree of satisfaction in providing skilled and empathetic care for a problem that afflicts a large number of individuals.

CLINICAL FEATURES

Sleep Physiology

On average, humans spend one-third of their lives asleep. Indeed, for all animal species sleep, or at least rest-activity variation, is an essential physiological adaptation. This supports the theory that sleep subserves important functions that are crucial to sustaining life and supporting optimal activity and productivity. It is surprising, therefore, to discover there are only primitive, poorly formed concepts about such basic questions as the purpose of sleep. Thus, much additional research is needed to define fundamental concepts in this field. With this limitation, a general overview of sleep is provided in the following, including some comments regarding basic regulatory mechanisms and hypotheses proposed for the function of sleep.

Patients often inquire about the amount of sleep they need. Although 8 h is the figure most often cited, some individuals may thrive on $4\frac{1}{2}$ h of sleep, and others appear to require $10\frac{1}{2}$ h to feel well and function at their best. Thus, the average amount of sleep needed is a median figure with a substantial standard deviation. Because individuals with a sleep regimen substantially below or above the median represent a very small population they might warrant evaluation for the presence of a sleep disorder.

Across species, the timing and pattern of sleep throughout a 24-h period varies considerably. For humans, sleep typically occurs during the night, with awakening most often coinciding with the onset of daylight hours (Minors and Waterhouse, 1981). The development of artificial lighting and the need for nighttime work have produced a population following a schedule that markedly deviates from the nighttime-rest, daytime-activity schedule.

Laboratory studies demonstrate that sleepiness is regulated by at least two factors: (1) the interval of prior wakefulness and (2) a circadian rhythm (Kribbs and Dinges, 1994). With respect to the latter, the primary period of peak sleepiness is in the late evening, coinciding with the time sleep normally occurs. A second peak of sleepiness occurs in early afternoon, coinciding with the traditional siesta hour

observed in many countries. The combination of postprandial fatigue with the circadian component of sleepiness in the afternoon represents a formidable challenge for many to remain awake and alert at this time of day.

Much of the information available on the timing and coordination of sleep, and its specific stages, is derived from studies using overnight sleep laboratory techniques [polysomnography (PSG)] (Guilleminault, 1982). Initially developed in the 1940s, PSG is widely used both for research studies on sleep physiology and as an important laboratory tool for diagnosing some primary sleep disorders. In the test, subjects typically report to a sleep laboratory in the early evening. A standard PSG involves the placement of at least two electrodes on the scalp, most often in a central and occipital position, two electrodes to identify eye movements, and one electrode on the submental muscle under the jaw to assess changes in muscle tone during the transition from wakefulness to sleep and during the different sleep stages. Additional detectors, or strain gauges, are employed to monitor airflow, respiratory effort, oxyhemoglobin saturation, an ECG, and limb movements. Other modifications of a polysomnographic study can be arranged to address specific questions. For example, EEG leads may be employed to assess the presence of nocturnal seizures. In some cases, a sleep study is videotaped to document movements or behaviors that might support the presence of disorders such as somnambulism or rapid eye movement (REM) behavior disorder. Such studies may be further customized to address diagnostic issues of relevance to specific sleep disorders, such as monitoring gastric acid secretion during sleep, or for assessing penile tumescence to aid in the diagnosis of impotence.

The subject is usually encouraged to initiate sleep at a customary bedtime hour (e.g., 11 P.M. to midnight). The interval between lights out and the initial onset of sleep is referred to as sleep latency, which is the period required to fall asleep. Although in some cases sleep occurs within a few minutes, more often, 15 to 30 min passes before sleep ensues. When more than 45 min is required, there are typically subjective complaints of trouble falling asleep. A well-known phenomenon in the sleep laboratory is the first night effect. Thus, for both patients with insomnia and for healthy volunteers with no history of sleep difficulties, the initial night in a sleep laboratory may be a stressful experience associated with a considerably prolonged sleep latency. Many people experience a comparable effect sleeping in an unfamiliar environment, such as a hotel room. Sleep latency is influenced by a number of factors, including stress, feeling uncomfortable in the bedroom environment, or having exercised or eaten a heavy meal too close to bedtime. Thus, complaints of difficulty falling asleep must be viewed in the context of the numerous factors that may influence this parameter.

Stage I sleep represents the transitional stage between wakefulness and sleep. Individuals in stage I may feel they are just dozing and will respond promptly to their name being called softly. Not considered to be particularly restful or restorative, stage I normally constitutes only 5 to 8% of total sleep. When stage I represents a substantially higher proportion of total sleep, there is normally a state of disrupted or nonrestorative sleep, as is seen in sleep apnea, periodic leg movements disorder, or some cases of depression.

The next stage of sleep typically encountered is stage II, which usually constitutes one-half to two-thirds of total sleep time. Stage II represents, in some respects, the core of sleep, and is considered to be a solid, well-consolidated phase of sleep. From an EEG perspective, stage II is characterized by two prominent waveforms: sleep spindles and K complexes.

In a typical night of sleep, the individual moves relatively quickly from stage II to stages III and IV, which are regarded as deep sleep. It is common practice to refer to stages III and IV combined as slow wave (SWS) or delta sleep. From an EEG perspective, slow wave sleep is characterized by prominent, large-amplitude, slow-frequency waves, which are referred to as delta waves. Muscle tone is reduced during slow wave sleep and autonomic functions (e.g., pulse, respiration) tend to be slow. An individual in slow wave sleep may be very difficult to arouse and, if wakened, may initially be dazed or confused. Slow wave sleep is thought to be crucial for a sense of restful, restorative sleep. In a typical night, the initial episode of slow wave sleep occurs within the first 30 to 40 min of sleep onset, and is generally the most prominent or intense of the night. Indeed, most slow wave sleep normally occurs within the first third of the sleep period.

The final stage is rapid-eye-movement (REM) sleep. It is widely known that REM sleep is associated with most dreaming activity, with only 10% of dreaming occurring during non-REM stages. The characteristics of dreaming are thought to differ as a function of sleep stage, with non-REM dreaming believed to be associated with a more amorphous sense or feeling, whereas REM-associated dreaming has more distinct images and plot lines. From a physiological perspective, REM is characterized by three prominent features: (1) low-voltage, fast activity, which is quite similar to the EEG pattern of alert wakefulness; (2) rapid eye movements; and (3) profound muscle atonia. The combination of an "activated brain" (low-voltage, fast EEG activity) in a "paralyzed body" (muscle atonia) has prompted some to refer to REM as paradoxical sleep and to suggest that this combination may represent an evolutionary adaptation to protect the organism from physically responding to dreams. Typically, REM occurs initially 70 to 90 min after sleep onset, with the interval between sleep onset and the first REM episode referred to as the REM latency. Normally, approximately 25% of total sleep time is composed of REM sleep.

After the first passage through the various sleep stages, the individual normally cycles through stage II, SWS, and REM sleep throughout the remainder of the night. As noted previously, most SWS is clustered in the first third of the sleep period. In contrast, REM sleep occurs more prominently, and in greater clusters, in the last third of the night.

In evaluating the results of an overnight laboratory sleep study, several types of variables are analyzed, including sleep onset latency, total sleep time, sleep efficiency (time asleep divided by total recording time), sleep continuity (awakenings and/or arousals, time awake after falling asleep), and sleep architecture (the composition and timing of the major sleep stages). In addition, data are provided regarding other physiological variables such as respiratory events (apneas and hypopneas), oxyhemoglobin saturation, periodic limb movements, and cardiac rhythm. Comments are provided about the impact of specific physiological events on sleep, such as when episodes of apnea disrupt sleep continuity.

Epidemiology of Sleep Disorders

A number of surveys have evaluated the prevalence of sleep complaints and sleep disorders in the general population. Polls conducted in the United States, Europe, and Australia have provided generally consistent findings that 30 to 40% of the adult population reported at least some degree of unsatisfactory, disturbed sleep on some occasions during the previous year. For example, a 1985 study examining over 3000 adults in the United States reported a 1-year prevalence rate for insomnia of 35%, with 17% of the population surveyed reporting serious or continuing problems with insomnia (Mellinger et al., 1985). It was also found that 85% of those with serious, persistent insomnia did not receive treatment for this condition.

The National Sleep Foundation commissioned surveys by the Gallup organization to assess the frequency and nature of sleep problems in the United States. Reports released in 1991 and 1995 described separate studies based on interviews with 1000 and 1027 participants, respectively (Sleep in America, 1991, 1995). The findings from the two surveys were generally comparable and included a number of interesting and important observations. Consistent with previous reports, between one-third and one-half of adults experience at least occasional sleep problems. It is striking that 9 to 12% of subjects reported regular or frequent problems with insomnia. The 1995 survey also found that adults with significant sleep problems reported a lower general physical health rating. Of course, this relationship may relate to several issues: (1) poor-quality sleep predisposes to impaired physical health; (2) chronic sleep problems predispose individuals to adopt a more negative view of their physical health status; and (3) poor physical health is likely to adversely affect the quality of sleep. Daytime napping was reported by about 4 of 10 adults, with 12% reporting dozing off during daytime activities. It is notable that only 30% of adults reporting difficulties sleeping indicated that they discussed their sleep problems with a physician or other health professional. Moreover, individuals with sleep problems reported they rarely make an appointment with a physician to discuss this issue. A separate study reported that only about one half of general physicians in an office practice obtain a comprehensive sleep history, even after a patient reports symptoms of poor-quality sleep. These results suggest that sleep problems are common in the general population and are inadequately recognized, diagnosed, and treated.

Although insomnia represents the most widespread and common sleep disorder, several other important conditions must also be considered when assessing the scope of sleep disorders. For example, obstructive sleep apnea, originally described in the early 1970s, is recognized as an important sleep disorder with a relatively high prevalence in the adult population that is associated with significant morbidity and mortality (Pack, 1994; Strollo and Rogers, 1996). The Wisconsin Sleep Cohort Study, an epidemiological investigation, reported, using fairly conservative criteria, a 2 to 4% incidence of obstructive sleep apnea in the adult population (Young et al., 1993).

Narcolepsy is a relatively low prevalence disorder, with some 125,000 to 250,000 total cases in the United States. However, it represents a substantial public health problem because of its chronicity and impact on daily functioning. Periodic limb movements during sleep (PLMS) disorder is another im-

portant category. Although the prevalence of PLMS disorder is difficult to ascertain, it is known to become more prevalent with age. In the 1995 Gallup survey, 18% of adults reported prominent leg movements or jerks during sleep.

Another category involves disorders of sleep schedule (i.e., circadian rhythm disorders). For example, problems with poor-quality sleep and sleepiness while awake are commonly encountered in individuals who do shift work. It has been reported that 26% of men and 18% of women are employed in jobs that require variable work shifts. Jet lag is another condition associated with poor-quality sleep and excessive daytime sleepiness. Given the increasingly complex conditions in the contemporary workplace, the prevalence of such occupationally generated sleep problems is likely to increase in the future.

Impact of Sleep Disorders

The impact of sleep disorders on overall health, quality of life, and broad economic variables has been estimated in several reports. Given the importance of sleep as a physiological function, it seems obvious that impaired sleep would have significant health consequences. However, the specific implications of sleep disruption have been difficult to identify, although a number of lines of evidence support the contention that poor-quality sleep is associated with deleterious consequences. As noted previously, respondents in the 1995 Gallup survey who reported persistent sleep difficulties were substantially more likely to rate their physical health as poor than were those who had limited or no sleep problems. Other insomnia studies have found substantial adverse effects on a number of quality-of-life issues, such as reduced satisfaction with life, impaired relationships, and difficulty at work. Studies aimed at examining the effects of sleep problems on functioning in the workplace have linked sleepiness to absenteeism, poor-quality performance, reduced productivity, and an increase in accident rates (Dinges, 1995). A particular category of accidents with immense public health consequence involves motor vehicles. Individuals with insomnia are reported to have a rate of motor vehicle accidents two to three times higher than is found in the general population. In a 1995 Gallup survey, 31% of adults reported they had dozed off while operating a motor vehicle. Moreover, 4% of adults indicated they had been involved in an automobile accident attributable to driving while sleepy.

A number of studies have attempted to link insomnia with a variety of illnesses (Briones, 1996). Insomnia has been correlated with increased risk for heart disease, hypertension, stroke, and diabetes. In the case of obstructive sleep apnea, the increased risk of hypertension and stroke is well established. An increased risk of mortality in patients suffering from insomnia has also been reported. It must be emphasized, however, that such associations do not prove causality, leaving a need for further studies to examine specific health consequences of disordered sleep.

Several investigators attempted to estimate the cost to society of sleeplessness and sleep disorders. Although such estimates are imprecise, they provide some perspective on the scope and impact of the problem. In one analysis the overall economic cost of insomnia was estimated to be approximately $100 billion (Stoller, 1994). Another analysis focusing on sleep-related accidents arrived at cost estimates of $50 billion (Leger, 1994).

DIAGNOSIS

The approach to sleep disorders described in this chapter is designed for the physician in an office practice setting. Recognizing that the generalist physician in contemporary practice has a waiting room full of patients, and a limited amount of time for each, it is still highly recommended that a few questions be asked to sample the areas of quality of sleep, daytime alertness, and functioning. When positive responses are elicited to broad screening questions, the physician must be prepared to follow up with a more comprehensive and thorough evaluation.

Initial Assessment of Sleep During an Office Visit

As noted previously, many individuals who suffer from significant and persistent sleep problems do not mention them during a visit with their physician. It is even more uncommon for patients to schedule an appointment to discuss such problems. Yet sleep problems are quite common and are associated with significant consequences for feeling and functioning well, quality of life, medical health, and emotional well-being. Considering these factors, it behooves the physician to assess pertinent issues relating to sleep problems concisely but thoroughly as a routine part of each office visit (Czeisler and Richardson, 1991).

An initial assessment of sleep quality should review several areas of relevance to common sleep disorders. By far the most frequently encountered sleep disorder is insomnia. It should be noted that insomnia is not a specific diagnosis, but rather the report that the sleep pattern or sleep quality is unsatisfactory. Symptoms of insomnia may have one or more of the following components:

1. Trouble falling asleep
2. Waking up frequently during the night (i.e., difficulty staying asleep)
3. Waking up too early in the morning (i.e., early-morning awakening)
4. Upon awakening, feeling the sleep has not been sufficiently restful or restorative

Therefore, in the assessment of insomnia, it may be appropriate to begin with a general, open-ended question about the overall quality of sleep, to be followed up by a few additional pointed questions to survey the general areas of potential symptomatology (Table 7-1).

Table 7-1

Questions to Survey Symptoms of Insomnia

How has your sleep been recently?
Do you have any problems falling asleep?
Do you often wake up during the night?
Do you tend to wake up too early in the morning?
Do you think that your sleep is restful and refreshing?

A second important manifestation of a prominent sleep disorder is excessive daytime somnolence. Several primary sleep disorders, including obstructive sleep apnea, PLMS disorder, and narcolepsy, often present with this symptom as a primary manifestation. In more severe presentation, patients will appear patently sleepy during an office visit and will have difficulty remaining awake throughout an interview. More typically, however, manifestations of excessive daytime somnolence are more subtle, with the patient reporting feeling fatigued or lacking in energy. As with insomnia, it is generally necessary to ask some specific, pointed questions to elicit symptoms of excessive daytime somnolence (Table 7-2).

Sleep problems may also be manifest by physiological symptoms or behaviors during sleep. Examples of common physical symptoms that may be indicative of a sleep disorder include prominent snoring; irregular breathing patterns or a choking, smothering sensation, which may be associated with obstructive sleep apnea; and frequent, repetitive leg jerks or kicks, which may indicate PLMS disorder. Elicitation of a history of prominent behaviors during sleep (parasomias) may indicate the presence of sleep disorders such as somnambulism or night terrors.

An additional category of sleep disorder involves alternations of sleep schedule. This category might involve an endogenous tendency to follow an unusual pattern of sleep and wakefulness. For example, individuals with advanced sleep phase syndrome tend to fall asleep early in the evening, then awaken early in the morning. In contrast, individuals with delayed sleep phase syndrome fall asleep very late at night and then sleep well into the day. In both cases, sleep tends to be sound and continuous during the sleep period, but falls outside of the more typical sleep-wake schedule. Other examples of sleep schedule (i.e., circadian rhythm) sleep disorders are related to occupational or behavioral factors. Common examples include jet-lag-related and shift-work-related sleep disorders.

Thus, an initial office evaluation of sleep should include several specific questions relating to sleep quality and manifestations of sleep disruption. It is also appropriate to inquire about daytime alertness and excessive daytime somnolence. Further evaluation can be directed to sleep-related physiological manifestations, including snoring, prominent leg movements, or behaviors associated with sleep. Finally, a question or two related to the characteristic time of sleep and wakefulness explores the area of circadian rhythm sleep disorders. This initial evaluation can be accomplished quickly with a limited number of appropriately directed questions. If these questions elicit significant positive findings, a more extensive evaluation of a possible sleep disorder should be conducted.

Comprehensive Evaluation of a Sleep Disorder

Once a symptom or multiple symptoms of sleep disturbance have been noted, it is appropriate to undertake a more extensive, systematic evaluation to obtain a specific diagnosis to identify, if possible, specific etiological factors so as to develop an appropriate treatment plan (Gillin and Byerley, 1990). This recommended approach is consistent with standard medical practice related to the evaluation of other symptoms (e.g., fever, chest pain) that might be related to a host of diagnostic possibilities and might require consideration of a range of treatments. In the case of sleep disorders, it is important to recall that insomnia is a symptom, not a diagnosis. All too often identification of insomnia triggers an immediate treatment recommendation, typically a prescription for a hypnotic, rather than stimulating a careful evalu-

Table 7-2

Questions to Elicit Symptoms of Excessive Daytime Somnolence

Do you feel excessively sleepy during the day?
Do you take naps frequently?
Do you tend to fall asleep while reading or watching TV?
Are there times when you fall asleep during other activities?
Is it occasionally difficult to stay awake while driving a car?

ation of underlying causative factors. Detailed in the following section is a recommended approach for the evaluation of a sleep disorder, using insomnia-related complaints as an example.

When a patient presents with symptoms of disturbed, poor-quality sleep, it is necessary to obtain additional information to put these symptoms into context. Thus, the physician must learn more about the nature of the symptoms, ask about other symptom categories that may be relevant to the insomnia complaints (in the manner of a review of systems analysis), and understand factors in the patient's life and environment that may be contributing to the sleep disruption. In undertaking this type of assessment it is often helpful to speak with the patient's spouse or bed partner who may be able to provide additional important information concerning, for example, snoring, irregular breathing, or leg movements that the patient is unable to describe.

Problems with insomnia can occur in the context of, or as the result of, a number of associated conditions. Thus it is important to move through a specific series of questions related to each of these areas. In this regard it is customary to obtain additional information about the nature and chronicity of sleep complaints. A typical categorization of insomnia duration describes transient insomnia as symptoms of disturbed sleep lasting for several days, short-term insomnia as difficulties lasting up to 3 weeks, and chronic insomnia as having a duration of more than 3 weeks. Assessment of the chronicity of the sleep problem is of importance in understanding the origin and etiology of the problem and appropriate therapy.

Many factors may precipitate alterations in sleep patterns. It is widely recognized that stress represents one of the most significant external variables that may impinge on the quality of sleep. In a 1995 Gallup survey, 46% of respondents who experienced problems with sleep attributed them to stress or worries. About a quarter of the respondents with sleep difficulties believed it is impossible to achieve success in a career without being sleep deprived. Thus, an effort must be made to establish whether some newly arising or more chronic, ongoing stressful circumstance is adversely affecting the sleep patterns. The process of discussing and clarifying the importance of stress-related factors may help the patient understand the origins of the sleep problem and encourage steps to modify these circumstances. In some cases, referral for counseling may be appropriate to help deal more effectively with stress.

Often aspects of the home environment and daily schedule and habits have a significant impact on sleep quality. The term sleep hygiene is routinely used to categorize this broad range of issues. Within the sleep hygiene framework it is often productive to examine the customary habits and patterns of the patient in times of retiring and arising, because irregular hours of sleep schedule may predispose some individuals to sleep problems. It is important to consider the condition of the bedroom's conduciveness to sleep. If the environment is too noisy, too warm or cold, or too bright, there may be negative effects on sleep. Additionally, consumption of a heavy or spicy meal close to bedtime, or exercising vigorously in the evening, may disrupt sleep. Thus, reviewing customary patterns of behavior that may influence sleep can be an illuminating and highly productive exercise. In this regard, it is sometimes helpful to have the patient maintain a sleep diary for a few weeks, charting timing and quality of nocturnal sleep, occurrence of daytime naps, feelings of alertness throughout the day, and other associated habits or behaviors. The process of charting often highlights critical factors contributing to sleep irregularities.

A number of substances or medications may affect sleep. Thus, although most know that caffeine has disruptive effects on sleep, many do not monitor the amount or timing of coffee consumption. Moreover, it is frequently overlooked that tea, cola products, and chocolate also contain appreciable amounts of caffeine. In addition, alcohol is a common cause of sleep disturbance. Although it has a sedative effect and is associated with a shortening of sleep latency, alcohol fragments sleep and disrupts sleep continuity. Many individuals consume alcohol to self-medicate in dealing with insomnia and associated anxiety or depression. This strategy is counterproductive in the long run because of its fragmenting effect on sleep. Additionally, after an individual becomes reliant on alcohol to fall asleep, efforts to discontinue its use may precipitate rebound insomnia, further reinforcing alcohol dependency.

A number of drugs prescribed for various medical and psychiatric indications have significant effects on sleep. Some, such as the antidepressant amitriptyline and a host of antihistamines, are markedly sedating and therefore must be considered in the differential diagnosis of patients presenting with manifestations of excessive daytime somnolence.

Medical Problems Associated with Sleep Disorders

A number of medical conditions or illnesses are commonly associated with disruption of sleep patterns (Winokur, 1997). Therefore, consideration of problems known to be linked to alterations in sleep is essential in the comprehensive assessment of sleep complaints. Examples include thyroid dysfunction (both hypothyroidism and hyperthyroidism), pulmonary disorders (e.g., asthma, chronic obstructive lung disease), gastrointestinal disorders (e.g., esophageal reflux), and neurological disorders (e.g., Parkinson's disease). Any condition associated with prominent pain can cause impaired sleep. For example, patients with fibromyositis, a condition characterized by muscular pain and specific tender points, often have problems with insomnia, polysomnographic studies revealing alpha intrusion into slow-wave sleep (referred to as alpha-delta sleep).

The comprehensive evaluation of a patient with symptoms of insomnia often includes a physical examination and laboratory tests to evaluate the presence of medical conditions that might cause or exacerbate disturbed sleep patterns. When possible, it is preferable to identify and treat an underlying medical condition rather than the insomnia itself.

Psychiatric Disorders and Sleep Disturbance

A wide range of psychiatric conditions is commonly associated with disturbances in sleep patterns, especially insomnia (Halaris, 1987). Thus, assessment of the presence of a major psychiatric disorder represents a critical area of exploration for a patient presenting with insomnia. Although psychiatric conditions, such as schizophrenia, or organic brain disorders, such as Alzheimer's disease, are often associated with prominent sleep problems, mood and anxiety disorders are of particular relevance because patients with depression and anxiety are encountered with greater frequency in general practice. Such individuals often manifest significant sleep disturbance, in some cases as a primary presenting complaint. In depression, complaints of insomnia are typically described in 70% or more of patients, with complaints of middle insomnia or early-morning awakening being especially characteristic (Winokur and Reynolds, 1994). In one study of sleep patterns in hospitalized patients with major depression, 90% had some form of EEG-verified sleep disturbance. Numerous PSG studies of sleep patterns in depressed patients have revealed characteristic alterations in sleep architecture, including disruptions in sleep continuity, alterations in REM sleep (e.g., a shortening of REM latency), and reductions in slow wave sleep.

In contrast to the more typical presentation of insomnia associated with depression, a substantial subset, perhaps 20%, of depressed patients suffer from hypersomnolence, often associated with daytime lethargy and fatigue. Patients with depression and hypersomnolence are often described as atypical depressives. Hypersomnolence has also been reported to be commonly observed in patients with bipolar depression or seasonal affective disorder.

The relationship between depression and sleep disturbance is complex. In some cases it is difficult to determine whether a disturbance in sleep represents a symptom of depression or an important etiological factor in the onset of the depressive episode. Many patients who present with depression and insomnia insist their depression would resolve promptly if they could simply get a few good nights of sleep. In fact, few studies have systematically evaluated the extent to which depression might be ameliorated by directly treating insomnia. Nevertheless, it is notable to emphasize that many cases of depression are not accurately diagnosed or treated because the patient or the physician focuses exclusively on the symptoms of insomnia and other somatic complaints commonly associated with clinical depression. It is generally believed that treating insomnia with a hypnotic without initiating treatment for the depression per se is an inadequate treatment strategy. Of particular concern in this regard is the association of clinical depression with a significant risk of suicide.

Perpetuating Factors for Insomnia

Because insomnia may be precipitated by a number of factors, it is important to identify, if possible, the variable(s) responsible for the sleep disturbance. Sleep experts also emphasize, however, that insomnia, once initiated, is often sustained by a series of reactions or perpetuating factors. Thus, an individual undergoing acute, severe disruption of sleep frequently develops pronounced anxiety about the prospect of being able to fall asleep. In many cases, a distinct physiological arousal pattern develops, sometimes triggered by entering the bedroom in preparation for sleep. The person may develop a set of worries and concerns about not being able to sleep adequately, and these may extend to an expectation of not being able to perform effectively at work and a belief that serious health problems will develop as a consequence of the disturbed sleep patterns. Additionally, the patient may demonstrate maladaptive behavioral patterns in attempting to deal with the sleep problem, such as napping during the day or using alcohol at night. This pattern of sleep disorder is referred to as psychophysiological insomnia. When manifestations of psychophysiological insomnia are identified, this problem must be dealt with in addition to the original precipitating factors.

Evaluation of Excessive Daytime Somnolence

Excessive daytime somnolence is a sleep disorder-related symptomatology that is commonly encountered in a general practice. As with insomnia, a systematic and comprehensive approach must be taken in evaluating this condition. Once initial symptoms are reported (Table 7-2), a number of possible disorders must be considered in the differential diagnosis of excessive daytime somnolence (Table 7-3).

The general evaluation of excessive daytime somnolence should include a comprehensive analysis

Table 7-3
Conditions and Disorders Associated with Excessive Daytime Somnolence

Sleep deprivation for any reason
Certain medical disorders (e.g., hypothyroidism)
Medications (e.g., sedating H_1 antihistamines, some antidepressant drugs, β blockers)
Depressive disorders (especially bipolar affective disorder, depressed and atypical depression)
Idiopathic CNS hypersomnolence
Periodic leg movement disorder
Obstructive sleep apnea
Narcolepsy

of symptoms and their severity. The circumstances under which these symptoms are manifest must be assessed, as should the extent to which the individual is hampered or incapacitated by the condition. A careful analysis of nocturnal sleep patterns may shed light on reasons for excessive daytime somnolence. A review of systems, a physical examination, and a battery of laboratory tests, as indicated, may reveal some underlying medical condition responsible for excessive daytime somnolence. In addition, a review of the patient's medication regimen may reveal drugs that cause sedation.

The primary sleep disorders most typically associated with symptoms of excessive daytime somnolence are narcolepsy and obstructive sleep apnea. Therefore, a detailed assessment of excessive daytime somnolence should include some questions specifically intended to elicit symptoms and findings characteristic of these conditions. Narcolepsy is characterized, in addition to excessive daytime somnolence, by a cluster of symptoms including cataplexy, a pronounced muscle weakness, typically triggered by intense emotion; sleep paralysis, a transient state of loss of motor control upon awakening, presumably related to a slightly prolonged state of REM-associated muscle atonia; and hypnagogic hallucinations, associated with either sleep onset or awakening. In the case of obstructive sleep apnea, subjects are frequently overweight, may present with a thick neck or other manifestation of upper airway obstruction, and typically have a history of prominent snoring. Additionally, patients with obstructive sleep apnea often describe fragmented, nonrestorative sleep, morning headaches and confusion, and, occasionally, choking or smothering sensations at night. For both narcolepsy and obstructive sleep apnea, PSG studies are required to confirm the diagnosis.

Use of Polysomnography in the Diagnosis of Sleep Disorders

An overnight laboratory sleep study is often needed to confirm the diagnosis of primary sleep disorders, including obstructive sleep apnea, narcolepsy, PLMS disorder, and REM behavior disorder; occasionally it is also needed in the general assessment of insomnia.

Because of the logistical problems and considerable expense involved in obtaining a PSG, it is not practical to obtain an overnight sleep study in a casual or indiscriminate manner. A PSG study does, however, represent an essential component of a diagnostic evaluation for sleep disorder. Therefore, the physician should have a clear understanding of instances in which a patient should be referred for a sleep study.

Obstructive sleep apnea represents the most frequent indication for a PSG study. Because obstructive sleep apnea is associated with a significant morbidity and mortality, it is an important disorder to recognize and diagnose accurately. Moreover, although obstructive sleep apnea can be suspected on the basis of clinical signs and symptoms, a definitive diagnosis requires PSG assessment. A laboratory assessment of suspected obstructive sleep apnea may involve one or two nights of study. In the two-night protocol, the first night is devoted to ascertaining the presence of obstructive sleep apnea, and the second is typically used to assess the effectiveness of a treatment for the condition referred to as nasal continuous positive airway pressure (CPAP) therapy. In the one-night "condensed" evaluation of obstructive sleep apnea, the first part of the night is used to confirm the presence of the condition, and the second part is used for CPAP titration. Characteristic PSG findings supporting the diagnosis of obstructive sleep apnea include repeated sleep-related respiratory events (apneas and hypopneas) throughout the night. The respiratory events are typically associated with arousals, thus representing a significant fragmentation of sleep, and with oxyhemaglobin desaturations. Although some debate exists regarding the number of apneas and hypopneas needed to confirm the diagnosis of obstructive sleep apnea, a commonly employed minimal figure for the respiratory disturbance index is ≥ 15 events per hour (Guilleminault, 1982; Pack, 1994). For many patients with this disorder, the frequency of respiratory events is considerably higher than this, reaching 100 events per hour or more. In light of the extent of sleep fragmentation produced, it is easy to understand why obstructive sleep apnea is typically associated with a pronounced degree of EDS. It is also important to note that the temporary cessation of airflow is associated with demonstrable respiratory effort as reflected by monitoring chest wall, diaphragmatic, and abdominal muscle activity. When cessation of airflow is coupled to lack of respiratory effort, a diagnosis of central apnea is made.

Narcolepsy is another primary sleep disorder for which PSG assessment is needed for diagnosis. The clinical profile for narcolepsy, including excessive daytime somnolence, cataplexy, sleep paralysis, and hypnagogic hallucinations, provides sufficient evidence to suspect the presence of this disorder. The laboratory evaluation of narcolepsy includes an overnight sleep study and a daytime test, the multiple sleep latency test (MSLT). This test is the most widely employed technique to

provide an objective and quantitative assessment of daytime sleepiness. In the evaluation of narcolepsy, the overnight PSG provides a general assessment of sleep quality and sleep architecture. Many patients with narcolepsy demonstrate a pattern of considerably fragmented nocturnal sleep. Additionally, patients with narcolepsy often enter REM sleep more rapidly after sleep onset than would normally be expected. In the multiple sleep latency test evaluation, conducted on the day after a nighttime PSG, subjects are asked to lie down and try to sleep at 2-h intervals (e.g., 9 A.M., 11 A.M., 1 P.M., and 3 P.M.). They are given 20 min to fall asleep and then are awakened and kept awake until the next nap interval. Results are evaluated by average time across the four nap opportunities to fall asleep and by the type of sleep that occurs in the nap opportunity. A mean latency to sleep onset of less than 5 min indicates the presence of pathological sleepiness. Although this type of sleep latency is typically seen in patients with narcolepsy, it is not diagnostic of the condition, as patients with obstructive sleep apnea, idiopathic CNS hypersomnolence, or pronounced sleep deprivation for other reasons can demonstrate very short mean sleep latencies. However, patients with narcolepsy typically demonstrate a second finding, short REM latency, on the multiple sleep latency test that helps establish the diagnosis. By established criteria for the diagnosis of narcolepsy, patients with this disorder will have two REM onsets among the four nap opportunities.

The PSG studies may be useful in the diagnosis of other sleep disorders as well. Periodic limb movements during sleep disorder is characterized by stereotyped, repetitive movements that occur at an interval of about 20 to 40 s. The limb movements can cause fragmented sleep, leading to complaints of disturbed, nonrestorative sleep or of EDS.

REM sleep behavior disorder is characterized by behaviors, some of which may be violent or aggressive, that appear to occur in concert with dream content. In REM sleep behavior disorder the behavioral episode is shown, on the basis of PSG monitoring, to arise from REM sleep. Moreover, patients with REM sleep behavior disorder typically manifest a loss of the usual muscle atonia associated with REM sleep, a circumstance that can be readily demonstrated by PSG techniques. In a patient with a history suggestive of REM sleep behavior disorder, the loss of muscle atonia during REM helps establish the diagnosis, even in the absence of behaviors during REM on the night of the study. Because REM sleep behavior disorder is reported to be associated with lesions of the midbrain or brain-stem regions, PSG findings consistent with REM sleep behavior disorder may be cause to consider some additional tests, such as neuroimaging of the brain.

Seizures are often associated with sleep and occasionally occur exclusively during sleep. When a PSG is requested to evaluate the presence of nocturnal seizures, a seizure montage is employed that involves additional scalp electrodes to identify seizure activity.

In general, PSG studies are not recommended for the routine assessment of symptoms of insomnia as these procedures are usually not informative in elucidating the etiology of most forms of this condition. Additionally, the use of PSG techniques for the evaluation of insomnia is not generally cost-effective. However, for some patients with chronic, severe insomnia who fail to respond to conventional thorough diagnostic and treatment efforts, a PSG evaluation may be appropriate. In such cases, it may be possible to demonstrate the presence of a primary sleep disorder that had not been suspected from the clinical evaluation. The definitive demonstration of a primary sleep disorder could open the way to more effective treatments.

Shown on Fig.7-1 is a representative algorithm for the evaluation of insomnia.

PHARMACOTHERAPY

Treatment of Insomnia

The term insomnia refers to a symptom of disturbed sleep, a symptom that can be associated with a number of different conditions or disorders. Thus, the first step in treating insomnia is to make a concerted effort to understand the reasons for the sleep disruption and identify, if possible, a specific etiology. When a cause for the insomnia is established, it is possible to develop strategies to deal most effectively with the underlying problem(s). Because a number of factors cause disrupted sleep patterns, the optimal treatment may be quite varied. In some cases, counseling or advice about stress management may be indicated. Patients often inadvertently develop maladaptive behavioral patterns that have an adverse impact on sleep. In such cases, reinforcement of proper sleep hygiene behaviors may be beneficial in restoring good-quality sleep. When a medical problem, substance abuse, or prescribed medication proves to be responsible for the sleep disorder, improvement can be achieved by addressing directly the underlying problem.

An example of a sleep disturbance being linked to a broader complicating variable is the co-occurrence of insomnia and a psychiatric illness, such as depression. When a patient is identified as having a major depressive disorder, it is common practice to evaluate carefully whether symptoms of insomnia are present. For example, the Hamilton Depression

Rating Scale, a standardizing rating scale for assessing the severity of depression, contains 3 discrete items from a total of 21 focusing on aspects of sleep disruption, including problems falling asleep, awakenings in the middle of the night, and early-morning awakenings. Equally important, the presence of insomnia should trigger careful investigation into the possible co-occurrence of depression. It is believed that as depression improves, so too will sleep. Although this pattern often appears to hold in clinical practice, few studies have systematically evaluated changes in sleep patterns with improvement in depression. In a recent study of depressed patients treated with interpersonal psychotherapy, but no medications, some variables, including sleep continuity and EEG delta sleep activity, actually worsened in those who demonstrated a positive response to therapy (Buysse et al., 1992). Additionally, recovered depressed patients with low delta sleep activity were found to be at higher risk for relapse. Thus, some data support the importance of considering the relationship between sleep physiology and depression during the course of treatment.

Recently a large number of new antidepressants have been approved by the FDA. Although these drugs are comparable with respect to efficacy, they exhibit a number of significant differences in pharmacological properties (Stahl, 1996). One site of action for antidepressants is the CNS neurotransmitters, particularly norepinephrine, serotonin, and dopamine. The majority of antidepressants modulate the activity of one or more of these neurotransmitters by blocking their reuptake at presynaptic sites.

A characteristic used to distinguish antidepressants is their selectivity. Some antidepressants, such as the tricyclics, display a broad pharmacological profile because of their ability to inhibit a number of neurotransmitter receptors in brain, including H_1 histamine receptors, muscarinic cholinergic receptors, and α_1-adrenergic receptors (Richelson, 1996). Many of the side effects associated with tricyclic antidepressants are due to these nonselective effects on the neurotransmitter receptor sites. For example, some of these drugs, such as amitriptyline and doxepin, are quite sedating, an effect attributable, at least in part, to potent histamine H_1 receptor blocking

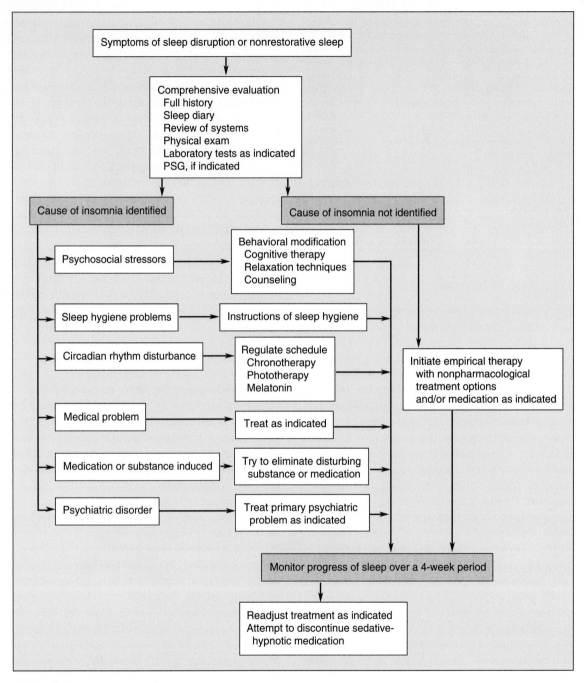

Figure 7–1.   *Assessment of insomnia.*

activity. The sedating tricyclics are often recommended for a subset of patients with depression and insomnia; some PSG studies confirm a shortening of sleep latency and an improvement in sleep continuity in subjects treated with these drugs.

Other antidepressants are highly selective in that their predominant action is on a single transmitter system. Examples include the selective serotonin reuptake inhibitors (SSRIs), such as fluoxetine. With SSRIs, insomnia is one of the most consistently reported side effects, typically occurring in some 20 to 25% of patients. A limited number of PSG studies with the SSRIs reported disruptive effects on sleep, including a reduction in sleep efficiency and an increase in the number of awakenings and arousals. The effects of the SSRIs on sleep are thought to be related to enhanced serotonin neurotransmission at the 5HT2 subtype of the serotonin receptor. This notion is reinforced by the finding that two antidepressants, nefazodone and mirtazapine, that enhance sleep in preclinical studies are potent inhibitors of the 5HT2 receptor. Limited information is available on the effects of mirtazapine on human sleep, but nefazodone has been studied extensively in both normal subjects and depressed patients. In one study patients with major depression with coexisting complaints of sleep disturbance were treated with either fluoxetine or nefazodone (Armitage et al., 1997). Their sleep patterns were evaluated on several occasions during treatment by PSG techniques. Both groups demonstrated a favorable and comparable antidepressant response. The changes in sleep pattern during the course of treatment, however, differed between the two. Thus, patients in the fluoxetine group had reduced sleep efficiency and a greater number of awakenings as compared with those receiving nefazodone.

These findings indicate that different antidepressants produce different effects on sleep physiology, even though they are of comparable efficacy with regard to depression. When considering treatment options for a patient with depression and insomnia, information should be reviewed for the various antidepressants for their effects on sleep architecture. Many clinicians favor combining an activating anti-depressant, such as fluoxetine, with a sedative-hypnotic compound to control insomnia in patients with coexisting depression and sleep disturbance. Although this practice is widespread and enthusiastically endorsed by many, data based on controlled prospective studies employing objective monitoring techniques, such as PSG, are lacking to assess the efficacy and safety of this approach. Another common clinical practice involves the adjunctive use of trazodone, a highly sedating antidepressant, typically in very low doses, in combination with an activating drug such as fluoxetine. Although the widespread use of this combination suggests that clinicians believe it is effective, there are no data to properly evaluate the suitability of this treatment strategy.

Pharmacological Treatment Options for Insomnia

For many patients with insomnia, medication represents an important, if not essential, therapy (Kupfer and Reynolds, 1997). Over the years, a number of drugs were employed in the treatment of insomnia. Historically, barbiturates, such as secobarbital, or barbituratelike hypnotics, such as chloral hydrate, were widely used for this condition. These drugs are now largely ignored because of their side effect profile and the substantial risk of dependence and withdrawal associated with their long-term use.

Sedating antidepressants such as amitriptyline or trazodone are now frequently used in the treatment of insomnia. With their role in treating patients who exhibit the combination of depression and insomnia being reasonably well established, many physicians have adopted the practice of prescribing sedating antidepressants in relatively low doses to subjects with insomnia but no depression. This seems intended, in part, to avoid the long-term use of hypnotics, which may carry a risk of dependence and withdrawal. A good deal of clinical experience suggests that low-dose antidepressant therapy can provide well-tolerated symptomatic relief for many chronic insomniacs. Studies are lacking, however, to demonstrate the efficacy and safety of the antidepressants when used in this way. It should also be noted that this class of drugs is associated with a significant risk of side effects, although they may be mild or negligible at the modest doses used for insomnia.

Benzodiazepines.   Currently, the most widely employed medications approved for the treatment of insomnia are the benzodiazepines, including triazolam, temazepam, quazepam, estazolam, and flurazepam, and the imidazopyridine zolpidem (Lader et al., 1985; Langtry and Benfield, 1990) (Table 7-4).

The benzodiazepine hypnotics differ from one another primarily in their onset of action, half-life, and number of active metabolites (Kupfer and Reynolds, 1997). Among the benzodiazepine hypnotics, triazolam, estazolam, and flurazepam have a rapid onset of action, quazepam has an intermediate or variable onset, and temazepam has a slow onset. In some cases this type of information is important for the proper management of insomnia. For example, for patients particularly disturbed with sleep onset

problems, a drug with a fast onset may be most effective and satisfactory. The patient must be informed about the rapid onset of the drug action because ingestion places the individual at risk for a fall or some other mishap if he or she does not retire immediately.

The half-life and active metabolites are also important with respect to the duration of action, pertaining both to efficacy in maintaining sleep and to the liability of experiencing side effects. The benzodiazepines are generally characterized as having short (5 h or less), intermediate (within a range of 6 to 24 h), or long (greater than 24 h) elimination half-lives. Based on this classification, triazolam is a short-acting compound, estazolam and temazepam are intermediate acting, and flurazepam and quazepam long-acting. Of course, active metabolites also contribute to the duration of action. Both quazepam and flurazepam, drugs classified as long-acting on the basis of the elimination half-lives of the parent

Table 7-4
Commonly Employed Drugs to Treat Insomnia

Medication	Brand name	Usual therapeutic dose (mg)	
		Adult	Elderly
Benzodiazepines			
Triazolam	Halcion	0.125–0.25	0.125
Estazolam	ProSom	1.0–2.0	0.5-1.0
Quazepam	Doral	7.5–15	7.5
Temazepam	Restoril	7.5–30	7.5–15
Flurazepam	Dalmane	7.5–30	7.5–15
Nonbenzodiazepines			
Zolpidem	Ambien	5.0–10	5.0
Antidepressant drugs (not an indication approved by the FDA)			
Amitriptyline	Elavil	10–100	10–50
Trazodone	Desyrel	50–150	25–100

compound, have active metabolites with considerably longer half-lives. As for flurazepam and quazepam, their long elimination half-lives and the presence of active metabolites with long half-lives raises the possibility that these drugs will accumulate with repeated administration.

Some general features have been identified that distinguish short-acting, as compared with long-acting, benzodiazepines when used in the treatment of insomnia. Thus, the short-acting compounds have a reduced liability for hangover, which includes daytime somnolence and impairment of psychomotor function or of memory and cognitive function. Moreover, short-acting agents have a minimal risk of accumulation with repeated administration. Limitations of the short-acting benzodiazepine hypnotics include lack of efficacy in controlling middle-of-the-night or early-morning awakenings, and some liability for the development of tolerance or rebound insomnia. The long-acting benzodiazepine hypnotics have greater efficacy in maintaining sleep throughout the night and convey some advantage in daytime anxiolytic effects. Moreover, the long-acting drugs are less likely to be associated with the development of tolerance or rebound insomnia. Potential drawbacks of long-acting benzodiazepines include an increased risk of daytime somnolence and impairment of memory, cognitive, and psychomotor function, and the potential for accumulation with repeated administration.

Benzodiazepines approved for use in the management of insomnia have all been examined extensively in prospective, controlled clinical trials, including studies employing PSG techniques (Parrino and Terzano, 1996). Patients with insomnia treated with a benzodiazepine in clinical trials generally report an improved quality of sleep, as reflected by shortened sleep latency, fewer awakenings during the night, and a sense that sleep is more restful and restorative. Adverse effects are related primarily to daytime somnolence, impairment of memory and cognitive or motor function, dizziness, and rebound insomnia. The likelihood that these side effects will occur appears to be highly correlated with the pharmacological profile of the benzodiazepine with respect to its half-life and the generation of active metabolites.

Using PSG techniques, benzodiazepines have been shown to shorten sleep latency and improve sleep continuity, including improved sleep efficiency, a reduced number of awakenings and arousals, and reduced time awake after sleep onset. Several changes in sleep physiology or sleep architecture have been reported following benzodiazepine administration. For example, the EEG profile of stage II sleep is altered, being characterized by a marked increase in sleep spindle activity. The clinical significance of this effect, if any, is not known. Chronic administration of a benzodiazepine is reported to suppress slow-wave sleep and REM sleep. It is unknown whether suppression of REM or slow wave sleep produces any deleterious consequences.

Rebound insomnia occurs with varying frequency upon abrupt termination of benzodiazepine therapy following chronic administration and has been convincingly demonstrated in studies using PSG techniques (Task Force Reports of the APA, 1996). Rebound insomnia is far more likely to ensue following discontinuation of a short-acting than a long-acting benzodiazepine. There is definite clinical significance to this response. Thus, a patient who is suffering from severe insomnia is likely to experience an improvement in symptoms when taking a benzodiazepine hypnotic. With continued use some degree of tolerance may develop, but overall improvement in the quality of sleep compared with the predrug state is likely to be maintained. If the patient decides to discontinue treatment suddenly, or inadvertently misses a dose, rebound insomnia may occur, particularly with the short-acting drugs. Although this precipitous alteration in sleep pattern represents a pharmacologically induced reaction, the patient often interprets this change as indicating that insomnia has returned, and, in fact, is quite severe in the absence of the medication. When the patient resumes taking the benzodiazepine, pronounced symptomatic improvement will occur almost immediately. Although this may largely represent the treatment of the withdrawal reaction, the patient may conclude there is the need to remain on medication to maintain satisfactory sleep. This series of events reinforces long-term use of hypnotics. Thus, in monitoring benzodiazepine therapy, it is important to educate the patient about the potential for rebound insomnia with a missed dose, to gradually taper the dose when discontinuing treatment after 3 to 4 weeks of continuous administration and, if possible, to encourage the development of more effective coping and adapting methods to deal with insomnia and minimize problems or discomfort if rebound insomnia should occur when the treatment regimen is terminated.

Patients must be warned about combining benzodiazepines with alcohol, as this combination has the potential to cause serious, if not lethal, complications, particularly with regard to respiratory function. Moreover, benzodiazepines must be used cautiously, if at all, in patients with obstructive sleep apnea, because these drugs may compromise further their respiratory function by suppressing the drive for respiration at the level of the brain stem and by enhancing muscle atonia during sleep, further accentuating the obstructive component. In addition, elderly patients are particularly prone to sleep disruptions during the night. If an elderly subject has taken a benzodiazepine hypnotic before retiring for the night and then awakens to use the bathroom, there is a risk the individual may be confused, suffer memory impairment, or become dizzy, increasing substantially the possibility of a fall. Additionally, elderly patients tend to take a number of different medications, enhancing the possibility of drug-drug interactions with the benzodiazepines. Drug classes that are particularly notable in this regard are the H_1 and H_2 histamine receptor antagonists and a number of the psychotropic agents. To cite one example, nefazodone, an antidepressant, which is metabolized through the CYPII D-4 hepatic microsomal enzyme system, has the potential to interact with the triazolobenzodiazepines, including triazolam, which are also metabolized by this enzyme.

The benzodiazepines act at a family of sites referred to as benzodiazepine receptors. The benzodiazepine receptor is a component of the γ-aminobutyric acid (GABA$_A$) receptor in brain. The benzodiazepine-GABA$_A$ macromolecular receptor complex contains binding sites for a number of neuroactive compounds, including ethanol, barbiturates, and the convulsant picrotoxin (Fig. 7-2). Activation of GABA$_A$ receptors increases the influx of Cl$^-$ ions, thereby hyperpolarizing the cell, which accounts for the inhibitory action of the amino acid neurotransmitter. Activation of the benzodiazepine site enhances the response to GABA, causing an even greater hyperpolarization of the neuron in the presence of a fixed amount of GABA. In the absence of GABA, or under conditions in which the GABA$_A$ receptor is inhibited, stimulation of a benzodiazepine receptor does not produce a physiological response, underscoring the importance of the interaction of these drugs with the GABA$_A$ receptor.

The benzodiazepine-GABA$_A$ receptor complex is composed of five distinct subunits. These can be arranged in different arrays, providing the molecular basis for a diverse population of benzodiazepine-GABA$_A$ receptors. From a pharmacological standpoint, several benzodiazepine receptor subtypes have been described. Thus, the benzodiazepine$_1$ receptor is highly localized in brain and is thought to mediate the anxiolytic and hypnotic effects of these drugs, whereas the benzodiazepine$_2$ receptor is concentrated in the spinal cord and is thought to be responsible for the muscle relaxant effects. The benzodiazepine$_3$ receptors, also referred to as the peripheral-type benzodiazepine site, are found in peripheral tissues and brain. Its role, if any, in mediating the psychotropic effects of these drugs is unknown.

Benzodiazepines produce a variety of behavioral effects in various animal species, including a dose-dependent sedation that led to their use as hypnotics. Benzodiazepines have been employed for a number of years as antianxiety agents, a use that was predicated on the basis of their anticonflict effects in animal models of stress. In addition, the benzodiazepines are anticonvulsants and skeletal muscle relaxants, and are used clinically for these purposes as well.

Nonbenzodiazepine hypnotics. Although some new hypnotics are considered nonbenzodiazepines, the response to these drugs is mediated by their attachment to a subtype of the benzodiazepine receptor. Thus, although these agents are nonbenzodiazepines in their chemical structure, their site of action is the same as the benzodiazepines. Nevertheless, the benzodiazepine and nonbenzodiazepine hypnotics are somewhat different in their mechanism of action. Thus, whereas benzodiazepines bind to virtually all the benzodiazepine receptors in brain, the nonbenzodiazepine hypnotics are highly selective for the benzodiazepine$_1$ receptor subtype. The potential physiological and clinical significance of this selectivity is supported by data showing that whereas benzodiazepines display comparable potencies in producing sleep and muscle relaxation, zolpidem, a nonbenzodiazepine hypnotic, is much more potent as a sedative than as a muscle relaxant. Moreover, the nonbenzodiazepines have a reduced side effect liability in comparison with the benzodiazepines. Because laboratory animal studies indicate that at high doses zolpidem does not retain its selectivity for sleep-inducing effects as compared with its muscle relaxant effects, its clinical selectivity will probably be most evident at low doses.

In clinical studies with nonbenzodiazepine hypnotics, including zolpidem, zaleplon (which is currently being studied in the United States), and zopiclone (which is available in Europe but not the United States), beneficial effects have been demonstrated in shortening sleep latency and, to a lesser extent, improving sleep continuity (Sanger et al., 1996). The nonbenzodiazepine hypnotics all display a rapid onset of action, short elimination half-lives (approximately 2.5 h for zolpidem), and no active metabolites. In contrast with the benzodiazepine hypnotics, zolpidem and zaleplon appear to exert minimal sup-

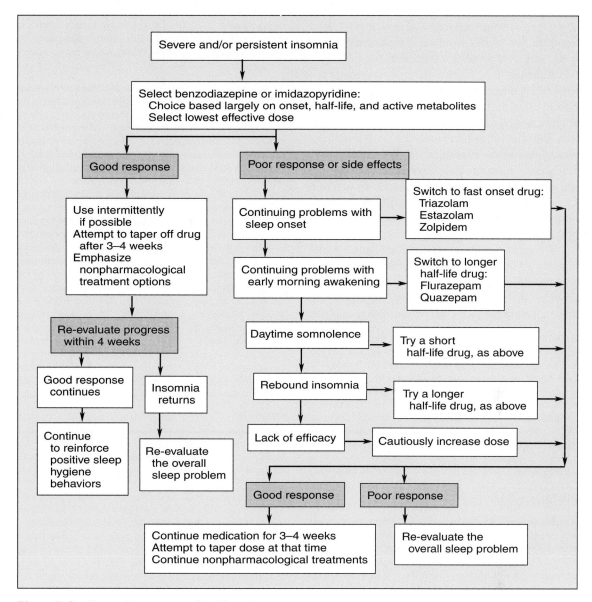

Figure 7–2. *Insomnia treatment algorithm.*

pressive effects on slow-wave and REM sleep, although there is some controversy on this matter.

Discontinuation of therapy with either zolpidem or zaleplon is associated with very little rebound insomnia (Sanger and Zivkovic, 1987). In one study patients with insomnia were treated for 4 weeks with either triazolam or zolpidem, after which all the subjects were given placebo (Monti et al., 1994). Patients who had received triazolam experienced significantly more rebound insomnia during the placebo phase than did those treated with zolpidem. If additional controlled studies demonstrate an advantage for the nonbenzodiazepine hypnotics in reducing rebound insomnia, this would represent a significant benefit in the management of this condition.

Although the nonbenzodiazepine hypnotics are particularly effective in inducing sleep, they are less effective than the benzodiazepines in sustaining sleep or preventing early-morning awakenings. In comparison with the benzodiazepines, the nonbenzodiazepine hypnotics have a reduced liability for hangover, attributable in part to their short duration of action, and are less likely to interact with alcohol or suppress respiration in patients with obstructive sleep apnea. Further studies are needed, however, to confirm these promising preliminary findings.

Shown in Fig. 7-2 is an algorithm listing guidelines for using hypnotics. Understanding the relevant pharmacological features of the various hypnotics provides the foundation necessary for employing these agents in the safest and most effective manner.

Barbiturates.   Some of the barbiturates, especially those in the intermediate- to longer-acting range, has secobarbital and amobarbital, have been used in the treatment of insomnia. As these drugs are quite sedating, they shorten sleep latency and improve sleep continuity. Most sleep specialists, however, advise that the barbiturates be employed only rarely for treating insomnia because of their highly unfavorable side effect profile. Significant disadvantages include a high probability for the development of tolerance and physical dependence, severe withdrawal reactions upon abrupt discontinuation of drug administration, significant potential for profound respiratory depression when taken with ethanol, and a serious risk of lethality in overdose.

Antihistamines.   Diphenhydramine and other antihistamines are commonly employed for treating insomnia. Indeed, many over-the-counter sleep aids contain an antihistamine as the main active ingredient. Inasmuch as a number of antihistamines are sedating, they may be of benefit in the treatment of insomnia and, indeed, in a limited number of clinical trials they displayed some efficacy in treating this condition. Tolerance to the hypnotic effects of antihistamines is quite common, however, and may develop within a few days. Moreover, there are significant side effects associated with their use including paradoxical agitation or excitement, and anticholingeric effects. These are particularly troubling for elderly patients, who frequently take other drugs with anticholingeric properties.

Antipsychotics.   A number of antipsychotics, such as chlorpromazine, have pronounced sedative effects. These sedating antipsychotics are often preferred for the management of patients who are actively psychotic, highly agitated, and experi-

encing patterns of disturbed sleep. Owing to their liability to produce serious side effects, such as tardive dyskinesia, the sedating antipsychotics are not recommended for the routine management of insomnia.

Tryptophan.   Tryptophan is an essential amino acid and the precursor of serotonin. Because serotonin is implicated in the regulation of sleep, including the initiation of sleep, interest has been expressed in the potential utility of tryptophan as an hypnotic. This interest intensified as a consequence of studies demonstrated that brain serotonin concentrations in laboratory animals are increased following the administration of large amounts of tryptophan. Thus, these studies suggested that the consumption of tryptophan could provide an effective strategy to increase the functional activity of brain serotonin systems and thereby produce a hypnotic response. In a limited number of clinical trials tryptophan was found to have modest efficacy in improving sleep in insomniacs, primarily by shortening sleep latency. Studies of this therapeutic option were precipitously interrupted in the United States several years ago following reports that administration of tryptophan may be associated with some serious side effects, including eosinophilia, myalgia, and, in rare instances, death. These adverse effects were subsequently traced to a contaminant in the tryptophan preparation and do not appear to have been due to any intrinsic effects of the amino acid itself. In the aftermath of this episode, the availability of tryptophan in the United States has diminished, although it may still be obtained in Europe where it is employed, to a limited extent, in the treatment of insomnia.

Melatonin.   Melatonin has received considerable attention in the lay press as a novel and effective treatment for insomnia. To date, only a limited number of controlled clinical studies have examined its efficacy and safety in this regard. Perhaps the most impressive study to date found that melatonin is effective in improving the sleep of elderly individuals with insomnia (Haimov et al., 1995). Because melatonin is available as a supplement and can be purchased in health food stores, individuals may choose to self-administer it without undergoing a proper evaluation to determine the cause of their insomnia. Caution must be employed in accepting efficacy claims for melatonin in the treatment of insomnia until more extensive and positive clinical data are forthcoming. Moreover, the fact that melatonin is available over the counter raises the possibility that some may be taking doses that exceed those used in controlled clinical trials.

Treatment of Chronic Insomnia

Although sleep specialists and expert panels consistently recommend that hypnotics be used only for a limited time, typically no more than 3 or 4 weeks, a subset of patients complains of insomnia on a chronic, long-term basis. These individuals may obtain some degree of relief upon initiation of a hypnotic. In many of these cases, return of insomnia occurs with discontinuation of therapy, even if adjunctive nonpharmacological treatments are instituted.

Thus, there is a real dilemma in treating such patients given the drawbacks of continued hypnotic therapy, which include a loss of efficacy over time and a possible alteration of sleep physiology that implies a worsening of the quality of sleep. Such concerns have been raised from studies with benzodiazepines; some patients develop tolerance to, and physical dependence on, these agents, and display rebound insomnia, and even distinct withdrawal reactions, upon termination of treatment.

Although there are a number of concerns associated with the long-term use of hypnotics, the clinician is frequently faced with the responsibility of caring for a patient who describes chronic problems with insomnia and experiences considerable emotional anguish and prominent difficulties in daily functioning as a consequence of impaired sleep. Moreover, persistent sleep problems may be associated with increased health risks. Therefore, careful clinical judgment must be exercised in determining the most advisable treatment plan for each patient. This is best practiced by being aware of the potential liabilities of the various hypnotics and by clearly informing the patient about potential risks and ways to avoid significant complications, such as being careful not to discontinue the drug abruptly or skip doses. There should also be continued encouragement of the use of nonpharmacological treatment options. Although limited data are available on the safety and efficacy of hypnotics following long-term use, some pertinent findings are emerging. In one study patients with insomnia were treated with zolpidem regularly for 360 days. In general, efficacy was maintained throughout the period and side effects, if present, were generally mild. As more data become available from long-term treatment, it will be easier to establish guidelines for the appropriate use of hypnotics in the treatment of chronic insomnia.

Treatment of Other Sleep Disorders

Disorders of excessive daytime somnolence. Symptoms of excessive daytime somnolence occur in patients with obstructive sleep apnea, narcolepsy, and idiopathic central nervous system hypersomnia, and in those experiencing disturbed sleep or limited sleep for any of a number of reasons.

Obstructive sleep apnea. Obstructive sleep apnea is a significant public health problem, but pharmacological approaches for its treatment are limited and not particularly effective. Several drugs have been proposed to be of value, including acetazolamide, nicotine, strychnine, medroxyprogesterone, and several antidepressants, particularly protriptyline; (Pack, 1994). Medroxyprogesterone was thought to be of benefit because of its stimulating effect on respiration. Antidepressants such as protriptyline are considered because of their potent REM suppressant effects because apneic events tend to be most prominent during REM sleep.

Unfortunately, clinical trials with these agents in obstructive sleep apnea have yielded disappointing results. To date, the most commonly employed treatment strategies for this condition include positional therapy, such as training the patient to avoid sleeping in the supine position; intraoral devices, including tongue retainers; surgical procedures, such as removal of the tonsils and adenoids, tracheostomy, uvulopalatopharyngoplasty, and nasal continuous positive airway pressure. This last modality probably represents the most widely employed, and most highly recommended, treatment for obstructive sleep apnea.

Basic research on the pathophysiology of sleep-disordered breathing has focused attention on the role of various neurotransmitters in the regulation of upper airway muscle activity. The demonstration that serotonin-containing neurons projecting from the caudal raphe area of the brain to upper airway motor neurons play an important role in regulating the activity of muscles supporting the upper airway raises the possibility that pharmacological agents with targeted effects on these serotonergic pathways may be of value in the treatment of this condition.

Narcolepsy. Narcolepsy is a disorder of excessive daytime somnolence associated with cataplexy and other characteristic symptoms. Treatment approaches for narcolepsy have involved the use of a central nervous system stimulant in combination with attempts to improve the quality of nighttime sleep, which is often impaired in the narcoleptic patient. Counseling should include recommendations for elective daytime naps and discussions about the advisability of driving and coping with work- or school-related responsibilities.

Stimulants used to treat this condition include dextroamphetamine, methylphenidate or pemoline, and an activating antidepressant, such as protriptyline or fluoxetine. Whereas the stimulants are of particular value in enhancing daytime alertness and diminishing excessive daytime somnolence or sleep attacks, they are of less consistent benefit in the management of cataplectic symptoms. Antidepressant drugs, on the other hand, control cataplexy but are of limited utility in treating the symptoms of excessive daytime somnolence.

Although stimulants offer considerable benefit in the treatment of narcolepsy and, in many cases, improve functioning and enhance the quality of life, they are associated with a number of significant limitations. Side effects associated with stimulants include cardiovascular responses, such as increases in pulse rate and blood pressure, insomnia, anxiety, agitation, restlessness, and, less commonly, psychiatric symptoms. In addition, chronic treatment with stimulants is associated with a risk for the development of tolerance and dependence, and can result in prominent withdrawal symptoms upon discontinuation of treatment. Efforts to limit the likelihood of tolerance sometimes involve tapering the dose of the stimulant at periodic intervals, such as every 2 to 3 months, in effect providing a drug holiday.

The range of problems associated with long-term administration of stimulants has enhanced interest in identifying alternative treatment options for narcolepsy. Modafinil is a novel agent currently available in some European countries and is, at the present time, under review in the United States. Controlled clinical trials conducted in this country and in Europe have demonstrated significant efficacy in reducing the symptoms of daytime sleepiness, although modafinil appears to have limited efficacy in controlling cataplexy. Therefore, modafinil may fill a niche in alleviating excessive sleepiness in narcoleptic patients who are not severely affected by cataplexy. Moreover, it is possible that combined therapy with

modafinil and another drug, such as protriptyline, that is effective for cataplexy will prove to be a common treatment strategy. Further clinical studies are needed, however, to establish the efficacy and safety of this type of combined treatment.

Modafinil appears to offer a significant advantage over stimulants in its side effect profile, with headaches and nausea being the most frequently reported events. Other notable advantages of modafinil over central nervous system stimulants include a reduced likelihood of cardiovascular effects and agitation, and a reduced liability for tolerance, dependance, and withdrawal (Touret et al., 1995).

The stimulants amphetamine and methylphenidate are believed to produce their effects by provoking the release of norepinephrine and dopamine in regions of the brain thought to be involved in maintaining arousal, the so-called wake-promoting centers (Simon et al., 1995). The enhancement of dopaminergic activity is also thought to explain the abuse potential of these drugs. In preclinical studies, modafinil was found to activate wake-promoting centers without producing significant effects on catecholamine neurotransmission, possibly explaining its lower abuse potential in comparison with stimulants. It should be noted that the primary mechanism of action for modafinil in promoting alertness remains unknown. In light of its clinical efficacy in reducing excessive daytime somnolence, there is considerable interest in identifying its mode of action.

Periodic limb movements during sleep. The prevalence of periodic limb movements during sleep disorder increases markedly with age, being relatively common in the elderly. This condition frequently occurs in conjunction with restless leg syndrome. Periodic limb movements can produce significant disruptions of sleep continuity and are associated with symptoms of insomnia, restlessness, disturbed sleep, and daytime sleepiness.

Several medications have been employed to treat periodic limb movements, with variable degrees of efficacy. Probably the most common strategy involves the use of a benzodiazepine, particularly a long-acting agent such as clonazepam. Clinical studies have yielded mixed results about the effectiveness of the benzodiazepines in reducing periodic limb movements, although clonazepam appears to reduce arousals and awakenings associated with this condition, improving subjective sleep quality and reducing daytime somnolence. Because daytime somnolence is a potential side effect of benzodiazepine therapy, however, patients with this condition must be monitored carefully when receiving a benzodiazepine to determine whether the benefits of therapy are offset by side effects.

Another pharmacological strategy employed in treating periodic limb movements involves the use of dopaminergic agents such as L-dopa or bromocriptine. Several studies have found that these drugs reduce periodic limb movements and ameliorate symptoms of restless leg syndrome. Potential problems with this approach include the development of rebound symptoms the day after drug administration, restlessness, agitation, and insomnia. Infrequently, patients on L-dopa develop psychotic symptoms.

Opioids are another treatment option for periodic limb movement during sleep disorder. These drugs have been reported to reduce periodic limb movements and provide relief from symptoms of restless leg syndrome. Because opioids are associated with a risk of abuse and addiction, however, they should be used with caution, being reserved only for those who fail to respond to benzodiazepines or L-dopa.

Sleep-related behaviors. A number of physiological and behavioral phenomena may occur episodically during sleep or be exacerbated by sleep. The term parasomnias refers to a group of non-rapid eye movement sleep-related behaviors including sleep walking (somnambulism) and sleep terrors. A REM sleep behavior disorder, as the name implies, refers to prominent behaviors, occasionally aggressive or violent, that arise during the REM phase and that are often linked to the content of a dream. Another differential diagnostic consideration for sleep-related behaviors is nocturnal seizures. The relationship of the sleep-related behaviors to seizure activity is usually not recognized until a PSG with a specially selected seizure montage is performed.

As is the case with most other sleep disorders, treatment of sleep-related behaviors is most effective when a specific diagnosis is made based on an underlying etiology. When the presence of nocturnal seizures is established, the therapy should be the most effective drug regimen for the identified form of epilepsy. In the case of REM sleep behavior disorder, clonazepam is quite efficacious. It is often necessary to evaluate patients with REM sleep behavior disorder for the presence of a midbrain or brain-stem lesion. When such a lesion is identified, treatment is focused on the proper management of the lesion. As for the parasomnias, medication generally is of limited value. Typically, counseling and behavior modification techniques are the most effective treatments.

Circadian rhythm sleep disorders. Included within the group of circadian rhythm sleep disorders are endogenous rhythm disorders, such as advanced and delayed sleep phase syndromes, irregular (non-24-h) sleep-wake pattern, and sleep difficulties related to disruption in sleep-wake schedule secondary to shift-work or travel across time zones.

Treatment of these sleep disorders has frequently emphasized counseling and behavioral adaptation strategies to optimize the capacity to cope with an irregular sleep schedule. Phototherapy has also been employed to deal with circadian rhythm sleep disorders. Light exposure is applied at selected times in the 24-h cycle in an attempt to alter rhythms in a desired direction. For example, light therapy applied at dusk is predicted to delay endogenous rhythms, whereas dawn light exposure should produce a phase advance. The effects of light exposure on endogenous circadian rhythms is thought to be mediated through alterations in melatonin secretion, with prominent phase-shifting effects of light exposure on melatonin secretion patterns having been demonstrated.

From a pharmacological standpoint, melatonin administration to alleviate circadian rhythm sleep disturbances represents a promising new strategy, although further studies are needed to establish its effectiveness. Melatonin has been shown to produce phase-shifting effects in both laboratory animal studies and clinical trials. Several preliminary reports have described beneficial effects of melatonin on subjects with sleep problems related to shift-work schedule or jet lag (Quera-Salva et al., 1996; Folkard et al., 1983). It should be noted that melatonin is reported to produce both phase-altering and direct hypnotic effects. How to optimize the balance between circadian and hypnotic effects is an issue that needs to be satisfactorily addressed. Chemical analogues of melatonin are also being evaluated in this regard because it is possible such a compound may offer some advantages with regard to selectivity, time course, safety, and side effects.

OTHER TREATMENTS

In perhaps 50% of patients with insomnia it is not possible to identify a reason for the sleep disorder, even after exhaustive evaluation. With such cases it is necessary to undertake a treatment plan for idiopathic insomnia, both to provide some symptomatic relief and to break a potentially escalating cycle of sleep disturbance. Most sleep specialists agree that hypnotic medications should be used cautiously and judiciously in the vast majority of cases. Recently, a number of treatments have been developed to serve either as an alternative, or a complement, to a medication regimen for insomnia (Winokur, 1997). Some of these are described in the following.

1. Sleep Hygiene Guidelines. Reviewing with the patient some of the basic elements of proper sleep hygiene can often encourage behavioral changes that may favorably effect sleep patterns. Discussion of sleep hygiene practices may often be conducted in the context of encouraging the patient to keep a detailed sleep diary for a period of time, after which the information is reviewed.

2. Stimulus Control. This involves behavior modification strategies designed to help reduce the likelihood of insomnia and provide the patient with simple coping methods to reduce the severity and frustration of episodes of insomnia. Examples of stimulus control include going to bed only when sleepy, getting out of bed and going to another room for a while if sleep does not ensue within a reasonable period of time, and avoiding napping during the day.

3. Relaxation Techniques. A variety of methods, including biofeedback, meditation, and deep muscle relaxation techniques, have elements in common for fostering a sense of relaxation in the face of potentially increased arousal levels. Learning an approach to relax more effectively and reliably may translate into an increased ability to relax and drift off to sleep at bedtime.

4. Cognitive Therapy. Although cognitive therapy techniques were initially developed for the treatment of depression, they have proved to be of considerable value for some patients with sleep disorders. Most patients with insomnia develop some exaggerated and negative thought about the meaning of their sleep problem that contributes to the perpetuation of insomnia. Aiding such patients in identifying their negative thoughts related to insomnia and in dealing with them more effectively can often be of substantial therapeutic benefit.

5. Sleep Restriction Therapy. A recently developed approach for the treatment of insomnia involves having the patient spend a selected, minimal time in bed at night, such as only from 1 A.M. to 6 A.M. Upon arising, the patient is to avoid any napping activity and continue going to bed only at 1 A.M., regardless of the amount of sleep achieved on the previous night. With this approach some degree of sleep debt will accumulate, presumably causing the patient to sleep more soundly and efficiently in the designated period. Once a constant pattern of sleep is achieved in the severely restricted period, the interval allowed for sleep is gradually extended. This approach, although grueling for the patient, is often quite effective.

6. Psychotherapy. For some individuals, insomnia occurs in the context of significant psychosocial stressors or personality problems. In such cases, referral for psychotherapy may represent an important component of the treatment strategy. The inability to identify and deal effectively with underlying stresses and psychological problems is likely to make the patient susceptible to repeated patterns of sleep difficulties.

It is useful for a physician to be familiar with the range of nonpharmacological treatments for the management of insomnia. There are a number of health and self-help books that provide considerable information about these techniques. In some cases it may be most appropriate to refer the patient to a therapist or sleep disorder specialist well versed in nonpharmacological strategies to treat the sleep disturbance in a more intensive manner.

For additional information on the drugs discussed in this chapter see chapters 10, 11, 17, 18, and 19 in *Goodman & Gilman's The Pharmacological Basis of Therapeutics* (Ninth Edition), McGraw-Hill, New York, 1996.

REFERENCES

Armitage R, Yonkers H, Cole D, Rush AJ: A multicenter, double-blind comparison of the effects of nefazodone and fluoxetine on sleep architecture and quality of sleep in depressed patients. *J Clin Psychopharm* 1997;17:161–168.

Benzodiazepine Dependence, Toxicity, and Abuse. A Task Force Report of the American Psychiatric Association, Washington, D.C., 1990.

Briones B, Adams N, Strauss M, et al: Relationship between sleepiness and general health status. *Sleep* 1996;19:583–588.

Buysse DJ, Frank E, Lowe KK, et al: Electroencephalographic sleep correlates of episode and vulnerability to recurrence in depression. *Biol Psych* 1997;41:406–418.

Czeisler CA, Richardson GS: Detection and assessment of insomnia. *Clin Therap* 1991;13:663–678.

Dinges DF: An overview of sleepiness and accidents. *J Sleep Res* 1995;4:4–14.

Folkard S, Arendt J, Clark M: Can melatonin improve shift workers' tolerance of the night shift? Some preliminary findings. *Chronobiol Int* 1983;10:315–320.

Gillin JC, Byerley WF: The diagnosis and management of insomnia. *N Eng J Med* 1990;322: 239–248.

Guilleminault C: *Sleeping and Waking Disorders: Indications and Techniques*. Boston, Butterworths, 1982.

Haimov I, Lavie P, Landon M, et al: Melatonin replacement therapy of elderly insomniacs. *Sleep* 1995;18:598–603.

Halaris A: *Chronobiology and Psychiatric Disorders*. New York, Elsevier, 1987.

Kribbs NB, Dinges DF: Vigilence decrement and sleepiness, in Harsh JR, Ogilvie RD (eds): *Sleep Onset Mechanisms*. Washington, D.C., American Psychological Association, 1994, pp 113–125.

Kupfer DJ, Reynolds III CF: Management of insomnia. *N Eng J Med* 1997;336:341–346.

Lader M, Lugarosi E, Richardson RG: The benzodiazepines and insomnia. *Clin Neuropharm* 1985;8:S1–S125.

Langtry HD, Benfield P: Zolpidem: A review of its pharmacodynamic and pharmacokinetic properties and therapeutic potential. *Drugs* 1990; 40:291–313.

Leger D: The cost of sleep-related accidents: A report for the National Commission on Sleep Disorders Research. *Sleep* 1994;17:84–93.

Mellinger GD, Balter MB, Uhlenhuth EH: Insomnia and its treatment prevalence and correlates. *Arch Gen Psych* 1985;42:225–232.

Minors DS, Waterhouse JM: *Circadian Rhythms and the Human*. Bristol, Wright PSG, 1981.

Monti JM, Attali P, Monti D, et al: Zolpidem and rebound insomnia-a double-blind, controlled polysomnographic study in chronic insomniac patients. *Pharmacopsych* 1994;27:166–175.

Pack AI: Obstructive sleep apnea. *Adv Intern Med* 1994;39:517–567.

Parrino L, Terzano MG: Polysomnographic effects of hypnotic drugs: A review. *Psychopharm* 1996;126:1–16.

Quera-Salva M, Defrance R, Claustrat B, et al: Rapid shift in sleep time and acrophase of melatonin secretion in short shift work schedule. *Sleep* 1996;19:539–543.

Richelson E: Synpatic effects of antidepressants. *J Clin Psychopharm* 1996;16:15–95.

Sanger DJ, Morel E, Ferrault G: Comparison of the pharmacological profiles of the hypnotic drugs zaleplon and zolpidem. *Eur J Pharm* 1996;313:35–42.

Sanger DJ, Zivkovic B: Investigation of the development of tolerance to the actions of zolpidem and midazolam. *Neuropharm* 1987;26:1513–1518.

Simon P, Hemet C, Ramassamy C, Costentin J: Non-amphetamine mechanism of stimulant locomotor effect of modafinil in mice. *Eur Neuropsychopharm* 1995;5:509–514.

Sleep in America. Conducted for the National Sleep Foundation. Prepared by: The Gallup Organization, 100 Palmer Square, Princeton, NJ, 08542, 1991.

Sleep in America. Conducted for the National Sleep Foundation. Prepared by: The Gallup Organization, 100 Palmer Square, Princeton, NJ 08542, 1995.

Stahl SM: *Essential Psychopharmacology*. Cambridge, England, Cambridge University Press, 1996.

Stoller MK: Economic effects of insomnia. *Clin Therap* 1994;16:873–897.

Strollo RJ, Rogers RM: Obstructive sleep apnea. *N Eng J Med* 1996;334:99–104.

Task Force Reports of the APA, 1996.

Touret M, Sallanon-Moulin M, Jouvet M: Awakening properties of modafinil without paradoxical sleep rebound: Comparative study with amphetamine in the rat. *Neurosci Lett* 1995;189:43–46.

Winokur A: Insomnia, in Rakel RE (ed): *Conn's Current Therapy*. Philadelphia, Saunders, 1997, pp 37–40.

Winokur A, Reynolds III CF: The effects of antidepressants on sleep physiology. *Primary Psych* 1994;1:22–27.

Young T, Palta M, Dempsey J, et al: The occurrence of sleep-disorderd breathing among middle-aged adults. *N Eng J Med* 1993;328:1271–1273.

ADDICTION AND SUBSTANCE ABUSE

Charles P. O'Brien

Addiction is a chronic, relapsing disorder that develops when certain drugs are taken in excess. The major addicting drugs are nicotine, alcohol, opioids, and stimulants such as cocaine. The transition from use to abuse to addiction depends on a range of variables: the susceptibility of the individual, the potency of the drug, and the enabling factors in the environment. The pharmacological aspects of addictive disorders are determined by the specific drugs chosen by the abuser. For example, opioid dependence is pharmacologically different from dependence on cocaine, alcohol, or nicotine. There are, however, features common to all addictive disorders, including loss of control of drug-taking and proneness to relapse even long after the last dose of the drug. Long-term, behaviorally-based treatment is necessary for addictive disorders. The results of treatment can be improved by specific medications that ease the symptoms of withdrawal and help to prevent relapse. When viewed as a chronic relapsing disorder, the goals of treatment are to improve the quality of life, reduce symptoms, and induce longer and longer periods of abstinence or at least periods of little drug use. From this perspective the results of treatment for addictive disorders are approximately in the range of the results achieved by medical treatments for other chronic disorders.

CLINICAL FEATURES

Addiction is a complex biopsychosocial problem that is largely misunderstood by the general public and much of the medical profession. The essential feature of this disorder is compulsive drug-taking behavior. Addiction (also called substance dependence) is diagnosed by applying behavioral criteria established by the American Psychiatric Association (Table 8-1). Intended to apply to all drugs of abuse, these criteria include potential behavioral symptoms related to drug taking and specify that three or more of these symptoms are required for the diagnosis of dependence. The behavioral symptoms consist of evidence of the intrusion of drug-taking behavior into normal activities. Although the presence of tolerance and withdrawal may be counted toward the diagnosis, they are not sufficient by themselves. Tolerance re-

fers to a need for markedly increased amounts of the substance to achieve the desired drug effect or a markedly diminished effect with continued use of the same amount of the substance. Withdrawal refers to a rebound of physiological effects that appear when, after regular use for a time that varies with the drug and the dose, the drug is abruptly discontinued. A withdrawal syndrome consists of symptoms that are generally the opposite of those produced by the drug. Substance abuse is essentially a less severe form of problematic drug taking and requires only one or two of the listed symptoms. If either tolerance or withdrawal is present along with behavioral symptoms, the diagnosis is advanced to the dependence category.

Confusion about these concepts exists for two reasons: First, it is commonly believed that tolerance and withdrawal are synonymous with addiction. In

Table 8-1

DSM-IV Diagnostic Criteria: Dependence

Pattern of substance use leading to clinically significant impairment or distress, as manifested by three (or more) of the following, occurring at any time in the same 12-month period:

1. Tolerance.
2. Withdrawal.
3. The substance is often taken in larger amounts or over a longer period than was intended.
4. There is a persistent desire or unsuccessful efforts to reduce or control substance use.
5. A great deal of time is spent in activities necessary to obtain the substance (e.g., visiting multiple doctors or driving long distances), use the substance (e.g., chain-smoking), or recover from its effects.
6. Important social, occupational, or recreational activities are abandoned or reduced because of substance use.
7. The substance use is continued despite knowledge of having a persistent or recurrent physical or psychological problem that is likely to have been caused or exacerbated by the substance (e.g., current cocaine use despite recognition of cocaine-induced depression, or continued drinking despite recognition that an ulcer was made worse by alcohol consumption).

reality, addiction is a behavior disorder that may or may not include tolerance and withdrawal. Prescribed medications for pain, anxiety, and even hypertension commonly produce tolerance and withdrawal symptoms on cessation. These are normal physiological adaptations to repeated use of many different kinds of medications. This distinction is important because patients with severe pain are sometimes deprived of adequate opioid medication simply because they show evidence of tolerance and exhibit withdrawal symptoms if the medication is abruptly stopped. In reality, patients given opioids for pain rarely develop the behavioral symptoms that would qualify them for a

diagnosis of addiction (dependence in DSM-IV). The term physical dependence is often applied to this nonaddiction situation, and must be distinguished from substance dependence as defined in DSM-IV, which is actually addiction.

A second reason for confusion is that drug-seeking behavior is usually not the only problem that requires treatment when a substance abuser seeks help. In most cases, there are important medical, psychiatric, social, occupational, and legal problems that may even overshadow the drug-taking behavior. Thus, addiction treatment programs must provide multimodality treatment. The prognosis of treatment may be less dependent on the quantity, frequency, or duration of drug use than on the coexisting problems, particularly psychiatric problems. The addiction treatment algorithm (Fig. 8-1) requires a full evaluation and treatment of any coexisting disorders.

ETIOLOGY OF ADDICTIVE DISORDERS

If drug abusers are asked why they take drugs, most will answer that they want to "get high," which generally refers to a kind of altered state of consciousness described as pleasurable or even euphoria. The type of high varies significantly across categories of drugs. Some abusers report they take the drug to relax, relieve tension, or relieve depression. A very small percentage will say that chronic headaches, backaches, or other types of pain was the original reason for taking analgesic drugs and then losing control. As each case is investigated more carefully, however, it is found to be far too complicated for any simple answer. In almost all cases, no single cause of addiction can be identified. As shown in Table 8-2, there are many variables that operate simultaneously to influence the likelihood of any given person becoming a drug abuser or addict. These variables can be organized into three categories: agent (drug), host (user), and environment. This is similar to the way in which the factors that determine who will contract an infectious disease are organized.

Agent (Drug) Variables

Drugs vary in their ability to produce immediate good feelings in the user. Those drugs that reliably produce intensely pleas-

Table 8-2

Multiple Simultaneous Variables Affecting Onset and Continuation of Drug Abuse and Addiction

Agent (Drug)

Availability
Cost
Purity and potency
Mode of administration
  Chewing (absorption via oral mucous membranes)
  Gastrointestinal
  Intranasal
  Intravenous (subcutaneous and intramuscular)
  Inhalation
  Speed of onset and offset of effects (pharmacokinetics: combination of agent and host)

Host (User)

Heredity
  Innate tolerance
  Speed of developing acquired tolerance
  Likelihood of experiencing intoxication as pleasure
Psychiatric symptoms
Prior experiences and expectations
Propensity for risk-taking behavior

Environment

Social setting
Community attitudes
  Peer influence, role models
Availability of other reinforcers (sources of pleasure or recreation)
Employment or educational opportunities
Conditioned stimuli: Environmental cues become associated with drugs after repeated use in the same environment.

measured in animals equipped with intravenous catheters connected to electric pumps that the animal can operate by a lever. Generally, animals such as rats and monkeys will work to obtain injections of the same drugs that humans tend to use excessively and in roughly the same order of potency. Thus medications can be screened for their abuse potential in humans by the use of animal models.

Reinforcing properties of drugs are associated with their ability to increase levels of the neurotransmitter dopamine in critical brain areas, particularly the nucleus accumbens (NAc). Cocaine, amphetamine, ethanol, opioids, and nicotine all reliably increase extracellular fluid dopamine levels in the NAc region. This can be measured in rats using brain microdialysis to obtain extracellular fluid while animals are freely moving or receiving drugs. Similar increases in dopamine in this brain structure are also observed when the rat is presented with sweet foods or an opportunity for coital activity. In contrast, drugs that block dopamine receptors generally produce unpleasant feelings (i.e., dysphoric effects). Neither animals nor humans spontaneously self-administer such drugs. While a causal relationship between dopamine and euphoria or dysphoria has not been established, the data are reasonably consistent for drugs of different classes.

Drugs with rapid onset of action tend to have greater abuse liability. Effects that occur soon after administration are more likely to initiate the chain of events that lead to loss of control over drug taking. The time that it takes the drug to reach critical receptor sites in the brain and the concentrations achieved can be influenced by the route of administration, rate of absorption, metabolism, and passage across the blood-brain barrier. The history of cocaine illustrates the changes in abuse liability of the same compound, depending on the chemical state and the route of administration. Use of this drug originated with the chewing of coca leaves, which causes cocaine in the alkaloidal state to be absorbed slowly into the circulation through the buccal mucosa. This results in low levels of cocaine gradually appearing in the brain. The mild stimulant effect produced by the chewing of coca leaves thus has a gradual onset; this practice has produced little, if any, abuse or dependence despite thousands of years of practice by natives of the Andes. In the late nineteenth century, chemists extracted cocaine from coca leaves, thus making pure cocaine available. Cocaine could be taken in higher doses by oral ingestion (gastrointestinal absorption) or by absorption through the nasal mucosa, yielding higher cocaine levels in the brain and a more rapid onset of action. Subsequently, it was found that a solution of cocaine hydrochloride could be injected intravenously, causing a very rapid onset of effects. With each "advance" in cocaine administration, there was an increment in blood level and speed of onset, and the drug became more likely to be abused. The advancements continued in the 1980s when crack cocaine was developed. Crack, which can be sold at a very low price on the street ($1 to $3 per dose), is alkaloidal cocaine (freebase) that can be readily vaporized by heating. Simply inhaling the vapors produces blood levels comparable to intravenous cocaine. The pulmo-

ant feelings (euphoria) are more likely to be taken repeatedly. Reinforcement refers to the ability of drugs to produce effects that make the user wish to take them again. The more strongly reinforcing a drug is, the greater the likelihood that the drug will be abused. Reinforcing properties of a drug can be reliably

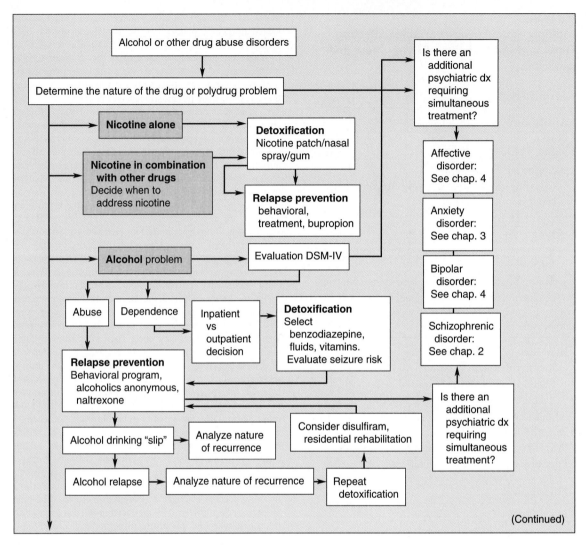

Figure 8–1. *Addiction treatment algorithm.*

nary route is highly effective because the lungs provide a large surface area for absorption into the pulmonary circulation. The cocaine-rich blood is returned to the left side of the heart where it is ejected into the arterial circulation without dilution by the systemic circulation. Thus arterial blood reaches a higher concentration than venous blood. This method rapidly delivers the drug to the brain and is also the preferred route for users of nicotine and cannabis. Inhalation of crack cocaine is therefore much more likely to produce addiction than chewing, drinking, or sniffing cocaine.

Although the characteristics of the drug are important, they do not completely explain the development of abuse and

addiction. Most of those who try abusable drugs do not become repetitive or compulsive users. Even experimentation with drugs that have a strong rewarding effect such as cocaine results in addiction in only a minority of cases (Table 8-2). The development of addiction, therefore, is also determined by two other class factors: host (user) and environment.

Host (User) Variables

In general, the effects of all drugs vary among individuals. Blood levels, for example, show wide variation when the same dose of a drug is administered to different people. This

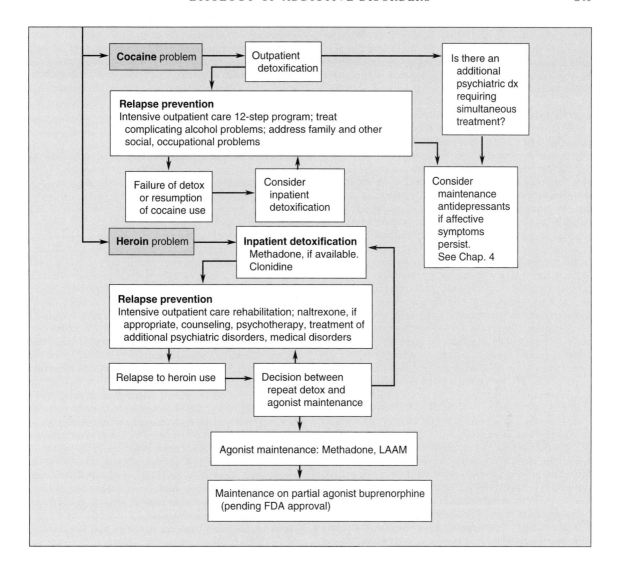

variation is due, in part, to genetically determined differences in absorption, metabolism, excretion, and receptor sensitivity. One of the results of these differences is that the subjective effects of a drug vary among individuals. In human subjects the separation of heredity from environmental influence is always very difficult. One line of research has followed individuals adopted at birth and raised in foster homes without contact with their biological parents (Schuckit, 1992). The biological children of alcoholics show an increased likelihood of developing alcoholism even when adopted at birth by nonalcoholic parents. The studies of genetic influences in this disorder show only an increased risk for developing alcoholism,

not a 100% determinism; this finding is consistent with a polygenic disorder that has multiple determinants. Even identical twins, who share the same genetic endowment, do not have 100% concordance when one twin is alcoholic. The concordance rate for identical twins, however, is significantly higher than that for fraternal twins. One biological trait that may influence the development of alcoholism (alcohol addiction) is innate tolerance to alcohol. Recent data (Schuckit et al., 1994) show that sons of alcoholics have reduced sensitivity to alcohol when compared with other young men of the same age (22) and drinking histories. Sensitivity was measured by studying the effects of two different doses of alcohol on motor performance and subjective feelings of intoxication. When the men were reexamined 10 years later, those who had been most tolerant (insensitive) to alcohol at age 22 were found to be most likely diagnosed as alcohol dependent. Although the presence of tolerance predicted the development of alcoholism even in the group without a family history of alcoholism, there were far fewer tolerant men in the negative family history group. Of course, having an innate tolerance to alcohol does not make a person an alcoholic, but it seems to increase significantly the probability for the disorder.

Studies suggest the opposite influence, a kind of "antialcoholism," can also be inherited. Ethanol is metabolized to acetaldehyde by alcohol dehydrogenase, which is then metabolized by a mitochondrial aldehyde dehydrogenase known as ALDH2. A common mutation occurs in the gene for ALDH2 resulting in a less effective enzyme. This allele has a high frequency of occurrence in Asian populations and results in an excess production of acetaldehyde, a noxious product of alcohol. The drinker with this allele experiences a very unpleasant facial flushing reaction 5 to 10 min after ingesting alcohol. The probability of becoming alcohol dependent is, therefore, reduced in people with this heredity, but the risk is not eliminated. Those who are strongly motivated to drink can endure the flushing to achieve the other effects of alcohol and thus become alcoholic. There are probably multiple genetic factors that can influence the probability of becoming alcohol dependent, but no single factor is determinant. Those who inherit a tolerance to alcohol, thereby having an increased probability of becoming alcoholic, may decide to remain abstinent; conversely, those who inherit the flushing reaction may continue to drink excessively.

Psychiatric disorders are another category of host variables, since drugs may produce immediate subjective effects that relieve preexisting mental symptoms. People with anxiety, depression, insomnia, or even subtle symptoms such as shyness may find, on experimentation or by accident, that certain drugs give them relief. The apparent beneficial effects are, however, transient. With repeated use of the drug, the person may develop tolerance and eventually compulsive, uncontrolled drug use. The process of self-medication is believed to be one mechanism whereby drug users become ensnared. The proportion of addicts who begin by the failed self-medication mechanism is unclear. Although psychiatric symptoms are commonly seen in drug abusers presenting for treatment, many of these symptoms begin after the person begins abusing drugs. Thus, drugs of abuse may produce more psychiatric symptoms than they relieve.

Environmental Variables

Initiating and continuing illicit drug use appear to be significantly influenced by societal norms and peer pressure. Taking drugs may be seen initially as a form of rebellion against authority. In some communities, drug users and drug dealers are role models who seem to be successful and respected; thus they are emulated by young people. There may also be a paucity of other options for pleasure or diversion. These factors are particularly important in communities where educational levels are low and job opportunities are scarce. Of course, these environmental factors do not operate alone. They interact with the agent and host variables described in the foregoing.

Pharmacological Phenomena

Although abuse and addiction are extremely complicated conditions involving many variables, there are a number of relevant pharmacological phenomena that occur independent of social and psychological dimensions. The first of these involves the changes in the way the body responds to a drug with repeated use. Tolerance is the most common response to repetitive use of the same drug. Tolerance can be defined as the reduction in response to the drug after repeated administrations. If a sensitive measurement of drug effects is used, tolerance to some effects begins with the first dose. Thus the second dose, even days later, produces a slightly smaller effect. With continued dose increases, enormous tolerance can be observed with certain drugs. Diazepam, for example, typically produces sedation at doses of 5 to 10 mg in a first-time user, but those who repeatedly use it to produce a kind of "high" may become tolerant to doses of several hundreds of milligrams and some abusers have had documented tolerance to more than 1000 mg per day.

Some drug effects provoke tolerance much more rapidly than other effects of the same drug. For example, tolerance develops rapidly to the euphoria produced by opioids such as heroin, and addicts tend to increase their dose to reexperience that elusive "high." In contrast, tolerance to the effects of opioids on the intestinal system (blocking smooth muscle contractions, constipation) develops more slowly. The discrepancy between tolerance to euphorigenic effects and tolerance to effects on vital functions such as respiration and blood pressure can lead to potentially fatal accidents in sedative abusers. Often these users are teenagers who take sedative drugs such as barbiturates or methaqualone. With repeated use, they require a larger and larger dose to obtain the groggy, drowsy state reported as high for this category of drugs. Unfortunately, tolerance to the effects of sedatives on vital brainstem functions develops much more slowly than tolerance for the high. This means that the therapeutic index (ratio of dose for toxic effects to dose for desired effects) decreases. Because the previous dose no longer produces a high experience, these young people may further increase the dose, which reduces the margin of safety. The next dose increment may be the dose that suppresses vital functions. When this happens, even an experienced user may suddenly lose blood pressure and respiratory functions while experiencing a potentially lethal overdose.

"Medical addict."   This is a term used to describe a patient in treatment for a medical disorder who has become "addicted" because he or she begins taking available prescribed drugs in excessive doses. This situation is rare in comparison to the large number of patients who receive medications capable of producing tolerance and physical dependence. An example would be a patient with chronic pain who begins using the prescribed medication more often than directed by the physician. If the physician restricts the prescriptions, the patient may begin seeing several doctors without the knowledge of the primary physician. Such patients may also visit emergency departments for the purpose of obtaining additional medication. Fear of producing such medical addicts results in needless suffering among patients with pain as physicians limit medications to avoid "creating an addict." Tolerance and physical dependence are inevitable consequences of chronic treatment with opioids and certain other drugs, but tolerance and physical dependence by themselves do not constitute addiction.

Addiction As a Brain Disorder

Repeated exposure to addicting drugs produces lasting changes in behavior as manifested by involuntary conditioned responses observed in addicts long after their last dose of the addicting drug (O'Brien et al., 1992). These conditioned responses or drug-related memories may play a role in relapse to compulsive drug taking. Wikler (1973) was the first to call attention to the role of conditioning in addictive disorders. More recently the neurochemical changes involved in the long-term changes produced by addicting drugs have been studied in animal models (Kalivas and Duffy, 1990) and at the level of gene transcription (Nestler and Aghajanian, 1997). The results of this improvement in understanding the nature of addiction is opening up new opportunities for treatment using medications (O'Brien, 1997) and approaches similar to those used for other chronic disorders.

THE COSTS
OF SUBSTANCE ABUSE

The four substances that currently produce the most important clinical problems in the United States are nicotine, ethyl alcohol, cocaine, and heroin. Nicotine derived from tobacco smoking has been linked to 450,000 deaths per year in the United States alone. Evidence is also accumulating to show that up to 50,000 nonsmokers die each year because of passive exposure to tobacco smoke. Thus nicotine is the most serious health problem. Alcohol costs society about $100 billion per year and about 100,000 lives including about 25,000 deaths on the highways. Illegal drugs such as heroin and cocaine, though linked to AIDS infection and crime, still cause far fewer deaths, in the range of 20,000 per year. The monetary and social costs of illegal drugs, however, are high. The government spends about $140 billion each year on the "War on Drugs," about 70% of which is spent on various types of law enforcement (i.e., supply reduction).

In this chapter, the major categories of drugs are discussed separately. Abusers frequently have favorites among these categories, but availability plays a large role in the selection of drug of abuse. Combinations across categories are very common. Alcohol is such a widely available drug that it is combined with practically all other categories. Some combinations are reportedly taken because of their interactive effects. An example is the combination of heroin and cocaine ("speedball") that is described in the opioid category. When confronted with a patient exhibiting signs of overdose or withdrawal, the physician must be aware of these possible combinations because each drug may require specific treatment. About 80% of alcoholics are also cigarette smokers, and probably an even larger proportion of heroin addicts smoke tobacco cigarettes. Thus there is usually a dual addiction to treat. The clinician must deal with the most urgent problem, which is generally the alcohol, heroin, or cocaine problem. During the course of treatment, however, there may be an appropriate time to address the nicotine problem. It is not fair to patients to simply ignore a serious dependence on nicotine just because the primary problem appears to be alcohol or illegal drugs.

ADDICTION SYNDROMES

Nicotine Dependence

Clinical description. The question of nicotine as the addicting component of cigarette smoking has been in the news throughout this decade. Evidence, both clinical and experimental, has accumulated demonstrating that nicotine meets all the criteria for an addicting substance. Although it is still being contested in court, the U.S. Food and Drug Administration (FDA) has acquired the authority to regulate nicotine as a drug partly in recognition of its addicting potential.

Nicotine has complex effects that result in its being self-administered by animals and humans. It is arguably the most important dependence-producing drug because the dependence is sustained by the smoking of cigarettes, the most common cause of preventable death and disease in the United States. The dependence produced by nicotine can be extremely durable as exemplified by the high failure rate among smokers who try to quit. Although over 80% of smokers express a desire to quit, only 35% try to stop each year and less than 5% are successful in unaided attempts to quit (APA, DSM-IV, 1994). Nicotine dependence (addiction) is a variable syndrome with some heavy smokers able to stop quickly, whereas others, despite dreadful symptoms such as emphysema with air hunger, continue compulsive smoking.

As with other addictions, nicotine addiction is influenced by multiple variables with no simple explanation that covers all cases. Nicotine itself produces positive reinforcement or reward. Users compare it to stimulants such as cocaine or amphetamine, though it is much less potent. In contrast, the majority of alcoholics and heroin addicts who also smoke report more difficulty giving up smoking than their other addiction. Whereas there are many casual users of alcohol and cocaine, the vast majority of nicotine addicts smoke regularly, and fewer than 10% smoke a small enough quantity of cigarettes (five or fewer per day) to avoid dependence.

Nicotine is readily absorbed through the skin, mucous membranes, and lungs. The pulmonary route produces discernible central nervous system effects in as little as 7 s. Thus each puff produces some discrete reinforcement. With 10 puffs per cigarette, the one-pack-per-day smoker reinforces the habit 200 times daily. The timing, setting, situation, and preparation of smoking all become associated repetitively with the effects of nicotine.

Nicotine has both stimulant and depressant-like actions. The smoker feels alert, yet there is some muscle relaxation. Nicotine activates the ventral tegmental area (VTA) to nucleus accumbens reward system in the brain; increased extracellular dopamine has been found in the NAc after nicotine injections in rats. Nicotine affects other systems as well, including endogenous opioids and glucocorticoids.

There is evidence for tolerance to the subjective effects of nicotine. Smokers typically report that the first cigarette of the day after a night of abstinence is most refreshing. Smokers who return to cigarettes after a period of abstinence lose tolerance because they may experience nausea if they return immediately to their previous dose. Persons naive to the effects of nicotine experience nausea at low nicotine blood levels, while smokers report nausea if nicotine levels are raised above their accustomed levels.

Negative reinforcement refers to the benefits obtained from the termination of an unpleasant state. In dependent smokers, there is evidence that some are smoking to avoid withdrawal symptoms because the urge to smoke occurs when nicotine levels drop. Some smokers even wake up during the night to have a cigarette, presumably to ameliorate the withdrawal symptoms brought on by low nicotine blood levels that have disrupted sleep. If the nicotine level is maintained artificially by a slow intravenous infusion, there is a decrease in the number of cigarettes smoked and in the number of puffs (Russell, 1987). Thus smokers may be smoking to achieve the reward of nicotine effects, avoid the pain of nicotine withdrawal, or, most likely, combine the two. Nicotine withdrawal symptoms are listed in Table 8-3.

While depressed mood (dysthymic disorder, affective disorder) is associated with nicotine dependence, it is not known whether depression predisposes one to begin smoking or whether depression develops during the course of nicotine dependence. There is some evidence that adolescents with depressive symptoms are more likely to become dependent smokers. Depression significantly increases during smoking withdrawal, which is cited as one reason for relapse. Another link to depression is the discovery that monoamine oxidase (MAO-B) inhibitory activity is found in a nonnicotine component of cigarette smoke (Fowler et al., 1996). The levels of inhibition of the enzyme are less than are found in antidepressant medication but may be enough to produce an antidepressant effect (and possibly also an antiparkinsonism effect). Thus smokers with a

Table 8-3

Symptoms of Nicotine Withdrawal Syndrome

Irritability, impatience, hostility
Anxiety
Dysphoric or depressed mood
Difficulty concentrating
Restlessness
Decreased heart rate
Increased appetite or weight gain

tendency toward depression may feel better while smoking, which makes quitting all the more difficult.

Pharmacotherapeutics. *Detoxification.* Nicotine replacement therapy is available in the form of skin patches, chewing gum, or nasal spray. Such replacement can ameliorate the symptoms of nicotine withdrawal, thus making it easier to quit smoking. Relapse, however, is quite high, particularly during the first 6 months of abstinence.

The blood nicotine concentrations achieved by different methods of nicotine delivery vary significantly, but none produces as high a peak arterial blood level as smoking tobacco cigarettes (Benowitz et al., 1988). Thus the rewarding effects in the brain of these nonsmoking alternatives are fewer. This also means that the alternative nicotine delivery systems have a low abuse potential because, unlike smoking, they do not produce a discernible high. These methods do, however, suppress the symptoms of nicotine withdrawal. Smokers should be able to transfer their dependence to the alternative delivery system and gradually reduce the daily nicotine dose with minimal withdrawal symptoms. More smokers can achieve abstinence with these methods, but over the ensuing weeks and months most of these quitters resume smoking. Comparisons with placebo treatment show large benefits for nicotine replacement at 6 weeks, but the effect diminishes with time. Longer-term studies of nicotine patch and nicotine chewing gum do show a small but significant advantage over placebo in abstinence rates at 6 and 12 months.

Anticraving medication. In 1997 the FDA approved bupropion as a medication to combat nicotine craving. This new indication for an established antidepressant was based on double-blind studies showing the benefits of bupropion in reducing craving and helping to maintain nicotine abstinence. The recommended program is for bupropion to be taken for a week before planned termination of smoking. The dosage is 150 mg per day for 3 days and then 150 mg twice per day. After 1 week, a nicotine patch is given to ease withdrawal symptoms and bupropion is continued along with behavioral treatment to reduce the risk of relapse. No long-term studies of this combined technique have yet been published.

The available studies for smoking cessation with nicotine patch or gum alone show verified abstinence rates at 12 months in the range of 20%. This is worse than the success rate for any other addiction. The poor success rate is due partly to the necessary goal of complete abstinence. When ex-smokers "slip" and begin smoking a little, they usually relapse quickly to their prior level of dependence. Thus complete abstinence is the criterion of success. Treatments that combine behavioral therapy and medication show the most promise.

Nicotine dependence in combination with other drugs. Most abusers of alcohol, cocaine, or heroin also smoke tobacco cigarettes. Because nicotine is a legal drug, many addiction treatment programs in the past have ignored the nicotine dependence and concentrated on alcohol or illegal drugs. In recent years, hospitals have begun banning smoking, forcing inpatients to use nicotine patches or suffer withdrawal. This can be a perfect opportunity to begin treatment of nicotine dependence even though it requires simultaneous attention to other drug problems. The same principles apply to outpatient treatment of substance abuse disorders. Nicotine dependence is a very damaging addiction and it should not be ignored. It may be necessary to begin by treating the most acute problem, but patients should be encouraged to address their dependence on nicotine and should be afforded the combination of medications described in the foregoing.

CENTRAL NERVOUS SYSTEM DEPRESSANTS

Alcohol

The use of ethyl alcohol prepared from the fermentation of sugars, starches, or other carbohydrates predates recorded history. Some experimentation with ethanol by people growing up in Western cultures is almost universal, and a high proportion of users find the experience pleasant. Approximately 70% of American adults occasionally use ethanol (alcohol), and the lifetime prevalence of alcohol abuse and alcohol addiction (alcoholism) in this society is 5 to

10% for men and 3 to 5% for women. Alcohol is classed as a depressant because it produces sedation and sleep. However, the initial effects of alcohol, particularly at lower doses, are often perceived as stimulation and are thought to be due to a suppression of inhibitory systems. Research volunteers who perceive only sedation after ingesting alcohol tend to choose not to drink in a choice test procedure (DeWit et al., 1989). There is considerable recent evidence indicating that alcohol enhances the actions of the inhibitory neurotransmitter γ-aminobutyric acid (GABA) at a subpopulation of GABA receptors (Harris et al., 1992). One of the effects of ethanol is an increase in activity of the dopaminergic pathway from the ventral tegmental area to the nucleus accumbens. This activation may be mediated by the effect on GABA receptors via a suppression of inhibitory interneurons, but the VTA activation results in an increase in extracellular dopamine in the NAc region. Further, there is evidence that this effect becomes learned as rats trained to self-administer alcohol begin to show an increase in NAc dopamine levels as soon as they are placed in the chamber where they have previously obtained alcohol (Weiss et al., 1993). Thus one of the pharmacological effects of alcohol is an increased level of extracellular dopamine in the NAc, similar to that seen with other drugs of abuse such as cocaine, heroin, and nicotine.

There is also evidence that the endogenous opioid system is involved in alcohol reinforcement based on a series of studies showing that alcohol self-administration in animals is blocked by opioid receptor antagonists such as naloxone and naltrexone. This concept is supported by recent human data showing that alcoholics report less euphoria when they drink alcohol while receiving the long-acting opioid receptor antagonist naltrexone (Volpicelli et al., 1992). Alcohol ingestion in the laboratory produced significant increases in peripheral β-endorphin levels in volunteers with a family history of alcoholism, but not in those without such history (Gianoulakis et al., 1992). Still another line of evidence points to an involvement of the serotonergic system in alcohol reinforcement (Naranjo, 1994). It is likely, therefore, that alcohol, a drug that reaches the central nervous system in relatively high concentrations and

affects cell membrane fluidity, produces effects at several neurotransmitter systems and thus has more than one mechanism for producing the pleasurable effects that lead to excessive use.

Alcohol impairs recent memory and in high doses produces the phenomenon of "blackouts" after which the drinker has no memory of his or her behavior while intoxicated. The effects on memory are unclear, but the evidence suggests that reports from patients about their reasons for drinking and their behavior during a binge are not reliable (Mello 1973). Alcohol-dependent persons often say that they drink to relieve anxiety or depression. When allowed to drink under observation, however, alcoholics typically become more dysphoric as drinking continues (Mendelson and Mello, 1979), thus contradicting the tension-reduction explanation.

Clinical description.   Mild intoxication by alcohol is familiar to almost everyone, but the symptoms vary among individuals. Some drinkers simply experience motor incoordination and sleepiness. Others initially become stimulated and garrulous. As the blood level increases, the sedating effects increase with eventual coma and death at high alcohol levels. The initial sensitivity (innate tolerance) to alcohol varies greatly among individuals and is related to family history of alcoholism (Schuckit et al., 1994). Those with low sensitivity for alcohol can tolerate high doses when first exposed to alcohol without experiencing incoordination and other signs of impairment. As indicated earlier, these people are also at greater risk for later developing alcoholism. Experience with alcohol can produce tolerance (acquired tolerance) such that extremely high blood levels (300 to 400 mg/dL) can be found in alcoholics who do not appear grossly sedated. In these cases, the lethal dose does not increase proportionately to the sedating dose, and thus the margin of safety (therapeutic index) is decreased.

Heavy consumers of alcohol not only acquire tolerance, but they also inevitably develop a state of physical dependence. This often leads to drinking in the morning to restore alcohol blood levels that fell as alcohol was metabolized during the night. Eventually these individuals may awaken during the night and drink to avoid the restlessness produced by low alcohol levels. The alcohol withdrawal syndrome (Table 8-4) generally depends on the size of the average daily dose and is usually treated by resumption of alcohol ingestion. Withdrawal symptoms are experienced frequently, but they are usually not severe or life threatening until they occur in conjunction with other problems such as infection, trauma, malnutrition, or electrolyte imbalance. In the setting of such complications, the syndrome of delirium tremens, or "DTs," (Table 8-4) may occur.

Alcohol produces cross tolerance to other sedatives and hypnotics such as the benzodiazepines. This means that the dose of a benzodiazepine to relieve anxiety will be higher than usual in an alcoholic. If, however, alcohol is taken along with the benzodiazepine, the combined effects are more dangerous than either alone. Benzodiazepines are relatively safe in overdose when taken separately, but they are potentially lethal in combination with alcohol.

The chronic use of alcohol and other CNS depressants is associated with the development of depression (McLellan et al., 1979), and the risk of suicide among alcoholics is one of the highest of any diagnostic category. Cognitive deficits have been reported in alcoholics tested while sober. These usually improve after weeks to months of abstinence (Grant, 1987). More severe impairment of recent memory is associated with specific brain damage caused by nutritional deficiencies, particularly lack of thiamine, common in alcoholics. Alcohol is toxic to many organ systems and it readily crosses the placental barrier, producing the fetal alcohol syndrome, a major cause of mental retardation.

Pharmacotherapeutics. *Detoxification.* A patient who presents with an alcohol withdrawal syndrome has a potentially lethal condition. Although most mild cases of alcohol withdrawal never come to medical attention, severe cases require general evaluation, attention to hydration and electrolytes, vitamins, especially high dose thiamine (100 mg IM to begin), and a sedating medication that has cross tolerance with alcohol so as to block withdrawal symptoms. Because of the likelihood of liver impairment, a short-acting benzodiazepine such as oxazepam can be given at doses sufficient to prevent or reduce the symptoms described in Table 8-4. For most alcoholics, oxazepam 30 to 45 mg four times per day and 45 mg at bedtime is the correct starting dosage, which can be adjusted depending on the patient's size and severity of symptoms and then tapered over 5 to 7 days. After medical evaluation, uncomplicated alcohol withdrawal can be effectively treated on an outpatient basis (Hayashida et al., 1989). When there are medical problems or a history of seizures, hospitalization is required. Attention to nutrition and vitamin supplements including thiamine is very important to prevent or reverse the development of memory problems.

Relapse prevention. Detoxification is only the first step of treatment. Complete abstinence is the objective of long-term treatment, and this is accomplished mainly by behavioral approaches. Medications that aid in this process are the focus of current research efforts.

Disulfiram. Disulfiram blocks the metabolism of alcohol, resulting in the accumulation of acetaldehyde, which produces an unpleasant flushing reaction shortly after alcohol is ingested. Knowledge of this unpleasant reaction helps the patient resist taking a

Table 8-4
Symptoms of Alcohol Withdrawal Syndrome

Alcohol craving
Tremor, irritability
Nausea
Sleep disturbance
Tachycardia, hypertension
Sweating
Perceptual distortion
Seizures (12–48 h after last drink)
Delirium tremens (rare in uncomplicated withdrawal)
   Severe agitation
   Confusion
   Visual hallucinations
   Fever, tachycardia, profuse sweating, dilated pupils
   Nausea, diarrhea

drink. Although pharmacologically quite effective, disulfiram has not been found to be clinically effective in controlled trials. In actual practice, many patients stop ingesting the medication either because they wish to resume drinking alcohol or because they believe that they no longer need the medication to remain sober. Disulfiram continues to be prescribed in conjunction with behavioral contracting or coercive efforts to ensure compliance with daily ingestion of the medication. It appears to be helpful in selected cases.

Naltrexone. Another medication available to prescribe as an adjunct in the treatment of alcoholism is naltrexone. Opioid antagonists were first developed for the treatment of opioid addiction. By blocking opioid receptors, they prevent the effects of heroin and other opioids. Subsequently, naloxone, a short-acting antagonist, and naltrexone were studied in animal models of alcohol dependence. These models included rats that were induced to drink alcohol by foot shock stress and rats that were selectively bred over several generations for alcohol preference. It was also found that certain monkeys readily learned to select alcohol in a choice paradigm; these animals were also tested with opioid receptor antagonists. Both naloxone and naltrexone were found to consistently decrease or block preference for alcohol in these models. Other studies have demonstrated that one of the actions of alcohol is to activate the endogenous opioid system. Blocking opioid receptors prevents the increase of dopamine produced by alcohol in the nucleus accumbens, thus interfering with the mechanism by which alcohol presumably produces its behavioral reward.

As a result of data obtained from these animal models, naltrexone was tested in a clinical trial in alcoholics engaged in a day hospital treatment program. Naloxone is a short-acting opioid antagonist with poor absorption by the oral route, but naltrexone is well absorbed from the gut and has high affinity for opioid receptors and a duration of action in brain of about 72 h. In the initial clinical trial (Volpicelli et al., 1990, 1992) naltrexone was found to block some of the reinforcing properties of alcohol and reduce craving for alcohol as compared with the alcoholics randomly assigned to placebo treatment.

Most significantly, the alcoholics assigned to naltrexone had a significantly decreased rate of relapse to alcohol drinking in this double-blind trial. The first clinical trial was replicated by others (O'Malley et al., 1992), and in 1995 the FDA approved naltrexone for the treatment of alcoholism. It should be emphasized, however, that alcoholism is a complex disorder and that naltrexone is at best an adjunct in a comprehensive rehabilitation program. In some patients, the medication helps substantially by reducing craving and limiting the effects of alcohol if the patient slips by taking a drink. Treatment should continue at least 3 to 6 months, and compliance with the ingestion of naltrexone should be encouraged and monitored.

Acamprosate. Another medication that may become available to aid in the treatment of alcoholism is acamprosate. This homotaurine derivative was found to be active in some animal models of alcoholism and in double-blind clinical trials. In preclinical studies, acamprosate acts on the GABA system and reduces postalcohol supersensitivity. It is unclear why this effect would be helpful in the treatment of alcoholism or whether indeed this is the critical effect of acamprosate. The data from large clinical trials, however, show a statistically significant advantage in the alcoholics randomly assigned to acamprosate compared with the group assigned to placebo. This medication is already available to clinicians in several European countries. The first multiclinic trial of acamprosate in the United States is currently under way, and it is hoped that this interesting compound will soon be available to American clinicians to aid in the treatment of alcoholism. It is interesting to note that because the mechanism of action of acamprosate appears to be completely different from that of naltrexone, an additive effect might be produced if the two treatments are prescribed in combination.

Benzodiazepines

Benzodiazepines are among the most commonly prescribed drugs throughout the world. They are used mainly for the treatment of anxiety disorders and insomnia (see Chaps. 3 and 7). Considering their widespread use, intentional abuse of prescription benzodiazepines is relatively rare. Currently there is a controversy relating to the development of tolerance to the beneficial effects of these medications and the occurrence of withdrawal symptoms when they are stopped. When a benzodiazepine is taken for up to several weeks, there is little tolerance and no difficulty in stopping the medication when the condition no longer warrants it. After several months, the proportion of patients who become tolerant increases, and reducing the dose or stopping the medication produces withdrawal symptoms (Table 8-5). It can be quite difficult to distinguish withdrawal symptoms from the reappearance of the anxiety symptoms that caused the benzodiazepine to be prescribed initially. Some patients may increase their dose over time because the benzodiazepine sedative effects definitely show tolerance. Many patients and their physicians, however, contend that the anxiety reduction produced by the medication continues to occur long after tolerance to the sedating effects. Moreover, these patients continue to take the medication for years according to medical directions without increasing the dose and are able to function very effectively as long as they take the benzodiazepine. The degree to which there is tolerance to the anxiolytic effects of benzodiazepines is a subject of controversy (Lader and File, 1987). There is, however, good evidence that significant tolerance does not develop to all benzodiazepine actions because some memory effects in response to acute doses persist in patients who have taken benzodiazepines for years

Table 8-5
Benzodiazepine Withdrawal Symptoms

Anxiety, agitation
Increased sensitivity to light and sound
Paresthesias, strange sensations
Muscle cramps
Myoclonic jerks
Sleep disturbance
Dizziness
Seizures
Delirium

(Lucki et al., 1986). The American Psychiatric Association formed a task force that reviewed the issues and published guidelines on the proper medical use of benzodiazepines (Benzodiazepine Task Force APA, 1990). Intermittent use when symptoms occur retards the development of tolerance and is, therefore, preferable to daily use. Patients with a history of alcohol or other drug abuse problems have an increased risk for the development of benzodiazepine abuse and should rarely if ever be treated with benzodiazepines on a chronic basis.

Although relatively few patients who receive benzodiazepines for medical indications begin to abuse their medication, there are individuals who specifically seek benzodiazepines for their ability to produce a high. Among these abusers there are differences in popularity with those benzodiazepines that have a rapid onset, diazepam and alprazolam, tending to be the most desirable. The drugs may be obtained by simulating a medical condition and deceiving physicians or simply through illicit channels. Illicit drug dealers provide benzodiazepines in most major cities at $1 to $2 per tablet. Such unsupervised use can lead to consumption of huge quantities and therefore tolerance to the benzodiazepine sedating effects. For example, whereas a dose of 5 to 20 mg per day of diazepam is typical for a patient receiving prescribed medication, abusers may take over 1000 mg per day and not experience gross sedation.

Abusers may combine benzodiazepines with other drugs to increase the desired effect. For example, it is part of the street lore that taking diazepam 30 min after an oral dose of methadone produces an augmented high not obtainable with either drug alone. Although there is some illicit use of benzodiazepines as a primary drug of abuse, most of the nonsupervised use is by abusers of other drugs who are attempting to self-medicate the side effects or withdrawal effects of their primary drug of abuse. Thus, cocaine addicts often take diazepam to relieve the irritability and agitation produced by cocaine binges, and opioid addicts find that diazepam and other benzodiazepines relieve the symptoms of opioid withdrawal when they are unable to obtain their preferred drug.

Pharmacological intervention. If patients receiving long-term benzodiazepine treatment by prescription wish to halt their medication, the process may take months of gradual dose reduction. Symptoms as listed in Table 8-5 may occur during this outpatient detoxification, but in most cases the symptoms are mild. If anxiety symptoms return, a nonbenzodiazepine such as buspirone may be prescribed, but this is usually less effective than benzodiazepines in these patients. Some authorities recommend transferring the patient to a long-half-life benzodiazepine such as clonazepam during detoxification; other medications recommended include the anticonvulsants carbamazepine and phenobarbital. Controlled studies comparing different treatment regimens are lacking. Because patients who have been on low-dose benzodiazepines for years usually have no adverse effects, the physician and patient should jointly decide whether detoxification and possible transfer to a new anxiolytic is worth the effort.

The specific benzodiazepine receptor antagonist flumazenil has been found useful in the treatment of overdose and in reversing the effects of long-acting benzodiazepines used in anesthesia. It has been tried in the treatment of persistent withdrawal symptoms after cessation of long-term benzodiazepine treatment. It was theorized that as an antagonist flumazenil might "reset" receptors after long-term agonist occupancy, but no clear benefits have yet been reported.

Deliberate abusers of benzodiazepines usually require inpatient detoxification. Frequently these drugs are part of a combined dependence involving alcohol, opioids, and cocaine. Detoxification can be a complex clinical pharmacological problem requiring knowledge of the pharmacology and pharmacokinetics of each drug. The patient's history may not be reliable, not simply because of lying, but also because the patient frequently doesn't know the true identity of drugs purchased on the street. Medication for detoxification should not be prescribed by the "cookbook" approach, but by careful titration and patient observation. The withdrawal syndrome from diazepam, for example, may not become evident until the patient develops a seizure in the second week of hospitalization.

Polydrug dependence. During a complex detoxification involving opioids and sedatives, a general rule is to stabilize the patient with respect to opioids by giving a level dose of methadone and then focus attention on the more life-threatening sedative withdrawal. The dose of methadone depends on the level of opioid dependence and can be adjusted beginning with a test dose of 20 mg. Opioid detoxification can begin after the more dangerous drugs are addressed. A long-acting benzodiazepine such as diazepam, clonazepam, or clorazepate or a long-acting barbiturate such as phenobarbital can be used to block the sedative withdrawal symptoms. The dose should be determined by a series of test doses and subsequent observations to determine the level of tolerance. Most complex detoxifications can be accomplished within 3 weeks, but some very high dose patients and those with additional psychiatric complications take even longer.

After detoxification, the prevention of relapse requires a long-term outpatient rehabilitation program similar to the treatment of alcoholism. No specific medications have been found useful in the rehabilitation of sedative abusers, but specific psychiatric disorders such as depression or schizophrenia, if present, require specific medications.

Barbiturates and Other Nonbenzodiazepines

The use of barbiturates and other nonbenzodiazepine sedating medications has declined greatly in recent years owing to the increased safety and efficacy of the newer medications. Abuse problems with barbiturates resemble in many ways those seen with benzodiazepines and should be approached by the treating physician in a similar way.

Because drugs in this category are frequently prescribed as hypnotics for patients complaining of insomnia, the physician should be aware of the problems that can develop. Insomnia should rarely be treated as a primary disorder except when produced by short-term stressful situations (see Chap. 7). Often sleep loss is a symptom of an underlying chronic problem such as depression or is only a relative decrease due to a change in sleep requirements with age. Prescription of sedative medications, however, can affect the patterns of sleep with subsequent tolerance to these medication effects. When the sedative is stopped, there is a rebound resulting in even worse symptoms of insomnia than existed before the medication (Kales et al., 1979). Such medication-induced insomnia requires detoxification by gradual dose reduction.

OPIOIDS

Opioids are used primarily for the treatment of pain. Some of the brain mechanisms involved in the perception of pain also produce a state of well-being, or euphoria. Thus, opioids are also taken outside medical channels to induce euphoria, or a high. The ability to produce euphoria, therefore, gives this group of drugs a great potential for abuse and has generated much research on separating the mechanisms of analgesia from that of euphoria. Thus far, no opioid has been discovered that produces analgesia without euphoria. The search for such a medication has, however, led to advances in understanding the physiology of pain. Drugs modeled after the endogenous opioid peptides may one day provide more specific treatment, but none of these is currently available to the clinician. Medications that do not act at opioid receptors, such as the nonsteroidal anti-inflammatory drugs (aspirin, ibuprofen, acetaminophen, etc.), have an important role in certain types of pain, especially chronic pain. However, opioids are still the best agents available for attenuating severe pain.

Opioids are most commonly used for the treatment of acute pain. Some patients in pain report liking the relaxing, anxiolytic, euphorigenic properties of opioids as much as the relief of pain. This is particularly true in high-anxiety situations, such as the crushing chest pain of a myocardial infarction. Normal volunteers with no pain given opioids in the laboratory may report the effects as unpleasant because of the side effects such as nausea, vomiting, and sedation. Patients with pain rarely develop abuse or addiction problems. Of course, patients receiving opioids develop tolerance routinely and if the medi-

cation is stopped abruptly they will show the signs of an opioid withdrawal syndrome. This means that they have become "physically dependent" but not addicted (i.e., not "dependent" according to the official psychiatric definition).

Opioids should never be withheld from patients with cancer out of fear of producing addiction. If chronic opioid medication is indicated, it is preferable to prescribe an orally active, slow-onset opioid with a long duration of action. These qualities reduce the likelihood of producing euphoria at onset or withdrawal symptoms as the medication quickly wears off. Methadone is an excellent choice for the management of chronic, severe pain. Another choice is MS Contin (oral morphine, controlled-release). Rapid-onset, short-duration opioids such as hydromorphone or oxycodone are excellent for acute, short-term use, such as during the postoperative period. As tolerance and physical dependence develop, however, the patient may experience the early symptoms of withdrawal between doses, and during withdrawal the threshold for pain decreases. Thus, for chronic administration, the long-acting analgesics are the superior treatment for most patients.

The major risk for opioid abuse or addiction occurs in patients complaining of pain with no clear physical explanation or with evidence of a chronic disorder that is not life threatening. An example would be chronic headaches, backaches, abdominal pain, or peripheral neuropathy. Even in these cases, an opioid might be considered as a brief emergency treatment, but long-term treatment with opioids is not advisable. In those relatively rare cases that develop abuse, the transition from legitimate use to abuse often begins with patients returning to their physician earlier than scheduled to get a new prescription or visiting emergency departments of different hospitals complaining of acute pain and asking for an opioid injection.

Heroin is the most widely abused opioid. There is no legal supply of heroin for clinical use in the United States. Some claim that heroin has unique analgesic properties for the treatment of severe pain, but this has not been supported by double-blind trials comparing it with other parenteral opioids. Heroin is widely available on the illicit market, however, and the price per milligram has dropped sharply in the

1990s. For many years heroin purchased on the street in the United States had very low potency. Each 100-mg bag had only 4 mg of heroin (range: 0 to 8 mg) and the rest was inert or toxic adulterants. In the mid-1990s, street heroin reached 45% purity in many large cities, with some samples testing as high as 85%. A higher average dose means that the level of physical dependence among heroin addicts will be higher and that users who interrupt regular dosing will develop more severe withdrawal symptoms. Whereas heroin previously required intravenous injection, the samples of heroin with greater purity can be smoked. This fact enables people to initiate heroin use who are reluctant to insert a needle into their veins.

While there is no accurate way to count the number of heroin addicts in the United States, based on extrapolation from overdose deaths, number of applicants for treatment, and number of heroin addicts arrested, the estimates range from 750,000 to 1 million. It is not known exactly how many more try heroin briefly but do not become regular users. A household survey (Anthony et al., 1994) reported that 1.5% of American adults had used heroin at some time in their lives, and of those 23% met the criteria for dependence.

Heroin Addiction

Injection of a heroin solution produces a variety of sensations described as warmth, taste, high, and intense pleasure ("rush") that is compared to sexual orgasm. There are some differences among the opioids in their acute effects, with morphine producing more of a histamine-releasing effect and meperidine producing more excitation.

Even experienced addicts, however, cannot distinguish between heroin and hydromorphone in double-blind tests. Further, there is no scientific evidence that heroin is more effective than hydromorphone in relieving severe pain, although some physicians in countries where heroin is available as an analgesic believe it to be superior. The popularity of heroin in the United States may be owing to its availability on the illicit market and to rapid onset of action.

After intravenous injection, the heroin response commences within 1 min. Heroin has high lipid solubility and thus it crosses the blood-brain barrier quickly and then is deacetylated to the active metabolites, 6-monoacetylmorphine and morphine. After the intense euphoria, which lasts from 45 s to several minutes, there is a period of sedation and tranquillity ("on the nod") lasting up to an hour. The effects of heroin wear off in 3 to 5 h depending on the dose. Experienced users may inject two to four times per day. Thus the heroin addict is constantly oscillating between being high and feeling the sickness of early withdrawal (Fig. 8-2). This produces many problems in the homeostatic systems regulated, at least in part, by endogenous opioids. For example, the hypothalamic-pituitary-gonadal axis and the hypothalamic-pituitary-adrenal axis are abnormal in heroin addicts. Women on heroin have irregular menses and men have a variety of

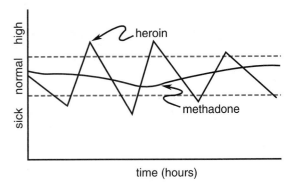

Figure 8–2.

sexual performance problems. Libido is low after a heroin injection, and premature ejaculation or even spontaneous emissions are problems during the withdrawal periods. Mood is also affected. Heroin addicts are relatively docile and compliant after taking heroin, but during withdrawal they become irritable and aggressive.

Based on patient reports, tolerance develops early to the euphoria-producing effects of opioids. There is also tolerance to the respiratory depressant, analgesic, sedative, and nausea effects. Heroin users tend to increase their daily dose depending on the availability of the drug and their ability to purchase it. If a supply is available, the dose can be progressively increased one hundred-fold. Even in highly tolerant individuals, the possibility of overdose remains if tolerance is exceeded. Overdose is likely to occur when potency of the street sample is unexpectedly high or when the heroin is mixed with a far more potent opioid such as fentanyl.

Treatment of Opioid Overdose

Opioid overdose consists of sedation or coma with very depressed respiration. This is often seen in the delivery room in a baby born to a mother who had received opioid analgesics during delivery. The same picture can also be seen in a heroin addict who injected a bag of opioid with much greater purity than usual or a bag containing a more potent opioid than heroin. This sometimes occurs when fentanyl is substituted for heroin by drug dealers.

Fortunately, there is an antidote for opioid overdose. Naloxone has high affinity for μ-opioid receptors, the site of action of morphine and other potent opioid agonists. Naloxone will displace the opioid from the receptor and thus promptly reverse the symptoms of overdose. Given intravenously, the effects begin in less than 1 min, but a subsequent injection may be required for full effect if the overdose is due to a very large dose of opioid. It is important to remember, however, that naloxone has a very short duration of action. If the overdose was caused by a longer-acting opioid, the patient will awaken after a naloxone injection and then 45 min later the overdose symptoms will return.

Clinical Picture of Opioid Addiction

Addiction to heroin or other short-acting opioids produces behavioral disruptions and usually becomes incompatible with a productive life. There is a significant risk for opioid abuse and dependence among physicians and other health care workers who have access to these drugs on a daily basis. Physicians often begin by assuming that they can manage their own dosage and they may rationalize their behavior based on the beneficial effects of the drug. For example, physicians with back pain may self-administer hydromorphone injections so that they can continue to be active and take care of their patients. Over time, however, the typical unsupervised opioid user loses control and behavioral changes are observed by family and coworkers. Apart from the behavioral changes and the risk of overdose, especially with very potent opioids, the chronic use of opioids is relatively nontoxic to organ systems.

Opioids are frequently used in combination with other drugs. A common combination is heroin and cocaine ("speedball"). Those who prefer this combination claim that it produces a more intense euphoria than is obtained with either drug alone. Heroin is sometimes used by addicts to "treat" the agitation and irritability that often follows a run of cocaine. Opioids and stimulants also interact in their pharmacological effects on the brain. Cocaine increases dynorphin levels in rats, and buprenorphine, which is a partial μ-opiate receptor agonist and kappa receptor antagonist, reduces cocaine self-administration in animals (Mello et al., 1989). Yet another related observation is that cocaine reduces the signs of opioid withdrawal in rats (Kosten, 1990). The clinical significance of these interactions between the opioid system and the effects of cocaine and other stimulants remains poorly understood.

Although opioids themselves are not toxic, the mortality rate among heroin addicts is quite high. These early deaths are frequently related to accidental overdoses, involvement in street crime, and risks of interactions with drug dealers. A large number of serious infections are associated with the use of unsterile drugs and sharing of injection paraphernalia. Infections common among heroin users include bacterial infections producing skin abscesses, pulmonary infections and endocarditis, and viral infections, especially HIV infection and hepatitis C. Intravenous drug use has become a major factor in the spread of HIV and hepatitis C, which typically lead to disability or early death.

Treatment of Opioid Addiction

As with other addictions, the first stage of treatment addresses physical dependence and consists of detoxification. The opioid withdrawal syndrome (Table 8-6) is very unpleasant, but rarely life threatening. It begins within 6 to 12 h of the last dose of a short-acting opioid and as long as 72 to 84 h after a very long acting opioid medication. Heroin addicts go through early stages of this syndrome frequently when heroin is scarce or expensive. Some therapeutic communities, as a matter of policy, elect not to treat withdrawal so that the addict can experience the suffering while being given group support. The duration and intensity of the syndrome are related to the kinetics of the individual drug. Heroin withdrawal is brief (5 to 10 days) and intense. Methadone withdrawal is slower in onset and lasts longer. The second stage of withdrawal, the protracted withdrawal syndrome (Table 8-6), is also likely to be longer in patients maintained on methadone.

Treatment of Opioid Withdrawal

Detoxification must be accomplished if the patient is scheduled for a drug-free residential program such as a therapeutic community or outpatient drug-free treatment. Unless there is a strong program to prevent

Table 8-6

Symptoms and Signs of Opioid Withdrawal

Symptoms	Signs
Craving for opioids	Pupillary dilatation
Restlessness, irritability	Sweating
Increased sensitivity to pain	Piloerection ("gooseflesh")
Nausea, vomiting, diarrhea, cramps	Tachycardia
Muscle aches	Increased blood pressure
Dysphoric mood	Yawning
Insomnia, anxiety	Fever

Protracted Withdrawal

Symptoms	Signs
Anxiety	Cyclic changes in
Insomnia	weight,
Drug craving	pupil size,
	respiratory center sensitivity

relapse, however, most detoxifications are followed by relapse to opioid use. Detoxification must also be accomplished if the patient is scheduled to be treated with the long-acting opioid receptor antagonist naltrexone to prevent relapse. If the patient is eligible for maintenance treatment and prefers this option, a detoxification is unnecessary. The patient can be transferred directly to methadone or l-α-acetyl methadol (LAAM) from heroin.

The most commonly used method for treating opioid withdrawal depends on cross tolerance and consists of transfer to a legal opioid medication and then gradual dose reduction. The principles of detoxification are the same for opioids as for other substances of physical dependence. It is convenient to change the patient from a short-acting opioid such as heroin to a long-acting one such as methadone. The initial dose of methadone is typically 20 mg. This is a test dose to determine the level needed to reduce withdrawal symptoms. The total dose on the first day of treatment can then be calculated depending on the response to this initial dose of metha-

done. If 20 mg produces no observable effect, the dose can be increased. The typical heroin user will be comfortable on 20 mg twice per day, with dose reductions of 20% per day during the course of detoxification. A larger initial dose of methadone is required for those taking higher daily doses of heroin.

A second approach to detoxification involves the use of clonidine, an antihypertensive medication. Clonidine is an α_2-adrenergic receptor agonist that activates presynaptic autoreceptors in the locus coeruleus, thus inhibiting adrenergic activity in the brain and periphery. Many of the autonomic symptoms of opioid withdrawal such as nausea, vomiting, cramps, sweating, tachycardia, and hypertension result from the loss of opioid suppression during the abstinence syndrome. Thus, because of its mechanism of action, clonidine is a nonopioid that alleviates many of the symptoms of opioid withdrawal. Because clonidine does not reduce the generalized aches and opioid craving characteristic of withdrawal, patients often complain during treatment with this drug. A limitation of this approach is that a dose of clonidine sufficient to reduce withdrawal symptoms also produces significant hypotension and dizziness.

A third treatment protocol for opioid withdrawal is theoretically but not practically useful; it involves activation of the endogenous opioid system without medication. The techniques proposed include acupuncture and several methods of CNS activation involving transcutaneous electrical stimulation. There are experiments showing that electrostimulation techniques can block signs of withdrawal in rats and produce evidence of increased endogenous opioid activity (Auriacombe et al., 1990).

Although stimulation of the endogenous opioid system would seem to be the most natural way to treat symptoms of opioid withdrawal, the effectiveness of this technique is difficult to demonstrate in controlled studies (Ellison, 1987). A fundamental problem is that patients in opioid withdrawal tend to be very suggestible, and the placebo effects caused by being connected to a mysterious box or having needles placed under the skin are formidable (Gariti et al., 1992).

Long-term management. If patients are simply discharged from the hospital after treatment of opioid withdrawal there is a high probability of a quick return to compulsive opioid use. Addiction is a chronic disorder that requires long-term treatment. Numerous factors influence relapse. One factor is that the withdrawal syndrome does not end in 5 to 7 days. There are subtle signs and symptoms often called the protracted withdrawal syndrome (Table 8-6) that persist for up to 6 months. These persistent changes tend to oscillate as though a new set point is being established (Martin and Jasinski, 1969), although the mechanism has not been elucidated. Following detoxification, outpatient drug-free treatment has a low probability of success; even when the patient has graduated from intensive treatment in a long-term therapeutic community, the relapse rate is high.

The most successful treatment for heroin addiction consists of stabilization on methadone. Patients who repeatedly relapse during drug-free treatment can be transferred directly to methadone without requiring detoxification. The dose of methadone must be sufficient to prevent withdrawal symptoms for at least 24 h. LAAM is another FDA-approved maintenance option that will block withdrawal for 72 h. Thus LAAM can be given to stable patients as infrequently as two to three times per week, thus eliminating the need for daily clinic attendance, which interferes with rehabilitation.

Agonist maintenance. Patients receiving methadone or LAAM will not experience the ups and downs experienced while on heroin (Fig. 8-2). Drug craving diminishes and may disappear. Neuroendocrine rhythms are eventually restored (Kreek, 1992). Because of cross tolerance (between methadone and heroin), patients who inject street heroin report a reduced effect from usual heroin doses. This cross-tolerance effect is dose-related so that higher methadone maintenance doses are more effective in preventing illicit opioid use as determined by random urine testing. Patients become tolerant to the sedating effects of methadone and thus are able to attend school or function in a job. Opioids also have a persistent mild stimulating effect noticeable after tolerance to the sedating effect such that reaction time is quicker and vigilance is increased while on a stable dose of methadone (Rothenberg et al., 1977).

Antagonist treatment. Another pharmacologic option is opioid antagonist treatment. Naltrexone is an antagonist similar to naloxone but with a long duration of action. It has a high affinity for μ receptors, and thus will competitively block the effects of heroin or other μ agonists. Naltrexone has almost no agonist effects and will not satisfy craving or relieve protracted withdrawal symptoms. For these reasons, naltrexone treatment does not appeal to the average heroin addict. It can be used after detoxification for patients with high motivation to remain opioid free. Physicians, nurses, and pharmacists who have frequent access to opioid drugs make excellent candidates for this treatment approach. Although originally developed for the treatment of opioid addiction, naltrexone is now more widely used throughout the world as a treatment for alcoholism.

New treatment options. There is currently much interest in developing new medications to aid in the treatment of addictive disorders. Buprenorphine is a μ-opioid partial agonist currently awaiting FDA approval (Johnson et al., 1992). It has minimal withdrawal symptoms, low potential for overdose, long duration of action, and ability to block heroin effects comparable to naltrexone. The formulation of buprenorphine that is expected to be approved is a combination with naloxone. The dose ratio is such that the naloxone antagonist properties would not significantly reduce the μ-agonist effects of buprenorphine when the combination is taken sublingually as directed. In contrast, if anyone injects the combination intravenously in an attempt to obtain euphoria, the antagonist naloxone, which has a high degree of intravenous potency, will effectively block the attempt. Because of its safety and low abuse potential in combination with naloxone, it is possible buprenorphine will be less strictly regulated than other opioids in the United States. This would permit the treatment of opioid addiction to become more like that of other medical disorders and would give appropriate patients the option of being treated in private physicians' offices rather than in large, inconvenient methadone clinics.

COCAINE AND OTHER PSYCHOSTIMULANTS

Epidemics of stimulant abuse tend to be cyclical in contrast to the relatively constant level of opioid abuse. Cocaine has had two periods of popularity in the United States during the past century. In the most recent period, usage peaked during 1985, reaching 8.6 million occasional users and 5.8 million regular users. More than 23 million Americans are estimated to have used cocaine at some time in their lives, but the number of current users has declined steadily to 2.9 million in 1988 and further to 1.3 million in 1992. The mid-1990s appears to be a late phase of the epidemic, but the number of frequent users (at least weekly) has remained steady since 1991 at about 640,000 persons. About 16% of those who try cocaine lose control at some point and become dependent. Some of the variables that influence the likelihood of progressing from use to abuse to

dependence are discussed at the beginning of this chapter. Availability and price are critical factors. Until the 1980s, cocaine hydrochloride suitable for intranasal or intravenous use was expensive and the only form available. The introduction of less costly cocaine alkaloidals (freebase, "crack") suitable for inhalation and easily purchased for as little as $2 to $5 in many major cities brought cocaine within reach of children and adolescents. Drug abuse on the whole is more common in males than in females, and for cocaine the ratio is about 2:1. Crack cocaine use, however, is particularly common in young women, approaching the proportion in males, and resulting in a significant amount of cocaine use during pregnancy.

The reinforcing effects of cocaine and cocaine analogues correlate best with their effectiveness in blocking the neuronal dopamine transporter or uptake site (Ritz et al., 1987). The transporter is a specialized membrane protein that recaptures dopamine that has been released by the presynaptic neuron, returning it to the intracellular stores of the neurotransmitter. Blockade of the transporter is believed to enhance dopaminergic activity at critical brain sites by prolonging the sojourn of the neurotrasmitter in the synaptic cleft. Cocaine, however, also blocks both norepinephrine (NE) and serotonin (5-HT) reuptake transporters, and chronic use of cocaine produces changes in these systems as well. Thus, neurotransmitters other than dopamine are likely to be involved in the physiological and psychological symptoms produced by cocaine.

The pharmacologic effects of cocaine in human subjects have been observed in the laboratory. Cocaine produces a dose-dependent increase in heart rate and blood pressure accompanied by increased arousal, improved performance at tasks of vigilance and alertness, and a sense of self-confidence and well-being. Higher doses produce euphoria that has a brief duration and is followed by a desire for more drug. Involuntary motor activity, stereotyped behavior, and paranoia may occur. Irritability and increased risk of violence are found among heavy chronic users. Studies of D2 dopamine receptors in hospitalized chronic cocaine users show a downregulation of these receptors that persists for months after the last dose of cocaine. The mechanism and consequences of this downregulation are poorly understood, but it is thought to be related to the depressive symptoms seen in former cocaine users and the high propensity to relapse to compulsive cocaine use.

The half-life of cocaine in plasma is about 50 min, but inhalant (crack) users typically desire more cocaine after 10 to 30 min. Intranasal and intravenous use also results in a high of shorter duration than would be predicted by plasma cocaine levels, suggesting that a declining plasma concentration is associated with termination of the high and resumption of cocaine seeking. This theory is supported by positron emission tomography (PET) imaging studies using ^{11}C-labeled cocaine showing that the time course of subjective euphoria parallels the uptake and displacement of the drug in the corpus striatum (Volkow et al., 1994).

Cocaine Abuse and Addiction

Addiction is the most common complication of cocaine use. Some users, especially of the intranasal type, can continue intermittent use for years. Others become compulsive users despite elaborate methods to maintain control. For example, a medical student may decide that he will only use cocaine on weekends or an attorney may resolve that she will never spend more on cocaine than the maximum that can be withdrawn from her bank's automatic teller machine. Gradually these techniques fail and the user begins taking cocaine more frequently than intended and spending more money on the drug. Stimulants tend to be used much more irregularly than opioids, nicotine, and alcohol. Binge use is very common, and a binge may last hours to days terminating only when supplies of the drug are exhausted.

The major route for cocaine metabolism involves hydrolysis of each of its two ester groups, resulting in loss of pharmacological activity. Benzoylecgonine, the demethylated form, is the major metabolite found in urine. Standard tests to detect cocaine use target the benzoylecgonine metabolite, which can be found in the urine for 2 to 5 days after a binge. Heavy users have been found to have positive urines for up to 10 days, and thus the urine test is only a marker of use in the past several days, but not necessarily recent use.

Cocaine is frequently taken in combination with other drugs. The cocaine-heroin combination was discussed earlier in the opioid section. Alcohol is another drug that cocaine users take to reduce the irritability experienced during heavy cocaine use. Some develop alcohol addiction in addition to their cocaine problem. An important metabolic interaction occurs when cocaine and alcohol are taken concurrently. Some cocaine is transesterified to cocaethylene, a metabolite that is equipotent to cocaine in blocking dopamine reuptake. Like cocaine, cocaethylene produces increased locomotor activity in rodents

and is readily self-administered by primates (Hearn et al., 1991).

Toxicity

Cocaine is directly toxic to organ systems. Effects include cardiac arrhythmias, myocardial ischemia, myocarditis, aortic dissection, cerebral vasoconstriction, and seizures. Pregnant cocaine users may experience premature labor and abruptio placentae (Chasnoff et al., 1989). Reports of developmental abnormalities in infants born to cocaine-using women are confounded by factors other than cocaine use such as prematurity, multiple drug exposure, and poor prenatal and postnatal care. Intravenous cocaine use increases the risk of a variety of needle-transmitted infections, but even crack smokers and intranasal users are found to have increased risk of sexually transmitted diseases including HIV.

Cocaine has been reported to produce a prolonged and intense orgasm if taken before intercourse. Its use is therefore associated with sexual activity, often compulsive and promiscuous. Long-term cocaine use, however, often results in reduced sexual drive, and complaints of sexual problems are common among cocaine users presenting for treatment. Psychiatric disorders are common in cocaine users who request treatment. They include anxiety, depression, and psychosis. Although some of these disorders undoubtedly existed before the stimulant use, many develop during the course of the drug abuse (McLellan et al., 1979).

Pharmacological Aspects of Cocaine Use

As described earlier, repeated use of a drug usually produces adaptations in the nervous system such that subsequent ingestions of the same dose produce a smaller effect. This is called tolerance. Acute tolerance or tachyphylaxis refers to a reduction in the effect when the drug is repeatedly taken on the same occasion. Acute tolerance has been observed in cocaine laboratory studies both in humans and in animals. With intermittent use, such as one dose per day over several days, the opposite change has been observed. In studies of stimulants such as cocaine and amphetamine using animal models, typically rats in a paradigm where behavioral activation is measured, the drug effects increase rather than decrease with repeated injections. This has been called sensitization and refers to an increased effect produced by repeated exposures to the same dose of the stimulant (Kalivas and Duffy, 1990). In human cocaine users, sensitization for the euphoria effect has not been reported by patients who request treatment for cocaine addiction. Sensitization has also not been observed in human laboratory studies, but experiments specifically searching for this phenomenon have not been attempted. To the contrary, some experienced users report that they require more cocaine over time to obtain euphoria (i.e., tolerance). In the laboratory, tachyphylaxis (rapid tolerance) has been observed with reduced effects when the same dose is given repeatedly in one session. Sensitization may involve behavioral conditioning (Post et al., 1987) and thus it is interesting to note that human cocaine users often report a strong response on seeing cocaine before it is taken into their bodies. This response has been measured in the laboratory when abstinent cocaine users are shown video scenes associated with cocaine use (O'Brien et al., 1992). The conditioned response consists of physiological arousal and increased drug craving.

Sensitization in humans has been linked to paranoid, psychotic manifestations of cocaine use. This phenomenon is based on the fact that binge-limited paranoia begins after long-term cocaine use (mean 35 months) in vulnerable users (Satel et al., 1991b). Thus repeated administration may be required to sensitize the patient to experience paranoia. The phenomenon of kindling has also been invoked to explain cocaine sensitization. Subconvulsive doses of cocaine given repeatedly will eventually produce seizures in rats (Weiss et al., 1989). This observation has been compared to electrical kindling of seizures and may underlie the gradual development of paranoia.

Because cocaine is typically used intermittently, even heavy users go through frequent periods of withdrawal, or "crash." The symptoms of withdrawal seen in users admitted to hospital are listed in Table 8-7. Careful studies of cocaine users during withdrawal (Satel et al., 1991) show gradual diminution of these symptoms over 1 to 3 weeks. Residual depression may be seen after cocaine withdrawal, and if it persists, antidepressant medication is indicated.

Medical Treatment

Because cocaine withdrawal is generally mild, treatment of withdrawal symptoms is usually not required. The major task in the management of cocaine addiction is not stopping the drug, but rather helping the patient to resist the urge to return to compulsive cocaine use. There is evidence that rehabilitation programs involving individual and group psychotherapy based on the principles of Alcoholics Anonymous and behavioral treatments based on reinforcing cocaine-free urine tests can result in significant improvement in the majority of cocaine users (Alterman

Table 8-7
Symptoms and Signs of Cocaine Withdrawal

Symptoms	Signs
Dysphoria, depression	Bradycardia
Sleepiness	
Fatigue	
Cocaine craving	

et al., 1992; Higgins et al., 1994). Nevertheless, there is great interest in finding a medication that can aid in the rehabilitation of cocaine addicts.

Desipramine (DMI) is a tricyclic antidepressant that has been tested in several double-blind trials involving cocaine addicts. Like cocaine, desipramine inhibits monoamine neurotransmitter reuptake, but its principal effects are on norepinephrine. It was hypothesized that DMI could relieve some of the symptoms of cocaine withdrawal and reduce desire for cocaine during the first month after stopping cocaine when the patient is most vulnerable to relapse. DMI showed significant efficacy early in the epidemic when given to a group of patients who were primarily white-collar, intranasal cocaine users (Gawin et al., 1989). Results of subsequent studies of DMI efficacy involving intravenous and crack cocaine users have been mixed. Other medications that have shown benefits include amantadine, a dopaminergic drug that may have short-term efficacy as an aid in detoxification (Alterman et al., 1992). Carbamazepine, an anticonvulsant, has been proposed as a treatment based on its ability to block kindling, a hypothetical mechanism in cocaine addiction. Several controlled studies in cocaine addicts, however, have failed to demonstrate any benefit from carbamazepine. Fluoxetine, a selective serotonin reuptake inhibitor, has been reported to produce a statistically significant reduction in cocaine use as measured by lower average urinary levels of the cocaine metabolite benzoylecgonine when compared with cocaine addicts assigned randomly to placebo treatment (Batki et al., 1991). Buprenorphine, a partial opioid agonist, has been found to reduce cocaine self-administration in monkeys (Mello et al., 1989), but a controlled study in patients dependent on both opioids and cocaine did not show a reduction in cocaine use. Thus far, all the studies of medications to help prevent relapse to cocaine dependence have described modest benefits at best. Even the small successes have been difficult to replicate, and there is general agreement that no medication is yet available that can reliably aid in the treatment of cocaine addiction.

OTHER STIMULANTS

Subjective effects similar to cocaine are produced by amphetamine, dextroamphetamine, methamphetamine, phenmetrazine, methylphenidate, and diethylproprion. Amphetamines increase dopamine activity primarily by stimulating presynaptic release rather than by blockade of dopamine reuptake, as is the case with cocaine. Intravenous or smoked methamphetamine is a primary drug of abuse in some parts of the United States; it produces an abuse and dependence syndrome similar to that of cocaine. A different picture arises when oral stimulants are prescribed in a weight reduction program. These drugs do reduce appetite with accompanying weight loss on a short-term basis, but the effects progressively diminish because of tolerance. There is evidence from studies in rodents of an appetite rebound when amphetamine is stopped, resulting in weight gain to a level above the preamphetamine baseline. Anorectic medications, therefore, are not considered to be a treatment for obesity by themselves, but rather as a short-term adjunct to behavioral treatment programs. A small proportion of patients introduced to these stimulants to facilitate weight reduction subsequently exhibit drug-seeking behavior to obtain the stimulant effects of the anorectic medication. These patients eventually may meet diagnostic criteria for abuse or addiction. Mazindol also reduces appetite, but it has less stimulant properties than amphetamine. In contrast, fenfluramine and phenylpropanolamine reduce appetite with no evidence of significant abuse potential. Unfortunately, fenfluramine (the racemic mixture) and dexfenfluramine have been associated with tragic cases of primary pulmonary hypertension and cardiac

valvular abnormalities. Also, animal studies have found depletion of serotonin granulation in the brains of monkeys and rats given fenfluramine, although the significance of this finding for humans is controversial. In 1997, the FDA banned the sale of both fenfluramine and dexfenfluramine because of these dangerous side effects.

Khat is a plant material chewed in East Africa and in Yemen because of its stimulant properties. It contains the alkaloid cathinone, which is similar to amphetamine. Recently, methcathinone, a congener with similar effects, has been synthesized in a string of clandestine laboratories throughout the midwestern United States. None of these stimulants has shown signs of reaching the epidemic proportions seen with cocaine during the 1980s.

Caffeine, a mild stimulant, is the most widely used psychoactive drug in the world. It is present in soft drinks, coffee, tea, cocoa, chocolate, and numerous prescription and over-the-counter drugs. Caffeine is absorbed from the gastrointestinal tract and is rapidly distributed throughout all tissues and easily crosses the placental barrier. Many of caffeine's effects are believed to occur by means of competitive antagonism at adenosine receptors. Adenosine, a constituent of adenosine triphosphate (ATP) and nucleic acids, is a neuromodulator that influences a number of metabolic functions in the CNS. Because adenosine generally reduces CNS activity, an antagonist such as caffeine displays stimulant properties.

Tolerance occurs rapidly to the stimulating effects of caffeine. Thus, a mild withdrawal syndrome can be produced by abrupt cessation of as little as one to two cups of coffee per day in double-blind studies. Caffeine withdrawal consists of feelings of fatigue and sedation. In high dose, headaches, nausea, and, rarely, vomiting, have been reported during withdrawal (Silverman et al., 1992). Although a withdrawal syndrome can be demonstrated, this does not imply addiction as discussed in the introduction to this chapter. Few caffeine users report loss of control of caffeine intake or difficulty in reducing or stopping caffeine if desired; thus caffeine is not listed in the category of addicting stimulants (DSM-IV).

Caffeine intoxication with high doses consists of nervousness, excitement, insomnia, diuresis, tachycardia, and muscle twitching. High levels of caffeine can aggravate existing anxiety disorders and can be the cause of insomnia. Thus a quantification of caffeine intake is an important part of the evaluation of patients with anxiety symptoms.

CANNABINOIDS (MARIJUANA)

The cannabis plant has been cultivated for centuries both for the production of hemp fiber and for its presumed medicinal and psychoactive properties. The smoke from burning cannabis contains many chemicals including 61 different cannabinoids that have been identified. One of these, Δ-9-tetrahydrocannabinol (THC), produces almost all the characteristic pharmacological effects of smoked marijuana.

Surveys have shown that marijuana is the most commonly used illicit drug in the United States. Usage peaked during the late 1970s when about 60% of high school seniors reported having used marijuana and nearly 11% reported daily use. This declined steadily in this cohort to about 40% lifetime use and 2% daily use in the mid-1990s. It must be noted that surveys among high school seniors tend to underestimate drug use because school dropouts are not surveyed. A recent development is the increased use of cannabis among eighth graders in the United States. The perception of marijuana as a dangerous drug has declined, and with it there has been an upswing in use, especially in the 10 to 15 year-old age group. Also, there has been a significant increase in the potency (THC content) of most marijuana samples obtained through illegal channels over this period.

In the past decade, a cannabinoid receptor has been identified in brain (Devane et al., 1988), and this receptor has been cloned (Matsuda et al, 1990). Although the physiological function of these receptors has not yet been elucidated, they are widely dispersed with high densities in the cerebral cortex, hippocampus, striatum, and cerebellum (Herkenham, 1993). The distribution of cannabinoid receptors is similar across several mammalian species, suggesting that these receptors have been conserved in evolution. An arachidonic acid derivative, anandimide, has been identified as an endogenous ligand for these sites (Devane et al., 1992). These exciting developments will likely have an impact on the understanding of marijuana abuse and dependence.

Clinical aspects of cannabis. The pharmacological effects of Δ-9-THC vary according to the dose, route of administration, experience of the user, vulnerability to psychoactive effects, and setting of use. Intoxication with marijuana produces changes in mood, perception, and motivation, but the effects sought after by most users are the "high" and "mellowing out." This is described as different from the stimulant high and the opioid high. The effects vary with dose, but the typical marijuana smoker experiences a high that lasts about 2 h. During this time there is impairment of cognitive functions, perception, reaction time, learning, and memory. Impairment of coordination and eye-tracking behavior has been reported to persist for several hours beyond the perception of high. These impairments have obvious implications for the operation of a motor vehicle or attendance at school.

Marijuana also produces complex behavioral changes such as giddiness and increased hunger. Some users have reported increased pleasure from sex and increased insight during a marijuana high. No studies have been reported that attempted to substantiate these claims.

Unpleasant reactions such as panic or hallucinations and even acute psychosis may occur. In several surveys, 50 to 60% of marijuana users have reported at least one such anxiety experience. They are seen more commonly with higher doses and with oral rather than smoked marijuana because smoking permits the regulation of dose according to the effects. Although there is no convincing evidence that marijuana can produce a schizophrenic-like syndrome, there are numerous clinical reports that marijuana use can precipitate a recurrence in people with a history of schizophrenia. Schizophrenics in remission appear to be particularly sensitive to the negative effects of marijuana on mental status.

One of the most controversial effects that has been claimed for marijuana is the production of an "amotivational syndrome." This syndrome is not an official diagnosis, but it has been used to describe young people who drop out of social activities and show little interest in school, work, or other goal-directed activity. When heavy marijuana use accompanies these symptoms, the drug is often cited as the cause. There are no data that demonstrate a causal relationship between marijuana and lack of motivation. There is no evidence that marijuana use damages brain cells or produces any permanent functional changes. There are animal data indicating impairment of maze learning that persists for weeks after the last dose, which is consistent with clinical reports of gradual improvement in mental state after cessation of chronic high-dose marijuana use.

Therapeutic benefits. Several medicinal effects of marijuana have been described. These include anti-nausea effects that have been applied to the side effects of anticancer chemotherapy, muscle relaxing effects, anticonvulsant effects and reduction of intraocular tension for the treatment of glaucoma. Patients suffering from AIDS have reported that smoked marijuana improves their appetite and helps to prevent the wasting syndrome seen in such patients and in terminal cancer patients. These medical benefits come at the cost of the psychoactive effects that often impair normal activities. Thus there is controversy over the question of whether marijuana is superior to conventional treatments for any of these disorders. Marinol (dronabinol) is a synthetic cannabinoid that can be taken orally for the treatment of nausea or wasting syndrome. Proponents of smoked marijuana (which is illegal) claim that the oral route does not permit adequate dose titration and thus dronabinol is not as effective as smoking the plant material. With the cloning of cannabinoid receptors and the discovery of an endogenous ligand for these receptors, it is hoped that medications can be developed that will target specific marijuana therapeutic effects without the psychoactive side effects.

Cannabinoid dependence syndrome. Tolerance develops to most of the effects of marijuana in both humans and laboratory animals (Jones, 1981). Tolerance can develop rapidly after only a few doses, but

it also disappears rapidly. Tolerance to large doses has been found to persist in experimental animals for long periods after cessation of drug use. Withdrawal symptoms and signs are not typically seen in clinical populations. In fact, relatively few patients ever request treatment for marijuana addiction. A withdrawal syndrome in human subjects has been described (Table 8-8). This syndrome has been demonstrated in marijuana users on a research ward who were given regular large oral doses. It is only seen clinically in persons who use marijuana on a daily basis and then stop. Compulsive or regular marijuana users do not appear to be motivated by fear of withdrawal symptoms although this has not been systematically studied. In 1997, surveys of substance abuse treatment programs show that approximately 100,000 persons were in treatment for marijuana dependence.

Treatment of marijuana dependence. Marijuana abuse and addiction have no specific treatments. Heavy users may suffer from accompanying depression and thus may respond to antidepressant medication, but this should be decided on an individual basis considering the severity of the affective symptoms after the marijuana effects have disappeared. The residual drug effects may continue for several weeks.

HALLUCINOGENIC DRUGS

Perceptual distortions that include hallucinations, illusions, and disorders of thinking such as paranoia

Table 8-8

Symptoms and Signs of Marijuana Withdrawal Syndrome

Restlessness
Irritability
Mild agitation
Insomnia
Sleep EEG disturbance
Nausea, cramping

can be produced by many drugs when they are taken in toxic doses. Perceptual distortions and hallucinations may also be seen during withdrawal from sedatives such as alcohol and barbiturates. Certain drugs, however, produce perceptual, thought, or mood disturbances at low doses with minimal effects on memory and orientation. These are commonly called hallucinogenic drugs, but their use does not always result in obvious hallucinations. In the United States, the most commonly used psychedelics are lysergic acid diethylamide (LSD), phencyclidine (PCP), MDMA (methylenedioxymethamphetamine, "ecstasy"), and a variety of anticholinergic drugs (atropine, benztropine). The use of these drugs received much public attention in the 1960s and 1970s, but their use waned in the 1980s. In 1989, the use of hallucinogenic drugs began to increase in the United States. By 1993, 11.8% of college students were reporting some use of these drugs during their lifetime, and the increase was most striking in younger cohorts beginning in the eighth grade.

Although psychedelic effects can be produced by a variety of different drugs, major psychedelic compounds come from two main categories. The indolamine hallucinogens include LSD, DMT (N,N-dimethyltryptamine), and psilocybin; the phenethylamines include mescaline, dimethoxymethamphetamine (DOM), methylenedioxyamphetamine (MDA), and MDMA. Both groups have a strong affinity for 5HT2 (serotonin) receptors (Titeler et al., 1988), but they differ in their affinity for certain other subtypes of 5-HT receptors. There is good correlation between the relative affinity of these compounds for 5-HT$_2$ receptors and their potency as hallucinogens in humans (Rivier and Pilet, 1971). The 5-HT$_2$ receptor is further implicated in the mechanism of hallucinations by the observation that antagonists of that receptor such as ritanserin are effective in blocking the behavioral and electrophysiological effects of hallucinogenic drugs in animal models. Recent binding studies on cloned 5-HT receptors, however, indicate that LSD interacts with many of the 14 subtypes of these receptors at nanomolar concentrations, and thus it is impossible to attribute the psychedelic effects to any single subtype (Peroutka, 1994). LSD is the most potent drug in this category, producing significant psychedelic effects with a total dose of as little as 25 to 50 µg. LSD, therefore, is over 3000 times more potent than mescaline.

LSD is sold on the illicit market in a variety of forms. A popular contemporary system involves postage stamp-sized papers impregnated with a varying dose of LSD (50 to 300 µg or more). While a majority of street samples sold as LSD actually contain LSD, the samples of mushrooms and other botanicals sold as psilocybin and other psyche-delics have a low probability of containing the advertised hallucinogen.

In human subjects the effects of hallucinogenic drugs are variable even in the same individual at different times. In addition to dose of the drug, individual variables and the setting in which the drug is given are important. LSD is rapidly absorbed after oral administration with onset of effects within 40 min, peaking at 2 to 4 h with gradual return to baseline over 6 to 8 h. At doses of 100 µg, LSD produces perceptual distortions and hallucinations; mood changes including elation, paranoia, or depression; intense arousal; and sometimes a feeling of panic. Signs of LSD ingestion include pupillary dilation, increased blood pressure and pulse, flushing, salivation, lacrimation, and hyperreflexia. Visual distortions are especially prominent with LSD. Colors seem more intense; shapes may appear altered, and the subject may focus attention on unusual items such as the pattern of hairs on the back of his hand.

Claims have been made about the potential of these drugs for enhancing psychotherapy and treating addictions and other mental disorders. These claims have not been supported by controlled treatment outcome studies; thus there is no current indication for these drugs as medications.

A "bad trip" usually consists of severe anxiety although at times it is marked by intense depression and suicidal thoughts. Visual disturbances are usually prominent. The "bad trip" from LSD may be difficult to distinguish from reactions to anticholinergic drugs and phencyclidine. There are no documented toxic fatalities from LSD use, but fatal accidents and suicides have occurred during or shortly after the trip. Prolonged psychotic reactions lasting 2 days or more may occur after the ingestion of a hallucinogen. Schizophrenic episodes may be precipitated in susceptible individuals, and there is some evidence that chronic use of these drugs is associated with the development of persistent psychotic disorders (McLellan et al., 1979). Frequent, repeated use of psychedelic drugs is unusual, and thus tolerance is not commonly seen. Tolerance does develop to the behavioral effects of LSD after three to four daily doses, but no withdrawal syndrome has been observed. Cross tolerance between LSD, mescaline, and psilocybin has been demonstrated in animal models.

Treatment of hallucinogen abuse. Because of the unpredictability of psychedelic drugs, any use carries some risk. Dependence and addiction do not occur, but users often require medical attention because of bad trips. The severe agitation seems to demand medication, although "talking down" by reassurance has been shown to be effective. Antipsychotic medications (dopamine receptor antagonists) may intensify the experience. Diazepam 20 mg orally has been found to be effective.

A particularly troubling aftereffect of the use of LSD and other similar drugs is the occurrence of episodic visual disturbances in a small proportion of former LSD users. These were originally called flashbacks and resembled the experiences of prior LSD trips. There is now an official diagnostic category called the hallucinogen persisting perception disorder (HPPD) (DSM-IV, 1994). The symptoms include false fleeting perceptions in the peripheral fields, flashes of color, geometric pseudohallucinations, and positive afterimages (Abraham and Aldridge, 1993). The visual disorder appears stable in half of the cases and thus represents an apparently permanent alteration of the visual apparatus. Precipitants include stress, fatigue, emergence into a dark environment, marijuana, antipsychotics, and anxiety states.

MDMA (Ecstasy). Both MDMA and MDA are phenylethylamines that have stimulant as well as psychedelic effects. MDMA became popular during the 1980s on some college campuses because of testimonials that it enhances insight and self-knowledge. It has also been recommended by some psychotherapists as an aid to the process of therapy although no data exist to support this contention. Acute effects are dose dependent and include tachycardia, dry mouth, jaw clenching, muscle aches, and, at higher doses, visual hallucinations, agitation, hyperthermia, and panic attacks.

MDA and MDMA produce degeneration of serotonergic nerve cells and axons in rats (Ricaurte et al., 1985). Although this has not been demonstrated in humans, the CSF of chronic MDMA users has been found to have low levels of serotonin metabolites. Thus there is possible neurotoxicity with no evidence that the claimed benefits of MDMA actually occur.

Phencyclidine. Phencyclidine has pharmacologic effects that are different from the psychedelics for which LSD is the prototype. It was originally developed as an anesthetic in the 1950s, but it was abandoned because of a high frequency of postoperative delirium with hallucinations. It was classed as a dissociative anesthetic because in the anesthetized state the patients remained conscious with staring gaze, flat facies, and rigid muscles. Abuse of this drug began in the 1970s, first in an oral form and then in

a smoked version enabling a better control over the dose. Researchers have given the drug to normal volunteers under controlled conditions and the effects have been carefully described. As little as 0.05 mg/kg produces emotional withdrawal, concrete thinking, and bizarre responses to projective testing. The symptoms produced by PCP include catatonic posturing and resemble the symptoms of schizophrenia. Abusers taking higher doses may appear to be reacting to hallucinations and exhibit hostile or assaultive behavior. Anesthetic effects increase with dosage; stupor or coma may occur with muscular rigidity, rhabdomyolysis, and hyperthermia. Intoxicated patients in the emergency department may progress from aggressive behavior to coma with elevated blood pressure and enlarged, nonreactive pupils.

PCP binds with high affinity to sites located in the cortex and limbic structures, resulting in blocking of N-methyl-D-aspartic acid (NMDA)-type glutamate receptors. Certain opioids and other drugs exhibit PCP-like activity in animal models and bind specifically to the same sites. There is evidence that NMDA receptors are involved in ischemic neuronal death caused by high levels of excitatory amino acids. Thus there is interest in analogues of PCP that also block NMDA channels but with fewer psychotogenic effects.

PCP is reinforcing in monkeys as evidenced by self-administration patterns that produce continuous intoxication (Balster et al., 1973). Humans tend to use PCP intermittently, but daily use is reported by about 7% of users in some surveys. There is evidence for tolerance to the behavioral effects of PCP in animals, but this has not been studied systematically in humans. Signs of a PCP withdrawal syndrome were observed in monkeys after interruption of daily access to the drug. These include somnolence, tremor, seizures, diarrhea, piloerection, bruxism, and vocalizations.

Treatment of phencyclidine abuse. Overdose must be treated by life support because there is no antagonist of PCP effects and no proven way to enhance excretion, although acidification of the urine has been proposed. PCP coma may last 7 to 10 days. The agitated or psychotic state produced by PCP can be treated with diazepam. Prolonged psychotic behavior requires antipsychotic medication such as haloperidol. Because of the anticholinergic activity of PCP, antipsychotics that have similar activity such as chlorpromazine should be avoided.

INHALANTS

Abused inhalants include several different categories of chemicals that are volatile at room temperature and produce abrupt changes in mental state when inhaled. Examples include toluene (from airplane glue), kerosene, gasoline, carbon tetrachloride, amyl nitrate, and nitrous oxide. Solvents such as toluene are typically used by children beginning at age 12. The material is usually placed in a plastic bag and the vapors inhaled. After several minutes of inhalation, dizziness and intoxication occur. Aerosol sprays containing fluorocarbon propellants are another source of solvent intoxication. Prolonged exposure or daily use may result in damage to several organ systems. Clinical problems include cardiac arrhythmias, bone marrow depression, cerebral degeneration, and damage to liver, kidney, and peripheral nerves. Death attributed to inhalant abuse is probably due to cardiac arrhythmias, especially accompanying exercise or upper airway obstruction.

Amyl nitrate produces dilation of smooth muscle and has been used in the past for the treatment of angina. It is a yellow, volatile, flammable liquid with a fruity odor. In recent years, amyl nitrate and butyl nitrate have been used to relax smooth muscle and enhance orgasm, particularly by male homosexuals. It is obtained in the form of room deodorizers and can produce a feeling of "rush," flushing, and dizziness. Adverse effects include palpitations, postural hypotension, and headache progressing to loss of consciousness.

Anesthetic gases such as nitrous oxide or halothane are sometimes used as intoxicants by medical personnel. Nitrous oxide is also abused by food service employees because it is supplied in disposable aluminum minitanks used as propellants for whipping cream canisters. Nitrous oxide produces euphoria and analgesia and then loss of consciousness. Compulsive use and chronic toxicity are rarely reported, but there are obvious risks of overdose associated with the abuse of this anesthetic.

TREATMENT OF ADDICTIVE DISORDERS

The management of drug abuse and addiction must be individualized on the basis of the drugs involved and the specific problems of the individual patient. The decision tree in Fig. 8-1 outlines the broad treatment options. Pharmacologic interventions have been described for each category when medications are available. An understanding of the pharmacology of the drug or combination of drugs ingested by the patient is essential to treatment. This is a matter of urgency in particular for the treatment of overdose or the detoxification of a patient who is experiencing withdrawal. It must be recognized, however, that the treatment of the underlying addictive disorder requires months or years of rehabilitation. The behavior patterns established during thousands of prior drug ingestions do not disappear with detoxification or even after a typical 28-day inpatient rehabilitation program. Long periods of outpatient treatment are necessary, with periods of relapse and remission. Although complete abstinence is the preferred goal, in reality most patients are at risk to reinitiate drug taking and require a period of retreatment. In this case, maintenance medication can be effective, such as methadone for opioid dependence. The process can best be compared to the treatment of other chronic disorders such as diabetes, asthma, or hypertension where long-term medication may be necessary, and complete cures unlikely. When viewed in the context of chronic disease, the available treatments for addiction are quite successful (McLellan et al., 1992; O'Brien, 1994). Long-term treatment is accompanied by improvements in physical status and in mental, social, and occupational function. Unfortunately, because there is general pessimism in the medical community about the benefits of treatment most of the therapeutic effort is directed at the complications of addiction such as pulmonary, cardiac, and hepatic dysfunction, rather than at addictive behavior itself. Prevention of these complications can best be accomplished by addressing the underlying addictive disorder, which requires a long-term rehabilitation program.

For additional information on the drugs discussed in this chapter see chapters 9, 10, 11, 17, 23, and 24 in *Goodman & Gilman's The Pharmacological Basis of Therapeutics* (Ninth Edition), McGraw-Hill, New York, 1996.

REFERENCES

Abraham HD, Aldridge A: Adverse consequences of lysergic acid diethylamide. *Addiction* 1993;88:1327.

Alterman AI, Droba M, Antelo RE, et al: Amantadine may facilitate detoxification of cocaine addicts. *Drug Alcohol Depend* 1992;31:19–29.

American Psychiatric Association: *Diagnostic and Statistical Manual of Mental Disorders,* 4th ed. Washington, DC, American Psychiatric Association, 1994.

Anthony JC, Warner LA, Kessler RC: Comparative epidemiology of dependence on tobacco, alcohol, controlled substances, and inhalants: Basic findings from the National Comorbidity Survey. *Exper Clin Psychopharmacol* 1994;2:244–268.

Auriacombe M, Tignol J, Le Moal M, Stinus L: Transcutaneous electrical stimulation with limoge current potentiates morphine analgesia and attenuates opiate abstinence syndrome. *Biolog Psychiat* 1990;28:650–656.

Balster RL, Johanson CE, Harris RT, Schuster CR: Phencyclidine self-administration in the rhesus monkey. *Pharmacol Biochem Behav* 1973;1:167–172.

Batki SL, Manfredi L, Jacob P III, Jones RT: Fluoxetine for cocaine dependence in methadone maintenance: Quantitative plasma and urine cocaine/benzoylecgonine concentrations. *J Clin Psychopharmacol* 1993;13:243–250.

Benowitz NL, Porchet H, Sheiner L, Jacob P III: Nicotine absorption and cardiovascular effects with smokeless tobacco use: Comparison with cigarettes and nicotine gum. *Clin Pharmacol Ther* 1988;42:2439–2445.

Benzodiazepine dependence, toxicity, and abuse. Task Force Report of the American Psychiatric Association, Washington D.C., 1990.

Chasnoff IJ, Griffith DR, MacGregor S, et al: Temporal patterns of cocaine use in pregnancy: Perinatal outcome. *JAMA* 1989;261:1741–1744.

Devane WA, Dysarz FA, Johnson MR, et al: Determination and characterization of a cannabinoid receptor in rat brain. *Mol Pharmacol* 1988;34:605–613.

Devane WA, Hanus L, Breuer A, et al: Isolation and structure of a brain constituent that binds to the cannabinoid receptor. *Science* 1992;258:1946–1949.

DeWit H, Pierri J, Johanson CE: Assessing individual differences in alcohol preference using a cumulative dosing procedure. *Psychopharmacology* 1989;98:113.

Ellison F, Ellison W, Daulouede JP, et al: Opiate withdrawal and electro stimulation. *L'Encéphale* 1987;XIII:225–229.

Fowler JS, Volkow ND, Wang G-J, et al: Inhibition of monoamine oxidase B in the brains of smokers. *Nature* 1996;379:733–736.

Gariti P, Auriacombe M, Incmikoski R, et al: A randomized double-blind study of neuroelectric therapy in opiate and cocaine detoxification. *J Substance Abuse* 1992;4:299–308.

Gawin FH, Kleber HD, Byck R, et al: Desipramine facilitation of initial cocaine abuse. *Arch Gen Psychiat* 1989;46(2):117–121.

Gianoulakis C, Angelogianni P, Meaney M, et al: Endorphins in individuals with high and low risk for development of alcoholism, in Reid LD (ed): *Opioids, Bulimia and Alcohol Abuse and Alcoholism.* New York, Springer-Verlag, 1990, pp 229–246.

Grant I: Alcohol and the brain: Neuropsychological correlates. *J Consult Clin Psychol* 1987;55:310–324.

Harris RA, Brodie MS, Dunwiddie TV: Possible substrates of ethanol reinforcement: GABA and dopamine, in Kalivas PW, Samson HH (eds): The neurobiology of drug and alcohol addiction. *Annals of the New York Academy of Sciences* 1992;654:61–69.

Hayashida M, Alterman A, McLellan AT, et al: Comparative effectiveness of inpatient and outpatient detoxification of patients with mild to moderate alcohol withdrawal syndrome. *N Engl J Med* 1989;320:358–365.

Hearn WL, Flynn DD, Hime GW, et al: Cocaethylene: A unique cocaine metabolite displays high affinity for the dopamine transporter. *J Neurochem* 1991;56:698–701.

Herkenham MA: Localization of cannabinoid receptors in brain: Relationship to motor and reward systems, in Korenman SG, Barchas JD (eds): *Biological Basis of Substance Abuse.* New York, Oxford University Press, 1993, pp 187–200.

Higgins ST, Budney AJ, Bickel WK, et al: Outpatient behavioral treatment for cocaine dependence: One-year outcome. *Exper Clin Psychopharmacol* 1995;3(2):205–212.

Johnson RE, Jaffe JH, Fudala PJ: A controlled trial of buprenorphine treatment for opioid dependence. *JAMA* 1992;267:2750–2755.

Jones RT, Benowitz NL, Herning RI: Clinical review of cannabis tolerance and dependence. *J Clin Pharmacol* 1981;21:143S–152S.

Kales A, Scharf MB, Kales JD, Soldatos CR: Rebound insomnia a potential hazard following withdrawal of certain benzodiazepines. *JAMA* 1979;241(16):1692–1695.

Kalivas PW, Duffy P: Effect of acute and daily cocaine treatment on extracellular dopamine in the nucleus accumbens. *Synapse* 1990;5:48–58.

Kosten TA: Cocaine attenuates the severity of naloxone precipitated opioid withdrawal. *Life Sciences* 1990;47:1617–1623.

Kreek MJ: Rationale for maintenance pharmacotherapy of opiate dependence, in O'Brien CP, Jaffe J (eds): *Addictive States.* New York, Raven Press, 1992, pp 205–230.

Lader M, File S: The biological basis of benzodiazepine dependence. *Psychol Med* 1987;17:539–547.

Lucki I, Rickels K, Geller AM: Chronic use of benzodiazepines and psychomotor and cognitive test performance. *Psychopharmacology* 1986;88:426-433.

Martin WR, Jasinski D: Psychological parameters of morphine in man: Tolerance, early abstinence, protracted abstinence. *J Psychiat Res* 1969;7:9–16.

Matsuda LA, Lolait SJ, Brownstein MJ, et al: Structure of a cannabinoid receptor and functional expression of the cloned cDNA. *Nature* 1990;346:561–564.

McLellan AT, O'Brien CP, Metzger D, et al: How effective is substance abuse treatment—compared to what? in O'Brien CP, Jaffe J (eds): *Addictive States.* New York, Raven Press, 1992, pp 231–252.

McLellan AT, Woody GE, O'Brien CP: Development of psychiatric illness in drug abusers. *N Engl J Med* 1979;301:1310–1314.

Mello NK: Short-term memory function in alcohol addicts during intoxication, in Gross MM (ed): *Alcohol Intoxication and Withdrawal: Experimental Studies, Proceedings of the 39th International Congress on Alcoholism and Drug Dependence.* New York, Plenum Press, 1973, pp 333.

Mello NK, Mendelson JH, Bree MP, Lukas SE: Buprenorphine suppresses cocaine self-administratoin by rhesus monkeys. *Science* 1989;245:859–862.

Mendelson JH, Mello NK: Biologic concomitants of alcoholism. *N Engl J Med* 1979;301:912–921.

Naranjo CA, Bremner KE: Serotonin-altering medications and desire, consumption and effects of alcohol-treatment implications, in Jansson B, Jörnvall H, Rydberg U, et al (eds): *Toward a Molecular Basis of Alcohol Use and Abuse.* Basel, Switzerland, Birkhuser Verlag, 1992, pp 209–229.

Nestler E, Aghajanian G: Moleuclar biology of addiction. *Science* 1997 (in press).

O'Brien CP: A range of research based pharmacotherapies for addiction. *Science* 1997 (in press).

O'Brien CP: Treatment of alcoholism as a chronic disorder, in Jansson B, Jörnvall H, Rydberg U, et al (eds): *Toward a Molecular Basis of Alcohol Use and Abuse.* Basel, Switzerland, Birkhäuser Verlag, 1994, pp 349–359.

O'Brien CP, Childress AR, McLellan AT, Ehrman R: Classical conditioning in drug-dependent humans, in Kalivas PW, Samson HH (eds): The neurobiology of drug and alcohol addiction. *Ann NY Acad Sci* 1992;654:400–415.

Peroutka SJ: 5-Hydroxytryptamine receptor interactions of *d*-lysergic acid diethylamide, in Pletscher A, Ladewig D (eds): *50 Years of LSD.* New York, Parthenon Publishing, 1994, pp 19–26.

Post RM, Weiss SRB, Pert A, et al: Chronic cocaine administration: Sensitization and kindling effects, in *Cocaine: Clinical and Biobehavioral Aspects.* New York, Oxford University Press, 1987, pp 109–173.

Ricuarte G, Byran G, Strauss L, et al: Hallucinogenic amphetamine selectively destroys brain serotonin nerve terminals. *Science* 1985;229:986–988.

Ritz MC, Lamb RJ, Goldberg SR, Kuhar MJ: Cocaine receptors on dopamine transporters are related to self-administration of cocaine. *Science* 1987;237:1219–1223.

Rivier L, Pilet PE: Composés hallucinogenes indoliques naturels. *Année Biol* 1971; 129–149.

Rothenberg S, Schottenfeld S, Meyer RE et al.: *Psychopharmacology* 1977;52:299.

Russell MAH: Nicotine intake and its regulation by smokers, in Martin WD, Van Loon GR, Iwamoto ET, Davis L (eds): *Tobacco Smoking and Nicotine.* New York, Plenum Press, 1987, p 25.

Satel SL, Price LH, Palumbo J. et al: Clinical phenomenology and neurobiology of cocaine abstinence: A prospective inpatient study. *Am J Psychiat* 1991;148:1712–1716.

Satel SL, Southwick SM, Gawin FH: Clinical features of cocaine induced paranoia. *Am J Psychiat* 1991;148:495–598.

Schuckit MA: Advances in understanding the vulnerability to alcoholism, in O'Brien CP, Jaffe J (eds): *Addictive States.* New York, Raven Press, 1992, pp 93–108.

Schuckit MA: *Drug and Alcohol Abuse: A Clinical Guide to Diagnosis and Treatment.* New York, Plenum Press, 1989, pp 85–86.

Schuckit MA: Low level of response to alcohol. *Am J Psychiat* 1994;151(2):184–189.

Siegel S: Morphine analgesic tolerance: Its situation specificity supports a pavlovian conditioning model. *Science* 1976;193:323–325.

Silverman K, Evans SM, Strain EC, Griffith RR: Withdrawal syndrome after the double-blind cessation of caffeine consumption. *N Engl J Med* 1992;327(16):1109–1114.

Srivastava ED, Russell MAH, Feyerabend C, et al: Sensitivity and tolerance to nicotine in smokers and nonsmokers. *Psychopharmacology* 1991;105:63–68.

Titeler M, Lyon RA, Glennon RA: Radioligand binding evidence implicates the brain 5-HT$_2$ receptor as a site of action for LSD and phenylisopropylamine hallucinogens. *Psychopharmacology* 1988;94:213–215.

Volkow ND, Fowler JS, Wolf AP: Use of PET to study cocaine in the human brain, in Rapaka R, Kuhar M (eds): *Emerging Techniques for Drug Abuse Research.* NIH Research Monograph Washington, D.C., 112:168–179, 1981.

Volpicelli JR, Alterman AI, Hayashida M, O'Brien CP: Naltrexone in the treatment of alcohol dependence. *Arch Gen Psychiat* 1992;49:876–880.

Weiss F, Lorang MT, Bloom FE, Koob GF: Oral alcohol self-administration stimulates dopamine release in the rat nucleus accumbens: Genetic and motivational determinants. *J Pharmacol Exper Therapeutics* 1993;267(1):250–267.

Weiss SRB, Post RM, Szele F, et al: Chronic carbamazepine inhibits the development of local anesthetic seizures kindled by cocaine and lidocaine. *Brain Research* 1989;497:72–79.

Wikler A: Conditioning of successive adaptive responses to the initial effects of drugs. *Conditional Reflex* 1973;8:193–210.

DEMENTIA AND DELIRIUM

Steven C. Samuels and Kenneth L. Davis

This chapter reviews the diagnosis, prognosis, and treatment strategies for dementia and delirium, with an emphasis on the pharmacologic treatment of these conditions. Pharmacologic management of the cognitive and behavioral aspects of Alzheimer's disease, vascular dementia, AIDS dementia, and dementia with Lewy bodies is at a variable stage of clinical development for each condition because of limitations in the understanding of the disease pathophysiology. Basic knowledge of Alzheimer's disease pathogenesis has led to the development of the cholinesterase inhibitors, tacrine and donepezil. Additional pharmacologic management with agents that putatively modify nerve injury and cell death is under investigation, as is management with muscarinic receptor agonists, adrenergic agents, anti-inflammatory agents, calcium modulators, estrogen, antioxidants and agents that modify processing of amyloid and tau. Depression, psychosis, sleep disorder, and anxiety are common behavioral disturbances associated with each dementia subtype, each of which can be managed with pharmacologic and environmental treatment strategies.

Delirium must be distinguished from dementia, and proper attribution of cause guides its treatment. Behavioral symptoms associated with delirium, such as sleep disturbance, psychosis, mood lability, anxiety, and psychomotor agitation often respond to pharmacologic and environmental therapies.

DEMENTIA

The major dementing disorders discussed in this chapter include Alzheimer dementia (AD), vascular dementia (VD), dementia with Lewy bodies (DLB), and AIDS dementia as these are the most common, accounting for over 80% of all dementias (Small et al., 1997). The conditions are described in terms of the clinical presentation, diagnosis, pathophysiology, and treatment strategies.

Definition and Clinical Description

Dementia is defined in *Diagnostic and Statistical Manual of Mental Disorders,* fourth edition (DSM-IV) as memory impairment with associated functional impairment accompanied by at least two of the following: aphasia, apraxia, agnosia, and impairment in higher executive functioning. The diagnosis is not made if delirium is present (American Psychiatric Association, 1994).

The most common dementia in the United States is AD, followed by VD and DLB. Other dementia subtypes include Parkinson's dementia, AIDS dementia, Pick's dementia, frontotemporal dementia, progressive supranuclear palsy, CJ dementia, Hallovorden-Spatz disease, substance-induced dementia, neurosyphilis, and alcohol dementia. Major psychiatric illnesses, such as schizophrenia, bipolar disease, depression, and delirium, may present with cognitive impairment. It is crucial to differentiate these conditions in establishing a diagnosis because the prognosis and treatment options differ among them.

Epidemiology

Prevalence estimates of dementia vary from 30.5/1000 per year for men and 48.2/1000 per year for women (Bachman, 1992). The incidence of dementia in 85- to 88-year-old Swedes was 90.1/1000 per year (61.3/1000 per year for men and 102.7/1000 per year for women). The incidence of Alzheimer's disease was 36.3/1000 per year, vascular dementia 39.0/1000 per year, while that of other dementias was 9.1/1000 per year (Aevarsson et al., 1996).

Presenting Symptoms

Dementia may present as increased forgetfulness, personality change, loss of initiative, impairment in judgment, difficulty performing familiar tasks, word finding difficulties, problems with abstract thinking, behavioral or mood changes (Alzheimer's Association, 1994). The noncognitive components of dementia include prominent behavioral disturbance, such as sleep disturbance, wandering, depression, or psychosis. The noncognitive symptoms often impede functioning and are a major reason for presentation to the physician.

Diagnostic Criteria

The imperative to correctly diagnose a dementia and classify the subtype stems from the different prognosis and treatment options among the various dementing disorders. In some dementias the definitive diagnosis is made with neuropathologic examination whereas with others, such as substance-induced dementia, there are no classic neuropathologic features on which to base the diagnostic decision.

Multiple classification systems assist in making the diagnosis of a dementia, with each dementia subtype possibly having more than one classification system. For example, there are DSM-IV and NINCDS/ADRDA criteria for AD. The DSM-IV diagnostic criteria are based on field trials and expert consensus, whereas the NINCDS/ADRDA criteria resulted from a working group that established uni-

form criteria for research purposes (McKhann et al., 1984) (Tables 9-1 and 9-2). Indeed, uniform diagnostic criteria facilitate the generalizability of clinical and research findings.

Dementia Evaluation

The evaluation for dementia is guided by practice guidelines and consensus statements (McKhann et al., 1984; Chiu et al., 1992; Roman et al., 1993; Chiesi et al., 1996; McKeith et al., 1996; American Psychiatric Association, 1997). Included are a careful historical review of presenting symptoms; past medical, surgical, psychiatric, family, social, and developmental histories; current and past use of prescription and over-the-counter medications, herbal remedies, and nontraditional treatments. The use of alcohol and illicit substances should be assessed. A thorough review of systems should be performed, with emphasis on head injury, seizure, incontinence, and motor and behavioral disturbances. Psychological testing to assess cognitive deficits and strengths contribute to diagnostic clarification and establishment of a treatment plan. Complete physical, neurological, and mental status examinations serve as a guide toward specialized diagnostic testing. Serum and urine should be assayed for infection, endocrine, renal, hepatic, electrolyte, and hematologic abnormalities. Vitamin deficiencies are assessed with serum studies. Moreover, an ECG and chest x-ray are standard during the evaluation. In patients at risk for sexually transmitted diseases, HIV and syphilis testing are appropriate. Indeed, even those most at risk may have been exposed to an infection while they were amnestic. Neuroimaging (CT, MRI) assesses for mass, bleed, and stroke. In special cases, functional neuroimaging (PET, SPECT, fMRI), CSF evaluation, and EEG may be useful. The goals of psychosocial assessment are to evaluate formal and informal supports and to develop an alliance with the patient and caregivers that will assist in implementing the treatment plan. Functional evaluation includes assessment of activities of daily living (ADLs) and instrumental activities of daily living

Table 9-1

NINCDS/ADRDA Criteria for Clinical Diagnosis of Alzheimer's Disease

1. Clinical diagnosis of possible Alzheimer's disease:

   May be made on the basis of the dementia syndrome, in the absence of other neurologic, psychiatric, or systemic disorders sufficient to cause dementia, and in the presence of variations in the onset, in the presentation, or in the clinical course;

   May be made in the presence of a second systemic or brain disorder sufficient to produce dementia, which is not considered to be the cause of the dementia; and

   Should be used in research studies when a single, gradually progressive severe cognitive deficit is identified in the absence of other identifiable cause.

2. Criteria for the clinical diagnosis of probable Alzheimer's disease include:

   Dementia established by clinical examination and documented by the Mini-Mental Test, Blessed Dementia Scale, or some similar examination, and confirmed by neuropsychological tests; deficits in two or more areas of cognition;

   Progressive worsening of memory and other cognitive functions;

   No disturbance of consciousness;

   Onset between ages 40 and 90, most often after age 65; and

   Absence of systemic disorders or other brain diseases that in and of themselves could account for the progressive deficits in memory and cognition.

3. Supporting evidence for diagnosis of probable Alzheimer's disease includes:

   Progressive deterioration of specific cognitive functions such as language (aphasia), motor skills (apraxia), and perception (agnosia);

   Impaired activities of daily living and altered patterns of behavior;

   Family history of similar disorders, particularly if confirmed neuropathologically; and

   Laboratory results of:

   > Normal lumbar puncture as evaluated by standard techniques,
   >
   > Normal pattern or nonspecific changes in EEG, such as increased slow-wave activity, and
   >
   > Evidence of cerebral atrophy on CT with progression documented by serial observation

4. Criteria for diagnosis of definite Alzheimer's disease are:

   The clinical criteria for probable Alzheimer's disease and

   histopathologic evidence obtained from a biopsy or autopsy

SOURCE Adapted from McKhann et al, 1984.

Table 9-2

DSM-IV Criteria for Dementia of the Alzheimer's Type

A. The development of multiple cognitive deficits manifested by both
   1. Memory impairment (impaired ability to learn new information or to re-call previously learned information).
   2. One (or more) of the following cognitive disturbances:
      a. Asphasia (language disturbance)
      b. Apraxia (impaired ability to carry out motor activities despite intact motor function)
      c. Agnosia (failure to recognize or identify objects despite intact sensory function)
      d. Disturbance in executive functioning (i.e., planning, organizing, sequencing, abstracting)

B. The cognitive deficits in Criteria A1 and A2 each cause significant impairment in social or occupational functioning and represent a significant decline from a previous level of functioning.

C. The course is characterized by gradual onset and continuing cognitive decline.

D. The cognitive deficits in Criteria A1 and A2 are not caused by any of the following:
   1. Other central nervous system conditions that cause progressive deficits in memory and cognition (e.g., cerbrovascular disease, Parkinson's disease, Huntington's disease, subdural hematoma, normal pressure hydrocephalus, brain tumor).
   2. Systemic conditions that are known to cause dementia (e.g., hypothyroidism, vitamin B_{12} or folic acid deficiency, niacin deficiency, hypercalcemia, neurosyphilis, HIV infection)
   3. Substance-induced conditions

E. The deficits do not occur exclusively during the course of a delirium.

F. The disturbance is not better accounted for by another Axis I disorder (e.g., Major Depressive Disorder, Schizophrenia).

SOURCE Adapted from American Psychiatric Association, 1994 (DSM-IV).

(IADLs) (Lawton, 1971) (Table 9-3). Additionally, a comprehensive review of patient safety issues is discussed, including wandering, driving, leaving the stove on unattended, or other behaviors that may place the patient or others at risk (Figure 9-1). Ideally, the patient should not be the sole informant and vigorous attempts should be made to obtain corrobo-rative information from others about history and to collaborate with others in developing a treatment plan.

Differential Diagnosis of Dementia

The comprehensive evaluation as described in the preceding makes it possible to clarify the diagnosis

Table 9-3
Functional Assessment

Is the patient independent, require some assistance, or dependent for each item?

Activities of Daily Living (ADL)
  Ambulation
  Transfer
  Dressing
  Toileting
  Feeding
  Grooming
  Bathing

Instrumental Activities of Daily Living (IADL)
  Using telephone
  Cooking
  Housekeeping
  Laundry
  Using transportation
  Finances
  Medications
  Shopping

SOURCE Adapted from Lawton, 1971.

(Table 9-4). Contributions from general medical conditions and substance use are aggressively explored since treatment of the medical condition, or elimination of the offending drug, may improve cognitive functioning.

Alzheimer's Dementia

The most common cause of dementia in the western hemisphere is AD, accounting for over 50% of the dementias. The prevalence increases with age and is more common in women. There are over 4 million AD patients in the United States (Brumback et al., 1994), with the direct and indirect costs of the disease approaching 90 billion dollars annually (Snow, 1996). Community prevalence of AD in those 65, 75, and 85 years old is 5, 15, and 50%, respectively (Evans et al., 1989).

Course and Outcome

The natural course of AD is a progressive decline with loss of cognitive and noncognitive function. Time from diagnosis until death averages 9 years, with a large individual variation (Walsh et al., 1990). Patients ultimately become bedridden and require total custodial care. Death often occurs from another condition, such as pneumonia. Factors associated with decreased survival include age, male gender, impairment in ADLs, and severity of dementia (Heyman et al., 1996) and severity of aphasia (Bracco et al., 1994). Race, marital status, and education do not significantly affect survival (Heyman et al., 1996). Predictive algorithms for time to death or placement in a long-term care facility based on clinical features of the disease have been developed and may assist in analyzing the effects of pharmacotherapy on survival and quality of life (Stern et al., 1997).

Table 9-4
Dementia Subtypes*

Alzheimer's dementia
Vascular dementia
Dementia with Lewy bodies
AIDS dementia
Parkinson's dementia
Pick's dementia
Frontotemporal dementia
Progressive supranuclear palsy
Huntington's dementia
Creutzfeldt-Jakob dementia
Normal-pressure hydrocephalus
Substance-induced dementia
Brain tumors
Endocrinopathies
Nutritional deficiencies
Neurosyphilis
Cryptococcus
Multiple sclerosis
Hallovorden-Spatz disease

* This list is not exhaustive, but rather representational of the more common dementia subtypes.

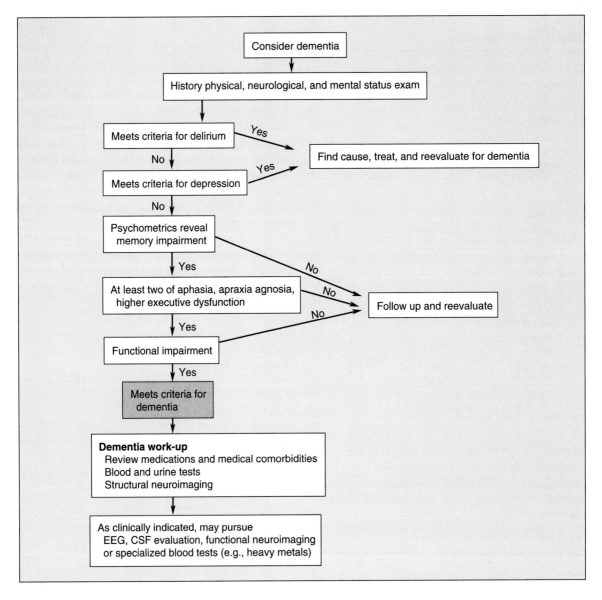

Figure 9–1. *Making a diagnosis of dementia.*

Genetics and Molecular Biology

Genetic mutations in Presenilin-1 (PS1), Presenilin-2 (PS2), and amyloid precursor protein (APP) are associated with AD (Murrell et al., 1991; Levy-Lahad et al., 1995; Sherrington et al., 1995). Other genotypes, such as APOE-ε4, place an individual at increased risk for the disorder AD (Strittmatter

et al., 1993). There are three isoforms of the APOE gene located on chromosome 19: APOE-ε2, APOE-ε3, and APOE-ε4. The APOE-ε4 allele correlates in a positive manner with cognitive impairment in very old nursing home residents (Altsteil et al., 1997). In some studies (Corder et al., 1993), but not others (Murphy et al., 1997), the presence of an APOE-ε4 allele in late-onset AD is related to increased risk of developing the disease, earlier age at death, earlier age at onset, and more severe disease.

Neuropathology

The gross pathologic changes in AD include generalized atrophy of the brain with reduction in gyral volume and widening of sulci. Histopathologically, plaques, tangles, and neuronal loss are characteristic of the disorder. Although some degree of atrophy, plaques, tangles, and neuronal loss may be found in the normal elderly, the quantity and location of the histopathologic changes in AD are standardized for diagnostic purposes (Khachaturian, 1985; Braak and Braak, 1997).

Cholinergic Function

Cholinergic function is altered in AD brain. Postmortem measures of choline acetyltransferase, the enzyme responsible for the synthesis of acetylcholine, demonstrate a negative correlation between enzyme activity and clinical dementia ratings prior to death (Perry et al., 1978; Bierer et al., 1995). There is preferential loss of cholinergic neurons in AD patients. Moreover, laboratory animals and humans receiving anticholinergic agents demonstrate impaired performance on memory tests. When given cholinergic enhancing agents, both laboratory animals and humans with structural deficits, or drug-induced cholinergic deficits, demonstrate an improvement in performance (Davis et al., 1982). In addition, clinical trials with inhibitors of cholinesterase, the enzyme responsible for the degradation of acetylcholine, support a role for cholinergic depletion in AD (Davis et al., 1992; Knapp et al., 1994; Rogers et al., 1996).

Adrenergic Function

The neurochemistry of AD is complex, and cholinergic activity may be potentiated by other neurotransmitter systems. Clonidine, an α_2-adrenergic receptor agonist, impairs frontal lobe function (Coull et al., 1995). α_2-Adrenergic receptor antagonists, such as idazoxan, increase norepinephrine by inhibiting presynaptic autoreceptors. Animal studies have demonstrated enhanced learning with cholinesterase inhibitors and have shown that presynaptic α_2-adrenergic receptor blockade may potentiate the effects of these drugs. Thus, laboratory animals given subthreshold doses of acetylcholinesterase inhibitors in combination with α_2-adrenergic receptor antagonists enhance learning (Camacho et al., 1996). Clinical trials testing this drug combination are currently underway.

Mechanisms of Neuronal Death

Excitatory amino acids. Excitatory amino acids (EAA) may play a role in the pathogenesis of AD. Thus, apoptosis, or programmed cell death, may result from alterations in glutaminergic function in brain. The hippocampus, cortico-cortical projections, and cortico-striatal connections contain high concentrations of glutamic and aspartic acids. Activation of glutamic acid receptors results in long-term potentiation, a correlate of memory production. Overstimulation of these receptors may also result in neurotoxicity. The three EAA-ionotropic receptor subtypes are classified as NMDA, AMPA, and kainate. The NMDA receptor, important in memory and learning, is stimulated by glutamic acid, aspartic acid, and NMDA, a chemical analogue of glutamic acid. The effects of glutamic acid on the NMDA receptor are modulated allosterically by polyamine and glycine receptor sites (Ito et al., 1990). The calcium channel associated with the NMDA receptor is blocked by magnesium in a voltage-dependent manner. Activity-dependent NMDA receptor antagonists also have a binding site within the ion channel. Both NMDA and AMPA receptor antagonists display neuroprotective properties in laboratory animals (Armstrong et al., 1994).

Oxidative stress. Oxidation, mediated by free radical formation, may be responsible, in part, for the neuronal damage associated with AD and other neurodegenerative disorders. Indeed, it has been suggested that Aβ neurotoxicity in AD is mediated by free radicals (Pike and Cotman, 1996). Free radical scavengers, or other agents that decrease the oxidation of neurons, such as immunosuppressants that inhibit transcription of factors that may be involved in neurodegeneration, may have a future therapeutic role in AD (Ogawa, 1996).

Calcium. Calcium is a chemical messenger that plays a vital role in neuronal function. Moreover, neuronal damage may be attributable to alterations in calcium homeostasis (Mattson et al., 1993). Both laboratory animal and human studies have suggested that nimodipine, but not other calcium channel blocking agents, improve memory and learning (Deyo et al., 1989; Ban et al., 1990; Tollefson, 1990; Parnetti et al., 1993; Besson et al., 1988).

Inflammation. Inflammatory mechanisms may contribute to the pathogenesis of AD as suggested by epidemiologic findings, the presence of inflammatory factors at the neurodegenerating sites, and causal in vitro and laboratory animal evidence. Thus, the prevalence of AD is decreased in patients taking nonsteroidal anti-inflammatory drugs (NSAIDs) and in those treated for rheumatoid arthritis (McGeer et al., 1996). The Baltimore Longitudinal Study revealed a decreased risk of developing AD in individuals who had taken NSAIDs for over 2 years compared with age-matched controls, with lower risk related to longer duration of NSAID use (Stewart et al., 1997). Additionally, in discordant sibling pairs at risk for AD, NSAID use was associated with decreased risk and delayed onset of the disorder (Breitner, 1995).

The inflammatory factors present at neurodegenerating sites in AD brains include interleukin Il-1 and Il-6, activated microglia, C1q, an early component of the complement cascade, and acute phase reactants (Aisen et al., 1994). *In vitro* tissue and laboratory animal data support the concept that inflammatory factors may be associated with the pathology of AD. For example, a transgenic mouse model that produces increased quantities of Il-6 causes neurodegeneration (Campbell et al., 1993), and Aβ toxicity is increased by C1q which interacts with it and cause increased Aβ aggregation (Webster et al., 1994). In different cell cultures, Il-1 increases the production of APP and augments the Aβ1-42 toxicity (Buxbaum et al., 1992; Fagarasan and Aisen, 1996).

Amyloid processing.   The amyloid cascade hypothesis, put forward by Selkoe, suggests that amyloid is an initiating event in the pathogenesis of AD (Selkoe, 1996). Neuritic plaques containing amyloid are present in AD brain areas involved in memory, with the density of plaques associated with the degree of cognitive impairment (Cummings, 1995). Moreover, the genes known to cause AD are associated with increased amyloid production or deposition (Citron et al., 1994, 1997; Greenberg et al., 1995; Scheuner et al., 1996). In addition, Down's syndrome patients who develop AD by age 50 have amyloid in their brains at an early age, even before they develop other neuropathologic AD lesions (Lemere et al., 1995; Querfurth, 1995). *In vitro*, Aβ damages neurons and activates microglia and inflammatory processes (Khoury et al., 1996), and blocking the formation of Aβ prevents toxicity (Masliah et al., 1996). Mice transgenic for human APP gene mutations produce many of the pathologic features of AD (Hsiao et al., 1996; Masliah et al., 1996). From a pharmacologic standpoint, each stage of the amyloid cascade is a potential site for therapeutic intervention in AD.

Tau processing.   Neurofibrillary tangles are another histopathologic hallmark of AD, although they are found in a number of other neurodegenerative diseases as well. Tangles contain paired helical filaments that are abnormal aggregations of tau proteins, and are found predominantly in axons. Abnormal phosphorylation of the tau protein appears to alter microtubule stability and may be involved in tangle formation (Trojanowski et al., 1990). Phosphorylated tau proteins are found in the hippocampus and the parietal and frontal cortices, areas involved in AD. Agents that modify tau processing may protect neurons from the destruction associated with tangle formation.

Pharmacologic Management

The current approved medications for mild to moderate AD include tacrine and donepezil, acetylcholinesterase inhibitors.

Tacrine.   Tacrine (9-amino-1,2,3,4-tetrahydroacridine) was the first cholinesterase inhibitor approved for the treatment of AD. It is a centrally acting, noncompetitive, reversible inhibitor of acetylcholinesterase and butyrylcholinesterase. Although originally synthesized in 1945, tacrine was not recognized as a cholinesterase inhibitor until 1953. While tacrine slows the apparent progression of AD in a subgroup of patients, several months of titration are required to attain the therapeutic dose. Tacrine use in AD is limited by qid dosing, potential hepatic toxicity, gastrointestinal side effects, and the need for frequent serum monitoring (Samuels et al., 1996).

Pharmacokinetics.   Tacrine is well absorbed, with bioavailability decreased 30 to 40% when it is taken with food. Peak plasma concentrations are attained 1 to 2 h after oral dosing. Steady-state concentrations are achieved 24 to 36 h after initiation or adjustment of dose. The volume of distribution for tacrine is 300 L/kg and the elimination half-life is 2 to 3 h. The drug is metabolized in the liver by CYP1A2 and CYP2D6 isozymes. It is hydroxylated and conjugated, with the primary metabolite being 1-hydroxy-tacrine. Since only a very small amount of tacrine is excreted by the kidney, dose adjustments are not necessary in patients with impaired renal function.

Pharmacodynamics.   Based on its mechanism of action, tacrine appears to work by increasing the availability of acetylcholine in brain. There is a nonlinear relationship between the plasma concentration of tacrine and oral dosing. The plasma concentration of tacrine in women is twice as high as in men, possibly owing to a lesser CYP1A2 activity in women. Because components of cigarette smoke induce CYP1A2, serum tacrine levels are one-third lower in smokers as compared to nonsmokers. Tacrine clearance does not appear to be related to age.

Clinical Trials.   There was significant variability in the methodological strength of clinical studies used to examine the efficacy of tacrine in AD. Thus, the very early studies showing promise were not well controlled, with subsequent work in the 1980s generating mixed results. These too were methodologically flawed, including the use of inadequate doses and treatment durations. Accordingly, generalizations about its effectiveness in AD were limited until the results of well-designed 12- and 30-week trials led to its approval (Davis et al., 1992; Knapp et al., 1994).

Prescribing Issues. A dose of at least 80 mg/day, and usually greater than 120 mg/day, appears necessary for a clinical response to tacrine, with 12 weeks being the minimal time required to titrate up to 120 mg/day. Gastrointestinal side effects or elevated transaminase levels may increase the titration interval. Tacrine administration should be discontinued if hepatic transaminase levels increase to five times the upper limit of normal. Patients may be rechallenged with tacrine after the transaminase levels normalize since a significant number of rechallenged patients may be successfully titrated to dosages greater than the original dosage. During clinical trials no deaths were associated with hepatitis in these patients. Tacrine should be used with caution in those with supraventricular cardiac arrhythmias and peptic ulcer disease because the drug enhances parasympathetic activity.

Precautions and adverse reactions. The most common side effects associated with tacrine are gastrointestinal, including dyspepsia, nausea, vomiting, diarrhea, anorexia, and abdominal pain. Serum monitoring of transaminases is required to screen for hepatic abnormalities, although they are most frequently asymptomatic. Although the rates of many adverse effects were similar in the tacrine and placebo groups, withdrawal from clinical trials occurred at a much higher rate with those taking the drug (Table 9-5).

Drug interactions. Coadministration of theophylline or cimetidine with tacrine increases serum concentrations of both since they are metabolized by the CYP1A2 enzyme. Tacrine inhibits butylcholinesterase, the enzyme responsible for degradation of succinylcholine, thereby prolonging the effect of the neuromuscular blocking agent.

Dosage and administration. Initiation of tacrine may proceed after a thorough physical examination and review of transaminase levels. Tacrine is started at 10 mg qid with the dose increased every 6 weeks by 10 mg until the target dosage of 40 mg qid is achieved. Titration may be limited by gastrointestinal side effects, evidence of elevated transaminases, or other adverse events. Gastrointestinal intolerance may be relieved by administering tacrine with food, although this decreases bioavailability by 30 to 40%. Elevations in transaminase preclude an increase in tacrine dosage and, in fact, may prompt a reduction in dose. If tacrine is discontinued for 4 weeks the drug may be administered once again beginning at 10 mg qid.

Hepatic monitoring and rechallenge. Patients who tolerate tacrine without significant elevations in hepatic transaminase levels (up to twice the upper limit of normal [ULN] of ALT [alanine aminotransferase]) are advised to have serum ALT monitoring every other week for 16 weeks, then monthly for 2 months, then once every 3 months. While patients with two to three times the ULN of ALT are advised to have weekly transaminase monitoring, those with ALT values three to five times the ULN should have their dose reduced 40 mg per day and should undergo weekly transaminase monitoring. When the ALT level normalizes in these patients the dosing titration may resume, with every other week transaminase monitoring. When ALT is five times the ULN drug administration should be terminated and the patient monitored for signs and symptoms of hepatitis. Evidence of clinical jaundice (total bilirubin greater than 3 mg/dL) or signs and symptoms of hypersensitivity, such as rash or fever, necessitate permanent cessation of tacrine without rechallenge. In a study of the hepatotoxic effects of tacrine, 88% of patients tolerated rechallenge and 72% were able to achieve higher tacrine doses than the initial one that resulted in discontinuation of the drug (Watkins et al., 1994).

Patients rechallenged with tacrine require weekly transaminase monitoring. After ALT values normalize, tacrine may be resumed at 10 mg qid. After 6 weeks the titration schedule may resume if there are no significant adverse symptoms and transaminase levels are less than three times the ULN. After transaminase values normalize, patients with initial elevations in ALT up to ten times the ULN may be rechallenged. Patients who develop hypersensitivity reactions to tacrine resulting in eosinophilia or granulomatous hepatitis should not be rechallenged.

Effects of tacrine. Tacrine may prolong the life of AD patients and reduce the likelihood of having to be placed in a nursing care facility (Knopman et al., 1996). Approximately 90% of the 663 patients in a 30-week clinical trial with tacrine were followed for

Table 9-5

Adverse Events Reported in Clinical Trials of Tacrine Compared with Placebo

	Tacrine (%) (n = 634)	Placebo (%) (n = 342)
Laboratory deviations		
Elevated transaminase	29	2
Digestive system		
Nausea and/or vomiting	28	9
Diarrhea	16	5
Dyspepsia	9	6
Anorexia	9	3
Abdominal pain	8	7
Flatulence	4	2
Constipation	4	2
Body as a whole		
Fatigue	4	3
Weight decrease	3	1
Musculoskeletal system		
Myalgia	9	5
Nervous system		
Dizziness	12	11
Ataxia	6	5
Insomnia	6	5
Somnolence	4	3
Tremor	2	<1
Psychobiological function		
Anxiety	3	2
Respiratory system		
Rhinitis	8	6

SOURCE Adapted from Warner Lambert, Tacrine package insert.

2 years, until they were placed in a nursing home, or died. The patients who received over 80 mg of tacrine per day were less likely to die during this time or to be placed in a nursing home compared with those receiving lower doses of the drug (odds ratio >2.7). While the absence of a drug-free control group limits the generalizability of these results, the dose-response nature of the findings are intriguing.

Donepezil. Donepezil hydrochloride (±2,3-dihydro-5,6-dimethoxy-2-[[1-(phenylmethyl)-4-piperidinyl]methyl]-1H-inden-1-one hydrochloride), introduced in the United States in December, 1996, was the second acetylcholinesterase inhibitor approved for treating AD. Advantages over tacrine include once daily dosing, lack of significant hepatotoxicity, no need for serum monitoring, and immediate dosing at therapeutic levels. *In vitro*, donepezil is more selective for acetylcholinesterase than butylcholinesterase.

Pharmacokinetics. Donepezil displays 100% oral availability which is unaffected by food. Peak plasma concentrations of donepazil occur 3 to 4 hours after oral dosing, with a steady-state volume of distribution at 12 L/kg. Donepezil is 96% bound to plasma proteins, predominantly albumin (75%) and α_1 acid glycoprotein (21%). Steady state is attained after multiple dosing in 15 days with a four- to sevenfold increase in donepezil concentration. Its elimination half-life is 70 h. Donepezil is metabolized in the liver by the CYP3D4 and CYP2D6 enzymes and undergoes glucuronidation. There are two active metabolites of donepezil, two major inactive metabolites, and multiple minor metabolites, all of which are excreted in urine. The manufacturer reports that patients with hepatic disease (stable alcoholic cirrhosis) displayed a 20% decreased hepatic clearance of the drug as compared to healthy controls. Patients with renal disease did not differ from healthy subjects in their clearance of donepezil.

Pharmacodynamics. Donepezil is a noncompetitive, reversible, inhibitor of the acetylcholine hydrolysis. As such, it presumably increases the synaptic concentration of this neurotransmitter in brain. Donepezil inhibits acetylcholinesterase more effectively than tacrine and is 1,250 times more selective as an inhibitor of acetylcholinesterase than butylcholinesterase. Oral daily dosage (1–10 mg) and plasma concentration are linearly correlated.

Clinical trials. Several clinical trials support the efficacy of donepezil in slowing the apparent progression of AD (Friedhoff et al., 1996; Rogers et al., 1996). In one 12-week, double-blind placebo-controlled study of probable AD patients, donepezil at 1-, 3-, and 5-mg, the 5-mg dose caused a statistically significant improvement in the ADAS cog compared with placebo. In another 12-week, double-blind placebo controlled study (5 mg, or 10 mg of donepezil) with a 3-week placebo washout period, the donepezil treated groups had statistically different means in ADAS cog scores compared with placebo. The differences between the 5- and 10-mg groups were not statistically significant. After 3 weeks of placebo washout the donepezil treated groups demonstrated loss of treatment effect. While the difference in ADAS cog scores between donepezil treated patients and placebo controls was about three units at 12 weeks, there is an expected change of nine points in untreated probable AD patients (Stern et al., 1994). At 12 weeks, patients receiving donepezil also displayed a statistically significant improvement compared to the placebo group in CIBIC plus scores, a clinician-based assessment of change after interview with the patient and caregiver.

A 30-week study with donepezil utilized the ADAS cog and CIBIC plus as outcome measures. The first 24 weeks included active, double-blind placebo controlled treatment, followed by 6 weeks of single-blind placebo-controlled washout. Patients were randomized to receive donepezil at 5 mg/day, 10 mg/day (after 1 week at 5 mg/day), or placebo. After 24 weeks, ADAS cog scores favored donepezil-treated patients as compared with the placebo group, although there was no statistically significant difference between the 5- and 10-mg donepezil groups. CIBIC plus scores at 24 weeks also statistically favored the donepezil-treated groups although, as with the ADAS cog scores, there was no difference between the donepezil groups receiving 5 and 10 mg per day. After the 6-week placebo washout the donepezil-treated and placebo groups were indistinguishable in ADAS cog scores, suggesting donepezil does not alter the underlying disease. There have been no clinical trials directly comparing tacrine and donepezil. However, at its best, the degree of improvement on the ADAS cog for donepezil is not as large as for tacrine at its best.

Prescribing issues. Donepezil does not appear to be hepatotoxic. Since donepezil may have vagotonic effects, patients with supraventricular cardiac arrhythmias, including "sick sinus syndrome" should be carefully monitored when taking the drug. The parasympathetic effects of donepezil may cause gastrointestinal disturbance and increased gastric acid secretion in some patients. Careful monitoring for gastrointestinal bleeding is required for those taking NSAIDs or with a history of active peptic ulcer disease who are administered donepezil. The 10-mg/day dosage is more commonly associated with nausea, diarrhea, and vomiting than the 5-mg/day dosage.

Precautions and Adverse Reactions. Diarrhea, nausea, insomnia, vomiting, muscle cramps, fatigue, and anorexia are the most common adverse effects reported with donepezil (Table 9-6). These are usually mild and resolved with continued treatment. Adverse events occurred more frequently in females and older patients. Nausea, diarrhea, and vomiting were the most common side effects associated with donepezil that led to discontinuation of treatment. Patients receiving 10 mg/day (titrated up from 5 mg after 1 week) had a higher discontinuation rate than the 5-mg/day group. In an open-label phase of treatment, the titration up to 10 mg/day was made at 6 weeks and the reported adverse events were lower than the more rapid titration group, and similar to the 5-mg/day donepezil group.

Table 9-6

Adverse Events Reported in Clinical Trials of Donepezil Compared with Placebo

Adverse event	Placebo ($n = 355$)	E2020 ($n = 747$)
Percent of patients with any adverse event	72	74
Body as a whole		
Headache	9	10
Pain, various locations	8	9
Accident	6	7
Fatigue	3	5
Cardiovascular system		
Syncope	1	2
Digestive system		
Nausea	6	11
Diarrhea	5	10
Vomiting	3	5
Anorexia	2	4
Hemic and lymphatic system		
Ecchymosis	3	4
Metabolic and nutritional systems		
Weight decrease	1	3
Musculoskeletal system		
Muscle cramps	2	6
Arthritis	1	2
Nervous system		
Insomnia	6	9
Dizziness	6	8
Depression	<1	3
Abnormal dreams	0	3
Somnolence	<1	2
Urogenital system		
Frequent urination	1	2

SOURCE Modified from 1996 donepezil package insert.

Drug interactions. *In vitro* studies suggest donepezil is highly bound to plasma proteins and will displace other drugs (furosemide, warfarin, digoxin) from these sites. Without *in vivo* studies, the implications of protein binding for potential drug interactions is unclear. This is a significant issue as the average AD patient is receiving a number of medications. Although the manufacturer reports that the binding of donepezil to albumin is unaffected by furosemide, warfarin, or digoxin, the effect of donepezil on malnourished or cachectic patients remains unclear. The company reports that donepezil has no significant pharmacokinetic effects on warfarin, theophylline, cimetidine, and digoxin, although no data are presented. Its effects on butylcholinesterase may increase the effects of succinylcholine. Agents that inhibit the CYP2D6 or CYP3A4 may inhibit the metabolism of donepezil, increasing the circulating levels of both compounds. Conversely, inducers of CYP2D6 or CYP3A4 may enhance the elimination of donepezil.

Dosage and administration. Donepezil is available in either 5- or 10-mg tablets as donezepil hydrochloride. The recommended starting dose is 5 mg/day. To minimize side effects that occur when the plasma concentration peaks, the medication is usually administered in the evening so the peak occurs during sleep. The clinical results provide little guidance on whether to increase the dosage from 5 to 10 mg/day. Although there were no statistically significant differences in outcomes between the two dosages, there was a trend favoring 10- to 5 mg/day. The patient and clinician need to discuss whether or not to increase the dosage to 10 mg/day. The half-life of donepezil is reported to be 70 h based on studies with younger patients since no half-life studies have been performed with the elderly. Because pharmacokinetic and pharmacodynamic changes in the elderly may lead to an increased half-life, it may be preferable to use 5 mg/day. Experience suggests it is best to increase the dose from 5 to 10 mg/day at 4 to 6 weeks while carefully monitoring for therapeutic and adverse effects.

Experimental Pharmacologic Approaches for AD

Cholinesterase inhibitors.

Physostigmine. Physostigmine is a reversible, short-acting cholinesterase inhibitor that requires frequent dosing. Its utility is limited by its peripheral cholinergic effects, such as nausea and vomiting. Dose finding optimizes patient response (Davis et al., 1978). A longer acting oral form of physostigmine salicylate has demonstrated benefit for AD patients in phase III trials, although it has not yet been approved for this use (Schwartz, 1996).

Eptastigmine. A long-acting form of physostigmine, eptastigmine (heptylphysostigmine) has demonstrated some benefit in the treatment of AD, although the dose response was an inverted U shape (Canal et al., 1996). Gastrointestinal side effects, and a report of agranulocytosis, must be considered when assessing the risk benefit ratio (Troetel et al., 1996).

ENA-713. ENA-713 is a "pseudo-irreversible" carbamate acetylcholinesterase inhibitor selective for the hippocampus and cerebral cortex. ENA-713 improves memory and global

measures as demonstrated in double-blind placebo controlled studies with AD patients. It is well tolerated in doses up to 6 mg bid and is awaiting review by the FDA (Anand et al., 1996).

Galanthamine. Galanthamine is a competitive, reversible inhibitor of acetylcholinesterase with no effect on butylcholinesterase. It also appears to enhance, in an allosteric manner, nicotinic cholinergic receptor activity. This drug is available in Austria. Multicenter trials in the United States and Europe have demonstrated a favorable response on the ADAS (Mohs and Cohen, 1988), a reliable measure of language, memory, and motor performance (Thomsen et al., 1995; Wilcock et al., 1996).

Metrifonate. Metrifonate is an irreversible inhibitor of acetylcholinesterase, similar to chemical warfare gases. Metrifonate has a preferential effect on acetylcholinesterase compared to butylcholinesterase (Unni et al., 1994). It is currently used to combat schistosomiasis (Cioli et al., 1995). *In vivo* the drug is converted to dichlorvos, a long-acting organic cholinesterase inhibitor. Laboratory animal studies and early clinical trials suggest this drug warrants further study as a treatment for AD (Cummings et al., 1996).

Muscarinic receptor agonists. Five different muscarinic receptors (M_1–M_5) have been identified that are involved in cognitive and postural modulation (Flynn et al., 1995). These receptors are coupled to G proteins and are found in brain and autonomic nervous system. The M_1 receptor is the most abundant in the brain regions responsible for memory and learning, and does not appear to be affected with AD progression (Flynn et al., 1995). The M_4 receptor is of interest because its density is increased in the cerebral cortical areas of AD brains (Flynn et al., 1995). When administered systemically, muscarinic receptor agonists do not mimic the normal, pulsatile stimulation of these sites, possibly resulting in the downregulation or desensitization of the receptors. There is evidence, however, that tonic stimulation may be important in attention and arousal (Flynn et al., 1991). Clinical trials with muscarinic receptor agonists have demonstrated some benefit. These agents may have more of a theoretical benefit in later disease, when presynaptic cholinergic neurons are greatly reduced or in combination with cholinesterase inhibitors (Flood et al., 1983, 1985).

Milameline. Milameline, a nonspecific, partial muscarinic receptor agonist, improves performance in animal models of cognition (M'Harzi et al., 1995). This drug has been shown to be well-tolerated by healthy controls and AD patients (Sedman et al., 1995). Although the doses of milameline required for stimulating central cholinergic activity are below those necessary to activate peripheral cholinergic systems, doselimiting side effects include nausea, vomiting, and severe abdominal cramping. A multicenter investigation of milameline for the treatment of AD is currently in progress.

Xanomeline. Xanomeline is a partial agonist at M_1 and M_4 receptors. Safety trials have demonstrated fair tolerability, with gastrointestinal side effects and hypotension leading a number of patients to discontinue the drug (Sramek et al., 1995). Xanomeline has been tested in a phase III trial where it displayed some benefit in noncognitive symptoms (Bodick et al., 1997). Transdermal delivery of the medication is also being investigated (Altsteil, 1996).

SB202026. SB202026 is a partial agonist at the M_1 receptor that has demonstrated tolerability and efficacy in a phase II clinical study (Kumar, 1996). The results of a phase III trial are not yet available (McCafferty, 1996).

Nicotine. Nicotinic cholinergic receptors also appear to play an important role in cognition (Nordberg, 1994). By binding to these presynaptic receptors, nicotine facilitates the release of acetylcholine and other neurotransmitters involved in learning and memory (Granon et al., 1995). Because of this, nicotinic receptor agonists may be effective in treating AD (Whitehouse and Kalaria, 1995).

In AD patients there is a decrease in the quantity of nicotinic receptors as measured by functional imaging and postmortem studies (Nordberg, 1992). When administered to AD patients nicotine decreases intrusion errors (Newhouse et al., 1988). Adverse effects on mood have been noted with nicotine (Sunderland et al., 1988). Nicotine may be administered by transdermal or intravenous routes. It is anticipated that advanced AD patients would display a decreasing benefit from nicotine over time as the quality and quantity of the nicotinic cholinergic receptors decline with disease progression.

Mechanisms of neuronal death.   Future treatments for AD will be aimed at modifying the mechanisms that contribute to neuronal injury and death.

Agents that modulate glutamatic acid. As reviewed in the preceding, glutaminergic dysfunction may contribute to apoptosis and cell death. For this reason, aniracetam and ampakines may be useful in the therapy of AD.

Aniracetam. Aniracetam is a pyrrolidine derivative that modulates metabotropic and AMPA-sensitive glutamatic acid receptors (Ito et al., 1990). The positive modulation of these receptors may result in facilitation of cholinergic transmission. Both laboratory animals and humans with experimentally induced cognitive impairments have improved performance when administered aniracetam. Clinical data support the cognitive enhancing effects of aniracetam in some studies (Parnetti et al., 1991; Senin et al., 1991; Lee and Benfield, 1994), but not others (Sorander et al., 1987). Confusion, unrest, anxiety, uneasiness, and insomnia are some adverse effects with the drug, but do not necessitate its discontinuation (Sorander et al., 1987). There has been no significant hepatic dysfunction associated with this agent.

Ampakines. Glutamic acid AMPA receptors appear to be decreased in AD brain, which may lead to alterations in calcium homeostasis and neuronal injury. Ampakines may increase AMPA receptor activity and facilitate learning and memory by enhancing long-term potentiation (Ito et al., 1990). Phase II clinical trials with ampakines demonstrated cognitive improvement in short-term recall in healthy adult men as compared with placebo (Lynch et al., 1997). An ampakine,

CX-516, is undergoing further investigation for efficacy and tolerability (Concar, 1996; Searching for Drugs that Combat Alzheimer's, 1996).

Agents that decrease oxidative stress. Free radical oxidation may be responsible for neuronal damage in AD and other neurodegenerative disorders. Moreover, free radicals may have a role in Aβ toxicity in AD (Pike and Cotman, 1996). Accordingly, free radical scavengers may display therapeutic benefit in AD.

Vitamin E and selegiline. Selegiline and vitamin E are antioxidants. A double-blind placebo-controlled trial compared the efficacy of each agent alone to a combination of vitamin E (2000 IU/day) and selegiline (10 mg/day) and placebo in moderately to severely affected AD patients (Sano et al., 1997). Outcome measures were changes from moderate to severe AD as measured with the Clinical Dementia Rating Scale (time to death, nursing home placement, loss of function on activities of daily living measures). Patients were followed for 2 years. The analysis covaried for baseline cognitive function as measured by the Mini Mental State Exam. All treatments were superior to placebo in delaying the onset of some measures. The combination of selegiline and vitamin E did not have an additive effect. None of the treatments improved cognitive function.

Idebenone. Idebenone is structurally related to ubiquinone, an intermediate in the oxidative phosphorylation pathway. Double-blind placebo-controlled trials of idebenone, at dose up to 360 mg/day, revealed this drug is efficacious in AD patients (Senin et al., 1992; Bergamasco et al., 1994; Weyer et al., 1996). Patients receiving idebenone had better performance at 6 and 12 months on ADAS total, ADAS cog, and CGI scores as compared to controls (Weyer et al., 1996, 1997). Idebenone is currently undergoing phase III clinical trials in the United States.

Calcium channel blockers. Because alterations in calcium homeostasis may cause neuronal injury and death (Mattson et al., 1993), calcium channel blockers have been studied in AD.

Nimodipine. There have been reports that nimodipine, a calcium channel blocker, improves learning and memory in humans and laboratory animals (Deyo et al., 1989; Ban et al., 1990; Tollefson, 1990; Parnetti et al., 1993), although others detected no benefit (Besson et al., 1988). There may be a selective dose response reflecting a functional selectivity of neurons to calcium levels. In one study, AD patients who received 90 mg, but not 180 mg, of nimodipine performed better than patients who received a placebo on a word list memory test (Tollefson, 1990).

Nerve Growth Factor. Nerve Growth Factor (NGF) is essential for the survival, regeneration, and function of cholinergic neurons. NGF is transported in a retrograde manner by neurons and binds to receptors in the basal forebrain, hippocampus, and cerebral cortex. It enhances acetylcholine synthesis by increasing the production of choline acetyltransferase, the enzyme responsible for the formation of this neurotransmitter (Dreyfus, 1989). NGF has exhibited a neuroprotective role in primates with experimentally placed neuronal lesions (Koliatsos et al., 1991). In one clinical study it was found to increase cerebral blood flow, improve verbal memory, and increase nicotinic receptor binding (Olson et al., 1992). There was evidence of improvement in cognitive functioning in two of three patients who received NGF by an intraventricular appliance. NGF appears to regulate nicotinic receptors and increase glucose metabolism in brain (Jonhagen et al., 1996). However, because NGF cannot cross the blood-brain barrier its clinical use is limited (Phelps et al., 1989). Agents that cross the blood-brain barrier and potentiate the action of endogenous NGF may have a role in the treatment of AD and other neurodegenerative conditions (Knuesel et al., 1992; Furukawa and Furukawa, 1990).

Estrogen. Estrogen may alter cerebral amyloid deposition and promote the survival and growth of cholinergic neurons (Honhjo et al., 1992; Jaffe et al., 1994). A placebo-controlled double-blind study of estrogen in AD is currently under way. A small number of subjects receiving 17-β estradiol for 5 weeks demonstrated some improvement in attention and verbal memory as compared with the placebo group (Asthana et al., 1996). Epidemiologic data support the potential beneficial effect of estrogen in delaying the onset of AD. In a large sample of women followed prospectively prior to the onset of AD, 12.5% took estrogen replacement therapy after menopause. Those who took estrogen developed AD at a later age than those who did not take the hormone. The relative risk of developing AD was almost three times higher in the nonestrogen women compared with those taking the hormone replacement even after adjusting for ethnic origin, education, and apolipoprotein E genotype (Tang et al., 1996). Additional support for the benefit of estrogen in AD comes from a retirement community where it was found that women taking estrogen had a decreased risk for developing the disorder as compared with those who were not receiving hormone replacement therapy. The positive results were dependent on the duration and dosage of estrogen (Paganini-Hill and Henderson, 1996). Women with AD receiving estrogen demonstrated a decrease in slow wave activity on EEG and an increase in cerebral blood flow in the motor area and lower frontal region on SPECT. Estrogen also improved MMSE score in these AD women at 3 and 6 weeks (Okhura et al., 1994).

Combination Treatments

Combined approaches to treatment are logical in AD since the pathogenesis appears to be multifactorial. Future treatments for AD may be similar to the multimodal approach used for controlling hypertension, cardiac disease, neoplastic disease, and AIDS. Although combination treatment with cholinesterase inhibitors and other agents has yet to be prospectively evaluated, a retrospective analysis of women receiving estrogen who were prescribed tacrine in the 30-week trial (Knapp et al., 1994), revealed improved functional and cognitive measures compared with those who were not receiving the hormone (Schneider et al., 1996). Prospective replication of these findings is required before combination treatment with estrogen and cholinesterase inhibitors can be recommended as a standard of care. Not all combination treatments will result in additive benefits as exemplified by the vitamin E and selegiline study where each was superior to placebo in the noncognitive outcome measures, but the drug combination displayed no additive effect (Sano et al., 1997). In addition to multiple drug therapy for AD, studies of psychosocial interventions in combination with medication need to be undertaken with respect to both the cognitive and noncognitive disturbances associated with AD.

Noncognitive Disturbances

Behavioral disturbances in dementia are common and may include psychosis, verbal and physical agitation, sleep disturbance, wandering, and personality changes. These complications contribute to patient suffering, caregiver stress, and increased utilization of health care resources. Moreover, they are often the primary reason a patient presents to an outpatient or emergency room setting. Behavioral disturbances are prevalent, heterogeneous, and vary in their longitudinal course (Devenand et al., 1997; Marin et al., 1997). Personality changes occur early in the disease and are often described as an amplification of preexisting personality traits. They may also take the form of irritability, apathy, withdrawal, and lack of relatedness to others (Rubin and Kinscherf, 1989). Later in the disease, personality change will occur in up to half of nursing home patients (Cohen-Mansfield et al., 1989).

Management of behavioral disturbances. The first step in managing these behavioral problems is defining them and understanding the antecedents and consequences of the behavior. A determination of the intensity, duration, and frequency of the behavior is useful in ascertaining whether a treatment approach is effective. Aggravating factors may include a caregiver's style of communication. For example, the patient may not understand comprehensive phrases with compound words. In this scenario, educating the caregiver to use short, simple phrases may be all that is required to change the behavior. Problem behavior may result in increased attention and decreased isolation for the patient. If a caregiver is made aware that the problem behavior is inadvertently being rewarded, then other techniques may be utilized to decrease the patient's isolation.

Attribution of the behavior to a basic need should be made if possible. For example, it is easy to attrib-

ute repetitive questioning about whether it is lunch time (no matter what time it actually is) to a patient's desire to eat. It may be more difficult to attribute urination in a plant to a patient's fear of going in the bathroom because every time he does and faces the mirror he sees someone else in the bathroom.

A general medical condition may be the cause for any problem. In demented patients, pain, constipation, infection, and medications are common culprits. Patients with dementia are often unable to describe the problem and express their discomfort with a behavioral change. Psychiatric illness may also cause behavioral changes in a demented patient.

Approaches to managing problem behaviors may include a change in the level of stimulation that the patient with dementia is receiving. Long-term memory may be spared, providing the opportunity for the patient with dementia to reminisce. Psychological testing, or careful bedside examination, may reveal areas of brain function that are still well preserved. Attempts to engage the patient should be geared toward the strengths that are retained. Often, behavioral disturbances decrease in demented patients when there is a routine with increased structure. Activities should be monitored to achieve an appropriate level of stimulation. In this regard, occupational therapy is an effective approach in older adults and has an empirical basis in managing behavioral disturbances in dementia (Clark et al., 1997).

Behavioral subtypes. *Psychosis.* Psychosis associated with dementia may be manifest in either delusions or hallucinations. The delusions most commonly involve "people stealing things." One possibility for this phenomenologic parsimony is that patients are attempting to make sense of their memory problems by confabulating. For example, after searching but not finding a misplaced item, the explanation is that the item was stolen. Misidentification is another common finding in patients with dementia. This behavior may be characterized by beliefs that "this house is not my home," or "my spouse is an imposter," or "there are other people in the room" when looking at the television or a reflection in the mirror. Misidentification may be explained by the visuospatial abnormalities found in AD. Organized delusional systems are less common in dementia, possibly because an ability to abstract with sufficient cognitive capacity is required to have a systemetized delusion. Visual hallucinations are more common than auditory hallucinations in AD.

Depressive Syndrome. Patients with dementia may have a preexisting depressive illness that recurs during the course of a dementia. Alternatively, depressive symptoms may have their debut during a dementia. In either case, recognition of the symptoms of depression is important as treatment may improve the quality of life for the patient and caregiver. Depressive symptoms may include dysphoria, irritability, anxiety, negativity, and uncontrolled crying. Although the mood disturbance may not reach criteria for DSM-IV diagnosis of coexisting major depression, bipolar disease, or other formal diagnostic criteria, the symptoms may contribute to patient and caregiver suffering. In this case, a trial of an antidepressant, mood stabilizer, or anxiolytic may be appropriate.

Sleep-wake disturbance. Sleep-wake disturbance may be another factor that negatively affects the quality of life for the patient and caregiver. If the patient does not sleep, both the patient and caregiver may become fatigued, leading to an exacerbation of other behavioral symptoms.

Nonpharmacologic approaches for managing sleep-wake disturbances include sleep hygiene and possibly phototherapy. A thorough medical review should search for the possibility of a treatable sleep disorder, such as restless leg syndrome or sleep apnea. Sleep hygiene includes eliminating daytime naps, using the bed only for sex and sleeping, and making certain that the bedroom is a comfortable temperature and free from extraneous noise and light. If the patient cannot fall asleep in 30 minutes, he or she is advised to leave the bedroom and only return to bed when sleepy again. Warm milk, or a warm bath, may be helpful prior to retiring. Medications should be carefully reviewed, with elimination of stimulants such as caffeine and dosing of activating drugs in the morning only. If the patient is already taking a hypnotic, the dose should be biased toward evening. Diuretics should be given early in the day and the patient should not have a heavy fluid intake

prior to sleep. Patients should attempt to retire in the evening and arise in the morning at the same time each day, regardless of the amount of sleep attained.

Phototherapy is of some benefit as a treatment for sleep disturbance. In a pilot study of 10 AD inpatients, those with sundowning and sleep disturbance were exposed to 2 hours per day of bright light therapy for 1 week. Clinical ratings demonstrated improvement in 8 of these patients (Satlin et al., 1992).

Pharmacologic management of a disturbed sleep-wake cycle may include the use of any conventional hypnotic, with the choice of medication based on side effect profile. The ideal agent would have fairly rapid onset of action and short duration of action to avoid hangover the next day and should not negatively affect cognitive function, nor be addictive.

Anxiety. Anxiety is commonly a manifestation of a medical illness, a medication-induced side effect, or a presentation of depression in the demented patient. After a thorough medical assessment and review of medications, consideration may be given to prescribing an anxiolytic or antidepressant. In some cases there may also be a role for mood stabilizers.

Wandering. Wandering is the type of behavioral disturbance that is location specific as to the degree of severity. Wandering unsupervised in an urban center near a busy highway places an AD patient at extreme risk. The same patient in a nursing home in a wandering garden with supervision may have virtually no risk. Wandering must be understood in a context of its cause. Walking and wandering may be an adverse effect of some medications. Others patients simply model behavior by following people out the door and around a building. Still others are drawn to the door or other objects that gain their attention in the distance. Placing the behavior in a proper perspective assists in developing a treatment plan. Nonpharmacologic approaches to manage wandering include supervision for safety and use of the Safe Return identification bracelets available through the Alzheimer's Association. Other management approaches take advantage of overlearned behaviors that are preserved in some patients with dementia. Stop signs, or facsimiles of the signs, posted on or near the exit doors may preclude wandering. The visuospatial problems in AD patients may be used to the advantage of decreasing wandering by changing markings on the floor near an exit. Dark markings near an exit may be misperceived as a pit or hole to be avoided. Other approaches include covering exit doors and locking doors with safety locks the patient is unable to open. Distraction may be temporarily useful for the wandering patient. This may take the form of food or an activity the patient enjoys. Music may be one example.

Medications for wandering should be used if nonpharmacologic approaches are not fully effective. Any class of medication may be helpful, with the choice often involving trial and error. Caution should be used with antipsychotic medications since these drugs may aggravate wandering by causing akathisia. Drugs which are sedating may increase the risk of a fall in the restless patient. There is preliminary evidence that cholinesterase inhibitors may decrease pacing behavior in a selective group of AD patients (Raskind et al., 1997).

Apathy/anergy. Apathy and anergy are other behavioral disturbances that may occur in dementia. Later stage patients with dementia often appear to be very withdrawn because of memory loss, language dysfunction, and an inability to care for themselves. Medical investigation into reversible causes of anergy should be considered, such as delirium. After establishing there is no immediate reversible contribution to the anergy or apathy, the possibility of a depressive syndrome that may be responsive to psychostimulants should be considered. Alternatively, antidepressants may be helpful, although they often have a longer response latency than psychostimulants.

Medication choices for behavioral disturbances. *Antipsychotics.* Schneider et al. performed a metanalysis of multiple inpatient antipsychotic studies for behavioral disturbances associated with various dementia syndromes. Compared to placebo, the antipsychotics were superior ($p < .05$, one tailed), with an effect size of 18% (Schneider et al., 1990). Limitations of the meta-analysis included a heterogeneous sample (any organic brain syndrome) and high placebo response rates. There are few outpatient studies utilizing antipsychotics to treat behavioral disturbance associated with dementia. Many of the studies already performed are limited because there was no placebo group and the samples are diagnostically heterogeneous.

The ideal choice of antipsychotic for behavioral disturbances cannot be determined from the current studies in the literature. Side effect profiles differ among antipsychotics, and the choice of agent may be guided by potential adverse effects. Lower potency antipsychotics are associated with an increased risk of sedation, orthostatic hypotension, and anticholinergic activity. The anticholinergic activity may worsen cognitive performance and aggravate urinary retention and constipation. With higher potency antipsychotics there is an increased risk of parkinsonism. With all antipsychotics there is a risk of tardive dyskinesia. Newer antipsychotics, such as risperdone, clozaril, olanzapine, quetiapine, and ziprasidone, may prove useful in the management of these behavioral disturbances, but all have their own set of potential adverse effects. Well-controlled studies of these newer agents for the treatment of noncognitive symptoms in AD have not yet been performed.

There is no information available to guide the clinician in determining the optimal dosage of antipsychotic agents for behavioral disturbances in dementia. In general, geriatric patients should be administered lower dosages and with slower titration schedules than others. Experience suggests it is best to start the frail patient with dementia and psychosis on a dosage of 0.25 to 0.5 mg haloperidol per day. Even at this dose such patients may develop severe parkinsonism. Hence, careful monitoring is required when a medication is started or dosage changed. An empirical trial of an antipsychotic for psychosis in a demented patient may take 6 to 12 weeks (Devenand, 1998).

Mood stabilizers. The utility of carbamazepine in behavioral disturbance associated with dementia is generally supported by case series and double-blind placebo-controlled studies in the nursing home setting. The modal dosage of carbamazepine in the 5-week treatment phase of the double-blind placebo-controlled study that demonstrated efficacy was 300 mg/day, which was well tolerated (Tariot et al.,

1994). The authors report that a follow-up study is "robustly positive" (Tariot et al., 1998).

Valproic acid is another mood stabilizer that may have utility in managing the noncognitive disturbances associated with dementia. However, the literature is limited to noncontrolled case series with heterogeneous samples. Sedation is reported as a possible dose-limiting side effect. Hepatic function and hematologic indices must be monitored in patients taking this drug. Dosages in the case series ranged from 240 to 1500 mg/day, with serum levels up to 90 ng/L.

Although there have been case reports that lithium displays some benefit in managing behavioral disturbances in demented individuals, it has not shown benefit in the majority of patients with behavioral disturbance. Its therapeutic index mandates cautious use in geriatric patients in general, and demented patients in particular. In general, lithium is not recommended in demented patients unless they also have clearly diagnosed bipolar disease.

Anxiolytics. Benzodiazepines have not been extensively studied in behavioral disturbances of dementia. These agents have attendant risks of dependence, sedation, amnesia, disinhibition, and falls. Target symptoms for which they may have utility are anxiety and sleep disturbance. Preference should be given to lorazepam and oxazepam because of their lack of active metabolites.

Buspirone is a nonbenzodiazepine anxiolytic with no risk of dependence, although its use may be associated with headache and dizziness. Controlled trials of buspirone are lacking in dementia patients with behavioral disturbance. In a trial comparing haloperidol (1.5 mg/day) and buspirone (15 mg/day) in 26 agitated nursing home residents, the buspirone group demonstrated benefit in anxiety and tension ratings (Cantillon et al., 1996). Both groups experienced behavioral improvement. There was no placebo group in this trial.

Zolpidem is a nonbenzodiazepine hypnotic. Case reports of patients with dementia have demonstrated improvement in agitation when treated with a low dose of this agent (Jackson et al., 1996). Controlled trials with zolpidem for behavioral disturbances have yet to be performed.

Antidepressants. Trazadone, an α_2-adrenergic and 5HT-2 receptor antagonist, is marketed as an antidepressant. Several case reports with dosage up to 400 mg/day suggest it is of benefit in attenuating agitation and aggression. A double-blind comparison trial between trazadone and haloperidol demonstrated that both are efficacious (Sultzer et al., 1997). Trazadone was more effective than haloperidol in decreasing resistance to care, and in reducing negativism, repetitive behaviors, and verbal aggression. Fewer patients taking trazadone dropped out of the trial than did those receiving haloperidol. There was no placebo group and some patients developed delirium while taking trazadone. Adverse effects limiting the utility of trazadone include orthostatic hypotension, sedation, and dizziness.

SSRIs. The serotonin selective reuptake inhibitors (SSRIs) have been used for behavioral disturbances associated with dementia. In particular they have been studied for their ability to reduce agitation. Alapracolate, citalopram, and sertraline have demonstrated positive effects in treating behavioral symptoms. Of these, only sertraline is available in the United States. Fluvoxamine and fluoxetine have not demonstrated benefit in treating behavioral disturbances associated with dementia. Further evaluation of these agents is required to determine the reason for the apparent selective benefit of some SSRIs over others. A multicenter trial with sertraline for behavioral disturbances in dementia is underway.

β-Adrenergic receptor antagonists. Case series support the benefit of using up to 520 mg/day of propanolol in managing agitation associated with organic brain syndromes (Greendyke et al., 1986). While bradycardia and hypotension may preclude dose escalation with propranolol, there is evidence that pindolol may provide benefit without the same limitations (Greendyke et al., 1989). β-Adrenergic receptor antagonists require further studies to replicate these findings, although careful use may be appropriate in the treatment of agitation associated with dementia.

Hormones. Case reports in a small group of demented men with physical aggression report some benefit when they were treated with conjugated estrogen or medroxyprogesterone acetate (Cooper, 1987; Kyomen et al., 1991).

Vascular Dementia

Clinical criteria. Vascular dementia (VD) is the second most common cause of dementia in the United States. In other regions of the world where stroke is very common, VD may exceed AD in prevalence. Recently, several criteria were proposed to diagnose vascular dementia. These include the NINDS-AIREN (Roman et al., 1993), the ADDTC (Chiu et al., 1992), DSM-IV (American Psychiatric Association, 1994), and ICD-10 (Wetterling et al., 1994). The DSM-IV (Table 9-7) and ICD-10 are diagnostic guidelines for clinical practice and have higher sensitivity than the guidelines developed for research studies (NINDS-AIREN).

The diagnostic criteria for vascular dementia are not uniform, with lack of consensus across criteria leading to variable diagnostic thresholds. Several authors have compared the criteria in their clinical samples and found that few patients meet diagnostic criteria for all sets (Amar et al., 1996; Verhey et al., 1996; Wetterling et al., 1996). The diagnostic criteria differ in sensitivity and specificity and are not interchangeable. Some studies require neuroimaging criteria in addition to clinical criteria. Few criteria have been neuropathologically validated. This lack of uniformity has clinical and research implications for differential diagnosis, epidemiology, prognosis, and treatment (Erkinjuntti et al., 1997).

The criteria to diagnose vascular dementia have traditionally relied on ischemia ratings such as the Hachinski Scale (Hachinski et al., 1975). This scale, when used alone, has low accuracy, sensitivity, and specificity according to neuropathologic confirmatory studies (O'Brien, 1988). The Hachinski scale

Table 9-7

Criteria for Vascular Dementia

A. The development of multiple cognitive deficits manifested by both
  1. Memory impairment (impaired ability to learn new information or to recall previously learned information).
  2. One (or more) of the following cognitive disturbances:
    a. Aphasia (language disturbance)
    b. Apraxia (impaired ability to carry out motor activities despite intact motor function)
    c. Agnosia (failure to recognize or identify objects despite intact sensory function)
    d. Disturbance in executive functioning (i.e., planning, organizing, sequencing, abstracting)

B. The cognitive deficits in Criteria A1 and A2 each cause significant impairment in social or occupational functioning and represent a significant decline from a previous level of functioning.
C. Focal neurological signs and symptoms (e.g., exaggeration of deep tendon reflexes, extensor plantar response, pseudobulbar palsy, gait abnormalities, weakness of an extremity) or laboratory evidence indicative of cerebrovascular disease (e.g., multiple infarctions involving cortex and underlying white matter) that are judged to be etiologically related to the disturbance.
D. The deficits do not occur exclusively during the course of a delirium.

SOURCE Adapted from American Psychiatric Association, 1994 (DSM-IV).

demonstrates the strongest level of discrimination between patients with medium- or large-sized clinical infarcts and patients with other related findings that are grouped together (lacunar infarcts, silent infarcts, chronic ischemic white matter changes, Binswanger's disease, mixtures of VD and AD, other vascular dementias than multi-infarct dementia) (O'Brien, 1988).

Vascular dementia appears to represent a heterogeneous group of entities with the common factor being a dementia, some disturbance in blood supply to the brain, and a relationship between the two. This diagnosis is ascertained by a careful history, clinical examination, and neuropsychological testing.

One of the commonly utilized criteria for VD is provided by the NINDS-AIREN International Workshop (Roman et al., 1993). In the NINDS-AIREN criteria, the supportive clinical features of VD are described as abrupt deterioration in cognitive function, gait disturbance or frequent falls, urinary frequency or incontinence, focal neurological findings (hemiparesis, lower facial weakness, sensory loss including visual field deficits, pseudobulbar syndrome, extrapyramidal signs), depression, mood lability, and psychiatric symptoms (Roman et al., 1993). The NINDS-AIREN criteria define dementia as cognitive deficits in memory plus two other domains. The cognitive deficits must cause functional impairment in ADLs but not be solely owing to the physical effects of stroke. Cases with disturbed consciousness, delirium, sensorimotor impairment, severe aphasia, and psychosis are excluded if the disturbance precludes completion of neuropsychological testing. The NINDS-AIREN criteria require focal signs consistent with a stroke on neurological examination. The criteria provide examples of different types of ischemic lesions that may relate to VD including multiple large-vessel strokes, a strategically placed infarct corresponding to the cognitive deficit, lacunar infarcts in the deep white and gray matter, extensive ischemic white matter changes, or combinations of these findings. The onset of the dementia must occur within 3 months of a recognized stroke, or be associated with a history of an abrupt decline in cognition, or fluctuating, stepwise progression of cognitive deficits.

Differentiating VD from AD is important because treatment approaches differ and there is an opportunity for primary and secondary prevention in VD. NINCDS-ADRDA definition of dementia require cognitive deficits in only two domains, and one of these does not have to be memory loss.

There are several subtypes of vascular dementia, with a recently published review describing eight (Konno et al., 1997) (Table 9-8). The first type was previously termed multiple infarct dementia. It is characterized by multiple large cerebral infarctions resulting from cardiogenic emboli. It has been proposed this subtype accounts for 27% of the vascular dementias. The second subtype of VD is a single infarct or several strategically placed infarcts (thalamus, frontal white matter, basal ganglia, angular gyrus), which accounts for 14% of the vascular dementias. The third subtype of VD is multiple subcortical lacunar infarctions that accumulate from atherosclerotic and degenerative changes within the walls of deep penetrating arterioles. This subtype is usually caused by hypertension and diabetes. Transient ischemic attacks, or stroke episodes, are often silent and may be gradually progressive, mimicking AD. Neuroimaging reveals the subcortical lacunar infarctions. Disconnection syndromes may result from the lacunar infarctions with a decrease in cerebral blood flow and functional metabolic changes in distant cortical and subcortical structures. This subtype is the most common of the vascular dementias, accounting for 30%.

The fourth subtype of VD is Binswanger's disease, or arteriosclerotic subcortical leukoencephalopathy. Binswanger's disease is characterized neuropathologically by

Table 9-8

Subtypes of Vascular Dementia

Multiple infarct dementia

Single infarct or several strategically placed infarcts

Multiple subcortical lacunar infarctions

Arteriosclerotic subcortical leukoencephalopathy

Mixture of large and small infarcts affecting cortical and subcortical structures

Hemorrhagic lesions

Subcortical lacunar infarcts from genitically determined arteriolopathies

Mixed vascular and Alzheimer's dementia

See text for details.
SOURCE Adapted from Konno et al., 1997.

decreased white matter density resulting from a partial loss of myelin sheaths, oligodendroglial cells, and axons. Small vessels supplying the white matter are occluded by fibrohyaline material. Clinically, patients present with dementia, limb rigidity, abulia, and urinary incontinence. AIDS, multiple sclerosis, and recent cranial radiation must also be considered in the differential diagnosis. The progression of Binswanger's disease is both gradual and stepwise, with development of neurological signs over several years. Multiple lacunar infarctions, periventricular white matter attenuation and hydrocephalus may be present on neuroimaging. This subtype accounts for only 3% of the vascular dementias.

The fifth subtype is a mixture of large and small infarcts affecting both the cortical and subcortical structures, whereas the sixth subtype results from hemorrhagic lesions, such as intracranial hematomas. Risk factors are uncontrolled hypertension, arteriovenous malformations, and intracranial aneurysms. The seventh type of VD is the genetically determined arteriolopathies that cause subcortical lacunar infarctions. Neuropathologically the lesions affect the small penetrating arteries of the basal ganglia and subcortical white matter. Examples include familial amyloid angiopathy, coagulopathies, and cerebral autosomal dominant arteriopathy with subcortical infarcts and leukoencephalopathy (Bousser and Tournier-Lasserve, 1993).

The eighth subtype of vascular dementia is mixed VD and AD. Usually this subgroup of VD patients has a family history of AD and risk factors for stroke. In neuroimaging, cortical atrophy and cerebral infarctions or hemorrhagic lesions are present. This subtype of VD also includes AD patients who develop intracerebral hemorrhage from an associated amyloid angiopathy.

Risk factors.   Risk factors for stroke are also risk factors for vascular dementia (Table 9-9). These include hypertension (Skoog et al., 1996; Lindsay et al., 1997), diabetes (You et al., 1995), atrial fibrillation (Wolf et al., 1978), cigarette smoking (You et al., 1995), coronary artery disease (Gorelick et al., 1993), congestive heart failure (Gorelick et al., 1993), carotid bruit (Gorelick et al., 1993), alcohol abuse (Lindsay et al., 1997), older age (Yoshitake et al., 1995), and male gender (Yoshitake et al., 1995). Additional risk factors for VD include decreased educational level (Tatemachi et al., 1994), occupation (Mortel et al., 1995a), presence of the apolipoprotein E epsilon 4 allele (APOE-ϵ4) (Gorelick, 1997), lack of estrogen replacement therapy after menopause (Mortel et al., 1995b), seizures (Moroney et al., 1996), cardiac arrhythmias (Moroney et al., 1996), and pneumonia (Moroney et al., 1996). The presence of these risk factors are supportive, but not necessary to make the

Table 9-9
Risk Factors for Vascular Dementia

Hypertension
Diabetes
Cigarette smoking
Coronary artery disease
Cardiac arrythmias
Congestive heart failure
Carotid bruit
Older age
Male
Decreased educational level
Occupation
APOE-ϵ4
Seizures
Lack of estrogen replacement therapy

diagnosis of VD. However, from a public health perspective, reduction of these risk factors may be one of the most significant treatments for VD.

Treatment.   The optimal treatment for vascular dementia is primary prevention. Education about improved control of the risk factors will result in decreased incidence of stroke and its sequelae, including vascular dementia. Once vascular dementia is present, optimal control of risk factors and comorbid medical conditions may decrease the rate of dementia progression. Aspirin therapy, warfarin, and ticlopidine have a role in selective cases.

Reduction of risk factors.   The reduction of risk factors for stroke may reduce the recurrence of cerebral infarctions. Control of hypertension with antihypertensives should be carefully monitored as overaggressive regulation of blood pressure may lead to a relative hypoperfusion, possibly further ischemia, malaise, confusion, and cognitive impairment. Cerebral embolic events are another treatable risk factor for stroke. Thorough evaluation for episodic cardiac arrhythmias with Holter monitoring and identification of the types of cerebral embolism with CT or MRI angiography, Doppler studies, and echocardiography are important. Atrial fibrillation that is not rate-controlled may lead to decreased cardiac output with decreased cerebral perfusion, resulting in ischemia and even infarction.

Current benefits of anticoagulation with warfarin or aspirin have been demonstrated with warfarin at doses producing INR at 2.0 to 4.5, and the dose of aspirin at 325 mg/day. To reduce the risk of stroke (and, inferentially, VD), patients with nonrheumatic atrial fibrillation, who can safely receive prophylactic antithrombotic therapy, should be given a trial of warfarin or aspirin (Stroke Prevention in Atrial Fibrillation Investigators, 1991). Anticoagulation therapy also reduces the risk of stroke after an MI (Van Bergen et al., 1994). The most serious potential complication from anticoagulant treatment is intracranial bleeding, which can be reduced by maintaining the INR less than or equal to 4 (Azar et al., 1996).

A systemic marker of inflammation, C-reactive protein was increased in men who developed MI or ischemic stroke (Ridker et al., 1997). Reduced levels of C-reactive protein were associated with reduced stroke and MI risk from aspirin, suggesting the potential benefit of anti-inflammatory agents in the prevention of ischemic stroke and MI (Ridker et al., 1997). Carotid endarterectomy is recommended for patients who demonstrate hemodynamically significant carotid artery stenosis (North American Symptomatic Carotid Endarterectomy Trial Collaborators, 1991) and those who present with ulcerated carotid plaques (Kistler et al., 1991). Poorly controlled diabetes mellitus and elevated plasma lipids may reduce cerebral perfusion by causing microangiopathy which may result in VD from lacunar infarctions. Thus, lowering triglyceride levels and regulation of blood sugar may improve cerebral blood flow and reduce the risk of further infarctions.

Cessation of cigarette smoking improves cerebral blood flow and cognitive performance (Rogers et al., 1985). All patients who smoke should be advised to abstain, regardless of whether they have already developed a VD. Gradual detoxification with transdermal nicotine may assist some in quitting (Cromwell et al., 1997).

Estrogen replacement therapy may be helpful as a prophylaxis in reducing the risk of VD (Mortel et al., 1995b). Estrogen replacement therapy is currently prescribed for osteoporosis, vasomotor menopausal symptoms, atrophic vaginitis, and hypoestrogenism. The beneficial effects of estrogen in cardiovascular disease, ischemic stroke, and VD may be supported by its ability to reduce platelet adhesion, decrease serum lipid levels, and reduce thrombolytic and vasoconstrictor effects of thromboxane A2 (Konno, et al., 1997).

Aspirin. Low-dose aspirin therapy is rational in that it reduces the formation of platelet aggregates and therefore thrombi formation. Aspirin also inhibits vasoconstrictor effects of thromboxane A2. While aspirin is beneficial in stroke prophylaxis and in reducing cardiovascular disease in men, it has not been well studied in women (Antiplatelet Trialists' Collaboration, 1988). In one study, aspirin 325 mg/day, combined with reduction of risk factors for stroke, improved or stabilized cerebral perfusion and neuropsychological performance in patients with mild to moderate multiple infarct dementia (Meyer et al., 1989). Although larger confirmatory studies are needed, low-dose aspirin is usually given to patients with VD who do not have a contraindication to its usage, such as a history of peptic ulcer disease or upper gastrointestinal bleeding.

Ticlopidine. Ticlopidine is a platelet antiaggregant that inhibits the adenosine diphosphate pathway of platelet aggregation. The Ticlopidine Aspirin Stroke Study (TASS) found that ticlopidine (250 mg bid) was more effective than aspirin (650 mg bid) in preventing fatal or nonfatal stroke (Hass et al., 1989). Beneficial effects of ticlopidine were observed in both women and men. Side effects associated with ticlopidine therapy are diarrhea, rash, bleeding, and severe neutropenia. The dermatologic and gastrointestinal side effects of ticlopidine are usually self-limiting. The possibility of neutropenia requires white blood cell monitoring.

Pentoxifylline. One 9-month double-blind placebo-controlled study of pentoxifylline in patients with DSM-III multi-infarct dementia (MID) found some improvement in cognitive and intellectual subscales of standardized assessment instruments as compared with placebo. The dosage of pentoxifylline was 400 mg tid (European Pentoxifylline Multi-Infarct Dementia Study, 1996).

Noncognitive Problems

Much of the research in this area is derived from the post-stroke literature. The general principles of pharmacologic and nonpharmacologic approaches outlined here are also applicable to other forms of dementia.

Post-stroke depression. Major depression has a prevalence rate of 10% in post-stroke patients. In a cross section of patients admitted for an acute stroke, 25% met criteria for major depression (Robinson et al., 1983). If the depressive symptoms are not rigorously limited to the threshold of major depression, the prevalence rate increases to 40% in patients followed for 2 years after a stroke (Robinson et al., 1987). Stroke in the left frontal cortex and basal ganglia are correlated with major depression (Robinson et al., 1984), with the severity of the depressive symptoms being correlated with the proximity of the lesion to the frontal pole (Robinson et al., 1981).

Unrecognized and untreated depressive symptoms have a negative effect on patients' participation and success in rehabilitation and recovery of function. This holds true even after the depression resolves (Parikh et al., 1990). Left hemispheric lesions associated with depression are more often associated with cognitive impairment than right hemispheric lesions (Bolla-Wilson et al., 1989).

An effort must be made to determine whether there are general medical conditions separate from the stroke that are causing the mood symptoms. Antidepressant medications have been found effective in post-stroke depressed patients. Thus, nortriptyline was superior to placebo in a 6-week double-blind placebo-controlled trial. Cautious use of this agent is recommended as there were a high rate of adverse effects, including delirium, syncope, dizziness, and oversedation (Lipsey et al., 1984). Trazadone has also been shown to be effective in a controlled study (Reding et al., 1986). Citalopram, a serotonin selective reuptake inhibitor, demonstrated benefit for post-stroke depression in a 6-week double-blind controlled trial (Andersen et al., 1994). The subgroup of patients who accounted for the difference between groups was mostly composed of later-onset de-

pressed patients (>7 weeks post-stroke). Many patients who develop depression early after a stroke experience spontaneous recovery. Other SSRIs have yet to be investigated in controlled trials.

Post-stroke anxiety. Anxiety seen post-stroke correlates highly with depression. One sample of patients with acute stroke found 27% met criteria for generalized anxiety disorder, with almost 75% having coexisting depressive symptoms (Castillo et al., 1993). This finding underscores the need to consider the diagnosis of depression and treat accordingly in patients who present with post-stroke anxiety. Medical conditions, or substances being taken that may be etiologically related to the anxiety should be identified and eliminated.

There are no systematic controlled pharmacologic trials of anxiety following stroke. Benzodiazepines are commonly utilized to treat anxiety in non-brain-injured patients and have a role in the care of post-stroke patients. Cautious use of short-acting agents that do not have active metabolites is recommended (e.g., lorazepam, oxazepam) to minimize adverse effects such as sedation, ataxia, confusion, and disinhibition. While buspirone may be useful in post-stroke anxiety, the onset of its effect takes several weeks to occur. There is no dependence, sedation, or substantial risk of increased falls with buspirone. Tricyclic antidepressants agents may benefit patients who present with generalized anxiety. Careful titration and monitoring for adverse anticholinergic effects are necessary with no controlled trials available to guide the choice of agent or dose. The SSRIs may be beneficial in some anxiety disorders, although they have not been studied in post-stroke patients. The SSRIs do not have the risk of tolerance, have a low abuse potential, and are useful in treating the comorbid depression that frequently accompanies post-stroke anxiety.

Post-stroke psychosis. Psychosis that occurs following a stroke may be caused by delirium, medication, or a general medical condition. There is a less than 1% prevalence of hallucinations after a stroke (Rabins et al., 1991). The psychosis post-stroke is commonly associated with right hemispheric lesions in the temporoparietal cortex and/or brain atrophy and seizures (Levine and Finklestein, 1982; Rabins et al., 1991).

The general principles of a delirium workup should be followed when determining the cause and choosing the treatment for the psychosis. First, the clinician searches for a general medical condition or consumption of a substance that is etiologically related to the symptoms. Thus, treatment includes dealing with an offending medical illness, removing any offending medications, and symptomatic treatment with an antipsychotic if the psychosis is interfering with functioning or participation in diagnostic testing or therapy.

Antipsychotics. There is a paucity of controlled studies on the use of antipsychotics for post-stroke patients with psychosis. General principles of antipsychotic choice, dosage, and titration are made from treating delirium and psychosis associated with AD. Antipsychotics should be initiated after a thorough review of the cause of psychosis. If the psychosis is interfering with the functioning or compliance with a treatment regimen, the benefit of antipsychotic medication may outweigh the risk. The choice of antipsychotic is based on side effect profile rather than efficacy. If a patient has preexisting parkinsonism, a mid-potency antipsychotic, such as, perphenazine or loxitane, may be started or a newer antipsychotic, such as risperdal, olanzapine, or seroquel, which have a substantially lower risk for extrapyramidal side effects, may be initiated. Caution should be exercised when prescribing antipsychotics that have anticholinergic effects, especially in patients with prostatic hypertrophy, orthostatic hypotension, or urinary retention. The anticholinergic effects of these drugs may also aggravate the cognitive deficits of the patient. When psychosis is associated with agitation, or a patient is unable to swallow, parenteral use of antipsychotic agents may become necessary. Many of the traditional antipsychotics are available in the intramuscular preparation, with some of the higher potency agents available for intravenous administration. Caution should be exercised with intravenous haloperidol as it has been associated with torsade de pointes (Metzger et al., 1993). Many of the newer antipsychotics are not available yet in parenteral form. The risk of tardive dyskinesia, and even the much less common tardive akathisia, should always be considered when prescribing an antipsychotic to a post-stroke patient with psychosis. Periodic attempts should be made to decrease or discontinue the antipsychotic.

Post-stroke mania. The prevalence of mania following stroke is very low, being less than 1% in one study (Robinson et al., 1988). Similar to other noncognitive disorders associated with dementia, a thorough investigation of the general medical condition and current medications is warranted as these may aggravate or cause the mania. Pharmacologic treatment of mania may include valproic acid, carbamazepine, gabapentin, or lithium.

Lithium. The use of lithium in post-stroke mania has not been well studied in a controlled manner. Some reports describe a poor response to lithium in secondary mania (Black et al., 1988). Caution must be exercised in treating post-stroke manic patients with lithium because of its low therapeutic index,

with patients with preexisting brain disease appearing to be more susceptible to the adverse effects. Lithium poisoning may take the form of neurological symptoms such as tremor, ataxia, dysarthria, extrapyramidal signs, cerebellar findings, nystagmus, delirium, or even mania (Nurnberger, 1985). Prior to initiating lithium therapy, an ECG, TSH, electrolytes, CBC, and renal function must be reviewed. A careful review of concurrent medications may reveal potential adverse drug interactions, such as increased lithium levels when given concurrently with certain diuretic agents and NSAIDs. During the course of continuation treatment, serum studies, ECG, and concurrent medications should be periodically reviewed. The serum lithium level should be monitored and, although the literature is not useful in suggesting therapeutic lithium levels in post-stroke manic patients, clinical experience suggests levels in the range of 0.5 to 0.7 mEq/L.

Carbamazepine. There have been no controlled efficacy studies with carbamazepine for post-stroke mania. Some evidence suggests that bipolar patients with associated organic conditions may be more responsive to carbamazepine than lithium (Himmelhoch and Garfinkel, 1986). Before initiation of carbamezepine CBC, platelet count, hepatic function tests, serum sodium, thyroid-stimulating hormone, and ECG should be obtained. Serum levels of other drugs metabolized by the CYP3A4 enzyme should be measured. Carbamazepine induces its own metabolism and therefore serum monitoring of carbamazepine is required for at least 6 months and whenever there is a change of dose or addition of another medication that may potentially interact with the drug. There are no guidelines regarding serum carbamazepine levels and clinical response in post-stroke patients with mania. Accordingly, dosing should be guided by clinical response. Adverse effects of carbamazepine include hyponatremia, bradycardia and atrioventricular block, leukopenia, thrombocytopenia, ataxia, nystagmus, confusion, and sedation. In theory, carbamazepine may be continued in patients with leukopenia as long as the WBC is greater than 3000/mm^3 (Tohen et al., 1995). Carbamazepine may be initiated at less than 100 mg in frail patients by using the liquid preparation. Dose titration should be made slowly as the post-stroke patient is often elderly, with decreased plasma protein resulting in an increased concentration of active drug and a decreased hepatic clearance.

Valproic acid. Valproic acid is another anticonvulsant agent that is used to treat post-stroke mania. However, there are no systematized controlled data to support its utility as a therapeutic agent for this condition. Pretreatment and treatment assessment requires hematologic and hepatic function measures. Potential adverse effects include sedation, ataxia, cognitive impairment, thrombocytopenia, elevation in hepatic transaminase, tremor, gastrointestinal side effects, and hair loss. Potential drug interactions may occur with other drugs that bind to plasma protein. Alopecia may be treated with vitamin supplements containing zinc and selenium. Dosing may continue as long as the WBC is greater than 3000/mm^3 and hepatic enzyme activity does not rise above three times the upper limit of normal. Valproic acid may inhibit its own metabolism and serum levels may increase on a stable dose of the drug. The serum levels of valproic acid that correspond to a beneficial clinical response are not currently identified for post-stroke patients with mania. Administration may be initiated with the liquid preparation at doses below 100 mg in the especially frail patients. Gradual titration may allow for tolerance to occur to the gastrointestinal side effects.

Gabapentin. Gabapentin, which enhances GABAergic activity, is being used to augment the effects of other anticonvulsants. There have been no controlled studies of gabapentin for post-stroke mania. A relatively safe agent, the chief side effect of gabapentin is sedation. There are no significant drug interactions with gabapentin and it does not produce active metabolites.

Others. Benzodiazepines and antipsychotics may also have a place in the management of post-stroke mania. These agents are discussed fully in the context of post-stroke anxiety and post-stroke psychosis.

AIDS DEMENTIA

Clinical Features and Epidemiology

AIDS dementia is characterized by cognitive disturbance, motor disturbance, and behavioral change. The cognitive symptoms present as a subcortical dementia with impaired short- and long-term memory, slowed thought processing, and decreased concentration (Navia et al., 1986). The motor symptoms include gait instability, poor balance, weakness, apraxia, and handwriting changes. Emotional lability, withdrawal, and apathy are common behavioral changes. The cognitive effects of AIDS on children include poor brain growth, developmental disabilities, neurological symptoms, and cognitive impairment (Mintz, 1996). The present discussion focuses on AIDS dementia in adults.

The diagnosis of AIDS dementia is one of exclusion as there is no definitive biologic marker for the disease, except for being HIV positive. Cerebrospinal fluid studies reveal markers of immune activation, pleocytosis, increased protein, and HIV-1 virus (Hollander et al., 1994). Neuroimaging may have an associated role in the diagnosis of AIDS dementia (Goodkin et al., 1997). Based on European epidemiology studies, risk factors for developing AIDS dementia include: increasing age, IV drug abuse, being a gay or bisexual man, and decreased CD4 count. AIDS dementia affects 15 to 20% of AIDS patients during the course of the illness, with the annual incidence being 7% after AIDS diagnosis (Chiesi et al., 1996). There is some evidence that patients who develop AIDS dementia have decreased survival compared to those AIDS patients who do not have dementia (Teira et al., 1996). Progression rates and symptom presentation are variable for AIDS dementia. Patients with AIDS dementia frequently develop psychiatric comorbidities and are sensitive to the potential adverse effects from the medications used to treat these conditions.

Pathologic Mechanisms

The proposed pathogenic mechanisms for AIDS dementia include neurovirulent strains of HIV, neurotoxicity of gp 120, nitric oxide mediation, injury by quinolonic acid, NMDA receptor–mediated damage, free radical mediation, apoptosis, immunologically mediated (cytokines, arachnoic acid metabolites) damage and altered blood-brain barrier permeability (Power and Johnson, 1995; Shi et al., 1996; Cunningham et al., 1997; Dewhurst and Whetter, 1997; Lipton, 1997; Yoshioka and Itoyama, 1997). One model of neuronal injury gaining favor is based on the hypothesis that inflammatory byproducts from the periphery penetrate the blood-brain barrier and overstimulate NMDA receptors. This leads to increasing levels of intracellular calcium that results in the release of glutamatic acid which overstimulates NMDA receptors on nearby neurons (Lipton and Gendleman, 1995). Accordingly, NMDA receptor antagonists and calcium channel blockers may be effective in treating this condition.

Neuroimaging

Structural and functional neuroimaging techniques are utilized to assist with diagnosis, prognosis, and therapeutics in AIDS dementia. An association has been demonstrated between HIV infection severity and atrophy of the basal ganglia, white matter lesions, and generalized atrophy on MRI or CT. However, there is a poor correlation between these measures and histopathologic findings. PET, SPECT, and magnetic resonance spectroscopy (MRS), with improved sensitivity, reveal basal ganglia abnormalities, bloodflow disturbance, and metabolite changes in HIV patients who do not have clinical evidence of infection (Kim et al., 1996). MRS may also play a role in the future in predicting responsiveness to certain pharmacotherapies (Salvan et al., 1997).

Evaluation

As with the management of other dementing disorders, it is important to search for aggravating medical conditions, such as abnormal thyroid status, electrolyte abnormalities, hematologic changes, and any infections, when AIDS dementia is suspected. Because cognitive impairment may be aggravated by the medications used to treat AIDS, the medication list requires careful review. The luxury of removing "nonessential" medications may be more limited in AIDS dementia since continuous dosing of antivirals and protease inhibitors may be necessary to enhance survival (Rabkin et al., 1997). Low vitamin B_{12} levels are common in AIDS patients. Recognition of this problem is imperative since vitamin supplementation may partially treat some of the cognitive deficits (Herzlich et al., 1993).

Pharmacologic Management

The literature supports the use of zidovidine, an antiviral, for AIDS dementia. One multicenter double-blind placebo-controlled study of 40 subjects with AIDS dementia demonstrated superiority of zidovidine 2000 mg/day to placebo after 16 weeks and the beneficial effects remained through a 16-week open-label extension (Sidtis et al., 1993). Zidovidine therapy is the current standard for AIDS patients with and without AIDS dementia since the medication, at high doses, may offer some protection against the development of AIDS dementia at 6 months to 1 year. The higher doses of zidovidine are limited by intolerable side effects in some patients (Melton et al., 1997).

The combination of zidovidine and didanosine was tested in an alternating and simultaneous dosing methodology for AIDS dementia. The randomized, but not blinded, trial demonstrated improvements in memory and selective attention measures in both regimens at 12 weeks. The improvements were more robust in patients with cognitive impairment at entry (Brouwers et al., 1997). In addition to zidovudine and didanosine, other reverse transcriptase inhibitors that are currently available are lamivudine, strvudine, and zalitabine. There are no clinical trial data with these other antivirals for AIDS dementia. Protease inhibitors, available as adjunctive therapy for HIV infection, have not been studied for efficacy in AIDS dementia.

Investigational Therapeutics

Ateverdine. Ateverdine is a non-nucleoside reverse transcriptase inhibitor that was tested in an open-label study in ten patients who failed or were intolerant to didanosine or zidovidine. The dose given was 1800 mg in divided doses over 12 weeks. Of the five patients who completed the study, 4 responded based on neuropsychological testing or SPECT. The drug was well tolerated (Brew et al., 1996). Further investigation of this compound is underway.

Pentoxyfylline. Pentoxyfylline decreases TNF α-activity and may have a role in treating AIDS or AIDS dementia, although controlled trials with this agent are lacking (Dezube et al., 1993).

NMDA receptor antagonists. Memantine, a congener of amantadine, is an NMDA receptor antagonist that has demonstrated a cytoprotective effects in cortical cell cultures infected with the HIV-1 coat protein, gp 120. Trials in laboratory animals and humans are needed (Muller et al., 1992). Likewise, while nitroglycerin may protect neurons from overstimulation of NMDA receptors, controlled studies have not been performed to assess its efficacy in this regard (Lipton, 1994).

Peptide T. Peptide T is an octapeptide under investigation for treatment of AIDS dementia. One patient receiving peptide T for 12 weeks had a functional change on FDG-PET, suggesting a possible role for further functional neuroimaging in evaluating the response to pharmacologic treatment for AIDS dementia (Villemagne et al., 1996). Clinical studies with peptide T are continuing (Bridge et al., 1991).

Nimodipine. Nimodipine is a calcium channel blocker that crosses the blood-brain barrier. Although there have been no clinical trials with nimodipine in AIDS dementia, it may attenuate neuronal damage by reducing the response to NMDA receptor stimulation by glutamic acid in brain.

OPC 14117. OPC-14117 is a lipophilic antioxidant that scavenges superoxide anion radicals. A double-blind, controlled, randomized clinical trial revealed that 240 mg/day of OPC-14117 is tolerated as well as placebo in a group of AIDS dementia patients (The Dana Consortium of HIV Dementia and Related Cognitive Disorders, 1997).

Behavioral Management

Common behavioral disturbances associated with AIDS dementia are mood symptoms (depressive, manic, or mixed), anxiety, apathy, anergy, demoralization, psychosis, insomnia, sleep-wake disturbance, and wandering. The approach to management involves concurrent pharmacologic and nonpharmacologic therapies after a thorough investigation and reversal of any aggravating comorbidities that may be contributing to the problem behavior. The general approaches and principles of treatment of the noncognitive disturbances in AIDS dementia are similar to those outlined for the noncognitive disturbances associated with AD.

Dementia with Lewy Bodies

Dementia with Lewy bodies (DLB) is another common form of dementia. The clinical features of this condition include a progressive decline in memory, language, praxis, and reasoning. Distinguishing clinical characteristics of DLB may include fluctuation in mental status with acute confusional states and hallucinations, most commonly visual, and increased sensitivity to antipsychotics. DLB is more common in men than women, and the progression may be more rapid than for AD.

DLB encompasses the pathologic diseases of Parkinson's disease (PD) with or without AD pathology, cortical Lewy bodies with plaques and cortical Lewy bodies without any concomitant AD pathology (Cummings, 1995). Dementia with Lewy bodies, a term proposed at the 1995 International Workshop on Lewy Body dementia, includes Lewy body dementia, diffuse Lewy body disease, senile dementia of the Lewy body type, and the Lewy body variant of Alzheimer's disease (McKeith et al., 1996).

Fifteen to 25% of elderly demented patients have cortical Lewy bodies, the defining pathologic characteristic of DLB (McKeith et al., 1996). Pathologic studies verifying the clinical diagnosis of AD found that DLB was often misdiagnosed clinically as AD (Galasko et al., 1994).

Differentiating DLB from AD and PD

APOE-ε4 may be a risk factor for DLB (Katzman et al., 1995). The prevalence of APOE-ε4 genotype in DLB is intermediate between AD and PD, suggesting that DLB may be the clinical co-occurrence of AD and PD (Hardy et al., 1994). The presence of APOE-ε4 does not appear to be altered in DLB (Morris et al., 1996).

Age at dementia onset is lower and presentation of parkinsonism that develops into a dementia is more common for patients with DLB (with no AD pathology) compared with patients with both DLB and AD pathology (Cercy et al., 1997). Patients with DLB perform worse on praxis testing, better on recall tests (Walker et al., 1997), and have increased fluctuation in consciousness compared with AD patients (Graham et al., 1997). Visual hallucinations are more common in DLB than AD, although this clinical finding has low sensitivity as a distinguishing characteristic (Ala et al., 1997). Lower cerebrospinal fluid homovanillic acid levels have been reported in DLB patients as compared with AD patients, probably reflecting alteration in dopamine metabolism (Weiner et al., 1996). DLB patients have a loss of cells in the substantia nigra that produce dopamine, similar to what is seen with PD patients.

The clinical severity of dementia in AD and DLB patients is correlated with Lewy body count, loss of choline acetyltransferase activity, neurofibrillary tangle, and neuritic plaque load. In contrast to AD patients, however, DLB patients do not demonstrate a correlation between the severity of clinical dementia and neurofibrillary tangle burden in the neocortex or antisynaptophysin activity, a measure of synaptic density (Samuel et al., 1997). DLB patients are less likely to have resting tremor or to present with a lateralized parkinsonism, but more likely to have more severe rigidity compared with PD patients (Gnanalingham et al., 1997).

Management of Parkinsonism

Antiparkinsonian drugs carry a risk of inducing psychosis in DLB patients. If the parkinsonism is interfering with functioning, the clinician may elect to treat the rigidity with baclofen (Moutoussis and Or-rell, 1996), or other parkinsonian features with L-dopa, although published experience with this approach is limited (Geroldi et al., 1997).

Management of Psychosis

If pharmacologic treatment is initiated for the hallucinations or delusions associated with DLB, consideration should be given to the fact these patients are known to be highly sensitive to the effects of antipsychotics. Traditional antipsychotics should be initiated at a lower dose, and titrated more slowly, in DLB patients than is the case with others. Clozapine may have a role in treating psychosis in DLB patients (Chacko et al., 1993); however, serum monitoring for hematologic abnormalities is required. Risperdone has been useful in treating psychosis in one case series (Allen et al., 1995), but not in another (McKeith et al., 1995). Olanzapine reduced psychosis in nondemented Parkinson's disease patients (Wolters et al., 1996), but response to olanzapine in DLB patients with psychosis has not yet been reported. To date there have been no controlled clinical trials of remoxipride, zotepine, mianserin, and ondansetron for psychosis in DLB.

Management of Depression

Up to 50% of DLB patients develop depression (Klatka et al., 1996). This rate is about five times greater than in AD patients, but approximates that found in PD. Depression is a treatable source of increased morbidity, utilization of health care services, functional impairment, and mortality (NIH Consensus Development Conference Statement, 1993; Samuels et al., 1996b). The goals in treating depression in demented patients are to improve cognition and diminish apathy (American Psychiatric Association, 1997).

Pharmacotherapy

The selection of antidepressants is based on side effect profile since superior efficacy has not been demonstrated for any one agent in DLB patients who are depressed. The APA Practice Guideline for Major Depression in Adults provides a useful summary of the literature on the efficacy of pharmacologic treatments for depression (American Psychiatric Association, 1993). Consideration should be given to anticholinergic effects, potential for drug interactions, sedation, and autonomic changes induced by antidepressants.

Electroconvulsive Therapy

There have been no clinical trials on the efficacy of electroconvulsive therapy (ECT) for the treatment of depression associated with DLB. However, ECT has been shown effective in treating the depression and improving the motor component in Parkinson's disease (Douyon et al., 1989) and the APA Practice Guidelines for Dementia endorse its use for treating depression associated with dementia (American Psychiatric Association, 1997). Thus, ECT should be considered for DLB patients with accompanying depression. Electrode placement, stimulus, and frequency of treatment should be adjusted to minimize cognitive side effects.

Cholinergic Changes in DLB

Although neocortical choline acetyltransferase levels are lower in neuropathologically confirmed DLB patients than AD patients, DLB patients sometimes respond to tacrine, a cholinesterase inhibitor (Perry et al., 1994). Since there are no established treatment modalities for the cognitive deficits associated with DLB, a trial with a cholinesterase inhibitor should be attempted with those patients having mild to moderate dementia.

Future Treatment Modalities for DLB

The common element of DLB pathology is the presence of Lewy bodies in the cerebral cortex and a clinical dementia. Since the cognitive decline in DLB does not appear due to Lewy bodies alone, therapeutic interventions must also address the associated plaques, tangles, or PD pathology. As criteria become more uniform in diagnosing DLB, clinical trials should be performed to determine whether some of the therapeutic agents being developed for the treatment of AD and PD will also modify the progression of DLB. Future treatments for DLB may include neurotransmitter replacement therapy, antioxidants, neuroprotective agents, drugs that interfere with amyloid metabolism, tau phosphorylation, tangle formation, APOE-ε4 gene products, anti-inflammatory agents, and glutamic acid receptor agonists.

DELIRIUM

Definition and Clinical Description

Delirium is defined in DSM-IV as "a disturbance in consciousness and a change in cognition that develops over a short period of time" (American Psychiatric Association, DSM-IV, p. 123). Patients with delirium are easily distractable, unable to sustain focused attention, have memory impairment, disorientation and aphasia. These cognitive deficits may be difficult to assess because of the inability of the patient to concentrate and symptom fluctuation over short time periods. Associated symptoms include affective disturbance, psychomotor agitation or retardation and perceptual disturbances such as illusions, hallucinations, or misinterpretations. Affective symptoms often fluctuate during the course of delirium and may include anxiety, fear, apathy, anger, euphoria, dysphoria, and irritability, all within short time periods. The perceptual changes are most frequently visual, but also occur in the auditory, tactile, or olfactory senses. These sensory problems, often disturbing to the patient, have been described as fragmented, poorly organized, dream, or nightmare-like. Additionally, confusion may lead to behavioral manifestations such as pulling at intravenous lines or other tubes.

Delirious patients are categorized on the basis of alertness and psychomotor activity. The hyperactive subtype is psychomotorly active, hypervigilant, restless, excitable, with loud or pressured speech, whereas the hypoactive subtype is psychomotorly slowed, quiet, withdrawn, with reduced alertness and decreased speech production. The loud patient gains the attention of others and is more likely to be diagnosed with delirium than the quiet patient who is not disturbing other patients or staff. Because delirium carries an increased risk of morbidity and mortality, the quietly delirious patient needs to be identified and appropriately treated. A concern with the loud, hyperactive delirious patient is the increased use of chemical or mechanical restraint with a risk that an appropriate diagnostic evaluation is neglected.

The etiology of a delirium may not be accurately assessed by activity level. Patients often present with alternating activity levels and may not fall neatly into one category. Thus, hyperactivity is commonly associated with anticholinergic toxicity, alcohol withdrawal, and hyperthyroidism, whereas hypoactivity is common in hepatic encephalopathy. This descriptive subtyping does not correspond reliably with EEG activity, cerebral blood flow, or ratings of fluctuations of consciousness. Additional subtypes of delirium include acute versus chronic, cortical versus subcortical, anterior versus posterior cortical, right versus left cortical, and psychotic versus nonpsychotic. These divisions are not universally accepted in the literature. The DSM-IV divides deliriums on the basis of etiology (Tables 9-10 through 9-13).

Table 9-10
Criteria for Delirium

A. Disturbance of consciousness (i.e., reduced clarity of awareness of the environment) with reduced ability to focus, sustain, or shift attention

B. A change in cognition (such as memory deficit, disorientation, language disturbance) or the development of a perceptual disturbance that is not better accounted for by a preexisting, established, or evolving dementia

C. The disturbance develops over a short period of time (usually hours to days) and tends to fluctuate during the course of the day

D. There is evidence from the history, physical examination, or laboratory findings that the disturbance is caused by the direct physiologic consequences of a general medical condition

SOURCE Adapted from American Psychiatric Association, 1994 (DSM-IV).

Table 9-11
Criteria for Substance Intoxication Delirium

A. Disturbance of consciousness (i.e., reduced clarity of awareness of the environment) with reduced ability to focus, sustain, or shift attention

B. A change in cognition (such as memory deficit, disorientation, language disturbance) or the development of a perceptual disturbance that is not better accounted for by a preexisting, established, or evolving dementia

C. The disturbance develops over a short period of time (usually hours to days) and tends to fluctuate during the course of the day

D. There is evidence from the history, physical examination, or laboratory findings of either (1) or (2):
  1. The symptoms in Criteria A and B developed during substance intoxication
  2. Medication use is etiologically related to the disturbance

SOURCE Adapted from American Psychiatric Association, 1994 (DSM-IV).

Significance

Delirium is a significant public health concern since this common syndrome is associated with increased morbidity and mortality. Patients with delirium remain in the hospital longer and are more commonly discharged to long-term care facilities. Behavioral manifestations of delirium may interfere with treatment compliance and are often precipitants for psychiatric consultation.

Epidemiology

In hospitalized inpatients, delirium has an incidence of 4 to 10% and a prevalence of 11 to 16% (Levkoff et al., 1991). One study found the highest prevalence of postoperative delirium in hip fracture (28–44%), followed by elective joint replacement (26%) and myocardial revascularization (6.8%) (Levkoff et al., 1991). Prevalence rates vary depending on patient and hospital characteristics. For example, delirium occurs more commonly in hospitals that perform complex surgical procedures or are tertiary referral centers for severely ill patients. Areas where AIDS is more common will have a higher prevalence rate of delirium related to AIDS-related illness or treatment. Substance abuse, another contributor to delirium, varies in community prevalence rates and substance choice and age predisposes patients to delirium. Delirium is present in 38.5% of patients over age 65 who are admitted to the hospital (Liptzin et al., 1991). Delirium was present in 1.1% of those in the community over age 55 in the Eastern Baltimore Mental Health Survey (Folstein MF et al., 1991).

Similarly, patients admitted to the hospital from a long-term care facility have a higher prevalence (64.9%) than patients admitted from the general community (24.2%) (Levkoff et al., 1991). This is not

Table 9-12
Criteria for Substance Withdrawal Delirium

A. Disturbance of consciousness (i.e., reduced clarity of awareness of the environment) with reduced ability to focus, sustain, or shift attention

B. A change in cognition (such as memory deficit, disorientation, language disturbance) or the development of a perceptual disturbance that is not better accounted for by a preexisting, established, or evolving dementia

C. The disturbance develops over a short period of time (usually hours to days) and tends to fluctuate during the course of the day

D. There is evidence from the history, physical examination, or laboratory findings that the symptoms in Criteria A and B developed during, or shortly after, a withdrawal syndrome

SOURCE Adapted from American Psychiatric Association, 1994 (DSM-IV).

Table 9-13
Criteria for Delirium Due to Multiple Etiologies

A. Disturbance of consciousness (i.e., reduced clarity of awareness of the environment) with reduced ability to focus, sustain, or shift attention

B. A change in cognition (such as memory deficit, disorientation, language disturbance) or the development of a perceptual disturbance that is not better accounted for by a preexisting, established, or evolving dementia

C. The disturbance develops over a short period of time (usually hours to days) and tends to fluctuate during the course of the day

D. There is evidence from the history, physical examination, or laboratory findings that the delirium has more than one etiology (e.g., more than one etiologic general medical condition, a general medical condition plus substance intoxication or medication side effect)

SOURCE Adapted from American Psychiatric Association, 1994 (DSM-IV).

surprising since the long-term care patients were older and more seriously ill. Changes in the pharmacokinetic and pharmacodynamic responses to drugs with age may explain, in part, the higher incidence of delirium in the elderly.

Risk Factors

Certain factors place patients at increased risk for developing delirium. Among these are preexisting cognitive impairment or brain injury, being old or very young, and medical comorbidity. In an attempt to quantify risk, one study of hospitalized inpatients found an 80% chance of developing delirium if there was one of the following: urinary tract infection (UTI) at any time during hospitalization; low albumin on admission and no UTI; increased WBC on admission but normal albumin and no UTI; proteinuria on admission but normal WBC; normal albumin and no UTI (Levkoff et al., 1991). Patients who have a history of delirium, alcohol dependence, cancer, diabetes, sensory impairment, or AIDS are at increased risk for developing delirium. Patient age may assist the clinician in determining the etiology of the delirium, with the very young and very old being more at risk for developing delirium from medical illnesses or toxic drug effects. Adolescents are at increased risk of abusing drugs and in sustaining traumatic head injury. Adult patients are at risk for cardiovascular, respiratory, and neoplastic disease and geriatric patients at risk for delirium superimposed on a dementing illness.

Course and Outcome

About half of the patients who develop delirium in the hospital will do so by the third hospital day (Bowman et al., 1992; Levkoff et al., 1994) and it may not completely resolve by the time of hospital discharge. Thus, one of six patients may have symptoms at 6 months after hospital discharge (Levkoff et al., 1992) and at 2 years follow-up, with the mortality risk and loss of functional independence in the community being increased in these subjects (Francis and Kapoor, 1992).

Evaluation

The diagnosis of a delirium is based on examination of the patient over a sufficient period of time so that alterations in the levels of consciousness and disturbances in cognition may be detected. One bedside examination for assessing orientation, memory, and concentration is the Short Orientation-Memory-Concentration Test of Cognitive Impairment (Katzman et al., 1983). Orientation is assessed by asking the patient's name, location, date, and time of day. To assess short-term memory, the patient is asked to register a name and address that is repeated until it can be recalled by the patient. Concentration is tested by having the patient count from 20 to 1 backwards followed by reciting the months of the year backwards. Finally, the patient is asked to recall the name and address. Scores are based on the number of errors. This examination, or selected portions of it, may be repeated several times a day and over several days to determine whether there are fluctuation in performance. The Mini Mental State Exam (MMSE) may also be used at the bedside to assess orientation, registration, concentration, recall, praxis, and the ability to name, repeat, and follow commands (Folstein et al., 1975) (Tables 9-14 and 9-15). Many instruments have been used to screen and diagnose delirium, although they suffer from limitations in reliability, validity, and ease of use. Many focus on cognition at the expense of noncognitive symptoms in delirium (Smith et al., 1994).

Because the delirious patient may not be a reliable informant the clinician should attempt to obtain corroborating information regarding premorbid course and presenting symptoms from family, friends, and clinical staff. Nursing progress notes documenting behavioral changes may provide useful clues about sleep duration and quality, confusion and perceptual disturbances.

Sleep disturbance is common among individuals with delirium, with the sleep-wake cycle often being out of synchronicity. Patients may demonstrate increased startle when awoken and frequently recount vivid dreams and nightmares. Sundowning, the worsening of a behavioral disturbance at night, is another frequent manifestation of delirium. While the prevalence of sundowning has not been studied in the hospital, it is present in one of eight patients over 60 years of age in the nursing home setting (Evans, 1987).

Perceptual disturbances may be assessed by allowing the patient to answer open-ended questions about how they are treated by others and whether any unusual events have occurred. This may be followed by more structured questions about hallucinations, such as, "Sometimes when people have this type of illness, their mind can play tricks on them. They can hear voices (or see things) that they do not usually hear (or see). Is this happening to you?" A patient picking at bedclothes or sheets may be experiencing hallucinations or illusions. At times, patients will be carrying on a conversation with themselves or turning their heads or moving their eyes, apparently responding to internal stimuli.

Mood disturbances such as depression may be assessed with the Hamilton Depression Scale (HAM-D) (Hamilton et al., 1969) or the Geriatric Depression Scale (GDS) (Yesavage et al., 1982).

Table 9-14
Short Memory-Orientation-Concentration Test

Items		Maximum error		Score		Weight
1	What *year* is it now?	1	___ ×	4	=	___
2	What *month* is it now?	1	___ ×	3	=	___
	(Memory phrase) Repeat this phrase after me: John Brown, 42 Market Street, Chicago					
3	About what *time* is it? (within 1 hour)	1	___ ×	3	=	___
4	*Count* backward 20 to 1	2	___ ×	2	=	___
5	Say the months in reverse order	2	___ ×	2	=	___
6	Repeat the memory phrase	5	___ ×	2	=	___

SOURCE Adapted from Katzman et al., 1983.

Table 9-15

Mini Mental State Exam

Items	Score
Orientation	
What is today's date?	____
What is the year?	____
What is the month?	____
What day is today?	____
What season is it?	____
What is the name of this hospital (clinic, place)?	____
What floor are we on?	____
What town or city are we in?	____
What county (district, borough, area) are we in?	____
What state are we in?	____
Immediate recall	
Ball	____
Flag	____
Tree	____
Attention and calculation	
D	____
L	____
R	____
O	____
W	____
Delayed recall	
Ball	____
Flag	____
Tree	____
Language	
Show the patient a wrist watch and ask to name it	____
Repeat for pencil	____
Ask the patient to repeat "No ifs, ands, or buts"	____
Take paper in right hand	____
Fold paper in half	____
Put paper on floor	____
"Close your eyes"	____
Write complete sentence	____
Draw intersecting pentagons	____

SOURCE Adapted from Folstein MF, Folstein SE, McHugh PR. Mini-mental state: a practical method for grading the cognitive state of patients for the clinician. *J Psychiatr Res* 1975;12:189–198.

The HAM-D is a clinician-based rating of various symptoms of depression. The GDS is a patient-centered instrument that is based on self-reported symptoms. The GDS does not include the overlapping symptoms that may be significantly influenced by medical illness, such as sleep and appetite disturbance. Manic symptoms may be assessed with the Young Mania rating scale (Young et al., 1978). One advantage of using a standardized scale as part of the evaluation is the improved validity and reliability of the resource as compared with the bedside clinical examination alone. Moreover, these scales are more objective than the bedside examination alone, yielding a numerical score. As a complement to the clinical exam, the scores may be followed over time to assess whether a treatment approach is effective.

Pathophysiology

Although delirium has been described in the medical literature for at least 2,500 years, the pathophysiology of the syndrome is not understood, although several theories have been proposed.

Neurochemical Changes

Because the cholinergic system is involved in attention, arousal, memory, and REM sleep, a reduction in cholinergic function has been implicated in the pathophysiology of delirium. Moreover, anticholinergic drugs impair memory and concentration and are associated with delirium and the serum levels of anticholinergic drugs increase with delirium and decrease when it resolves. When atropine is administered to laboratory animals it causes behavioral and EEG changes, supporting an important cholinergic role in delirium. Anticholinergic cognitive impairment may be reduced with the acetylcholinesterase inhibitors physostigmine, donepezil or ENA-713 (see dementia section) (Milam and Bennett, 1987).

The dopaminergic system may also play a role in the pathogenesis of delirium. Antipsychotic agents decrease dopamine and provide symptomatic relief in delirious patients. Agents that increase dopamine such as sinemet, buproprion, and amantadine, cause delirium as a side effect. Hypoxia, which can also induce delirium, increases extracellular dopamine.

Cerebrospinal fluid somatostatin-like reactivity and beta endorphin are decreased in delirious patients as ompared to age-matched controls. This decrease in protein concentration persisted at 1 year follow up. A potential confounding factor is that these patients had some degree of dementia that may have better accounted for the decreased CSF levels of beta endorphin and somatostatin.

Neuronal Injury

Alterations in oxidative metabolism may result in neuronal injury. In one report, EEG findings in delirium were reversed when treating hypoxic patients with oxygen, hypoglycemic patients with glucose, and anemic patients with transfusions (Engel et al., 1945). Further studies entailing more direct measures of oxidative metabolism have yet to be performed. Hypoxia and hypoxemia decrease the synthesis and release of acetylcholine, possibly explaining how alteration in oxidative metabolism contributes to delirium.

Modifications in glutamic acid neurotransmission in brain may be involved in apoptosis and neuronal injury. Thus, excessive activation of NMDA receptors causes cell death and phencyclidine may produce delirium by blocking this receptor. Ketamine, which also blocks the NMDA receptor, alters levels of consciousness. Future therapeutic agents for delirium, such as glutamic acid receptor agonists, may target the NMDA receptor.

Damage to the blood-brain barrier may result in neuronal injury and delirium. Animal studies following the intraventricular administration of interleukin-1 revealed clinical and EEG manifestations of delirium. Delirium is common in patients receiving chemotherapy with interleukin-2, lymphokine-activated killer cells, or α-interferon. A proposed mechanism involves damage to capillary endothelia that may disrupt the blood-brain barrier.

The delirium associated with hepatic encephalopathy may give clues to the pathogenesis of the condition (Riordan et al., 1997). These include accumulation of unmetabolized ammonia, production of false neurotransmitters, activation of GABA receptors, changes in cerebral metabolism, and an alteration of Na^+/K^+-ATPase activity. Other mechanisms include deposition of mangenese in the basal ganglia, zinc deficiency, and altered activity of the urea-cycle enzymes. The most successful approaches for treating hepatic encephalopathy entail increasing ammonia metabolism or decreasing ammonia production.

Causes of Delirium

The etiology of delirium is based on a clinician interpretation of available data (Figure 9-2). The common categories that should be systematically reviewed as potential causes include infections, metabolic or endocrine disorders, traumatic, nutritional or environmental insults, neoplastia, and medication or substance abuse. The DSM-IV divides the causes of delirium into general medical conditions, substance intoxication or withdrawal, and multiple etiologies. Most frequently, there are many aggravating factors that contribute to a delirium. Not all causes of delirium are reversible or even known.

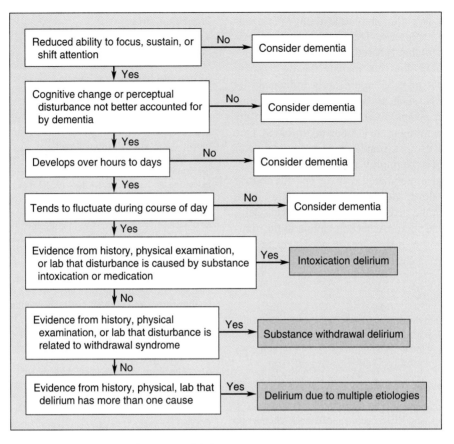

Figure 9–2. *Making a diagnosis of delirium.*

Substance Intoxication and Withdrawal-Induced Delirium

The diagnosis of a substance-induced delirium is made when a medication or other chemical agent is thought to be etiologically related to the conditon. The goal of treatment is to remove the offending agent. The responsible substance may be determined from clinical history, physical exam, and laboratory tests, such as a toxicology screen. Familiarity with the common toxic syndromes is useful as it may guide the investigation to include screening for additional agents. Assistance is available through the local Poison Control Center that has a database describing responses to most prescription and nonprescription agents, herbs, chemicals, and plants. Once

the offending agent is identified, appropriate treatment may be initiated. Established procedures are available for the treatment of overdose of substances such as acetaminophen, aspirin, organic solvents, ethylene glycol, opioids, benzodiazepines, barbiturates, and anticholinergic agents (Goldfrank et al., 1994). Familiarity with common substances of abuse as delirium-inducing agents is also recommended. These include cocaine, phencylodine, heroin, alcohol, nitrous oxide, speed, marijuana, and ecstasy. Opioid-induced delirium may be reversed with naloxone, an opioid receptor antagonist. The effects are often temporary and may precipitate drug withdrawal. Patients who abuse opioids may be at risk of HIV infection from sharing needles or from having sex while delirious or intoxicated.

Benzodiazepine intoxication may precipitate a delirium. In addition to supportive measures, the benzodiazepine receptor antagonist flumenezil may be helpful. Precautions must be taken to guard against withdrawal in the case of benzodiazepines, alcohol, or opioid overdose since withdrawal may cause delirium itself. The treatment entails controlled detoxification to prevent a worsening of the delirium or even death from withdrawal.

Alcohol and benzodiazepine withdrawal are treated by replacing the offending agent with a benzodiazepine and gradually reducing the dosage of the medication. The dose of benzodiazepine should be titrated to prevent autonomic hyperactivity. In addition, thiamine, folate, and multiple vitamins are administered to patients in alcohol withdrawal. Benzodiazepine detoxification is often performed at a slower rate than alcohol detoxification. Opioid withdrawal presents with flulike symptoms and may be accompanied by delirium. Gradual tapering of the opioid, or replacement with a longer-acting opioid, such as methadone, may be successful. The treatment of substance abuse and dependence also has a non-pharmacologic component such as the 12-step programs cited by Alcoholics Anonymous and Narcotics Anonymous.

Laboratory Workup

Laboratory data assist in determining the etiology of the delirium (Table 9-16). After a thorough history and careful physical examination, serum studies to be considered include: CBC with differential; electrolytes; renal and liver function tests; glucose; thyroid studies; RPR; HIV antibody; calcium; magnesium; folate; B_{12} and sedimentation rate. Urinalysis and urine toxicology may also be helpful as may arterial blood gas, chest x-ray, and ECG. In selective cases, an EEG, lumbar puncture, body fluid cultures, and neuroimaging may be necessary. There is no general panel of tests that will consistently determine the etiology of a delirium. While a broadly cast net will yield more information, it is more costly. The primary care physician may choose to involve consultants to assist in determining the appropriate diagnostic workup and optimal treatment.

Table 9-16

Suggested Laboratory Workup for Delirium

CBC with differential
Electrolytes
Renal function
Liver function
Glucose
Thyroid function
RPR
HIV
Ca
Mg
Folate
B_{12}
ESR
Urinalysis
Urine toxicology
ABG
Chest x-ray
ECG
EEG
LP
Neuroimaging

Diagnostic Tools

EEG. The EEG may have utility as a diagnostic tool for delirium. Over 50 years ago, Romano and Engel found a correlation between decreased arousal and background frequency and disorganization of the EEG (Romano and Engel, 1944). Later they proposed the expression "acute brain failure" to describe what is now called delirium. Quantitative EEG has been used to distinguish delirium from dementia in elderly subjects with an unclear differential diagnosis. An increase in the amount of theta activity correctly classified delirium 89% of the time, with only 6% falsely classified as having a dementia (Jacobson et al. 1993).

Brain imaging. MRI has revealed structural lesions in the basal ganglia of patients taking antidepressants who were more likely to develop delirium

(Figiel et al., 1989). Moderate to severe white matter lesions have also been identified in patients who developed delirium during a course of electroconvulsive therapy (Figiel et al., 1990). A CT scan revealed focal changes in the association areas of the right hemisphere, cortical atrophy, and ventricular dilatation as being more common in patients who developed delirium as compared with a control group (Kaponen et al., 1989). Case reports using SPECT describe patients with potential causes of delirium such as hypoxic brain injury, alcohol withdrawal, and postcardiotomy (Caspari et al., 1993; Doyle and Warden, 1996; Rupright et al., 1996).

Differential Diagnosis

The DSM-IV divides deliriums on the basis of etiology. The differential diagnosis for delirium is the differential diagnosis for psychosis. This includes dementia, schizophrenia, mood disorder with psychosis, general medical conditions, substance intoxication, and substance withdrawal. Often the causes of a delirium are multifactorial.

Distinguishing Dementia from Delirium

Memory impairment is common to both dementia and delirium, however, a patient with early dementia is usually alert without fluctuations in levels of consciousness. Because the patient with dementia is susceptible to superimposed delirium, alterations in levels of attention and concentration, combined with cognitive impairment, should not be attributed solely to the natural history of a dementing illness. In fact, patients with dementia should be carefully assessed for delirium. Often these patients are unable to communicate the acute discomfort that may occur with a worsening of a chronic medical condition or the development of acute symptoms of an infection. Patients with dementia and behavioral disturbances may have a delirium that explains the alteration in their behavioral state. Physical examination, serum and urine studies, chest x-ray, and ECG should be considered as the onset of the delirium may reflect a serious intercurrent medical illness. In addition, careful review may identify nonessential medications

used to treat either the comorbid medical illnesses or the behavioral disturbances associated with the dementia. These medications may actually be causing the delirium.

Some cases of delirium appear to be harbingers for dementia, or may allow for the recognition of a cognitive impairment that was previously unnoticed. The brief time period within which delirium develops differentiates it from dementia (Table 9-17).

Schizophrenia

The medical history will often assist in differentiating delirium from schizophrenia or schizophreniform psychosis. For example, in delirium the inability to appropriately maintain and shift attention differentiates from schizophrenia and memory problems and disorientation are usually absent in schizophrenia. There is a subset of schizophrenic patients with dementing illness, with the differential points discussed earlier being applicable when considering these patients. In delirium, current medications, concurrent medical illness, chemical intoxication, or withdrawal often assist in distinguishing delirium from schizophrenia. The delusions in delirium are usually not as bizarre or as well-systematized as in schizophrenia. However, schizophrenia and delirium are not mutually exclusive since schizophrenics may develop a superimposed delirium.

Antipsychotics used to treat schizophrenia may cause delirium. Adverse effects of antipsychotics that are associated with delirium include neuroleptic malignant syndrome (NMS), which constitutes a medical emergency, and akathisia, a subjective feeling of restlessness with frequent psychomotor agitation. Features of NMS include fever, rigidity, autonomic hyperactivity, increased CPK, and leukocytosis. Additionally, many antipsychotics possess anticholinergic effects that may contribute to delirium.

Mood Disorders with Psychosis

Mood disorders such as depression or mania with psychosis may be confused with delirium. It is important to differentiate mood disturbance with psychotic features from delirium because of the differing

Table 9-17
Differential Diagnosis of Delirium and Dementia

Feature	Delirium	Dementia
Onset	Acute, often at night	Insidious
Course	Fluctuating, with lucid intervals during the day; worse at night	Stable over the course of the day
Duration	Hours to weeks	Months or years
Awareness	Reduced	Clear
Alertness	Abnormally low or high	Usually normal
Attention	Lacks direction and sensitivity; distractibility; fluctuation over the course of the day	Relatively unaffected
Orientation	Usually impaired for time; tendency to mistake unfamiliar for familiar places and persons	Often impaired
Memory	Immediate and recent impaired	Recent and remote impaired
Thinking	Disorganized	Impoverished
Perception	Illusions and hallucinations, usually visual and common	Often absent
Speech	Incoherent, hesitant, slow, or rapid	Difficulty in finding words
Sleep-wake cycle	Always disrupted	Fragmented sleep
Physical illness or drug toxicity	Either or both present	Often absent, especially in Alzheimer's disease

SOURCE Adapted from Lipowski ZJ: *Delirium: Acute Confusional State.* New York, Oxford University Press, 1990, 192.

prognosis and treatments and an unrecognized and untreated depression is associated with increased morbidity, disability, utilization of health resources, and mortality (Samuels et al., 1996b; Lebowitz et al., 1997). Mania is also associated with disability and morbidity (Rice and Miller, 1995). The mood component is not as predominant in delirium as in the mood disorders, although dysphoria, expansive mood, or mood lability may be associated with delirium. Patients with mood disorders more frequently have a history of mood disturbance. The theme of the psychosis in mood disturbances is often consistent with depression or mania including delusions of guilt, death, or worthlessness for depression, and grandiose delusions in mania. In contrast, the delusions in delirium are usually more fragmented. Persistence of mood abnormalities is more common in mood disturbance than delirium. Disruption in attention and the cognitive disturbance helps differentiate delirium from mood disorders with psychosis. Careful cognitive examination should aid in properly diagnosing either disorder. Depression with psychosis is ideally treated with antidepressants and antipsychotics or ECT. Bipolar patients who are manic with psychosis are treated with a mood stabilizer, an antipsychotic, or ECT. A delirium that is misidentified as a mood disorder with psychosis will often worsen since the drugs used to treat the mood disorder may enhance confusion, leaving undiagnosed and untreated the underlying cause of the delirium.

Treatments

The treatment of delirium has two principal components (Table 9-18). The first priority is identifying, if possible, and reversing the underlying cause, whereas the second priority is the symptomatic treatment of behavioral disturbances. Common behavioral problems that may respond to pharmacologic and psychotherapeutic management include sleep disturbance, psychosis, mood lability, psychomotor agitation, confusion, and anxiety.

Sleep disturbance.   Delirium may be associated with changes in the quality or quantity of sleep. Medically ill patients in the hospital setting may have their sleep interrupted for diagnostic procedures, vital signs, and other ward activities. Treatments aimed at improving the quality of sleep will minimize unnecessary interventions and adjust the level of stimulation to that appropriate for the given patient. Foods, medications, and exhaustion may aggravate insomnia or produce over-sedation. A review of medications may lead to the identification of nonessential drugs that can be decreased or discontinued, a general principle in delirium management.

Because day-night reversal may occur in a delirious patient, one who is getting inadequate sleep may benefit from decreased stimulation and elimination of activating medications. Existing medications that are sedating may be administered at night in an at-

Table 9-18
Managing Delirium

Determine underlying cause

Treat/reverse underlying cause

Eliminate any nonessential medications

Maximize/optimize control of medical illness

Provide safe environment

Provide appropriate level of stimulation

Reorient patient

Educate patient and caregiver about diagnosis, treatment, and prognosis

tempt to improve the quality of sleep. Alternatively, trazadone at a low dose, zolpidem, or a small amount of a benzodiazepine may be attempted to reset the circadian sleep cycle. Antipsychotics may be considered if psychosis accompanies the interruption of sleep. Any agent that causes sedation should be used with caution when treating delirium. The patient who is over sedated has an increased risk of falls and aspiration, and is unable to assist with his or her own ADLs. Occasionally, oversedation may be confused with anergy, withdrawal, demoralization, and depression. Patients who present with these symptoms unassociated with the use of sedatives, may benefit from a trial with a psychostimulant such as methylphenidate or dextroamphetamine. Use of the psychostimulants require close monitoring of the vital signs for evidence of autonomic hyperactivity. These drugs also carry a risk of inducing psychosis and worsening delirium.

Psychoses.   Hallucinations or delusions that accompany a delirium may be managed with antipsychotics. High-potency agents, such as haloperidol, are preferred to chlorpromazine or thioridazine because the latter are more powerful anticholinergics. More recently, the atypical antipsychotics clozapine, risperdone, and olanzapine have become available. While clozapine carries an increased risk of seizure, sedation, and agranulocytosis, it may have a role in treating patients with severe parkinsonism who are also psychotic. Risperdone is reported to be less likely to induce extrapyramidal side effects than traditional antipsychotics. This agent has not been carefully studied in delirium, however, and is available only in oral form. Clinical experience suggests that parkinsonism, a potential adverse effect, may develop after several weeks to months of treatment with risperdone. Because olanzapine is less prone to causing parkinsonism, it may have a role in treating the psychosis associated with delirium. Side effects of olanzapine include sedation and hypotension. Quetiapine, another atypical antipsychotic has not been studied in treating psychosis associated with delirium. Its side effects include sedation, dizziness, and orthostatic hypotension. After the delirium resolves, antipsychotic administration should be discontinued to reduce patient exposure to the potential adverse effects of these agents.

Mood lability. Although labile mood is a common feature of delirium, it is generally not necessary to add a mood stabilizer or antidepressant to the pharmacotherapeutic regimen during the course of a delirium unless a mood disorder is present. Effective strategies to manage lability of mood include keeping the patient safe, explain illness and treatment options, and reorienting and assuring the patient that he or she is not "crazy." Often an explanation that properly attributes behavioral changes to delirium is beneficial to patients, their families, and caregivers.

Psychomotor agitation. The visibly agitated delirious patient demands increased staff time and is apt to receive more "prn" medication than the quietly delirious patient who is picking at his or her sheets but not yelling or thrashing. Although physical restraints may be necessary to protect a patient from injury, they should be a method of last resort after less restrictive approaches have been attempted. Restraints often increase agitation, and improper use has been associated with injury, including death (Miles, 1996). Physical agitation may preclude completion of diagnostic tests that are necessary to determine the etiology of the delirium. Companions may accompany patients to these tests, offering calm support, simple redirection, and reassurance. To provide appropriate assistance, family members, friends, and paid caregivers require education about the nature and course of delirium, as well as the specifics about each phase of diagnosis and treatment.

Low-dosage, high-potency antipsychotics may be required to treat psychomotor agitation associated with psychosis. Haloperidol may be given orally, intramuscularly, or intravenously. Intravenous haloperidol must be used with caution as it has been associated with cardiac arrythmias, including torsades de pointes. The QTc duration has been useful as a predictive marker of arrhythmia in some studies of iv butyrophenones. The combination of an antipsy-chotic and a benzodiazepine is often used in treating psychomotor agitation because of the additive sedative effect. A companion who stays with the patient continuously and provides supportive treatments can often reduce the necessity for physical restraints or medication.

Confusion. A fluctuation in concentration and frequent disorientation is a hallmark of delirium. Behavioral interventions that assist the confused patient include frequent orientation clues such as a large visible clock, calendar, lighting, familiar objects, and a companion. There is no specific pharmacotherapy for confusion. The general principles of searching for the cause of the delirium, keeping the patient safe, and decreasing or terminating any nonessential medications should be heeded.

Anxiety. Extreme anxiety, panic, and posttraumatic stress disorder symptoms have been associated with different stages of delirium. The patient, unaware of what is occurring, is frequently disoriented, often psychotic and commonly sleep deprived. After the delirium has resolved, time-limited supportive psychotherapy may assist in integrating the experience of the delirium into a less fearful and anxiety-provoking memory. This may prove challenging since memory for the delirious episode is often patchy. Pharmacotherapeutic interventions include benzodiazepines and antipsychotics if there is psychosis accompanying the presentation of anxiety.

MEDICATION LIST

The currently available medications discussed in this chapter are listed in Table 9-19. Please see the text for dosages of medications being used in clinical trials.

ACKNOWLEDGMENT

Adam M. Brickman's technical assistance in the preparation of this manuscript is greatly appreciated.

Table 9-19

Drug List

Cholinesterase inhibitors
  Tacrine (Cognex) (10, 20, 30, 40 mg)
  Donepezil (Aricept) (5, 10 mg)

Anticoagulants
  Aspirin
  Ticlopidine (Ticlid) (250 mg)
  Pentoxyfylline (Trental) (400 mg)
  Warfarin (Coumadin) (1, 2, 2.5, 4, 5, 7.5,
    10 mg)

Anticonvulsants
  Valproic acid
    (Depakene) (250 mg)
    (Depakote) (125, 250, 500 mg)
  Carbamazepine (Tegretol) (100, 200, 400 mg)
  Gabapentin (Neurontin) (100, 300, 400 mg)

Antipsychotics
  Haloperidol (Haldol) (0.5, 1, 2, 5, 10, 20 mg)
  Fluphenazine (Prolixin) (1, 2.5, 5, 10 mg)
  Thiothixane (Navane) (1, 2, 5, 10, 20 mg)
  Loxipine (Loxitane) (5, 10, 25, 50 mg)
  Perphenazine (Trilafon) (2, 4, 8, 16 mg)
  Thioridazine (Mellaril) (10, 15, 25, 50, 100,
    150, 200 mg)
  Molindone (Moban) (5, 10, 25, 50, 100 mg)
  Chlorpromazine (Thorazine)
  Clozapine (Clozaril) (25, 100 mg)
  Risperdone (Risperidal) (1, 2, 3, 4 mg liquid
    1 mg/mL, 100 mg/bottle)
  Olanzapine (Ziprexa) (2.5, 5, 10 mg)
  Quetiapine (Seroquel) (25, 100, 200 mg)
  Ziprasidone

Hypnotics
  Zolpidem (Ambien) (5, 10 mg)

Opioid receptor antagonists
  Naloxone (Talwin) (50 mg)
  Naltrexone (ReVia) (50 mg)

Vitamins
  Thiamine (100 mg PO or IM)
  Folate (1 mg)

Antidepressants
  Serotonin selective reuptake inhibitors (SSRI)
    Sertraline (Zoloft) (50, 100 mg)
    Fluvoxamine (Luvox) (50, 100 mg)
    Fluoxetine
      (Prozac) (10, 20 mg)
      (Prozac liquid) (20 mg/5 cc))
    Citalopram
    Alaproclate
  Other antidepressant
    Trazadone (Desyrel) (50, 100, 150, 300 mg)

Anxiolytics
  Buspirone (BuSpar) (5, 10 mg)

Benzodiazepines
  Lorazepam (Ativan) (0.5, 1, 2 mg)
  Oxazepam (Serax) (10, 15, 30 mg)
  Clonazepam (Klonopin) (0.5, 1, 2 mg)

Benzodiazepine receptor antagonist
  Flumazenil (Romazicon) (0.1 mg/mL; 5 mL
    or 10 mL vials)

Stimulants
  Methylphenidate (Ritalin) (5, 10, 20 mg)
  Dextroamphetamine
    (Dextrostat) (5, 10 mg)
    (Dexadrine) (5, 10, 15 mg)

β-Adrenergic receptor antagonists
  Pindolol (Visken) (5, 10 mg)
  Propanolol (Inderol) (10, 20, 40, 60, 80 mg)

Mood stabilizers
  Lithium (Lithonate) (150, 300 mg)

Hormones
  Estrogen (Premarin) (0.3, 0.625, 0.9, 1.25,
    2.5 mg)
  Medroxyprogesterone acetate
    (Amen) (10 mg)
    (Cycrin) (2.5, 5, 10 mg)

For additional information on the drugs discussed in this chapter see chapters 8, 10, 17, 18, 19, 23, 54, 57, and 62, in *Goodman and Gilman's The Pharmacological Basis of Therapeutics* (Ninth Edition), McGraw-Hill, New York, 1996.

REFERENCES

Aevarsson O, Skoog I. A population-based study on the incidence of dementia disorders between 85 and 88 years of age. *J Am Geriatr Soc* 44(12):1455–1460.

Aisen PS, Davis KL. Inflammatory mechanisms in Alzheimer's Disease: Implications for therapy. *Am J Psychiatry* 1994;151:1105–1113.

Ala TA, Yang KH, Sung JH, Frey WH 2nd. Hallucinations and signs of parkinsonism help distinguish patients with dementia and cortical Lewy bodies from patients with Alzheimer's disease at presentation: a clinicopathological study. *Neurosurg Psychiatry* 1997;62(1):16–21.

Allen RL, Walker Z, D'Ath PJ, Katona CL Risperidone for psychotic and behavioural symptoms in Lewy body dementia [letter]. *Lancet* 1995;346(8968):185.

Altsteil L: Cholinomimetic Therapy in Alzheimer's Disease: Experience with the Muscarinic Agonist Xanomeline. Second Annual Conference on the Therapeutics of Alzheimer's Disease. June 3–4, 1996; Garden City, New York.

Altsteil LD, Greenberg DA, Marin D et al.: Apolipoprotein E genotype and cognition in the very old. Lancet 1997;349:1451.

Amar K, Wilcock GK, Scott M: The diagnosis of vascular dementia in the light of the new criteria. *Age Ageing* 1996;25(1):51–55.

American Psychiatric Association: Practice guideline for major depressive disorder in adults. *Am J Psychiatry* 1993;150(4 suppl):1–26.

American Psychiatric Association: Practice guideline for the treatment of patients with Alzheimer's disease and other dementias of late life. *Am J Psychiatry* 1997;154(5 Suppl):1–39.

American Psychiatric Association: *Diagnostic and Statistical Manual of Mental Disorders*, 4th ed. (DSM-IV). Washington, DC, APA, 1994.

Anand R, Garabawi G, Enz A: Efficacy and safety results of the early phase studies with Exelon (TM) (ENA-713) in Alzheimer's disease: An overview. *J Drug Dev Clin Pract* 1996;8:109–116.

Andersen G, Vestergaard K, Lauritzen L: Effective treatment of poststroke depression with the selective serotonin reuptake inhibitor citalopram. *Stroke* 1994;25:1099–1104.

Antiplatelet Trialists' Collaboration. Secondary prevention of vascular disease by prolonged antiplatelet treatment. *Br Med J* 1988;296:320-331.

Armstrong DM, Ikonomovic MD, Sheffield R, Wenthold RJ: Glutamate receptor subtype immunoreactivity in the entorhinal cortex of non-demented elderly and patients with Alzheimer's disease. *Brain Res* 1994;639:207–216.

Asthana S, Craft S, Baker LD, et al.: Transdermal estrogen improves memory in women with Alzheimer's disease [Abstract]. Society for Neuroscience Abstracts: Vol 22, part 1: Page 200. 26th Annual Meeting. Washington, DC, Nov 16–21, 1996.

Azar AJ, Koudstaal PJ, Wintzen AR, et al: Risk of stroke during long-term anticoagulant therapy in patients after myocardial infarction. *Ann Neurol* 1996;39:973–975.

Bachman DL, Wolf PA, Linn R, et al.: Prevalence of dementia and probable senile dementia of the Alzheimer type in the Framingham Study. *Neurology* 42(1):115–119 (Jan 1992).

Ban TA, Morey L. Aguglia E, et al.: Nimodipine in the treatment of old age dementias. *Prog Neuro Psychopharmacol Biol Psychiatry*. 1990;14:525–551.

Bergamasco B, Scarzella L, La Commare P: Idebenone, a new drug for the treatment of cognitive impairment in patients with dementia of the Alzheimer's type. *Funct Neurol.* 1994;9:161–168.

Besson JAO, Palin AN, Ebmeier KP, et al. Calcium antagonists and multi-infarct dementia: a trial involving sequential NMR and psychometric assessment. *Int J Geriatr Psychiatry* 1988;3:99–105.

Bierer LM, Haroutunian V, Gabriel S, et al.: Neurochemical correlates of dementia severity in Alzheimer's disease: relative importance of the cholinergic deficits. *J Neurochem* 1995;64:749–760.

Black DW, Winokur G, Bell S, et al.: Complicated mania. *Arch Gen Psychiatry* 1988;45:232–236.

Bodick NC, Offen WW, Levey AI, et al.: Effects of Xanomeline, a selective muscarinic receptor agonist, on cognitive function and behavioral symptoms in Alzheimer disease. *Arch Neurol* 1997;465–473.

Bolla-Wilson K, Robinson RG, Starkstein SE, et al.: Lateralization of dementia of depression in stroke patients. *Am J Psychiatry* 1989;146:627–634.

Bousser MG, Tournier-Lasserve E: Summary of the proceedings of the first international workshop on CADASIL, Paris, May 19–21, 1993. *Stroke* 1994;25:704–705.

Braak H, Braak E: Diagnostic criteria for neuropathologic assessment of Alzheimer's disease. *Neurobiol Aging* 1997;18(4 Suppl):S85–S88.

Bracco L, Gallato R, Grigoletto F, et al.: Factors affecting course and survival in Alzheimer's disease. A 9-year longitudinal study. *Arch Neurol* 1994;51(12):1213–1219.

Breitner JC, Welsh KA, Helms MJ, et al.: Delayed onset of Alzheimer's disease with nonsteroidal anti-inflammatory and histamine H2 blocking drugs. *Neurobiol Aging* 1995;16(4):523–530.

Brew BJ, Dunbar N, Druett JA, et al.: Pilot study of the efficacy of atevirdine in the treatment of AIDS dementia complex. *AIDS* 1996;10(12):1357–1360.

Bridge TP, Haseltine PN, Parker ES, et al.: Results of extended peptide T administration in AIDS and ARC patients. *Psychopharmacol Bull* 1991;27:237–245.

Brouwers P, Hendricks M, Lietzau JA, et al.: Effect of combination therapy with zidovudine and didanosine on neuropsychological functioning in patients with symptomatic HIV disease: a comparison of simultaneous and alternating regimens. *AIDS* 1997;11(1):59–66.

Brumback RA, Leech RW. Alzheimer's disease, pathophysiology and the hope for therapy. *J Okla State Med Assoc* 1994;87:103–111.

Buxbaum JD, Oishi M, Chen HI, et al. Cholinergic agonists and interleukin 1 regulate processing and secretion of the Alzheimer beta/A4 amyloid protein precursor. *PNAS USA* 1992;89:10075–10078.

Camacho F, Smith CP, Vargas HM, Winslow JT: α-2-Adrenoreceptor antagonists potentiate acetylcholinesterase inhibitor effects on passive avoidance learning in the rat. *Psychopharmacology* 1996;124:347–354.

Campbell IL, Abraham CR, Masliah E, et al.: Neurologic disease induced in transgenic mice by cerebral overexpression of interleukin 6. *PNAS USA* 1993;90:10061–10065.

Canal N, Imbimbo BP, Bassi S, et al.: Relationship between pharmacodynamic activity and cognitive effects of eptastigmine in patients with Alzheimer's disease. *Clin Pharmacol Therapeut* 1996;60:218–228.

Cantillon M, Brunswick R, Molina D, et al.: Buspirone vs haloperidol: a double blind trial for agitation in a nursing home population with Alzheimer's disease. *Am J Geriatr Psychiatry* 1996;4:263–267.

Caspari D, Trabert W, Heinz G, et al.: The pattern of regional cerebral blood flow during alcohol withdrawal—a single photon emission tomography study with 99mTc-HMPAO. *Acta Psychiatr Scand* 1993;87(6):414–417.

Castillo CS, Starkstein SE, Federoff JP, et al.: Generalized anxiety disorder following stroke. *J Nerv Ment Disord* 1993;181:100–106.

Chacko RC, Hurley RA, Jankovic J: Clozapine use in diffuse Lewy body disease. *J Neuropsychiatry Clin Neurosci* 1993;5(2)206–208.

Chiesi A, Vella S, Dally LG, et al.: Epidemiology of AIDS dementia complex in Europe. AIDS in Europe Study Group. *J Acquir Immune Defic Syndr Hum Retrovirol* 1996;11(1):39–44.

Chiu HC, Victoroff JI, Margolin DM, et al.: Criteria for the diagnosis of ischemic vascular dementia proposed by the State of California Alzheimer's Disease Diagnostic and Treatment Centers. *Neurology* 1992;42:473–480.

Cioli D, Pica-Mattoccia L, Archer S: Antischistosomal drugs: past, present and future? *Pharmacol Ther* 1995;68:35–85.

Citron M, Vigo-Pelfrey C, Teplow DB, et al.: Excessive production of amyloid beta protein by peripheral cells of symptomatic and presymptomatic patients carrying the Swedish familial Alzheimer disease mutation. *PNAS* 1994;91:11993–11997.

Citron M, Westaway D, Xia W, et al.: Mutant presenilins of Alzheimer's disease increase production of 42-residue amyloid beta-protein in both transfected cells and transgenic mice. *Nat Med* 1997;3:67–72.

Clark F, Azen SP, Zemke R, et al.: Occupational therapy for independent-living older adults: a randomized controlled trial. *JAMA* 1997;278(16):1321–1326.

Cohen-Mansfield J, Marx MS, Rosenthal AS. A description of agitation in the nursing home. *Gerontology* 1989;3:M77–M84.

Concar D: Here's a drug to remember. New Scientist: November 23, 1996: p14.

Cooper AJ: Medroxyprogesterone acetate (MPA) treatment of sexual acting out in men suffering from dementia. *J Clin Psychiatry* 1987;48:368–370.

Corder EH, Saunders AM, Strittmatter WJ, et al.: Gene dose of apolipoprotein E type 4 allele and the risk of Alzheimer's disease in late onset families. *Science* 1993;261:921–923.

Coull JT, Middleton HC, Robbins TW, Sahakian BJ: Contrasting effects of clonidine and diazepam on tests of working memory and planning. *Psychopharmacol Berl* 1995;120(3):311–321.

Cromwell J, Bartosch WJ, Fiore MC, et al.: Cost-effectiveness of the clinical practice recommendations in the AHCPR guideline for smoking cessation. Agency for Health Care Policy and Research. *JAMA* 1997;278(21):1759–1766.

Cummings BJ, Cotman CW: Image analysis of beta-amyloid in Alzheimer's disease and relation to dementia severity. *Lancet* 1995;346:1524–1528.

Cummings JL. Lewy body diseases with dementia: pathophysiology and treatment. *Brain Cogn* 1995;28(3):266–280.

Cummings J, Bieber F, Mas J, et al.: Metrifonate in Alzheimer's disease—results of a dose finding study: Abstract at Fifth International Conference on Alzheimer's Disease and Related Disorders. July 26–29, 1996. Osaka, Japan.

Cunningham AL, Naif H, Saksena N, et al.: HIV infection of macrophages and pathogenesis of AIDS dementia complex: interaction of the host cell and viral genotype. *J Leukoc Biol* 1997;62(1):117–125.

The Dana Consortium on the Therapy of HIV Dementia and Related Cognitive Disorders: Safety and tolerability of the antioxidant OPC-14117 in HIV-associated cognitive impairment. *Neurology* 1997;49(1):42–146.

Davis KL, Mohs RC: Enhancement of memory processing in Alzheimer's disease with multiple-dose intravenous physostigmine. *Am J Psychiatry* 1982;139:1421–1424.

Davis KL, Mohs RC, Tinkleberg JR, et al.: Physostigmine: Improvement in long term memory processes in humans. *Science* 1978;201:272–274.

Davis KL, Thal LJ, Gamzu ER, et al.: A double-blind, placebo controlled multicenter study of Tacrine for Alzheimer's disease. *N Eng J Med* 1992;327:1253–1259.

Devenand DP: Neuroleptics for behavioral complications of dementia, in Nelson JC (ed): *Geriatric Psychopharmacology*. New York, Marcel Dekker, 1998, 405–426.

Devenand DP, Jacobs DM, Tang M-X, et al.: The course of psychopathology in mild to moderate Alzheimer's disease. *Arch Gen Psychiatry* 1997;54:257–263.

Dewhurst S, Whetter L: Pathogenesis and treatment of HIV-1 infection: recent developments. *Front Biosci* 1997;2:D147–D159.

Deyo RA, Staube KT, Disterhoft JF: Nimodipine facilitates associative learning in aging rabbits. *Science* 1989;243:809–811.

Dezube BJ, Pardee AB, Chapman B, et al.: Pentoxifylline decreases tumor necrosis factor expression and serum triglycerides in people with AIDS: NIAID AIDS Clinical Trials Group. *J Acquir Immune Defic Syndr* 1993;6(7):787–794.

Diagnosis and treatment of depression in late life: The NIH Consensus Development Conference Statement. *Psychopharmacol Bull* 1993;29(1):87–100.

Douyon R, Serby M, Klutchko B, Rotrosen J. ECT and Parkinson's disease revisited: a "naturalistic" study. *Am J Psychiatry* 1989;146(11):1451–1455.

Doyle M, Warden D: Use of SPECT to evaluate postcardiotomy delirium. [letter]. *Am J Psychiatry* 1996;153(6):838–839.

Dreyfus CF: Effects of nerve growth factor on cholinergic brain neurons. *Trends Pharmacol Sci* 1989;10:145–149.

Engel GL, Webb JP, Ferris EB: Quantitative electroencephalographic studies of anoxia in humans: comparison with acute alcohol intoxication and hypoglycemia. *J Clin Invest* 1945;24:691–697.

Erkinjuntti T, Ostbye, T, Steenhuis R, et al.: The effect of different diagnostic criteria on the prevalence of dementia. *NEJM* 1997;337:1667–1674.

European Pentoxifylline Multi-infarct Dementia Study. *Eur Neurol* 1996;36(5):315–321.

Evans DA, Funkenstein HH, Albert MS, et al.: Prevalence of Alzheimer's disease in a community population of older persons: higher than previously reported. *JAMA* 1989;262(18):2551–2556.

Evans LK: Sundown syndrome in institutionalized elderly. *J Am Geriatr Soc* 1987;35(2):101–108.

Fagarasan MO, Aisen PS: Il-1 and anti-inflammatory drugs modulate A-beta cytotoxicity in PC12 cells. *Brain Res* 1996;723:231–234.

Figiel GS, Krishnan KRR, Breitner JC, et al.: Radiologic correlates of antidepressant-induced delirium: the possible significance of basal ganglia lesions. *J Neuropsychiatry Clin Neurosci* 1989;2:188–190.

Figiel GS, Krishnan KRR, Doraiswamy PM: Subcortical structural changes in ECT-induced delirium. *J Geriatr Psychiatry Neurol* 1990;3:172–176.

Flood JF, Smith GE, Cherkin A: Memory retention: potentiation of cholinergic drug combinations in mice. *Neurobiol Aging* 1983;4(1):37–43.

Flood JF, Smith GE, Cherkin A: Memory enhancement: supraadditive effect of subcutaneous cholinergic drug combinations in mice. *Psychopharmacology (Berl)* 1985;86(1–2):61–67.

Flynn DD, Ferrari KiLeo G, Mash DC, Levey AI: Differential regulation of molecular subtypes of muscarinic receptors in Alzheimer's disease. *J Neurochem* 1995;64(4):1888–1891.

Flynn DD, Weinstein A, Mash DC: Loss of high-affinity agonist binding to M1 receptors in Alzheimer's disease: implications for the failure of the cholinergic replacement therapies. *Ann Neurol* 1991;29:256–262.

Folstein MF, Bassett SS, Romanoski AJ, et al.: The epidemiology of delirium in the community: the Eastern Baltimore Mental health Survey. *Int Psychogeriatr* 1991;3:169–176.

Folstein MF, Folstein SE, McHugh PR: Mini-mental state: a practical method for grading the cognitive state of patients for the clinician. *J Psychiatr Res* 1975;12:189–198.

Francis J, Kapoor WN: Prognosis after hospital discharge of older medical patients with delirium. *J Am Geriatr Soc* 1992;40(6):601–606.

Friedhoff LT, Farlow MR, Mohs RC, Rogers SL: Donepezil (E2020) demonstrates significant improvement in cognitive and global function in patients in mild-to-moderately severe Alzheimer's disease. *ACNP*, December 9–13, 1996, San Juan, Puerto Rico.

Furukawa S, Furukawa Y. Nerve growth factor synthesis and its regulatory mechanisms: an approach to therapeutic induction of nerve growth factor synthesis. *Cerebrovasc Brain Metab Rev* 1990;1:328–344.

Galasko D, Hansen LA, Katzman R, et al.: Clinical-neuropathological correlations in Alzheimer's disease and related dementias. *Arch Neurol*, 1994;51;888–895.

Geroldi C, Frisoni GB, Bianchetti A, Trabucchi M: Drug treatment in Lewy body dementia. *Dement Geriatr Cogn Disord* 1997;8(3):188–197.

Gnanalingham KK, Byrne EJ, Thornton A, et al.: Motor and cognitive function in Lewy body dementia: comparison with Alzheimer's and Parkinson's diseases. *J Neurol Neurosurg Psychiatry* 1997;62(3):243–252.

Goldfrank LR, Flomenbaum NF, Lewin NA, et al. *Goldfrank's Toxicologic Emergencies*, 5th ed., Norwalk, CT, Appleton & Lange, 1994.

Goodkin K, Wilkie FL, Concha M, et al.: Subtle neuropsychological impairment and minor cognitive-motor disorder in HIV-1 infection. Neuroradiological, neurophysiological, neuroimmunological, and virological correlates. *Neuroimaging Clin N Am* 1997;7(3):561–579.

Gorelick PB. Status of risk factors for dementia associated with stroke. *Stroke* 1997;28:459–463.

Gorelick PB, Brody J, Cohen D, et al.: Risk factors for dementia associated with multiple cerebral infarcts: a case-control analysis in predominantly African-American hospital based patients. *Arch Neurol* 1993;50:714–720.

Graham C, Ballard C, Saad K: Variables which distinguish patients fulfilling clinical criteria for dementia with Lewy bodies from those with Alzheimer's disease. *Int J Geriatr Psychiatry* 1997;12(3):314–318.

Granon S, Poucet B, Thinus-Blanc C, et al.: Nicotinic and muscarinic receptors in the rat prefrontal cortex: differential roles in working memory, response selection and effortful processing. *Psychopharmacology (Berl)* 1995;119(2):139–144.

Greenberg SM, Rebeck GW, Vonsattel JP, et al.: Apolipoprotein E epsilon 4 and cerebral hemorrhage associated with amyloid angiopathy. *Ann Neurol* 1995;38:254–259.

Greendyke RM, Berkner JP, Webster JC, et al.: Treatment of behavioral problems with pindolol. *Psychosomatics* 1989;30:161–165.

Greendyke RM, Kantor DR, Schuster DB, et al.: Propanolol treatment of assaultive patients with organic brain disease: a double blind crossover, placebo-controlled study. *J Nerv Ment Dis* 1986;174:290–294.

Hachinski VC, Lliff LD, Zilhka E, et al: Cerebral blood flow in dementia. *Arch Neurol* 1975;32:632–637.

Hamilton M: Standardized assessment and recording of depressive symptoms. *Psychiatr Neurol Neurochir* 1969;72(2):201–205.

Hardy J, Crook R, Prihar G, et al.: Senile dementia of the Lewy body type has an apolipoprotein E epsilon 4 allele frequency intermediate between controls and Alzheimer's disease. *Neurosci Lett* 1994;182(1):1–2.

Hass WK, Easton JD, Adams HP, et al.: A randomized trial comparing ticlopidine hydrochloride with aspirin for the prevention of stroke in high-risk patients. *N Engl J Med* 1989;321:501–507.

Herzlich BC, Schiano TD: Reversal of apparent AIDS dementia complex following treatment with vitamin B12. *J Intern Med* 1993;233(6):495–497.

Heyman A, Peterson B, Fillenbaum G, Pieper C: The consortium to establish a registry for Alzheimer's disease (CERAD). Part XIV: Demographic and clinical predictors of survival in patients with Alzheimer's disease. *Neurology* 1996;46(3):656–660.

Himmelhoch JM, Garfinkel ME: Sources of lithium resistance in mixed mania. *Psychopharmacol Bull* 1986;22:613–620.

Hollander H, McGuire D, Burack JH: Diagnostic lumbar puncture in HIV-infected patients: analysis of 138 cases. *Am J Med* 1994;96(3):223–228.

Honhjo H, Tamura T, Matsumoto Y, et al.: Estrogen as a growth factor to central nervous cells. Estrogen treatment promotes development of acetylcholine-positive basal forebrain neurons transplanted in the anterior eye chamber. *J Steroid Biochem Mol Biol* 1992;41:633–635.

Hsiao K, Chapman P, Nilson S, et al.: Correlative memory deficits, A beta elevation, and amyloid plaques in transgenic mice. *Science* 1996;274:99–102.

Ito I, Tanabe S, Kohda A, Sugiyama H.: Allosteric potentiation of quisqualate receptors by a nootropic drug aniracetam. *J Physiol* 1990;424:533–543.

Jackson CW, Pitner JK, Mintzer JE: Zolpidem for the treatment of agitation in elderly agitated patients. *J Clin Psychiatry* 1996; 57(8):372–373.

Jacobson SA, Leuchter AF, Walter DO: Conventional and quantitative EEG in the diagnosis of delirium among the elderly. *J Neurol Neurosurg Psychiatry* 1993;56:153–158.

Jaffe AB, Toran Allerand CD, Greengard P, Gandy SE: Estrogen regulates metabolism of Alzheimer's amyloid beta precursor protein. *J Biol Chem* 1994;269:13065–13068.

Jonhagen M, Wahlund LO, Amberla K, et al.: Nerve Growth Factors as a treatment of Alzheimer's Disease: Abstract 645: Osaka Fifth International Conference on Alzheimer's Disease. July 24–29, 1996.

Kaponen H, Hurri L, Stenback U, et al.: Computed tomography findings in delirium. *J Nerv Ment Dis* 1989;4:226–231.

Katzman R, Brown T, Fuld P, Peck A, Schechter R, Schimmel H: Validation of a short Orientation-Memory-Concentration Test of cognitive impairment. *Am J Psychiatry* 1983;140(6):734–739.

Katzman R, Galasko D, Saitoh T, et al.: Genetic evidence that the Lewy body variant is indeed a phenotypic variant of Alzheimer's disease. *Brain Cogn* 1995;28(3):259–265.

Khachaturian ZS: Diagnosis of Alzheimer's disease. *Arch Neurol* 1985;42(11):1097–1105.

Khoury JE, Hickman SE, Thomas CA, et al.: Scavenger receptor-mediated adhesion of microglia to beta-amyloid fibrils. *Nature* 1996;382:716–719.

Kistler JP, Buonanno FS, Gress DR: Carotid endarterectomy: specific therapy based on pathophysiology. *NEJM* 1991;325:505–507.

Klatka LA, Louis ED, Schiffer RB: Psychiatric features in diffuse Lewy body disease: a clinicopathologic study using Alzheimer's disease and Parkinson's disease comparison groups. *Neurology* 1996;47(5):1148–1152.

Knapp MJ, Knopman DS, Soloman PR, et al.: A 30-week randomized controlled trial of high dose Tacrine in patients with Alzheimer's disease. *JAMA* 1994;271:985–991.

Knopman D, Schneider L, Davis K, et al.: Long-term tacrine (Cognex) treatment: effects on nursing home placement and mortality. *Neurology* 1996;47:166–177.

Knuesel B, Kaplan DR, Winslow JW, et al.: K-252b selectively potentiates cellular actions and trk tyrosine phosphorylation mediated by neurotrophin-3. *J Neurochem* 1992;59:715–722.

Koliatsos VE, Clatterbuck RE, Nauta HJW, et al.: Human nerve growth factor prevents degeneration of basal forebrain cholinergic neurons in primates. *Ann Neurol* 1991;30:831–840.

Konno S, Meyer JS, Terayama Y, et al.: Classification, diagnosis and treatment of vascular dementia. *Drugs Aging* 1997;11:361–373.

Kumar R: Efficacy and safety of SB202026 as a symptomatic treatment for Alzheimer's Disease. *Ann Neurol* 1996; 40:504.

Kyomen HH, Nobel KW, Wei JY: The use of estrogen to decrease aggressive physical behavior in elderly men with dementia. *J Am Geriatr Soc* 1991;39:1110–1112.

Lawton MP: The functional assessment of elderly people. *J Am Geriatr Soc* 1971;19(6):465–481.

Lebowitz BD, Pearson JL, Schneider LS, et al.: Diagnosis and treatment of depression in late life: consensus statement update. *JAMA* 1997;278(14):1186–1190.

Lee CR, Benfield P: Aniracetam: an overview of its pharmacodynamic and pharmacokinetic properties, and a review of its therapeutic potential in senile cognitive disorders. *Drugs Aging* 1994;4(3):257–273.

Lemere CA, Lopera F, Kosik KS, et al.: The E280A presenilin 1 Alzheimer's mutation produces A beta 42 deposition in severe cerebellar pathology. *Neurobiol Dis* 1996;3:16–32.

Levine DN, Finklestein S: Delayed psychosis after right temporoparietal stroke or trauma: relation to epilepsy. *Neurology* 1982;32:267–273.

Levkoff SE, Evans DA, Liptzin B, et al.: Delirium: the occurrence and persistence of symptoms among elderly hospitalized patients. *Arch Intern Med* 1992;152(2):334–340.

Levkoff SE, Cleary PD, Liptzin B, et al.: Epidemiology of delirium: an overview of research issues and findings. *Int Psychogeriatr* 1991;3:149–167.

Levkoff SE, Safran C, Cleary PD, et al.: Identification of factors associated with the diagnosis of delirium in elderly hospitalized patients. *J Am Geriatr Soc* 1988;36:1099–1104.

Levkoff SE, Liptzin B, Evans DA, et al.: Progression and resolution of delirium in elderly patients hospitalized for acute care. *Am J Geriatr Psychiatry* 1994;2:230–238.

Levy-Lahad E, Wasco W, Poorkaj P, et al.: Candidate gene for the chromosome 1 familial Alzheimer's disease locus. *Science* 1995;269(226):973–977.

Lindsay J, Hebert R, Rockwood K: The Canadian study of health and aging: risk factors for vascular dementia. *Stroke* 1997;28:526–553.

Lipowski ZJ. *Delirium: Acute Confusional State.* New York, Oxford University Press, 1990.

Lipsey JR, Robinson RG, Pearlson GD, et al.: Nortriptyline treatment of poststroke depression: a double blind treatment trial. *Lancet* 1984;1:297–300.

Lipton SA: Neuropathogenesis of acquired immunodeficiency syndrome dementia. *Curr Opin Neurol* 1997;10(3):247–253.

Lipton SA: Neuronal injury associated with HIV-1 and potential treatment with calcium-channel and NMDA antagonists. *Dev Neurosci* 1994;16:145–151.

Lipton SA, Gendleman HF: Seminars in medicine of the Beth Israel Hospital, Boston. Dementia associated with acquired immunodeficiency syndrome. *N Engl J Med* 1995;322:934–940.

Liptzin B, Levkoff SE, Cleary PD, et al.: An empirical study of diagnostic criteria for delirium. *Am J Psychiatry* 1991;148:454–457.

Lynch G, Granger R, Ambros-Ingerson J, et al.: Evidence that a positive modulator of AMPA-type glutamate receptors improves delayed recall in aged humans. *Exp Neurol* 1997;145(1):89–92.

M'Harzi M, Palou AM, Oberlander C, Barzaghi F: Antagonism of scopolamine-induced memory impairments in rats by the muscarinic agonist RU 35,926 (CI-979). *Pharmacol Biochem Behav* 1995;51:119–124.

Marin DB, Green CR, Schmeidler J, et al.: Noncognitive disturbances in Alzheimer's disease: frequency, longitudinal course, and relationship to cognitive symptoms. *J Am Geriatr Soc* 1997;45(11):1331–1338.

Marx J: Searching for Drugs that Combat Alzheimer's [News]. *Science* 1996;273:50–53.

Masliah E, Sisk A, Mallory M, et al.: Comparison of neurodegenerative pathology in transgenic mice overexpressing V717F beta-amyloid precursor protein and Alzheimer's disease. *J Neurosci* 1996;16(18):5795–5811.

Mattson MP, Barger SW, Cheng B, et al.: beta-Amyloid precursor protein metabolites and loss of neuronal Ca2⁺ homeostasis in Alzheimer's disease. *Trends Neurosci* 1993;(10):409–414.

McCafferty J. SB2020226 Muscarinic Partial Agonist. Second Annual Conference on the Therapeutics of Alzheimer's Disease. June 3–4, 1996, Garden City, New York.

McGeer PL, Shulzer M, McGeer EM: Evidence supporting the inflammatory hypothesis of AD: Abstract 807: Osaka Fifth International Conference on Alzheimer's Disease. July 24–29, 1996.

McKeith IG, Ballard CG, Harrison RW: Neuroleptic sensitivity to risperidone in Lewy body dementia [letter]. *Lancet* 1995;346(8976):699.

McKeith LG, Galasko D, Kosaka K, et al.: Consensus guidelines for the clinical and pathologic diagnosis of dementia with Lewy bodies (DLB): report of the consortium on DLB international workshop. *Neurology* 1996;47(5):1113–1124.

McKhann G, Drachman D, Folstein M, et al.: Clinical diagnosis of Alzheimer's disease: report of the NINCDS-ADRDA Work Group under the auspices of Department of Health and Human Services Task Force on Alzheimer's Disease. *Neurology* 1984;34(7):939–944.

Melton ST, Kirkwood CK, Ghaermi SN: Pharmacotherapy of HIV dementia. *Ann Pharmacother* 1997;31:457–473.

Metzger E, Friedman R. Prolongation of the corrected QT and torsades de pointes cardiac arrhythmia associated with intravenous haloperidol in the medically ill. *J Clin Psychopharmacol* 1993;13(2):128–132.

Meyer JS, Rogers RL, McClintic K, et al.: Randomized clinical trial of daily aspirin therapy in multi-infarct dementia. *JAGS* 1989;37:549–555.

Milam SB, Bennett CR: Physostigmine reversal of drug induced paradoxical excitement. *Int J Oral Maxillofac Surg* 1987;16:190–193.

Miles S. A case of death by physical restraint: new lessons from a photograph. *J Am Geriatr Soc* 1996;44(3):291–292.

Mintz M: Neurological and developmental problems in pediatric HIV infection. *J Nutr* 1996;126(10 Suppl):2663S–2673S.

Mohs RC, Cohen L: Alzheimer's Disease Assessment Scale (ADAS). *Psychopharmacol Bull* 1988;24:627–628.

Moroney JT, Bagiella E, Desmond DW, et al.: Risk factors for incident dementia after stroke: role of hypoxic and ischemic disorders. *Stroke* 1996;27:1283–1289.

Morris CM, Massey HM, Benjamin R, et al.: Molecular biology of APO E alleles in Alzheimer's and non-Alzheimer's dementias. *J Neural Transm Suppl* 1996;47:205–218.

Mortel KF, Meyer JS, Herod B, et al.: Education and occupation as risk factors for dementias of the Alzheimer and ischemic vascular types. *Dementia* 1995a;6:55–62.

Mortel KF, Meyer JS. Lack of postmenopausal replacement therapy and the risk of dementia. *J Neuropsychiatry Clin Neurosci* 1995b;7:334–337.

Moutoussis M, Orrell W: Baclofen therapy for rigidity associated with Lewy body dementia [letter]. *Br J Psychiatry* 1996;169(6):795.

Muller WE, Schroder HC, Ushijima H, et al.: gp120 of HIV-1 induces apoptosis in rat cortical cell cultures: prevention by memantine. *Eur J Pharmacol* 1992;226(3):209–214.

Murphy GM Jr, Taylor J, Kraemer HC, et al. No association between apolipoprotein E epsilon 4 allele and rate of decline in Alzheimer's disease. *Am J Psychiatry* 1997;154(5):603–608.

Murrell J, Farlow M, Ghetti B, Benson MD: A mutation in the amyloid precursor protein associated with hereditary Alzheimer's disease. *Science* 1991;254(5028):97–99.

Navia BA, Jordan BD, Price RW: The AIDS dementia complex: 1: Clinical features. *Ann Neurol* 1986;19:517–524.

Newhouse PA, Sunderland T, Tariot PN, et al.: Intravenous nicotine in Alzheimer's disease: a pilot study. *Psychopharmacology (Berl)* 1988;95:171–175.

Nordberg A: Neuroreceptor changes in Alzheimer's disease. *Cerebrovasc Brain Metab Rev* 1992;4:303–382.

Nordberg A: Human nicotinic receptors: their role in aging and dementia. *Neurochem Int* 1994;25(1):93–97.

North American Symptomatic Carotid Endarterectomy Trial Collaborators: Beneficial effect of carotid endarterectomy in symptomatic patients with high grade carotid stenosis. *NEJM* 1991;325:445–453.

Nurnberger JI: Diuretic induced lithium toxicity presenting as mania. *J Nerv Ment Disord* 1985;173:316–318.

O'Brien MD: Vascular dementia is underdiagnosed. *Arch Neurol* 1988;45:797–798.

Ogawa N: Neuronal death and immunosuppressant-immunophilin-transcription systems. Abstract 167. Osaka Fifth International Conference on Alzheimer's Disease. July 24–29, 1996.

Ohkura T, Isse K, Akazawa K, et al.: Evaluation of estrogen treatment in female patients with dementia of the Alzheimer type. *Endocr J* 1994;41:361–371.

Olson L, Nordberg A, von Holst H, et al.: Nerve growth factor affects C-nicotine binding, blood flow, EEG, and verbal episodic memory in an Alzheimer's disease patient. *J Neural Transm* 1992;4:79–95.

Paganini-Hill A, Henderson VW: Estrogen replacement therapy and risk of Alzheimer disease. *Arch Intern Med* 1996;156(19):2213–2217.

Parikh RM, Robinson RG, Lipsey JR, et al.: The impact of post stroke depression on recovery in activities of daily living over two year follow-up. *Arch Neurol* 1990;47:785–789.

Parnetti L, Bartorelli L, Bainiouto S, et al.: Aniracetam (Ro 13-5057) for the treatment of senile dementia of the Alzheimer's type: results of a multicentre clinical study. *Dementia* 1991;2:262–267.

Parnetti L, Senin U, Carosi M, et al.: Mental deterioration in old age: results of two multicenter, clinical trials with nimodipine. *Clin Ther* 1993;15:394:406.

Perry EK, Haroutunian V, Davis KL, et al.: Neocortical cholinergic activities differentiate Lewy body dementia from classical Alzheimer's disease. *Neuroreport* 1994;5(7):747–749.

Perry EK, Tomlinson BE, Blessed G, et al.: Correlation of cholinergic abnormalities with senile plaques and mental test scores in senile dementia. *Br Med J* 1978;2(6150):1457–1459.

Phelps CH, Gage FH, Growden JH, et al.: Potential use of nerve growth factor to treat Alzheimer's disease. *Neurobiol Aging* 1989;10:205–207.

Pike CJ, Cotman CW: Beta-amyloid neurotoxicity in vitro: Examination of potential contributions from oxidative pathways. Abstract 423. Osaka Fifth International Conference on Alzheimer's Disease. July 24–29, 1996.

Power C, Johnson RT HIV-1 associated dementia: clinical features and pathogenesis. *Can J Neurol Sci* 1995;22(2):92–100).

Querfurth HW. Beta APP mRNA transcription is increased in cultured fibroblasts from the familial Alzheimer's disease-1 family. *Mol Brain Res* 1995;28:319–337.

Rabins PV, Starkstein SE, Robinson RG: Risk factors for developing atypical (schizophreniform) psychosis following stroke. *J Neuropsychiatry Clin Neurosci* 1991;3:6–9.

Rabkin JG, Ferrando S: A "second life" agenda: psychiatric research issues raised by protease inhibitor treatments for people with the human immunodeficiency virus or the acquired immunodeficiency syndrome. *Arch Gen Psychiatry* 1997;54(11):1049–1053.

Raskind MA, Sadowsky CH, Sigmund WR, et al.: Effect of tacrine on language, praxis, and noncognitive behavioral problems in Alzheimer disease. *Arch Neurol* 1997;54(7):836–840.

Reding MJ, Orto LA, Winton SW, et al.: Antidepressant therapy after stroke: a double blind trial. *Arch Neurol* 1986;43:763–765.

Rice DP, Miller LS: The economic burden of affective disorders. *Br J Psychiatry* 1995;27 (suppl):34–42.

Ridker PM, Cushman M, Stampfer MJ, et al.: Inflammation, aspirin, and the risk of cardiovascular disease in apparently healthy men. *NEJM* 1997;336:973–979.

Riordan SM, Williams R: Treatment of hepatic encephalopathy. *N Engl J Med* 1997;337(7):473–479.

Robinson RG, Bolduc P, Price TR. A two year longitudinal study of post stroke depression: diagnosis and outcome at one- and two-year follow-up. *Stroke* 1987;18:837–843.

Robinson RG, Boston JD, Starkstein SE, Price TR. Comparison of mania with depression following brain injury: causal factors. *Am J Psychiatry* 1988;145:172–178.

Robinson RG, Kubos KL, Starr LB, et al.: Mood disorders in stroke patients: importance of location of lesion. *Brain* 1984;107:81–93.

Robinson RG, Starr LB, Kubos KL, et al. A two year longitudinal study of post stroke mood disorders: findings during the initial evaluation. *Stroke* 1983;14:736–744.

Robinson RG, Szetela B: Mood changes following left hemispheric brain injury. *Ann Neurol* 1981;9:447–453.

Rogers SL, Friedhoff LT: The efficacy and safety of donepezil in patients with Alzheimer's disease: results of a US multicentre, randomized, double-blind, placebo controlled trial. *Dementia* 1996;293–303.

Rogers RL, Meyer JS, Judd BW, et al.: Abstention from cigarette smoking improves cerebral perfusion among elderly chronic smokers. *JAMA* 1985;253:2970–2974.

Roman GC, Tatemichi TK, Erkinjuntti T, et al.: Vascular dementia: Diagnostic Criteria for research studies. Report on the NINDS-AIREN international workshop. *Neurology* 1993;43:250–260.

Romano J, Engel GL: Studies of delirium, I: electroencephalographic data. *Arch Neurol Psychiatry* 1944;51:356–377.

Rubin EH, Kinscherf DA: Psychopathology of very mild dementia of the Alzheimer type. *Am J Psychiatry* 1989;146:1017–1021.

Rupright J, Woods EA, Singh A: Hypoxic brain injury: evaluation by single photon emission computed tomography. *Arch Phys Med Rehabil* 1996;77(11):1205–1208.

Salvan AM, Vion-Dury J, Confort-Gouny S, et al.: Brain proton magnetic resonance spectroscopy in HIV-related encephalopathy: identification of evolving metabolic patterns in relation to dementia and therapy. *AIDS Res Hum Retroviruses* 1997;13(12):1055–1066.

Samuel W, Alford M, Hofstetter CR, Hansen L: Dementia with Lewy bodies versus pure Alzheimer disease: differences in cognition, neuropathology, cholinergic dysfunction, and synapse density. *J Neuropathol Exp Neurol* 1997;56(5):499–508.

Samuels SC, Davis KL: A risk benefit assessment of tacrine for the treatment of Alzheimer's Disease. *Drug Safety* 1996;16(1):66–77.

Samuels SC, Katz IR, Parmelee PA, et al.: Use of the Hamilton and Montgomery Asberg Depression Scales in institutionalized elder patients. *Am J Geriatr Psychiatry* 1996b;4(3):237–246.

Sano M, Ernesto C, Thomas RG, et al.: A controlled trial of selegiline, alpha-tocopherol, or both as treatment for Alzheimer's disease. *N Engl J Med* 1997;336:1216–1222.

Satlin A, Volicer L, Ross V, et al.: Bright light treatment of behavioral and sleep disturbances in patients with Alzheimer's disease. *Am J Psychiatry* 1992;149:1028–1032.

Scheuner D, Eckman C, Jensen M, et al.: Secreted amyloid beta-protein similar to that in the senile plaques of Alzheimer's disease is increased in vivo by the presenilin 1 and 2 and APP mutations linked to familial Alzheimer's disease. *Nature Med* 1996;2:864–870.

Schneider LS, Farlow MR, Henderson VW, Pogoda JM: Effects of estrogen replacement therapy on response to tacrine in patients with Alzheimer's disease. *Neurology* 1996;46:1580–1584.

Schneider LS, Pollock VE, Lyness SA: A meta-analysis of controlled trials of neuroleptic treatment in dementia. *J Am Geriatr Soc* 1990;38:553–563.

Schwartz G: Results of extended release physostigmine in the treatment of Alzheimer's disease. ACNP. December 9–13, 1996 San Juan, Puerto Rico.

Sedman AJ, Bockbrader H, Schwarz RD: Preclinical and phase 1 clinical characterization of CI-979/RU35926, a novel muscarinic agonist for the treatment of Alzheimer's disease. *Life Sci* 1995;56:877–882.

Selkoe DJ: Amyloidosis of A beta42 as the common pathogenetic mechanism of all forms of Alzheimer's disease. Abstract 146. Fifth International Conference on Alzheimer's Disease and Related Disorders. July 26–29, 1996. Osaka, Japan.

Senin U, Abeate G, Fieschi C, et al.: Aniracetam (Ro13-5057) in the treatment of senile dementia of the Alzheimer type (SDAT): results of a placebo controlled multicentre clinical trial. *Eur Neuropsychopharmacol* 1991;1:511–517.

Senin U, Parnetti L, Barbagallo-Sangiorgi G, et al.: Idebenone in senile dementia of the Alzheimer's type: a multicentre study. *Arch Gerontol Geriatr* 1992;15:249–260.

Sherrington R, Rogaev EI, Liang Y, et al.: Cloning of a gene bearing missense mutations in early-onset familial Alzheimer's disease. *Nature* 1995;375(6534):754–760.

Shi B, De Girolami U, He J, et al.: Apoptosis induced by HIV-1 infection of the central nervous system. *J Clin Invest* 1996;98(9):1979–1990.

Sidtis JJ, Gatsonis C, Price RW, et al.: Zidovudine treatment of the AIDS dementia complex: results of a placebo-controlled trial: AIDS Clinical Trials Group. *Ann Neurol* 1993;33(4):343–349.

Skoog I, Lernfelt B, Landahl S, et al. 15-year longitudinal study of blood pressure and dementia. *Lancet* 1996;347:1141–1145.

Small GW, Rabins PV, Barry PP, et al.: Diagnosis and treatment of Alzheimer disease and related disorders: consensus statement of the American Association for Geriatric Psychiatry, the Alzheimer's Association, and the American Geriatrics Society. *JAMA* 1997;278(16):1363–1371.

Smith MJ, Breitbart WS, Platt MM: A critique of instruments and methods to detect, diagnose, and rate delirium. *J Pain Symptom Manage* 1994;10:35–77.

Snow C. Medicare HMOs develop plan for future of Alzheimer's programing. *Modern Healthcare* 1996:67–70.

Sorander LB, Portin R, Molsa P, et al.: Senile dementia of the Alzheimer's type treated with aniracetam: a new nootropic agent. *Psychopharmacology* 1987;91:90–95.

Sramek JJ, Hurley DJ, Wardle TS, et al.: The safety and tolerance of xanomeline tartrate in patient's with Alzheimer's disease. *J Clin Pharmacol* 1995;35:800–806.

Stern RG, Mohs RC, Davidson M, et al.: A longitudinal study of Alzheimer's disease: measurement, rate, and predictors of cognitive deterioration. *Am J Psychiatry* 1994;151(3):390–396.

Stern Y, Tang MX, Albert MS, et al.: Predicting time to nursing home care and death in individuals with Alzheimer disease. *JAMA* 1997;277(10):806–812.

Stewart WF, Kawas C, Corrada M, Metter EJ: Risk of Alzheimer's disease and duration of NSAID use. *Neurology* 1997;48:626–632.

Strittmatter WJ, Saunders AM, Schmechel D, et al.: High-avidity binding to beta-amyloid and increased frequency of type 4 allele in late-onset familial Alzheimer disease. *Proc Natl Acad Sci USA* 1993;90(5):1977–1981.

Stroke Prevention in Atrial Fibrillation Investigators: Stroke prevention in atrial fibrillation study: final results. *Circulation* 1991;84:527–534.

Sultzer DL, Gray KF, Gunay I, et al.: A double-blind comparison of trazadone and haloperidol for treatment of agitation in patients with dementia. *Am J Geriatr Psychiatry* 1997;5:60–69.

Sunderland T, Tariot PN, Newhouse PA: Differential responsivity of mood, behavior and cognition to cholinergic agents in elderly neuropsychiatric populations. *Brain Res* 1988;472:371–389.

Tang MX, Jacobs D, Stern Y, et al.: Effect of oestrogen during menopause on risk and age at onset of Alzheimer's disease. *Lancet* 1996;348:429–432.

Tariot PN, Erb R, Leibovici, et al.: Carbamazepine treatment of agitation in nursing home patients with dementia: a preliminary study. *J Am Geriatr Soc* 1994;42:1160–1166.

Tariot PN, Schneider LS: Nonneuroleptic treatment of complications of dementia: applying clinical research to practice, in Nelson JC (ed): *Geriatric Psychopharmacology* New York: Marcel Dekker, 1998:427–454.

Tatemachi TK, Paik M, Bagiella MS, et al.: Risk of dementia after stroke in a hospitalized cohort: result of a longitudinal study. *Neurology* 1994;44:1885–1891.

Teira R, Uriarte E, Munoz J, et al.: Prognostic factors and survival of patients with the AIDS dementia complex. *Int Conf AIDS* 1996;11:296.

Thomsen T, Bickel U, Fischer JP, et al.: Galanthamine hydrobromide is a long-term treatment of Alzheimer's disease: selectivity toward human brain acetylcholinesterase compared with butyrylcholinesterase. *J Pharmacol Exp Ther* 1995;274(2):767-770.

Tollefson GD. Short term effects of the calcium channel blocker nimodipine (Bay-e-9736) in the management of primary degenerative dementia. *Biol Psychiatry* 1990;27:1133–1142.

Tohen M, Castillo-Ruiz J, Baldeessarini RJ, et al.: Blood dyscrasias with carbamazepine and valproate: a pharmacoepidemiological study of 2,228 cases at risk. *Am J Psychiatry* 1995;152:413–418.

Troetel WM, Imbimbo BP: Overview of the Development of Eptastigmine, a long acting cholinesterase inhibitor. Fifth International Conference on Alzheimer's Disease and Related Disorders. July 24–29, 1996. Osaka, Japan.

Trojanowski JQ, Schmidt ML, Otvos L, et al.: Vulnerability of the neuronal cytoskeleton in aging and Alzheimer's disease: widespread involvement of all three major filament systems. *Ann Rev Gerontol Geriatr* 1990;10:167–182.

Unni LK, Womack C, Hannant ME, Becker RE: Pharmacokinetics and pharmacodynamics of metrifonate in humans. *Methods Find Exp Clin Pharmacol* 1994;16:285–289.

Van Bergen PFMM, Jonker JJC, van der Meer, et al.: Anticoagulants in the secondary prevention of events in coronary thrombosis (ASPECT) research group: effect of long term anticoagulant treatment on mortality and cardiovascular morbidity after myocardial infarction. *Lancet* 1994;313:499–503.

Verhey FRJ, Lodder J, Rozendaal N, Jolles J: Comparison of seven sets of criteria used for the diagnosis of vascular dementia. *Neuroepidemiology* 1996;15:166–172.

Villemagne VL, Phillips RL, Liu X, et al.: Peptide T and glucose metabolism in AIDS dementia complex. *J Nucl Med* 1996;37(7):1177–1180.

Walker Z, Allen RL, Shergill S, Katona CL: Neuropsychological performance in Lewy body dementia and Alzheimer's disease. *Br J Psychiatry* 1997;170:156–158.

Walsh JS, Welch HG, Larson EB: Survival of outpatients with Alzheimer-type dementia. *Ann Intern Med* 1990;113(6):429–434.

Watkins PB, Zimmerman HJ, Knapp MJ, et al.: Hepatotoxic effects of tacrine administration in patients with Alzheimer's disease. *JAMA* 1994;271:992–998.

Webster S, O'Barr S, Rogers J: Enhanced aggregation and beta structure of amyloid beta peptide after coincubation with C1q. *J Neurosci Res* 1994;39:448–456.

Weiner MF, Risser RC, Cullum CM, et al.: Alzheimer's disease and its Lewy body variant: a clinical analysis of postmortem verified cases. *Am J Psychiatry* 1996;153(10):1269–1273.

Wetterling T, Kanitz RD, Borgis KJ: The ICD-10 criteria for vascular dementia. *Dementia* 1994;5:185–188.

Wetterling T, Kanitz RD, Borgis KJ: Comparison of different diagnostic criteria for vascular dementia (ADDTC, DSM-IV, ICD-10, NINDS-AIREN). *Stroke* 1996;27(1):30–36.

Weyer G, Babej-Dolle RM, Hadler D, et al.: A controlled study of 2 doses of idebenone in the treatment of Alzheimer's disease. *Neuropsychobiology* 1997;36(2):73–82.

Weyer G, Erzigkeit H, Hadler D, Kubicki S: Efficacy and safety of idebenone in the long-term treatment of Alzheimer's disease: a double-blind, placebo controlled multicentre study. *Hum Psychopharmacol* 1996;11:53–65.

Whitehouse PJ, Kalaria RN: Nicotinic receptors and neurodegenerative dementing diseases: basic research and clinical implications. *Alzheimer Dis Assoc Disord* 1995;9(suppl 2):3–5.

Wilcock G, Wilkinson D: Galanthamine hydrobromide: interim results of a group comparative, placebo controlled, study of efficacy and safety in patients with a diagnosis of senile dementia of the Alzheimer's Type. Abstract at Fifth International Conference on Alzheimer's Disease and Related Disorders. July 26–29, 1996. Osaka, Japan.

Wolf PA, Dawber TR, Thomas HE, et al.: Epidemiologic assessment of chronic atrial fibrillation and risk of stroke: The Framingham Study. *Neurology* 1978;28:973–977.

Wolters EC, Jansen EN, Tuynman-Qua HG, Bergmans PL: Olanzapine in the treatment of dopaminomimetic psychosis in patients with Parkinson's disease. *Neurology* 1996;47(4):1085–1087.

Yesavage JA, Brink TL, Rose TL, et al.: Development and validation of a geriatric depression screening scale: a preliminary report. *J Psychiatr Res* 1982;17(1):37–49.

Yoshitake T, Kiyohara Y, Kato I, et al.: Incidence and risk factor of vascular dementia and Alzheimer's disease in a defined elderly Japanese population. *Neurology* 1995;45:1161–1168.

Yoshioka M, Itoyama Y: Pathogenesis of HIV-1-associated-neurologic diseases. *Nippon Rinsho* 1997;55(4):897–903.

You R, McNeil JJ, O'Malley HM, et al.: Risk factors for lacunar infarction syndromes. *Neurology* 1995;45:1483–1487.

Young RC, Biggs JT, Ziegler VE, Meyer DA: A rating scale for mania: reliability, validity and sensitivity. *Br J Psychiatry* 1978;133:429–435.

NEUROMUSCULAR DISORDERS

Stanley H. Appel

Neuromuscular diseases are disabling disorders of peripheral nerves, the neuromuscular junction, and muscle caused by a wide range of pathologies. Many of the disorders of peripheral nerve, neuromuscular junction and muscles are due to inherited traits with recent advances made in defining these genetic characteristics. Moreover the last decade has witnessed tremendous progress in treating the large number of neuromuscular disorders that are acquired. The most significant advances have been made in treating inflammatory conditions associated with immune-mediated pathologies, a focus of this chapter. Emphasis is placed on Guillain-Barré syndrome and chronic inflammatory demyelinating polyneuropathy, examples of inflammatory neuropathies; myasthenia gravis and Lambert-Eaton myasthenic syndrome, examples of immune-mediated neuromuscular junction abnormalities; and dermatomyositis, polymyositis, and inclusion body myositis, examples of inflammatory myopathies. To a variable extent, the pathogenesis of these disorders appears to result from immune-mediated injury and, to a variable extent, they respond to immunosuppressive therapies.

DISEASES OF PERIPHERAL NERVES

Peripheral nerves may be compromised by a wide range of pathologies, and can be clinically characterized by the fiber types affected, the time course of symptomatic development, which may include motor, sensory and autonomic dysfunction, and the pathophysiologic process involved. Damage to a single nerve, termed mononeuropathy, may result from trauma, infection, or other causes. Damage to multiple nerves affected individually, mononeuropathy multiplex, may result from vasculitis, other inflammatory or dysimmune processes, genetic causes, or diabetes. As for polyneuropathies, or damage to multiple nerves, most are relatively symmetric and generalized, usually compromise distal more than proximal musculature, and result in paresthesias, dysesthesias, and burning sensations (positive symptoms), as well as numbness and sensory loss (negative symptoms).

These distal manifestations are not only due to impaired impulse conduction following demyelination or other causes, but also to the vulnerability to disease of axons and nerve terminals dependent on axoplasmic flow and the synthetic machinery of neuronal cell bodies in the far-removed dorsal root ganglia, spinal cord, or brain stem. Some polyneuropathies are predominantly sensory; others are predominantly motor. The polyneuropathies are also classified on whether they are of acute or chronic onset. The focus of the present text is on a treatable, important example from each category: acute inflammatory demyelinating polyneuropathy (AIDP), which is also known as the Guillain-Barré syndrome (GBS), and chronic inflammatory demyelinating polyneuropathy (CIDP)

Guillain-Barré Syndrome

Guillain-Barré syndrome is one of the most important neurological disorders and gratifying to treat, owing to the dramatic response of patients to the care provided in hospital intensive care units and the effectiveness of the newer immunomodulatory therapies. The clinical syndrome consists of rapidly developing weakness occurring days to weeks after an upper respiratory tract infection, with at least 30% of patients having no antecedent infection. Sensory symptoms, such as paresthesias of the feet, may be present early. Although sensory signs are commonly present, they are usually mild. Deep aching back pain and dysesthetic leg pain, however, can also be an early and disabling symptom in GBS (Moulin et al., 1997). Weakness may begin in the lower extremities and then involve the upper extremities, and facial, bulbar, and respiratory musculature, ascending within hours to days. The presentation of GBS can be quite variable, with weakness beginning in facial musculature and upper extremities, then descending to involve the lower extremities. The onset is usually symmetric, with the weakness accompanied by absent or diminished tendon reflexes. Autonomic neuropathy is a common component of GBS, occurring in approximately 50% of cases, although sphincter muscles are unaffected. The course of the disease is monophasic, with worsening occurring over several days to several weeks, followed by a plateau for days to months, and then improvement, usually over several months. While there was slightly increased incidence of GBS following the 1976 to 1977 immunization with swine influenza vaccine (Schonberger et al., 1979), no such problem has been associated with influenza vaccine formulations used from 1980 to 1988 (Roscelli et al., 1991).

The age-specific incidence and the U.S. morbidity and mortality burden for GBS were recently compiled (Prevots et al., 1997). The estimated annual incidence for GBS is 3.0/100,000, with the incidence increasing with age from 1.5/100,000 at less than 15 years old, to 8.6/100,000 in persons 70 to 79 years old. The estimated number of GBS-related deaths averages about 600 per year. Thus, GBS is a significant health burden among older adults in the United States, with a marked increase in incidence after age 40.

In its classical presentation with motor, sensory, and autonomic symptoms and signs due to a demyelinating polyradiculoneuropathy, GBS is quite distinctive, and the diagnosis relatively straightforward. Variants of GBS can also present as axonal polyneuropathies with motor symptoms and signs, acute motor axonal neuropathy, or with motor and sensory symptoms and signs, acute motor and sensory axonal neuropathy. The acute axonal form is usually associated with more severe dysfunction and a poorer prognosis (Feasby et al., 1986). The presence of ophthalmoplegia, ataxia, and areflexia is a GBS variant known as the Miller Fisher syndrome. From a diagnostic perspective, in the absence of cranial nerve involvement, even with preservation of sphincter function, it is important to rule out by neuroimaging spinal cord compression as a cause of these symptoms. In the differential diagnosis it is also important to eliminate acute intermittent porphyria or metal intoxications as causes of the acute neuropathy, as well as systemic illnesses such as infectious mononucleosis, paraneoplastic syndromes, or various metabolic syndromes. Patients with human immunodeficiency virus (HIV) are at risk for developing polyneuropathy or polyradiculoneuropathy, which could be due to GBS, cytomegalovirus polyradiculoneuropathy, or even lymphoma associated with HIV infection (Miller et al., 1988; Said et al., 1991). Although these syndromes may often be difficult to differentiate on the basis of the clinical manifestations per se, the spinal fluid examination in the HIV-related polyradiculoneuropathy syndromes usually reveals the presence of polymorphonuclear leukocytes and evidence of the virus.

Autonomic dysfunction, including visual blurring, abdominal pain, chest pain, hypotension, and tachycardia, can lead to serious difficulties and may account for the previously poor prognosis in GBS. In a recent study employing tests of autonomic function, subclinical autonomic involvement of both parasympathetic and sympathetic functions was present in the vast majority of patients (Flachenecker et al., 1997).

Laboratory Findings

In GBS, electromyography (EMG) and nerve conduction velocity, as well as spinal fluid examination, are of significant diagnostic assistance. Three to 7 days after onset, EMG and nerve conductions demonstrate slowing of motor, and to a lesser extent sensory, conduction velocities, prolonged distal latencies and F-wave latencies, reduced amplitude of compound muscle action potentials and possibly sensory action potentials, as well as focal and asymmetrical conduction block as evidence of a segmental demyelinating polyneuropathy. On the other hand, acute motor axonal neuropathies have normal sensory nerve action potentials and conduction velocities, with reduced compound muscle action potentials and only a slight reduction in conduction velocities. When both motor and sensory function are impaired, both compound muscle action potentials and sensory nerve action potentials may be severely compromised, with distal latencies and conduction velocities difficult to measure, suggesting the presence of severe motor and sensory axonopathy. In the Miller Fisher syndrome, despite the ataxia, ophthalmoplegia, and areflexia, general strength is preserved and EMG and nerve conduction velocities may be normal in the extremities.

The cerebrospinal fluid examination can be of important diagnostic value in GBS, with the protein usually elevated to greater than 60 mg/dL and the number of cells normal (five or less per μL). Very early in the course of disease the cerebrospinal fluid protein may be normal, and elevation of cells to 30 does not exclude the diagnosis.

Because biopsies of sural nerves may not demonstrate inflammation or demyelination, they are not a routine part of most clinical evaluations in GBS, although they may be of value for research purposes. In pathologic studies, proximal nerves and nerve roots are prominently affected (Asbury et al., 1969), with edema, segmental demyelination, and infiltration of the endoneurium with mononuclear cells, including macrophages. The mononuclear cells appear to interact both with Schwann cells and the myelin sheath. Although GBS is a polyradiculoneuropathy, pathology may also be present within the central nervous system (CNS). In 13 autopsied cases, mononuclear infiltrates of lymphocytes and activated macrophages were present within the spinal cord, medulla oblongata and pons in the majority of cases (Maier et al., 1997). No primary demyelination was noted within the CNS. In cases with protracted clini-

cal courses, activated macrophages were the predominant cell type in both central and peripheral nervous systems as well as the presence of CD4 + and CD8 + T lymphocytes.

Pathogenesis. Demyelination and inflammatory infiltrates in nerve roots and proximal nerves can account for the symptoms and signs of GBS, and both humoral and cell-mediated immunity have been implicated. The presence of lymphocytes and macrophages in a perivenous distribution, and in association with myelinated axons, first suggested the potential role of autoimmune reactions in the demyelinative process (Asbury et al., 1969). This examination of human acute inflammatory demyelinating neuropathy was prompted by the earlier demonstration (Waksman and Adams, 1955) that immunization of laboratory animals with peripheral nerve myelin and adjuvant produces an experimental allergic neuritis. Subsequently, although purified myelin proteins, such as the P2 myelin basic protein or peptide fragments of the P2 (Rostami et al., 1990) and PO protein (Milner et al., 1987) were demonstrated to induce experimental neuropathy, antibodies to these constituents are not commonly detected in GBS. The T-cell lines derived from the spleen and lymph nodes of rats immunized with P2 synthetic peptide 53-78 can adoptively transfer severe experimental allergic neuritis to naive syngeneic rats (Rostami and Gregorian, 1991). Thus, cell-mediated, and possibly humoral immune mechanisms, can contribute to an experimental model of peripheral nerve inflammatory injury.

Most recent studies on GBS have focused on glycoconjugates and lipopolysaccharides of the myelin sheath, the Schwann cell membrane, or the axonal membrane as the major antigens initiating the inflammatory/immune reaction in GBS. In a detailed study from Japan, 31 isolates from patients with GBS were serotyped for *Campylobacter jejuni* antigens (Yuki et al., 1997). In this typing, the Penner method uses heat-stable lipopolysaccharides, whereas the Lior method uses heat-labile protein antigens. The PEN 19 and LIO 7 antigens of *C. jejuni* were isolated more frequently from GBS patients (52% and 45%, respectively) than from sporadic *C. jejuni* enteritis patients (5% and 3%, respectively), and were associated with an increase in anti-GM1 antibodies possibly due to a GM1-like lipopolysaccharide antigen. In reports from other countries, the incidence of *C. jejuni* infections preceding the development of GBS is much lower. In addition, the percentage of patients with antiganglioside antibodies is much more variable, ranging from a low of 5% to a high of 60% (reviewed in Hartung et al., 1995). However, no correlation has been found between the presence of GM1 antibodies and clinical or electrophysiologic features of the disease (Enders et al., 1993; Vriesendorp et al., 1993).

In the Miller Fisher syndrome, anti-GQ1b antibodies have been commonly detected (Chiba et al., 1993; Willison et al., 1993). These are clearly detectable at paranodal regions by immunohistochemistry of human cranial nerves innervating the eye (Chiba et al., 1993). It has also been found that antibodies to GQ1b may block transmission in a mouse neuromuscular system (Roberts et al., 1994).

In the acute motor axonal neuropathy form of GBS, antecedent infection with *C. jejuni* may be more common, and anti-GM1 antibodies and the complement activation product C3d may be bound to the axolemma of motor fibers (Hafer-Macko et al., 1996).

The anti-GM1 antibodies can also bind at the nodes of Ranvier, thereby interfering with nerve conduction. These antibodies might also be involved in degeneration of motor nerve terminals and intramuscular axons, as demonstrated in a recent case of GBS presenting with acute motor axonal neuropathy (Ho et al., 1997). The *C. jejuni* enteritis leading to GBS may also enhance generation of gamma delta T lymphocytes, which could actively participate in the inflammatory/immune process (Ben-Smith et al., 1997). High serum levels of the cytokine, tumor necrosis factor-alpha, but not interleukin-1 beta or the soluble interleukin-2 receptor, appeared to correlate with the electrodiagnostic abnormalities in GBS (Sharief et al., 1997). Autopsy specimens suggest that complement may be involved in at least some cases of the classical acute inflammatory demyelinating form of GBS based on the demonstration of both C3d and the C5b-9 membrane attack complex on the outer surface of Schwann cells (Hafer-Macko et al., 1996).

Thus, most constituents present in immune-mediated disorders are present in GBS. Although antibodies against glycoconjugates may participate in the pathogenesis of several of the different clinical forms of the GBS syndromes, their exact role is unclear. Even when anti-GM1 antibodies are present, their reactivity may not be with GM1 per se but with glycolipids or glycoproteins possessing similar, or related, carbohydrate moieties. As a result, the specific antigens within the Schwann cell and axonal membrane that are targets of the inflammatory/immune response, and the specific role of immunoglobulins, await clarification. Further, in many cases of GBS, there is no evidence of prior or concomitant *C. jejuni* infection, no evidence of anti-GM1 antibodies, and no indication as to the organism whose constituents may initiate the immune reaction, possibly by molecular mimicry (Jahnke et al., 1992).

Careful studies of nerve biopsy and autopsy tissue indicate that cell-mediated mechanisms may contribute to the pathogenesis of GBS. Lymphocytes and macrophages are present from nerve root to motor terminals in severe GBS, with activated macrophages in close proximity to, and phagocytosing, myelin (Hall et al., 1992). Although evidence from the experimental model of inflammatory neuropathy provides mechanisms whereby T lymphocytes could participate in the neuropathic process, there are no convincing data to suggest these are operative in GBS. At the present time, the scientific evidence suggests the involvement of activated T cells crossing the blood-nerve barrier and initiating demyelination in conjunction with antibodies specific for nerve antigens, cytokines, such as tumor necrosis factor (TNF)-α and interferon-γ, the components of complement, possibly including the membrane attack complex, and activated macrophages. More work is required, however, to determine whether each of these components is absolutely required, and in what specific sequence, in the pathogenesis of GBS.

Therapy. Treatment of the acute and rapidly evolving symptoms and signs of GBS requires supportive critical care, usually within a hospital intensive care unit (ICU), and immunosuppresive measures directed at the mechanisms responsible for the disease (Fig. 10-1). Patients with GBS should be admitted to the hospital for close monitoring of respiratory and autonomic function. The more rapid the evolution of weakness, the greater the likelihood respiratory support will be needed. Careful and repeated neurologic evaluation is required as are frequent vital capacity measurements and frequent suctioning. It is difficult to feel secure in the early stages of disease because even in the presence of marginal but adequate repiratory and bulbar function, slight aspiration may aggravate autonomic dysfunction and precipitate respiratory failure.

The primary reason for the improved prognosis and decrease in mortality with GBS in recent years is the early transfer of patients to an ICU. A vital capacity below 20 mL/kg and difficulty clearing secretions are indications for transfer to an ICU, and for considering intubation. The goal is to avoid emergency intubation in the setting of frank respiratory failure, with wide swings in blood pressure and heart rate often precipitating myocardial dysfunction and infarction. The most important issues in supportive care involve preventing and rapidly treating pulmonary and bladder infections and, with the use of subcutaneous heparin (5000 units q12h), preventing venous thrombosis in the legs and subsequent pulmo-

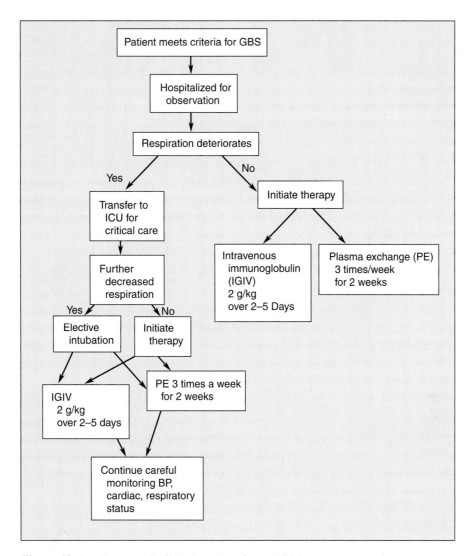

Figure 10–1. *Treating Guillain-Barré syndrome (GBS)*

nary embolism. There should also be carefully monitoring of nutrition and bowel function. Because autonomic dysfunction can contribute signficantly to mortality, continuous assessment of cardiac status and blood pressure is imperative.

One often overlooked component of ICU care of GBS is the severe anxiety associated with complete paralysis when intellectual function is intact. Thus, psychological support is of great importance. All aspects of the disease need to be carefully explained,

including the likelihood for progression and how each phase will be treated. The patient should be reassured that the prognosis for complete recovery is excellent, even if he or she is respirator-dependent at the time. Establishing a means of communication with eye movements can help lessen the patient's feeling of isolation. In our experience, the use of 0.5 mg lorazepam q 4 to 6 h may be helpful with nocturnal hallucinations, 0.5 mg risperidone or 2.5 mg olanzapine may be of value.

The treatment of GBS has undergone revolutionary change over the last decade. For example, plasma exchange is now recognized as an effective therapy. While the mechanism for its beneficial effects are unknown, it is thought to be related to the removal of antibodies, cytokines, complement and other inflammatory/immune mediators. In an open, multicentered North American trial comparing plasma exchange with no treatment, it was found that five consecutive daily exchanges resulted in a shorter hospitalization and more dramatic improvement than was seen in untreated controls (Guillain-Barré Syndrome Study Group, 1985). Treatment was most effective when initiated within the first week after onset of symptoms. This study was confirmed by the French Cooperative Group, demonstrating a more rapid recovery in 220 patients in a randomized multicenter trial with four plasma exchanges (French Cooperative Group, 1987). In a 1-year assessment of these patients, 71% in the plasma exchange group demonstrated full muscle strength recovery compared with 52% in the control group (French Cooperative Group, 1992). The appropriate number of exchanges at mild and moderate stages of weakness was evaluated in 556 GBS patients randomized according to severity and number of exchanges (French Cooperative Group, 1997). In the mild group, two plasma exchanges were more effective than none; in the moderate group, four plasma exchanges were more beneficial than two. Six plasma exchanges were no more beneficial than four in either moderate or severe groups. At present, most centers experienced in the management of GBS still employ five to six exchanges via a Shiley catheter over a period of 8 to 10 days to avoid the stress of daily plasma exchanges. Plasmapheresis also diminishes morbidity in childhood GBS by shortening the interval until recovery of independent ambulation (Epstein et al., 1990). Although plasma exchange is relatively safe, it still requires careful monitoring in GBS because of the autonomic dysfunction and the low threshold for infections.

High-dose intravenous immunoglobulin (IGIV) has also become a mainstay of therapy for GBS, significantly shortening the duration and severity of the disease. As with plasma exchange, the mechanism of the beneficial affect of IGIV is unknown.

Some possibilities include eliminating pathogenic antibodies with antiidiotype antibodies, blocking Fc components of antibodies on target cells, inhibiting the deposition of complement, dissolving immune complexes, downregulating lymphocyte functions, or interfering with cytokine production or function. A total dose of 2 g/kg of immunoglobulin is administered over a 2- to 5-day period. A randomized trial comparing IGIV and plasma exchange demonstrated a median time to improvement of 41 days with plasma exchange and 27 days with immunoglobulin therapy (van der Meche et al., 1992). In addition, immunoglobulin therapy was associated with significantly fewer complications and less need for mechanical ventilation. The major factor adversely affecting prognosis was older age. A subsequent randomized multicenter trial of plasma exchange and IGIV in 383 patients during the 2 weeks after neuropathic symptoms onset documented that the two had equivalent efficacy, and that the combination did not confer a significant advantage (Plasma Exchange/Sandoglobulin Guillain-Barré Syndrome Trial Group, 1997).

Immunoglobulin therapy has also demonstrated efficacy and safety in severe pediatric GBS, with doses of 2 g/kg over a 2-day period (Shahar et al., 1997). Side effects are usually mild and infrequent. Headache may occur, especially in patients with migraine, and may also be accompanied by aseptic meningitis and spinal fluid pleocytosis. Chills, fever, and myalgia are also sometimes encountered, as is acute renal dysfunction, including renal failure. Anaphylactic reactions may occur with IGIV, especially in patients with IgA deficiencies (Thornton et al., 1993). The main disadvantage of both IGIV and plasma exchange is the cost. However, this is clearly outweighed by the benefits of these therapies, even in this era of managed care.

High-dose intravenous corticosteroids (methylprednisolone at 500 mg per day for 5 days) has been studied in a double-blind, placebo-controlled, multicenter trial with 242 patients. No significant difference was noted in any outcome measure or in relapse rate (Guillain-Barré Syndrome Steroid Trial Group, 1993). A subsequent open trial, however, studied 25 patients with GBS treated for 5 days with

IGIV (0.4 g/kg per day) and 500 mg methylprednisolone intravenously per day, and compared them with historical controls receiving IGIV only. The group treated with both steroids and IGIV fared better, with 76% improving by one or more functional grades after 4 weeks compared with 53% in the historical controls treated only with IGIV (The Dutch Guillain-Barré Study Group, 1994). This raises the possibility that corticosteroids may have a role in the therapy of GBS. Clearly, a randomized clinical trial is required to determine whether the addition of IV corticosteroids to either plasma exchange or IGIV therapy will significantly improve prognosis.

Chronic Inflammatory Demyelinating Polyneuropathy

Chronic inflammatory demyelinating polyneuropathy (CIDP) is a symmetric polyneuropathy or polyradiculoneuropathy presenting with weakness, sensory deficits, and paresthesias. Typically it evolves over at least 2 or more months in a steadily progressive, stepwise progressive, or relapsing fashion. In some patients the course may be progressive to death; in others it may continue to fluctuate with multiple exacerbations and remissions (Dyck et al., 1975). Both proximal and distal muscles may weaken, with reflexes decreased to absent. Infrequently, the cranial nerves, including oculomotor, trochlear, and abducent nerves, may be affected. In a study of 67 consecutive patients conforming to clinical and electrophysiologic definitions of CIDP, 51% had a variant presentation, 10% a pure motor syndrome, 12% a sensory ataxic syndrome, 9% a mononeuritis multiplex pattern, 4% a paraparetic pattern, and 16% a relapsing acute Guillain-Barré–like syndrome (Gorson et al., 1997). In this same series pain was more frequent than in previous reports (42%). Diabetic patients may also develop a progressive, moderately severe, predominantly motor neuropathy involving the legs that meets the electrophysiologic as well as clinical criteria of CIDP (Stewart et al., 1996).

CIDP has been reported to be relatively rare in childhood. In a study of 13 children 1.5 to 16 years of age, the disease was monophasic in three (23%) with a single relapse in four (30%), and multiple relapses in six (46%) (Nevo et al., 1996). In children antecedent events are uncommon, the onset of symptoms more precipitous, and gait abnormalities a more frequent presenting symptom (Simmons et al., 1997).

Laboratory Findings

In CIDP, as in GBS, EMG and nerve conduction velocities, as well as spinal fluid examination, are of diagnostic importance. Serum blood chemistries are also helpful in ruling out metabolic neuropathies that may simulate aspects of CIDP such as diabetic, uremic, hepatic, and hypothyroid-mediated nerve damage, as well as polyneuropathies associated with HIV or Lyme disease. Serum protein electrophoresis is of value to rule out monoclonal gammopathy, which may occur in the setting of myeloma or as monoclonal gammopathy of undetermined significance (MGUS). The presence of monoclonal gammopathy should prompt a search for osteosclerotic myeloma or isolated plasmacytoma with a skeletal bone survey, urine examination for monoclonal protein, and possible bone marrow examination

On EMG, motor unit potentials have characteristic findings of denervation and a variable degree of fibrillation depending on the duration and severity of the lesions. Motor and sensory nerve conduction velocities in upper and lower extremities are usually slowed by more than 20%, unless the demyelinating process is largely confined to nerve roots and proximal nerves. A variable degree of nerve conduction block may be present, as well as a variable degree of dispersion of the compound muscle or nerve action potential. Distal latencies and fissures are usually prolonged in this condition. Proximal nerve segments may have greater slowing of conduction velocity than distal nerve segments. The electrodiagnostic criterion of partial conduction block in CIDP is a greater than 20% drop in compound muscle action potential between proximal and distal sites (e.g., elbow and wrist). Multifocal motor neuropathy is considered to be a clinical entity distinct from CIDP. The presence of partial motor conduction block in CIDP, however, has suggested that aspects of the clinical and electrophysiologic spectrum of multifocal motor neuropathy may overlap with CIDP (deCarvalho et al., 1997).

On spinal fluid examination, the protein is generally elevated to greater than 60 mg/dL, and cells are usually five or less. The local IgG synthesis rate may be increased, and the Q albumin may be elevated indicating breakdown in the blood-nerve or blood-brain barrier.

Sural nerve biopsy may be of considerable diagnostic help showing evidence of inflammation and demyelination, or even marked edema of the myelin sheath. On teased fiber examination, segmental demyelination may be apparent and, in some cases, axonal degeneration may predominate.

Recently a number of reports have suggested that magnetic resonance imaging (MRI) may provide insight into the ongoing inflammatory process in CIDP. Indeed, MRI of brachial plexus lesions demonstrated symmetrically enhanced signal densities on T2-weighted images (Van Es et al., 1997). Massive nerve root enlargement in the cauda equina in the lumbosacral region has also been detected by MRI (Schady et al., 1996). In addition, in CIDP nerve enlargement with high signal intensity has been reported with proton or T2-weighted images at sites of demyelination that were defined electrophysiologically (Kuwabara et al., 1997). Of interest is the fact that as the patients improved clinically, the gadolinium enhancement of the lesions disappeared, suggesting that the focal conduction abnormalities may correlate with inflammatory lesions, compromising the blood-nerve barrier

Pathogenesis.   As in GBS, inflammation and demyelination of nerve roots and proximal nerves suggest that the clinical course and neuropathology is best explained by a series of immune-mediated reactions. As a result, the importance of T and B lymphocytes, antibodies specific for nerve antigens, activated macrophages, cytokines such as TNF-α, and complement components have all been implicated. In CIDP, however, the immunologic cascade is even less defined than with GBS. What is even more obscure are the specific immunologic mechanisms that define CIDP as a more protracted chronic disorder with fewer spontaneous remissions than GBS. Answering this question may reveal that GBS and CIDP are acute and chronic variants of the same process differentiated only by specific immune response mechanisms.

Experimental allergic neuritis (EAN) provides the best circumstantial evidence for the importance of immune mechanisms in CIDP and the possible relationship of acute and chronic inflammatory demyelinating polyradiculoneuropathy. When rabbits are immunized with a single large multiportal dose of peripheral myelin, they consistently develop EAN with a chronic progressive or relapsing course. The clinical, electrophysiologic, and pathologic features of this condition are identical to human CIDP. Although antimyelin antibodies are present, T-cell responses have not yet been defined (reviewed in Hahn, 1996). Injection of Lewis rats with myelin or myelin proteins P2 and PO results in a more acute EAN, which can be adoptively transferred to syngeneic animals with antigen-specific (P2 and PO) T cells. Humoral mechanisms may also play a role if myelin antibodies could penetrate the blood-nerve barrier. Alteration of the blood nerve barrier is, in fact, produced experimentally by systemic transfer of ovalbumin-specific activated T cells followed by intraneural injection of ovalbumin. Following these inoculations, endoneurial perivenous inflammation with T cells and macrophages develops, leading to conduction block and mild demyelination, which can be markedly enhanced by the cotransfer of antimyelin immunoglobulins (Harvey et al., 1995). Thus, in experimental models, activated T cells accumulate in peripheral nerves, alter the blood-nerve barrier, and, together with antimyelin antibodies, orchestrate primary demyelination in a dose-dependent manner.

In human CIDP the participating elements in the immune attack are not as well characterized as with GBS and experimental models. In sural nerve biopsies with CIDP, endoneurial infiltration of CD3+ T cells was found in 10 of 13 cases, epineurial T cells were present in 11 of 13 cases and CD68+ macrophages often occurred in endoneurial perivascular clusters (Schmidt et al., 1996). Although cytokines are increased in GBS, they do not appear to be increased in the cerebrospinal fluid in CIDP (Sivieriet et al., 1997); nor is the cytokine TNF-α increased in the serum (Melendez-Vasquez et al., 1997).

The presence and role of a prevalent group of circulating antibodies is less clear in CIDP than in GBS. The IgM antibodies to GM1 ganglioside were present in only 15% of patients with CIDP, with none having IgG antibodies to GM1 (Melendez-Vasquez et al., 1997). Further, only 10% of CIDP cases had serologic evidence of *C. jejuni* infection. IgG and IgM antibodies to other gangliosides, chondroitin sulphate, sulfatides, or myelin proteins were found in fewer than 10% of cases. Several CIDP patients with slowly progressive disease and electrophyiologic findings consistent with demyelination were reported to have IgM monoclonal antibodies that bound to human brain tubulin (Connolly et al., 1997). However, in a much larger series of CIDP patients β-tubulin antibodies were present in only 10.5% as measured by immunoblot techniques (Manfredini et al., 1995). Thus, unlike GBS, CIDP is not associated with any specific infections, nor is there an increased incidence of antibodies to myelin autoantigens or glycoconjugates. Clearly, additional studies are required to clarify the triggering events for CIPD and to determine the sequence of specific steps involved in its pathogenesis.

Therapy. Treatment with immunosuppressive regimens continues to evolve as a therapy for CIDP (Fig. 10-2). Until recently, corticosteroids were considered the treatment of choice based on a randomized, controlled study (Dyck et al., 1982). In this case, prednisone is initiated at doses of 60 to 80 mg per day taken in the morning for 8 weeks, and then tapered slowly by 10 mg per month, and subsequently switched to alternate-day dosing. Improvement in strength usually first appears after several months, and continues for 6 to 8 months before the maximal benefit is obtained. Relapses may occur when the steroids are tapered or discontinued, requiring the doses to be readjusted upward, or alternative treatments instituted. The major problem with chronic oral steroids are weight gain, cushingoid features, hypertension, glucose intolerance, agitation and irritability, insomnia, osteoporosis, aseptic necrosis of the hip, and cataracts. These side effects can be quite

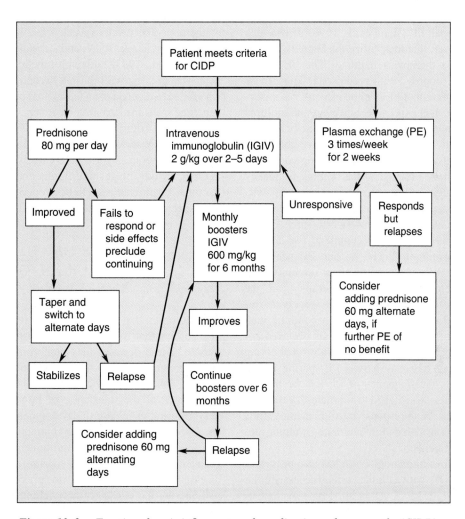

Figure 10–2. *Treating chronic inflammatory demyelinating polyneuropathy (CIDP)*

problematic, especially at high doses, and warrant consideration of alternative therapies.

Plasma exchange (PE) has proven to be an effective therapy for CIDP patients. In an early study, a prospective, double-blind, sham-controlled trial of plasma exchange provided significant improvement for approximately one third of patients with the condition (Dyck et al., 1986). In a recent confirmation, 18 untreated CIDP patients were randomized prospectively to receive 10 PE or sham PE over 4 weeks in a double-blind trial. The results showed that 80% of the treated subjects improved substantially in all clinical outcome measures. When PE administration was stopped, 66% relapsed, and all improved with subsequent open PE (Hahn et al., 1996). It was also found, however, that to stabilize the benefits, immunosuppressive therapy is required. The PE nonresponders did improve with prednisone. Thus, these data demonstrate that PE is quite effective as a therapy for CIDP. It is expensive, however, and multiple exchanges must be conducted either alone or in combination with other immunosuppressive therapies, such as prednisone. Because there are no controlled studies that have established the optimal frequency of PE either alone or in combination with prednisone, many different regimens have been developed empirically. Some have started with two to three PE per week for 6 weeks; others recommend two PE per week for 3 weeks followed by one PE per week for 3 weeks. Following improvement in clinical and electrophysiologic parameters therapy can be stopped and the patient monitored weekly or biweekly. Alternatively, treatment can continue with less frequent PEs. If improvement has occurred but frequent PEs are still required, the addition of 50 mg prednisone per day may have a PE-sparing effect. Subsequently, the frequency of PE can be tapered and the prednisone switched to alternate-day therapy. If the patients are unresponsive to PE therapy, they should be considered for alternate immunosuppressive treatments.

Intravenous immunoglobulin has also proven of benefit in CIDP, with a clinical effectiveness similar to that seen with PE (Dyck et al., 1994). A double-blind, placebo-controlled, prospective cross-over trial was conducted with 25 patients completing both treatment periods and receiving 400 mg/kg immunoglobulin or placebo on 5 consecutive days (Hahn et al., 1996). Significant differences in favor of IGIV were observed for all the clinical end points, with benefit most likely in patients having had the disease for 1 year or less. In 10 IGIV responders with relapsing CIDP, improvement lasted a median time of 6 weeks. In this case all 10 patients were maintained and stabilized with IGIV "pulse" therapy of 1 g/kg immunoglobulin. Thus, IGIV is also beneficial in CIDP with an efficacy similar to PE. As indicated previously, IGIV therapy is expensive and side effects are relatively minor. A study consisting of 67 patients was undertaken to compare the three modes of therapy. The results revealed the response rates of plasma exchange, IGIV, and steroids were similar (Gorson et al., 1997), although functional improvement was greatest with plasma exchange. Of the 26 who failed to respond to an initial therapy, nine (35%) benefited from an alternative treatment, and of the 11 who required a third modality, three (27%) improved. Overall in this series, 66% responded to one of the three main therapies for CIDP. Clearly, in CIDP as in GBS, the advantages of different combinations of the three treatments need to be properly assessed in a prospectively controlled clinical trial.

DISEASES OF THE NEUROMUSCULAR JUNCTION

The neuromuscular junction is the target of a number of disorders that impair transmission from nerve to muscle. These diseases may compromise the postsynaptic junction and the acetylcholine receptor (AChR). With a deficiency of the AChR, there is an impairment of the translation of information from neurotransmitter release to development of the muscle action potential and muscle contraction. Myasthenia gravis (MG) is the most prominent example of such a postsynaptic disease. Neuromuscular junction diseases may also compromise the presynaptic terminal, altering the release of acetylcholine (ACh) and thereby decreasing its availability to interact with the AChR to intiate muscle contraction. The Lambert-

Eaton myasthenic syndrome (LEMS) is the best-known example of such a presynaptic disease. Whether the pathology is pre- or postsynaptic, the result is a significant weakness with sparing of sensory function, with the most common presentation being as an autoimmune disease generally responsive to immunosuppressive medication.

Myasthenia Gravis

Myasthenia gravis (MG) is an acquired autoimmune disorder characterized by weakness and fatigability of skeletal muscles. The incidence of MG is less than 1 per 100,000, with a prevalence of 10 to 15 per 100,000 (Sorensen and Holm, 1989; Oosterhuis, 1989). The disease is more common among females in the first several decades of life, and among males over the age of 50 (Grob et al., 1981).

The clinical syndrome is characterized by variable weakness and fatigability, which may fluctuate throughout the day and from day to day. Increase in weakness may occur as the day progresses or with exertion, and improvement may develop with rest. The extraocular and eyelid muscles can be affected early and usually asymetrically, giving rise to double vision and ptosis. While in a small percentage (10–15%) of cases the disease remains confined to the eyes, more typically it gradually becomes more generalized, involving the limbs, especially the proximal musculature such as the iliopsoas and the deltoids. The triceps muscle and finger flexors and extensors are also involved. Swallowing difficulty, secondary to compromise of the pharyngeal muscles, can lead to choking and, with laryngeal weakness, to aspiration of food and secretions. The major concern is weakness of the respiratory muscles leading to impairment of breathing and respiratory myasthenic crises. Exacerbations can be provoked by emotional stress, infections, altered hormonal states (especially hypothyroidism and hyperthyroidism), and various medications, such as aminoglycoside antibiotics, anti-arrhythmics, diuretics, magnesium salts, and β-adrenergic receptor blocking agents.

Transient neonatal MG with weak sucking and crying, and impaired swallowing and respiration, develop in about 12% of infants born to myasthenic mothers (Namba et al., 1970). The signs usually appear within the first several hours after birth and may last from several weeks to 2 months, with no recurrence in later life. There is usually no correlation between the severity of disease in mother and infant, even though it is most likely caused by the transplacental passage of AChR antibodies. MG may also appear in infancy and childhood as a sporadic acquired autoimmune disease. In this case it is quite similar to adult MG. It may also appear at birth, in infancy, in childhood, or in adulthood as a congenital myasthenic syndrome, which consists of a number of genetically mediated abnormalities of presynaptic or postsynaptic structures that impair neuromuscular transmission. These conditions are usually inherited as autosomal recessive traits. In different syndromes, clinical weakness ranging from diplopia and ptosis to more generalized weakness has been described (Engel et al., 1994).

Laboratory Findings

Bedside pharmacologic tests may be of value in MG because inhibiting the enzyme acetylcholinesterase (AChE), which catalyzes the breakdown of ACh, may improve symptomatology. Edrophonium (Tensilon), a short-acting AChE inhibitor, when injected intravenously may improve the performance of a muscle group that fatigues on examination, such as the eyelid levators, the deltoid, or the iliopsoas. Initially, 2 mg of edrophonium is injected and the muscle strength monitored after 1 min. In the absence of improvement, injections of an additional 3 mg, followed by 5 mg, can be performed. Some patients may be sensitive to small amounts of edrophonium chloride, precipitating a respiratory crisis. Thus, a resuscitator should be available to breathe for the patient in such an emergency. Any beneficial effects in response to edrophonium usually last for only a few minutes. A positive test provides support for the diagnosis of MG, although it is not specific for this condition, occurring in patients with peripheral neuropathies, brain stem lesions, ALS, and poliomyelitis as well.

EMG is usually of diagnostic value in MG. In the majority of patients with generalized MG, a decrementing response of greater than 10% is found after stimulation at 3 Hz. This decrementing response is a consequence of the reduced safety margin of neuromuscular transmission and results from the decreased number of AChR on the muscle membrane, the widened intersynaptic cleft, and the decreased amount of ACh released following the first 5 to 10 low-frequency stimuli. When two or more distal and two or more proximal muscles are examined, 95% of MG patients display a positive response in at least one muscle (Ozdemir et al., 1976). When only a single distal muscle is tested, however, only 50% of patients have positive decrementing responses. Proximal limb muscles are more likely to demonstrate the decrementing response than those in the distal limb. In patients with ocular MG, less than one half have a significant decrementing response. Single-fiber EMG may also be useful in defining neuromuscular dysfunction by measuring the mean interpotential interval between two fibers since, in MG, this interval is usually prolonged. Although this measure is not specific for MG, it may indicate the involvement of the neuromuscular junction when the diagnosis is in doubt.

While 80% of patients with acquired, autoimmune MG have serum antibodies against the AChR (Tindall et al., 1981), more than 50% of patients with ocular MG do not. In generalized MG the titer of AChR antibodies is usually elevated, whereas in ocular MG it is lower. The AChR antibodies can bind to different sites on the AChR, with the majority attaching to a region of the alpha subunit designated the main immunogenic region (Tzartos et al., 1988), that is separate from the ACh binding site. Although a number of functional assays for these main immunogenic region AChR antibodies have been developed, none of the antibody specificities correlate with the clinical state or duration of disease (Tzartos et al., 1982). In general, the antibody titer correlates poorly with the severity of MG. In the patient with improvement in clinical state following immunosuppressive therapy, however, reduced AChR antibody titers are noted over the long term (Oosterhuis et al., 1983). Antibodies that bind to striated muscle (striational antibodies) are also present in MG, especially in patients with thymoma, with one study showing that such antibodies are present in 84% of thymoma patients (Limburg et al., 1983).

Pathogenesis.   MG is considered a classical example of an autoantibody-mediated and T-cell–dependent autoimmune disease. The major physiologic and morphologic changes in MG are at the neuromuscular junction and result primarily from AChR antibodies decreasing the number of AChR on the muscle postsynaptic membrane. IgG and complement are deposited at the neuromuscular junction in MG as assayed by immunoelectron microscopy (Engel et al., 1977).

In extracts of MG muscle, IgG was found to be complexed to AChR. In MG, the number of AChR decreased (Fambrough et al., 1973), the postsynaptic membrane is markedly simplified, and the membrane surface available for insertion of new AChR reduced (Engel et al., 1981). This pathology could be produced either by antibody-mediated increases in AChR internalization and degradation (antigenic modulation), or by antibody- and complement-mediated destruction of the postsynaptic architecture. Evidence exists that both processes may participate in the alterations of the neuromuscular junction. The complement membrane attack complex is present at the neuromuscular junction in MG, with vesicles containing the membrane attack complex being shed into a widened intersynaptic space (Sahashi et al., 1980; Engel et al., 1981). This continuous shedding could reduce the number of AChR and also simplify the junctional folds. Antibody-mediated cross-linking of AChR followed by internalization and degradation have also been implicated as a process for decreasing the number of AChR (Fumagalli et al., 1982; Stanley and Drachman, 1978). Thus, both antigenic modulation and complement-mediated injury may combine to produce the neuromuscular alterations in MG. The passive transfer of MG from man to mouse supports the important role of humoral mechanisms in the pathogenesis of MG by revealing that the antibodies themselves can initiate neuromuscular dysfunction (Toyka et al., 1977).

The triggers for production of AChR antibodies are unknown. The possibility of molecular mimicry has been raised by the demonstration of shared epitopes between human AChR and a number of bacterial and viral constituents (Stefannson et al., 1986; Schwimbeck et al., 1989). In MG, however, the AChR antibodies are polyclonal (Tzartos et al., 1982), and attempts to isolate a virus or identify specific reactivity with microbial antigens have been unsuccesful. Thus, molecular mimicry of a single epitope is unlikely to explain the findings in MG. It is known that production of AChR antibodies requires both CD4 + T helper lymphocytes and B lymphocytes (Hohlfeld et al., 1986). Experimental models of MG suggest that the immunopathology is initiated by the presentation of AChR to T lymphocytes (Lennon et al., 1976). There is no question the thymus is involved in MG, with 70% of patients having thymic hyperplasia with germinal centers, and 15% a thymoma at the time of diagnosis or during the course of the illness (Castleman, 1966). Thus, it is possible that the initial steps in the pathogenesis of MG take place within an abnormal thymic microenvironment. Additional studies are needed, however, to determine whether the thymus provides both the source of the AChR antigen (possibly from thymus myoid cells) and the T cells that drive B cells to produce AChR antibodies. No single immunodominant T-cell AChR epitope has been identified in MG, and the ability of AChR epitopes to stimulate normal as well as MG T cells suggests the possible role of altered immunosuppression in initiating the immuno-pathogenesis of MG.

Therapy. Treament of MG consists of symptom-atic therapy with AChE inhibitors, and attempts to influence the natural history with thymectomy and immunosuppression with corticosteroids, azathio-prine, and/or cyclosporine, as well as plasmapheresis and intravenous immunoglobulins (Fig. 10-3). Al-though the detailed understanding of the pathophys-iology of MG has certainly helped explain some of the beneficial effects of such regimens, it is discon-certing that no large, double-blind, controlled trials have been conducted to determine which therapies are most appropriate in a given patient at a particular time. As a result, different regimens are preferred by experienced clinicians.

Anticholinesterase medications can improve muscle strength by prolonging the half-life of ACh at the neuromuscular junction thus allowing the neu-rotransmitter to cross the widened intersynaptic cleft to interact with the decreased number of AChR on the muscle membrane. Pyridostigmine bromide is the most widely used AChE inhibitor. The usual initial dose is 60 mg as often as every 4 to 6 h during the day. A sustained-release form of pyridostigmine (180 mg) is available for administration at bedtime to improve strength in the early morning sufficient to allow the patient to swallow the morning dose of medication. The pharmacologic action of the 60-mg dose begins within 30 to 60 min, peaks at 2 to 3 h, and declines over the next 2 to 3 h. Muscles may respond in a variable manner, and the dose and timing may have to be increased to improve strength, al-though it is rarely necessary to exceed 120 mg every 3 h. It is important to note that some muscles may be improving in strength as the dose of AChE inhibi-tors is increased, whereas other muscles may be los-ing strength. At all times respiration must be moni-tored carefully to note whether improvement in some muscles takes place at the expense of precipitous drops in pulmonary function. Side effects of AChE inhibitors include diarrhea, cramps, and increased bronchial secretions, most of which can be readily treated. Because AChE inhibitors provide only symp-tomatic relief, more definitive treatment with immu-nosuppressive intervention is usually required.

Corticosteroids have proven quite effective in the therapy of MG, with different regimens providing benefit when used by experienced clinicians. The specific mechanism of action of steroids in the treat-ment of MG, while presumably involving the modi-fication of the immune response, is unclear. As in other immune-mediated disorders, initiating therapy with high-dose corticosteroids may be more effective in a shorter period of time than low-dose corticoste-roids. Side effects are, however, often the major limi-tation in determining the duration of corticosteroid therapy (Sghirlanzoni et al., 1984) . These adverse effects include diabetes, gastric ulcers, hypertension, weight gain and fluid retention, aseptic necrosis of bone, osteoporosis, and cataracts. Recurrent infec-tions are always a concern with steroids as with most immunosuppressive regimens. If any of these conditions are already present (e.g., diabetes, gastric ulcers), steroids would be contraindicated.

Steroids carry a special risk in MG because high doses may precipitate a relatively rapid exacerbation of weakness, especially of the respiratory muscula-ture. Depending on the dose and the route of adminis-tration, this exacerbation may occur from 4 to 7 days after initiating therapy. Therefore, high-dose corticosteroids should only be employed when the patient can be carefully monitored. When there is significant oropharyngeal and respiratory muscle weakness, hospitalization is usually required to mon-itor the neurological and respiratory status and the response to medication. For the severe generalized MG patient with swallowing difficulty, mild to mod-erate respiratory compromise, and no contraindica-tions, high-dose intravenous methylprednisolone (1000 mg per day for 5 days) can be employed while carefully monitoring blood sugar, salts, blood pres-sure, and respiratory function. Calcium and hista-

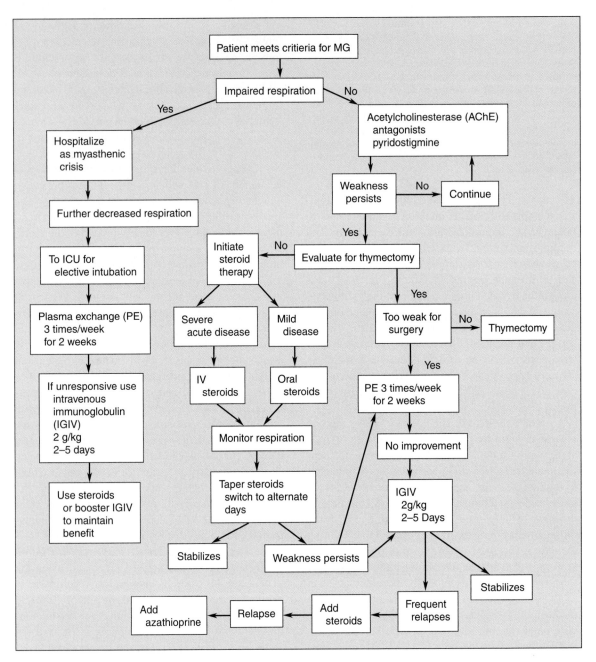

Figure 10–3.   *Treating myasthenia gravis (MS)*

mine H2 receptor antagonists are also added. In the presence of deteriorating respiratory function the patient should be moved to an ICU and other immunosuppressive modalities, such as plasma exchange or IGIV, considered. As symptoms improve, oral prednisone can be administered using an alternate-day regimen. Some have successfully employed IV methylprednisolone with slightly different dosing schedules (Arsura et al., 1985).

Patients with mild weakness can have their treatment initiated as outpatients starting with 60 mg per day, followed several weeks later by an alternate-day regimen, decreasing the doses by 10 mg per month to the lowest dose that can sustain clinical improvement. This is usually 15 to 20 mg on alternate days. Even at doses of 60 mg per day, however, some patients may experience a sudden exacerbation of weakness. As a result, some clinicians intiate therapy at doses of 20 mg per day and then increase doses by 10 mg per week until a dose of 60 mg per day is achieved. Thereafter, patients can be switched to alternate-day dosing. By slowly increasing the steroid dose, sudden respiratory difficulty can be avoided, although this may delay intial beneficial effects on muscle strength without postponing the onset of side effects. Gradual reduction of steroids must be dictated by balancing the improvement in strength with the increase in side effects. Reducing corticosteroids too quickly, however, may exacerbate myasthenic weakness.

Azathioprine, in doses of 2 to 3 mg/kg per day, can provide clinical benefit in a large percentage (70 to 90%) of MG patients (Mantegazza et al., 1988). In this same series, patient responsiveness did not differ when prednisone alone, azathioprine alone, or prednisone and azathioprine combined were compared. In severe disease refractory to prednisone alone, the combination of prednisone and azathioprine may be beneficial (Gajdos et al., 1993). A limitation of azathioprine is that the clinical benefit may be delayed as long as 3 to 6 months. The initial dose is usually 50 mg per day, increased by 50 mg per day every 3 days to a total dose of 150 to 200 mg per day. Special attention must be paid to the possible appearance of hematologic and hepatic side effects. Gastrointestinal irritation can be avoided by

administering azathioprine in divided doses after meals. Potential mutagenic side effects may preclude its use in females with childbearing potential. The use of azathioprine may also be limited by its cost.

Cyclosporine has been found to induce significant improvement in MG patients not previously treated with an immunosuppressive agent (Tindall et al., 1987). Cyclosporine treatment can begin at 5 mg/kg per day in two divided doses taken 12 h apart, with serum concentrations monitored at trough levels. The major limitation to the use of cyclosporine is its cost and its potential side effects, including nephrotoxicity, hypertension, and hepatotoxicity, which can be eliminated by lowering the dose. However, its cost and side effect potential have discouraged most clinicians from considering cyclosporine a drug of choice for MG.

Plasma exchange can provide significant benefit for patients who experience sudden worsening of myasthenic weakness, for those who need improved strength before surgery, and patients for whom corticosteroid side effects or ineffectiveness mandate other therapeutic approaches. Improvement with PE may be limited to only days or may last many weeks. A general protocol is six PEs of 2 L over a 9-day period, with oral prednisone, 30 mg per day, and cyclophosphamide, 100 mg per day, administered daily after the exhanges to limit rebound. At the termination of the exchanges the prednisone is switched to 50 mg alternating with 10 mg every other day and gradually tapered. The cyclophosphamide is continued for 1 month and then halted. The combination of these immunosuppressive medications and PE may well prolong the usual limited benefit by several months because many patients treated with this regimen may not require repeat exchanges for at least 1 year. Adverse reactions to this regimen have been relatively minimal. Of greater concern are its high cost and potential complications, such as pain and infections associated with the shunts placed to maintain vascular access.

Intravenous immunoglobulins have been successfully employed in MG. Although the benefit of IGIV may appear within several days and last for weeks, the response is quite variable among patients. In cases where corticosteroids and PE are contraindicated, IGIV may be the treatment of choice. The usual dose is similar to that employed in other neuromuscular disorders, namely, 2 g/kg of immunoglobulin administered intravenously in divided doses over a 2- to 5-day period. Intravenous pulse therapy of a single dose of 600 mg/kg on a monthly basis may be required to sustain the therapeutic benefit. While the mechanisms of the beneficial action of IGIV in MG are not clear, they are probably the same as those suggested in other disorders, namely, the presence of anti-idiotype antibodies, blocking Fc components of antibodies and altering complement deposition, complement action, immune responses, or cytokines. The side effects of chills, headache, and fever associated with IGIV were elaborated upon earlier. The major drawback to this therapy is its cost. In a recent study, 87 patients with an exacerbation of MG were randomized to receive either three PEs or IGIV (400 mg/kg) for 3 or 5 days. Both PE and IGIV were found to be effective, with IGIV displaying slightly fewer side effects (Gajdos et al., 1997). The sample size was small, however, and a much larger, properly controlled study is still needed to determine the comparative benefits and optimal dosing and frequency of PE and IGIV.

Thymectomy is of proven value in the treatment of MG. The benefit continues to increase for 7 to 10 years following surgery, with a remission rate of approximately 50% (Penn et al., 1981; Papatestas et al., 1987). Both men and women show improvement, but females with early disease, thymic hyperplasia, and high AChR antibody titers may show an earlier, but not necessarily greater, benefit over the long term. Beyond the age of 60, little thymus tissue may be present and therefore the benefit of thymectomy may be less (Lanska, 1990). Optimal preparation of MG patients with PE or immunosuppression may be required for those with significant weakness. In the hands of a skilled surgeon, a sternum-splitting transthoracic approach permits the best opportunity for maximal removal of thymic tissue; postoperative management with an experienced intensive critical care team provides the best outcomes. The presence of thymoma as detected with computed tomography of the anterior mediastinum mandates surgical exploration and thymectomy (Morgenthaler et al., 1993). Inasmuch as thymectomy patients may become extremely sensitive to AChE inhibitors immediately after surgery, caution should be exercised in using such medications for the first 24 to 36 h postoperatively.

Significant impairment of respiration and swallowing can lead to a myasthenic crisis, which requires emergency hospital admission. Decreasing vital capacity below 2 L should prompt transfer of the patient to an ICU experienced in the management of respiratory insufficiency. With further deterioration of respiratory function below 1 L or 25% of predicted vital capacity, prompt intubation and ventilatory support must be instituted, and careful attention paid to fluid and electrolyte balance and to the possible presence of infection. In the ICU setting, in the absence of infection, PE may be useful in enhancing recovery. With infection, IGIV may be helpful, along with appropriate antibiotic therapy. Although immunosuppressive medication has been of value, the availability of skilled critical care teams and ventilatory care expertise is probably more responsible for the significant improvement in the prognosis of the MG patient in crisis. Currently, the outlook for patients with MG has improved dramatically, with more than 90% returning to meaningful, productive lives.

Lambert-Eaton Myasthenic Syndrome

The Lambert-Eaton myasthenic syndrome (LEMS) is characterized by weakness and fatigability on exertion, most marked in the proximal lower extremity and truncal muscles, and is occasionally accompanied by myalgias (Eaton et al., 1957). Involvement of the upper extremities and exocular muscles is much less common with LEMS than MG. Patients with LEMS often demonstrate difficulty rising from a sitting or reclining position. A brief period of maximal voluntary muscle contraction will, however, temporarily improve the function of relaxed muscles. Although severe respiratory muscle compromise is uncommon with LEMS, recognition that it may occur as a primary manifestation can be life-saving (Nicolle et al., 1996). Autonomic system abnormalities are present in the majority of LEMS patients and include decreased salivation, decreased sweating, loss of pupillary light reflexes, orthostatic hypotension, and impotence (Rubenstein et al., 1979). Deep tendon reflexes are decreased or absent in most patients, but they may become normal for a brief time after a short period of maximal exercise of the muscles associated with the tendons being tapped.

LEMS occurs more frequently in males than females (O'Neill et al., 1988). Approximately two thirds of patients, mostly males over the age of 40, have an associated malignancy. Close to 80% of these neoplasms are small-cell carcinomas of the lung that may become apparent at the time of diagnosis of LEMS or only several years later. The minority of LEMS cases not associated with neoplasms may occur at any age, often in females, and are associated with autoimmune disorders such as thyroid disease, pernicious anemia, juvenile-onset diabetes, and MG (Gutmann et al., 1972; Newsom-Davis et al., 1991). The pattern of muscle weakness is usually sufficient to differentiate LEMS from MG, although the pattern of LEMS may simulate motor neuropathy or even motor neuron disease. Laboratory examinations are often necessary to make a definitive diagnosis and rule out other neuromuscular disorders.

Laboratory Findings

EMG is extremely helpful in establishing the diagnosis of LEMS. The counterpart to the brief clinical improvement in strength following maximal exercise is apparent on EMG as an increase in the compound muscle action potential (CMAP) with maximal voluntary activity (Lambert et al., 1961). The amplitude of the CMAP is usually reduced with a single supramaximal nerve stimulus, consistent with compromised ACh release that is insufficient to generate action potentials at many neuromuscular junctions. The CMAP will then increase after maximal voluntary activity for 10 to 20 s as a reflection of increased ACh release. Stimulation greater than 10 Hz for 5 to 10 s can also produce a temporary increase in CMAP. Stimulation at 2 to 3 Hz may show a decrement in addition to the decrease in CMAP amplitude, with postexercise recovery and amplitude facilitation

of 10 to 300%. Needle EMG may reveal low-amplitude, short-duration motor unit potentials and variably increased polyphasic potentials. With single-fiber EMG the mean interpotential interval may be increased as evidence of involvement of the neuromuscular junction, even in clinically normal muscles. These maximal exercise- and stimulation-dependent EMG findings help differentiate LEMS from motor neuropathy, motor neuron disease, and MG.

The muscle biopsy in LEMS is usually normal, with occasional nonspecific findings such as type-2 atrophy. Despite extensive evidence implicating the neuromuscular junction, especially the presynaptic terminal, in the pathophysiology of LEMS, routine electron microscopic studies are negative. Only sophisticated freeze-fracture electron microscopic analyses (Engel et al., 1982) have demonstrated specific changes. This technique is not routinely available in diagnostic laboratories.

Pathogenesis. Experimental studies have suggested that decreased release of ACh from the motor nerve terminal at the neuromuscular junction is responsible for the impaired neuromuscular transmission and weakness characteristic of LEMS. The pathologic process is thought to be triggered by autoimmune mechanisms in which antibodies against the voltage-gated calcium channel, or associated proteins, alter the membrane morphology, number of calcium channels, and rates of calcium entry.

The importance of immune mechanisms in the pathogenesis of LEMS was initially based on circumstantial evidence, that is, the increased incidence of autoimmune diseases in patients without associated malignancy and the suggestion of immune-mediated paraneoplastic disease in patients with malignancy. The first cogent evidence for the importance of immune-mediated mechanisms was the passive transfer of physiologic deficits with LEMS IgG (Lang et al., 1981). Following the injection of mice with LEMS IgG for approximately 1 to 3 months, the mean quantal content of ACh released from nerve terminals was reduced, similar to what had been observed in LEMS intercostal muscle biopsies (Elmqvist et al., 1968). The pathophysiologic effects of passive transfer were noted whether quantal ACh release was evoked by electrical stimulation or by potassium-induced depolarization. Because no postsynaptic changes were detected, the effects were attributed to alterations at the presynaptic motor terminal.

Following passive transfer of LEMS IgG, changes in the extracellular calcium concentrations could increase ACh release from motor nerve terminals to normal levels, suggesting the IgG altered calcium entry through specific voltage-gated calcium channels (VGCC) in the presynaptic membrane. Because such VGCC are components of active zone particles, the demonstration of altered morphology with freeze-fracture studies of the active-zone particles in both LEMS motor nerve terminals (Fukunaga et al., 1982) and mouse motor nerve terminals following the passive transfer of LEMS IgG (Fukunaga et al., 1983) suggested that the VGCC could be the target of the LEMS antibody-mediated attack. Further studies have suggested that LEMS IgG depletes presynaptic membrane active-zone particles by antigenic modulation (Nagel et al., 1988). LEMS IgG can also impair transmitter release in sympathetic and parasympathetic nerves by reducing the function of one or more subtypes of VGCC (Waterman et al., 1997).

LEMS IgG diminishes the function of VGCC in small-cell carcinoma in vitro suggesting a possible link between VGCC antibodies and small-cell carcinoma-induced LEMS (Lang et al., 1989). The VGCC that influence ACh release in the mammalian presynaptic terminal are predominantly P or Q type (Uchitel et al., 1992). Thus, although LEMS IgG react with multiple types of calcium channels in small-cell carcinoma (Meriney et al., 1996), the reactivity with P-type VGCC probably more directly relates to the altered ACh release from motor terminals in LEMS (Viglione et al., 1995).

Using an immunoprecipitation assay with human cerebellar extract with I-125–labeled P- or Q-type ligand (omega-conotoxin MVIIC), 66 of 72 LEMS serum samples (91%) were positive for the presence of VGCC antibodies (Motomura et al., 1997), whereas only 24 of 72 (33%) were positive for N-type VGCC. Thus, anti-P- or Q-type VGCC antibodies are present in an extremely high percentage of LEMS patients and are therefore likely candidates for mediating the physiologic alterations at the neuromuscular junction. However, the results of using an immunoprecipitation assay with labeled crude extracts raises the possibility that tightly associated proteins rather than the VGCC itself might be the true target. The most straightforward way to refute this suggestion was to demonstrate reactivity with specific peptide constituents of the VGCC, which was undertaken. Antibodies to one or both of two synthetic peptides of the alpha 1 subunit of the P- or Q-type VGCC were demonstrated in 13 of 30 LEMS patients (Takamori et al., 1997). Among 30 LEMS sera, 9 reacted with one epitope, and 6 with the other; 2 of the 15 positive sera reacted with both epitopes. Thus, the data are becoming more convincing that the P- or Q-type VGCC may be the primary target of the immune attack. The antibodies and epitopes which give rise to the altered pathophysiology of LEMS remain to be determined.

As in other autoimmune diseases, antibodies may be present to several proteins. In LEMS, antibodies to synaptotagmin have been found (Lang et al., 1993) which may induce an immune-mediated model of LEMS following immunization of rats (Takamori et al., 1994). Synaptotagmin antibodies are only present, however, in a small number of LEMS patients (Lang et al., 1993). Further studies are needed to determine whether antisynaptotagmin antibodies play any role in the pathophysiology of even the small number of patients in which they are present, or whether they are a manifestation of "determinant spread" with antibody production to proteins closely associated with VGCC, and of no pathophysiologic significance.

Therapy. In LEMS patients with an associated neoplasm, therapy should be directed primarily toward eliminating the tumor (Fig. 10-4). Such treatment may trigger a remission both in the small-cell carcinoma and in the neuromuscular symptoms and signs (Jenkyn et al., 1980). In LEMS unassociated with malignancy, initial efforts should be directed toward treating the immune process and attempting to increase the entry of calcium into the presynaptic terminal, thereby enhancing ACh release. In the short term, increasing the entry of calcium might be accomplished by a blockade of the outward potassium current at the presynaptic terminal. The compound 3,4-diaminopyridine, which has just such a physiologic effect, has been found to improve motor and autonomic signs and symptoms in LEMS (McEvoy et al., 1989; Sanders et al., 1993). Dosages of 3,4-diaminopyridine range from 15 to 45 mg per day, with doses over 60 mg possibly being associated with seizures. Side effects at the lower doses include paresthesias, increased bronchial secretions, diarrhea, and palpitations. At the present time, this drug is not available for routine clinical use.

Guanidine hydrochloride is known to provide symptomatic relief for LEMS patients but is extremely toxic. A recent report suggests that low-dose guanidine (below 1000 mg per day) together with pyridostigmine may be a safe and effective treatment for prolonged symptomatic treatment of LEMS (Oh et al., 1997).

Over the longer term, LEMS therapy should be directed toward the cause of the decreased entry of calcium, namely, the immune-mediated process and the antibodies directed against presynaptic terminal VGCC. Corticosteroids, PE (Newsom-Davis et al., 1984), and IGIV have all been used successfully

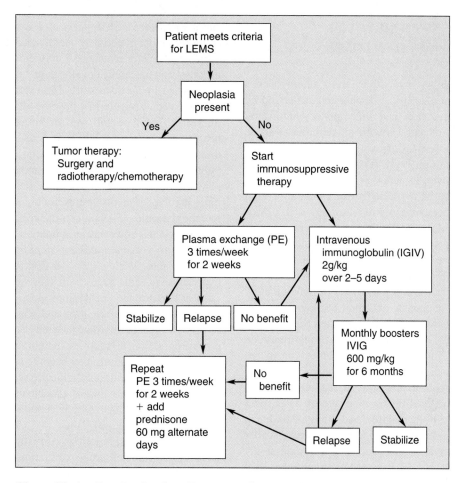

Figure 10–4. *Treating Lambert-Eaton myasthenic syndrome (LEMS)*

in treating LEMS patients, although the number of subjects in each of the trials has been relatively small, and no preferred mode of therapy scientifically established. In a randomized, double-blind, placebo-controlled crossover trial in nine patients over 8 weeks, IGIV (2 g/kg over 2 days) caused an improvement by 2 to 4 weeks which had declined by 8 weeks (Bain et al., 1996). Interestingly, a reduction in VGCC antibodies accompanied the short-term improvement. However, this decrease took place over such a short period of time it is possible that IGIV directly or indirectly neutralized the VGCC antibodies and thereby improved clinical function. Delayed anti-idiotype antibody action or some other mechanisms could not be excluded. In one report, monthly courses of IGIV therapy (2 g/kg over 5 days) administered to a LEMS patient without detectable malignancy produced long-lasting clinical benefit (Muchnik et al., 1997). As discussed earlier, side effects of IGIV are relatively minor. The major problem with IGIV, as with PE, is its cost and relatively temporary benefit realized unless repeated treatments are conducted. It is entirely possible that oral corticosteroids, combined with IGIV, may provide a synergistic effect and eliminate the necessity for frequent boosters to sustain benefit.

INFLAMMATORY MYOPATHIES

The inflammatory myopathies are a heterogeneous group of acquired muscle diseases characterized by muscle degeneration and inflammatory infiltrates. The majority of patients with inflammatory muscle disease have dermatomyositis (DM), polymyositis (PM), or inclusion body myositis (IBM). It is important, however, to note that inflammatory myopathies may also be associated with parasitic or viral infectious processes; systemic disorders such as vasculitis, sarcoidosis, and polymyalgia rheumatica; or the "overlap syndromes" of rheumatoid arthritis, mixed connective tissue disease, systemic lupus erythematosus, Sjögren's syndrome, or scleroderma. Because they all are characterized by inflammatory involvement of muscle and their etiologies are unknown, DM, PM, and IBM have often been lumped together in past clinical studies, obscuring important information. These disorders should be considered distinctive since there is little evidence suggesting they are variable expressions of the same disease. The three usually differ in their age of onset, with DM affecting both children and adults, PM being uncommon in childhood and most typically seen after the second decade of life, and IBM most commonly occurring after age 40. In fact, data suggest that IBM may be the most common myopathy of older age. The disorders also may differ in their association with malignancy, particularly for DM (Barnes et al., 1976) with males over the age of 40 (Devere et al., 1975; Tymms et al., 1985). The clinical presentation, the character and location of the inflammatory infiltrates, and the responsiveness to immunosuppressive drugs, such as corticosteroids, may also differ among the three conditions.

Clinical Features

In DM, especially in childhood, the disease may commence with systemic symptoms including fever and malaise. A characteristic rash follows that accompanies or, more commonly, precedes proximal muscle weakness. The cheeks may appear flushed, and a violaceous rash appears on the eyelids, especially the upper eyelids, frequently accompanied by edema and telangiectasia. An erythematous rash of the chest and neck may develop in an area that would be exposed by an open shirt. The extensor surfaces of the knees and elbows become discolored and thickened, and the skin over the knuckles can also become erythematous. The nail beds may develop discoloration, followed by telangiectasia and edema. Subsequently, weakness becomes apparent, accompanied by pain and stiffness. Proximal muscles are more involved than distal muscles in both upper and lower extremities. Flexion contractures at the ankles can also occur, however, in childhood DM.

The progression and duration of the disease are quite variable. With childhood DM, patients may experience an acute attack with subsequent recovery even in the absence of immunosuppressive therapy. Others may follow a remitting and relapsing course, or may evolve into a chronic progressive illness. With rapid progression, all muscles, including swallowing, speech, and respiration, may become compromised. In up to 70% of children, calcifications may be present in subcutaneous tissues (Pachman, 1988). The mortality of childhood DM is reported to be 5 to 10% (Sullivan et al., 1977).

In adult DM, skin lesions consisting of a malar rash, periorbital heliotrope coloration and edema, and erythema of the knees, elbows, and the anterior neck and chest are similar to those of childhood DM, and may progress to brawny thickening and depigmentation. The skin lesions are usually accompanied by or precede the appearance of proximal muscle weakness, although the presence of the characteristic DM skin lesions has also been reported in the absence of muscle involvement (Euwer and Sontheimer, 1993).

An associated malignancy has been reported in up to 40% of adult patients with DM, whereas the incidence of an associated malignancy with PM is considerably lower (Callen, 1988). The malignancy may precede or follow the onset of disease, and its removal, such as ovarian tumors, may improve muscle weakness. Clearly, the major problem in this case is that the cancer itself can be life-threatening. At present the true incidence of malignancy associated with either PM or DM is unknown because of the relatively small numbers of patients involved in the reported studies, and because tumor detection may follow or precede the onset of muscle involvement by 1 or more years.

In PM, the pattern of muscle weakness is similar to DM, although PM does not share the distinct clinical characteristics of DM. The onset of PM is usually gradual, evolving over weeks to months, compromising proximal muscles of the upper and lower extremities. However, weakness may also begin with surprising suddenness. The onset is typically after the second decade of life, being rarely seen in childhood. The disease usually spares eye and facial muscles. Dysphagia may be a common symptom. The characteristic DM rash is usually absent, but other systemic involvement, such as arthritis, has been reported in up to 50% of patients with PM (Schumacher et al., 1979). Impaired respiratory function may also be present in PM as well as DM as a consequence of respiratory muscle weakness, aspiration pneumonia due to dysphagia, and interstitial lung disease (Wiedemann et al., 1989). Cardiac involvement, including alterations of the conduction system, cardiomyopathy, and cardiac failure have also been reported in both PM and DM (Gottdiener et al., 1978; Askari, 1988).

IBM usually presents as a generalized weakness, most commonly over the age of 50, and in males more often than females. The diagnosis is often delayed because of the clinical similarities between IBM and PM. A helpful distinguishing clinical characteristic may be an early involvement of the distal musculature of the upper extremities, with weakness of the finger flexors and atrophy of the forearm muscles, and the proximal and distal musculature of the lower extremities with weakness of the quadriceps and ankle dorsiflexors. A recent study of 21 randomly selected patients with histologically confirmed IBM supports the specificity of forearm flexor muscle involvement, and suggests the potential, albeit expensive, usefulness of MRI. Twenty of the 21 IBM patients demonstrated a relatively specific "marbled brightness" of the flexor digitorum profundus musculature of the upper extremities with T1-weighted MR images (Sekul et al., 1997).

IBM is often difficult to diagnose from clinical features alone. As with PM, IBM may present in the second to fourth decades and may also compromise shoulder girdle and facial musculature. Transient myalgias may occur early in the course of the disease. Clinical features of peripheral neuropathy may be present with decreased tendon reflexes. There has been no reported increased association of IBM with malignancy. Even with an asymmetrical involvement of finger flexors and knee extensors, the most important clinical feature distinguishing IBM from DM and PM remains the relative unresponsiveness of IBM to immunosuppressive therapy (Amato et al., 1996). Although most cases of IBM are sporadic, familial IBM has been described (Massa et al., 1991), with some resembling familial distal myopathies (Sunohara et al., 1989). While various types of hereditary IBM map to chromosome 9p1-q1, the specific gene defect is not yet known (Argov et al., 1997).

Laboratory Findings

The erythrocyte sedimentation rate (ESR) is usually elevated in DM and PM, but not in IBM. The ESR is normal in almost 50% of DM and PM cases, however, and does not correlate with muscle weakness, nor is it useful for monitoring the effectiveness of therapy. Serum creatine phosphokinase (CPK) is a sensitive indicator of muscle injury in DM and PM. Usually the skeletal muscle isoenzyme of CPK (MM) is elevated. The central nervous system isozyme (BB) may also be elevated because of ongoing muscle regeneration. Other enzymes, such as aldolase and lactic dehydrogenase, may be increased in DM and PM, but CPK is still a more sensitive index of muscle degeneration and membrane leakiness and therefore a more useful measure of disease progression and therapeutic efficacy. Serum myoglobin may also be increased in DM and PM, and can also be employed to monitor disease progression and guide treatment regimens. When serum enzyme levels do not appear to correlate with the clinical state, however, especially following immunosuppressive therapy such as plasmapheresis, clinical parameters such as muscle strength are still the most relevant indices of disease progression and therapeutic efficacy. In IBM, CPK is usually normal and is therefore not helpful as a therapeutic guide. Serum antibodies against tRNA synthetases, especially against the histidyl tRNA synthetase (Jo-1 antibody), have been described in 20% of patients with PM, most prominently in association with inflammatory arthritis and to a lesser extent with Raynaud's phenomenon (Targoff, 1993). Other antibodies, such as the Mi-2 antibody against a nuclear helicase and the SRP (signal recognition particle) antibody against a cytoplasmic constituent, appear to correlate with rates of disease progression, although their direct relevance to pathogenesis is unclear (Mimori, 1996).

EMG is an extremely useful, although not very specific, diagnostic test in the inflammatory myopathies. In both DM and PM the motor unit potentials are reduced in amplitude and duration and short-duration polyphasic motor unit potentials are usually present, especially in proximal muscles. Further, insertional activity is increased, and fibrillation potentials and positive sharp waves noted. Similar findings of short duration, polyphasic motor unit potentials with fibrillation potentials, positive sharp waves, and increased electrical irritability are also seen in IBM with both proximal and distal distributions which are often asymmetrical. A mixed pattern of short-duration myopathic units together with long-duration, high-amplitude neurogenic motor unit potentials should raise the possibility of IBM, as should a mixed pattern of myopathic EMG features in some muscles and neuropathic features in other muscles. The EMG pattern itself, however, is not sufficiently specific to distinguish IBM from PM and DM.

Muscle biopsy is an important procedure to help establish the diagnosis and define the character and extent of inflammation. Evidence for myopathy in all three conditions are a variation in muscle fiber diameter, the presence of necrotic as well as regenerating fibers, and an increase in connective tissue. Prominent changes in DM include perivascular inflammation with diffusely scattered inflammatory cells in the perimysium, and less inflammation in the endomysium. The inflammatory lymphocytes cells are B and CD4 + T lymphocytes with highest concentrations at perivascular sites, and lowest at endomysial sites (Arahata and Engel, 1984; Engel and Arahata, 1984). One of the striking features of DM is that endothelial cells of intramuscular blood vessels undergo degenerative and regenerative changes, and, in ultrastructural studies, demonstrate characteristic microtubular inclusions. Both type 1 and type 2 muscle fibers in DM, but not in PM or IBM, often demonstrate atrophy in a perifascicular distribution (Engel et al., 1994).

In PM, the inflammatory cells also occur at perivascular, perimysial, and endomysial locations, although the process involving the endomysium is more marked, and macrophages and lymphocytes are CD8 + T lymphocytes with few B lymphocytes surrounding nonnecrotic muscle fibers (Engel et al., 1994). In PM, there are fewer B cells and T helper lymphocytes in perimysium and endomysium than in DM, and there is no significant vasculopathy, endothelial cell alterations, or perifascicular atrophy. For PM patients unresponsive to immunosuppressive therapy, repeat muscle biopsy has often demonstrated histologic features of IBM (Amato et al., 1996).

In IBM, angular fibers and variation in muscle fiber diameter may be present and the extent of inflammation may be quite variable. Endomysial inflammatory infiltrates resemble the infiltrates of PM with activated CD8 + T lymphocytes and macrophages, but no B lymphocytes (Arahata and Engel, 1986; Arahata and Engel, 1988B; Arahata and Engel, 1988A). The muscle fiber lesions in IBM may, however, be quite distinctive with the presence of cytoplasmic rimmed vacuoles surrounded by basophilic material (Yunis and Samaha, 1971; Carpenter et al., 1978). An interesting feature of the muscle pathology in IBM is its striking similarity to what is seen with Alzheimer's disease brain (Mirabella et al., 1996A). Eosinophilic inclusions are often present in proximity to the vacuoles. These inclusions are congophilic and react with antibodies for beta amyloid, the beta amyloid precursor protein, ubiquitin (Mendell et al., 1991; Askanas et al., 1992) and apolipoprotein E (Mirabella et al., 1996B). Paired helical filaments are also present and react with the antibodies for hyperphosphorylated tau as noted in Alzheimer brain. In muscle biopsies from patients with hereditary IBM, rimmed vacuoles and congophilia are usually present (Murakarmi et al., 1995), although the immunoreactivity for phosphorylated tau in hereditary IBM differs from sporadic IBM (Mirabella et al., 1996A).

It is important to note that the myopathology of IBM is not specific. Chronic dystrophies, such as oculopharyngeal dystrophy, also demonstrate cytoplasmic deposits that stain positively for amyloid and ubiquitin (Villanova et al., 1993), and rimmed vacuoles have been described in Welander's distal myopathy (Lindberg et al., 1991). The presence of rimmed vacuoles, inflammation, and typical cytoplasmic and nuclear filamentous inclusions, however, may also occur in IBM patients with atypical clinical presentations. Four patients have been described, one with a scapuloperoneal syndrome, one with postpolio-like syndrome, and two with associated immune-mediated diseases (Schlesinger et al., 1996). Two of these responded to high-dose steroid therapy, suggesting we have much to learn about the spectrum of IBM.

Pathogenesis

The presence of inflammatory infiltrates in DM, PM, and IBM, albeit circumstantial, first suggested the importance of autoimmune mechanisms in disease pathogenesis. Studies of HLA antigens have demonstrated an increased association of DM and PM with HLA-DR3 in linkage disequilibrium with HLA-B8 (Plotz et al., 1989). In none of the three conditions, however, has an antigen been described with sufficient specificity to meet the criteria for an autoimmune etiology.

In DM, a severe muscle angiopathy is present with prominent infiltration of B lymphocytes, and, within perimysial vessel walls, immunoglobulins and the C3 component of complement can be detected (Emslie-Smith and Engel, 1990). Components of the complement membrane attack complex (MAC) C5b-9 can also be detected by light and electron microscopic immunohistochemistry (Kissel et al., 1986). Macrophages and cytotoxic T cells are also present, albeit to a lesser extent. These studies suggest a complement-dependent injury of intramuscular capillaries mediated by immunoglobulins or immune complexes, possibly leading to a reduction in capillary number with subsequent ischemia, microinfarcts, and further inflammation. In DM, but not in PM, distinctive local cytokine activity can be demonstrated by monitoring the expression of the signal transducer and activator of transcription 1 (STAT1). This reactivity is especially prominent in atrophic perifascicular muscle fibers. Because interferon-γ is known to activate STAT1 in vitro, it could possibly be involved with ischemia in the perifascicular muscle fiber pathology in DM (Illa et al., 1997).

In PM, in contrast with DM, humoral immune mechanisms appear to be less relevant than cell-mediated immune mechanisms, and the endomysium rather than the perimysium appears to be the critical site of attack. Nonnecrotic muscle fibers are surrounded and infiltrated by CD8 + cytotoxic lymphocytes, which are oligoclonal by T-cell receptor typing (Mantegazza et al., 1993). B lymphocytes, CD4 + T lymphocytes, and macrophages are less common at these endomysial locations. These data suggest that muscle fiber injury in PM is mediated by an antigen-driven reaction in which cytotoxic CD8 + T lymphocytes recognize antigenic peptides presented by MHC I expressed on the surface of the muscle fiber. One mechanism by which cytotoxic cells may induce injury is by the mediator perforin. In studies of DM and PM muscle using semiquantitative PCR, immunohistochemistry, and confocal

laser microscopy, perforin was vectorially oriented toward the target muscle fiber in almost 50% of CD8 + T cells that contacted a muscle fiber in PM (Goebels et al., 1996). In DM, perforin was distributed randomly in the cytoplasm of the inflammatory T cells. Thus, the T-cell receptor-antigen interaction on the muscle fiber surface in PM may initiate a perforin- and secretion-dependent mechanism responsible for muscle fiber injury.

Another potential mechanism of muscle fiber injury could involve activation of Fas, initiating a programmed cell death cascade (apoptosis). This was investigated in three patients with DM, five with PM, four with IBM, and three with Duchenne muscular dystrophy (DMD) (Behrens et al., 1997). Fas was not detected in control muscle, but was expressed in muscle fibers and inflammatory cells in all four conditions. Expression was especially elevated in a higher percentage of muscle fibers in PM and IBM than in DM and DMD. Bcl2, however, which can protect cells from apoptosis, was also expressed in a significantly greater number of cells in PM and IBM, suggesting that the potential susceptibility to Fas-induced apoptosis may be countered by enhanced Bcl2 protection. In fact, there is no evidence to support an apoptotic cascade either in muscle fibers or inflammatory cells in PM, DM, or IBM (Schneider et al., 1996).

Necrotic muscle fiber injury may also occur in PM albeit to a slightly lesser extent than nonnecrotic fiber injury (Arahata and Engel, 1988A). In this setting macrophages may predominate, and cytotoxic CD8 + T lymphocytes are far less frequent. This suggests that even in PM a humoral immune process may be operative in which an antibody-mediated, and possibly complement-dependent, injury of muscle may occur in the absence of T lymphocyte-dependent cytotoxicity.

The nature of the antigen initiating the immune response in PM is presently unknown. Although numerous viruses have been implicated, all efforts to isolate specific viral antigens in PM muscle have been unsuccessful. Nevertheless, viruses could still be responsible for triggering an autoimmune reaction against muscle antigens in a susceptible host. The inclusions in IBM were originally thought to be "myxovirus-like structures" (Chou, 1967), but there has been no subsequent evidence to support a viral origin of IBM inclusions or filaments. As with PM, however, viruses could still be responsible for triggering a host response leading to the myopathology of IBM.

An autoimmune etiology of IBM has been the prevailing hypothesis given the inflammatory myopathy and clinical similarities to PM. The relative unresponsiveness to immunosuppressive therapy, and the unexpected presence of beta amyloid, paired helical filaments, and hyperphosphorylated tau in muscle fibers, however, have raised the possibility that the pathogenesis of IBM may be similar to the pathogenesis of Alzheimer's disease, and that altered amyloid metabolism may play a significant role. Even though IBM may be the most common myopathy of older age, the simultaneous presence of Alzheimer's disease and IBM is rare. Furthermore, in documented IBM, nonnecrotic muscle fibers invaded by cyto-toxic T cells are several times more frequent than fibers demon-strating congophilic amyloid inclusions (Pruitt et al., 1996). In addition, the myopathology of IBM is not absolutely specific with the membranous whorls and filamentous inclusions hav-ing been described in oculopharyngeal dystrophy. Thus, an autoimmune reaction as an initiating event in IBM is still more likely than a specific perturbation in amyloid metabolism as the cause of muscle injury as may be the case for neuronal injury in Alzheimer brain.

In accord with an autoimmune etiology is the report of seven patients with inflammatory IBM with CD8+ cells invading nonnecrotic, MHC-1–expressing fibers. All seven patients expressed the DR3 allele (Sivakumar et al., 1997). In another report, the restricted usage of V alpha and V beta families of T-cell receptors was demonstrated in muscle com-pared with peripheral blood lymphocytes, indicating a selec-tive homing or local proliferation of T lymphocytes in the inflammatory lesions in IBM (Fyhr et al., 1996). An increased incidence of paraproteinemia (22.8%) has also been demon-strated in IBM (Dalakas et al., 1997A). Nevertheless, in IBM muscle, many constituents of the amyloid plaque of Alz-heimer's disease are present and require explanation. Direct transfer of the beta amyloid precursor protein gene into cul-tured normal human muscle was able to induce congophilia, beta amyloid-positive filaments, and nuclear tubulofilamen-tous inclusions, suggesting that increased amyloid expression could contribute to the pathologic cascade (Askanas et al., 1997). Furthermore, most of the proteins that accumulate in IBM (including beta amyloid and tau) are present as constit-uents of the human neuromuscular junction (Askanas and Engel, 1995).

Thus, autoimmunity and altered amyloid metabolism are not mutually exclusive since autoimmune reactions could initi-ate a pathologic process that could subsequently be aggravated by an overexpression of amyloid. While the nonresponsiveness of most IBM patients to immunosuppressive therapy does not invalidate the hypothesis of an autoimmune trigger, it might suggest that the pathologic cascade involving amyloid, once initiated by an immunologic process, continues independently. For example, 75% of IBM vacuolated muscle fibers contain inclusions that stain positively for neuronal and inducible nitric oxide synthases and nitrotyrosine (Yang et al., 1996), suggesting the generation of free radicals, which would not be responsive to immunosuppressant therapy, may be involved as well. Free radical stress might also contribute to the multiple mitochondrial DNA deletions in IBM (Santorelli et al., 1996). Even assuming that the process is antigen-driven, the unknown nature of the putative antigen summoning cytotoxic T cells, and the lack of understanding as to how amyloid becomes involved, suggest that neither the autoimmune nor the amyloid-overex-pression theories themselves, provide convincing explanations for the pathogenesis of IBM. Thus, these potential mechanisms of pathology cannot serve as the basis for a rational therapeutic approach for the treatment of this condition.

Therapy

Most therapies for the treatment of inflammatory myopathies are empirical, with large double-blind, placebo-controlled trials lacking (Fig. 10-5). Further-more, the failure to separate various subgroups of DM and PM in many clinical studies has obscured natural history data and the true benefit of various therapeutic modalities in the distinct syndromes. Thus, current treatment regimens are often based on anecdotal experience. Despite these limitations, most agree that immunosuppressive therapy is bene-ficial for many patients with inflammatory myopa-thies. As a result, it will be difficult to conduct large-scale, appropriately controlled studies with these compounds in the future. Such studies would be of considerable value, however, as new, more specific approaches are devised to target many of the immunologic problems of the inflammatory myopathies that are not currently being addressed, such as the complement-mediated humoral attack of perimysial vasculature in DM, or the oligoclo-nal cytotoxic T-lymphocyte attack of muscle fibers in PM.

Corticosteroids are usually the initial therapeutic choice in DM and PM. Although beginning regimens for oral therapy vary between 30 and 100 mg per day, an aggressive approach is preferable, especially because the higher the total dose the better the clinical response over the first few months (Henriksson and Lindvall, 1990). In addition, the earlier therapy is instituted the better, because delaying therapy may limit responsiveness (Joffe et al., 1993). Oral doses of 80 to 100 mg per day of prednisone (or 1 mg/kg per day) taken as a single dose in the morning should be taken for 4 to 6 weeks until the muscle strength begins to improve and/or the CPK begins to decrease. Although reports suggest that CPK will decline be-fore improvement in muscle strength (Oddis and Medsger, 1989), we have followed a number of pa-tients in whom the decrease in CPK lagged behind the improvement in strength. Thus, it is suggested that both measurements be made, but that the pa-tient's clinical response, rather than any specific chemical improvement, be used as the more relevant guide for modifying the steroid dose.

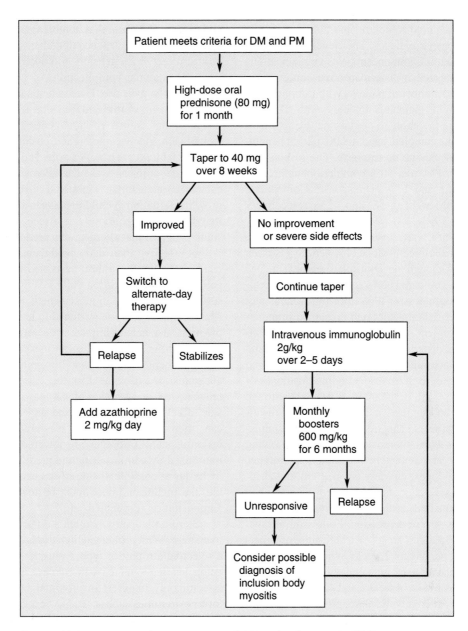

Figure 10–5. *Treating dermatomyositis (DM) and polymyositis (PM)*

With a favorable response, and in the absence of untoward side effects, the dose of prednisone can be gradually reduced by 20 mg every 3 to 4 weeks until a maintenance dose of 15 to 20 mg per day or 30 mg every other day is reached by 4 to 6 months.

Reductions from this point should be executed very slowly by 2.5 mg (for daily dosages) or 5 mg (for alternate-day dosages) every 4 to 6 weeks as long as strength is improving or maintained. Often, alternate-day maintenance doses of 10 to 20 mg for many months are required to control the disease, even in steroid-responsive patients. The benefit of prednisone and other oral immunosuppressive medications has been analyzed in a retrospective cohort study with a limited number of patients with inflammatory myopathy (113 patients). Patients with DM responded more favorably to prednisone therapy, with 30% achieving complete benefit, 60% partial benefit, and only 10% having no response. The response of patients with PM was 10% complete benefit, 73% partial benefit, and 17% no response. Comparable figures in IBM were 0, 58, and 42%, respectively (Joffe et al., 1993).

In patients with severe disease, intravenous, high-dose methylprednisolone (1 g per day) is often employed. Although no controlled studies in DM and PM have compared oral versus intravenous treatments, the usefulness of high-dose intravenous steroids in other inflammatory and presumed immune-mediated disorders, such as the vasculitides and connective tissue disorders, prompted its use in DM and PM. Experience suggests that a 3- to 5-day regimen of 1 g per day of intravenous methylprednisolone administered over 2 h in the morning accords with the goal of early and aggressive therapy to combat the inflammatory process. This treatment can be administered in a closely monitored outpatient unit, following general clinical parameters including electrolytes, glucose, vital signs, and any adverse emotional responses. On several occasions high-dose therapy had to be terminated because of severe hyperactivity or, the converse, severe depression. Following intravenous therapy, patients are given a high-dose oral therapy of 80 mg per day for 2 weeks, which is reduced in a stepwise manner to 60 mg per day for 3 to 4 weeks, 50 mg per day for 3 to 4 weeks, and 40 mg per day for 3 to 4 weeks. Alternatively, although far more expensive and less practical, patients can be maintained on boosters of intravenous methylprednisolone every 3 to 4 weeks. If patients have not objectively shown any improvement after 3 months of oral or intravenous therapy (as monitored by assessment of muscle strength), they should be considered unresponsive to prednisone, and tapering should be accelerated.

When initiating therapy with corticosteroids it is imperative to evaluate carefully the possibility of underlying disorders that might aggravate steroid side effects. In the presence of diabetes, gastritis and gastric ulcers, hypertension, osteoporosis, or infection, the potential complications of corticosteroids may preclude their use. Even when such conditions are not present, steroid-induced side effects may develop in the course of treatment. These include weight gain, glucose intolerance, cushingoid appearance, high blood pressure, gastritis and gastric ulceration, osteoporosis, avascular necrosis of the hip, cataracts, glaucoma, emotional irritability, and growth retardation in children. Alternate-day therapy may help minimize these side effects. Although no studies suggest that alternate-day prednisone therapy is less effective than daily prednisone, most clinicians, including the author, have the impression that patients do better using a daily dosing regimen for several months until clinical benefit is established. Thereafter, patients are switched to an alternate-day program. To help minimize side effects, antacids such as Tums, which is also an inexpensive source of supplemental calcium, and histamine H_2-receptor antagonists are of value. Limiting caloric intake and reducing the consumption of salt may also minimize side effects. Facial flushing and general irritability can often be tolerated with reassurance they will lessen as steroid dosages are lowered. Insomnia is minimized by administering the prednisone as early in the day as possible. If side effects become intolerable, the prednisone dose must be lowered or drug administration terminated.

Steroid myopathy is often a difficult side effect to manage. With prolonged high doses of prednisone, a selective atrophy of type 2 muscle fibers can develop, leading to increased weakness. This weakness is commonly manifest in proximal muscles of the lower extremities such as the hip flexors. These same muscles are affected with exacerbations of DM and PM, however, making it difficult to differentiate steroid myopathy from worsening inflammatory myopathy. The continued presence of fibrillations and positive sharp waves on EMG would favor inflammatory myopathy. From a practical management point of view, weakness due to worsening disease is often the more likely explanation, and the appropriate treatment would be to increase the prednisone dose. Each situation must be carefully evaluated, however, and a determination must be made of systemic illness or infections that could exacerbate disease, of recent history of prednisone dosages, and the specific muscle groups in which the weakness has increased. If, for example, neck flexor weakness and swallowing difficulties worsen along with proximal leg weakness, then steroid-induced weakness is less likely. On the other hand, steroid myopathy and exacerbating disease can coexist, and the appropriate management may require lowering the steroid dosages, or seeking the "steroid-sparing" effects of other immunosuppressants.

Azathioprine is commonly used in combination with corticosteroids, either to permit a lowering of the prednisone dosages to limit its side effects, or as primary therapy in patients with DM or PM who are unresponsive to the steroid (Bohan et al., 1977; Henriksson and Lindvall, 1990). There is little evidence suggesting that azathioprine should be used before initiating treatment with steroids. The dosage of azathioprine is 2 mg/kg, although some clinicians will use up to 3 mg/kg. The major side effects of azathioprine are usually dose-dependent and therefore can be reversed by lowering the dose of the medication. Included are bone marrow suppression with leukopenia, thrombocytopenia, and anemia, as well as liver toxicity (Kissel et al., 1986). A significant drawback to azathioprine therapy is that it takes 3 to 6 months for the drug to become effective, which limits its utility if relatively immediate therapeutic benefit is required. Therefore, azathioprine should be added to the therapeutic regimen only when it becomes evident that steroids alone may not ameliorate the condition.

Methotrexate has been reported to be of benefit in steroid-resistant patients with inflammatory myopathies (Metzger et al., 1974; Joffe et al., 1993). Methotrexate has a more rapid onset of action than azathioprine, although its oral absorption is more variable. Side effects of methotrexate include hepatotoxicity, stomatitis, bone marrow suppression, and pneumonitis. Methotrexate can be administered orally beginning at 5 to 10 mg weekly for the first 3 weeks (approximately 2.5 mg every 12 h) with dosages increasing by 2.5 mg per week up to a total of 20 to 25 mg weekly. It can also be administered intravenously with weekly doses of 0.4 to 0.8 mg/kg. In general, most neurologists have more experience with other immunosuppressants in the inflammatory myopathies, and therefore methotrexate is not commonly employed in neurologic practice.

Intravenous immunoglobulin is being used more frequently to treat inflammatory myopathies when patients do not respond to corticosteroid therapy. In children, the elderly, or others with increased risk factors for developing complications of corticosteroid therapy, IGIV is often the first immunosuppressant therapy employed. In combined studies, 20 of 23 patients with DM and 11 of 14 patients with PM demonstrated significant benefit on IGIV treatment (Dalakas et al., 1993). IGIV improved strength, the rash, and the underlying immunopathology, while increasing capillary density, decreasing vascular MAC, and decreasing MHC-I expression on muscle fibers in DM patients. No controlled studies of differing regimens have been published, but, empirically, the starting dose of 2 gm/kg immunoglobulin administered over 2 to 5 days is effective, followed by monthly boosters for several months. The benefit of IGIV is usually limited to only 4 to 8 weeks, making boosters important. If the patient fails to respond in 3 to 4 months, it is unlikely any improvement will be forthcoming by continuing the monthly boosters. The combination of low-dose oral corticosteroids and IGIV may well be synergisitic, but controlled studies are needed to establish this benefit.

The major disadvantages of IGIV therapy are its cost and the necessity for repeated boosters to maintain therapeutic benefit. Side effects to IGIV are usually minimal provided infusion rates do not exceed 200 cc/h or 0.08 mL/kg. Adverse reactions include headache, chills, malaise, myalgias, and chest discomfort as well as increased blood pressure, which most often responds to lowering the rate of infusion. Anaphylactic reactions are rare, but may occur in a setting of the combination of low IgA in the patient (possibly due to anti-IgA antibodies) and a small IgA present in the Ig preparation (Thornton and Ballow, 1993). Renal toxicity is also a concern, especially in those with underlying renal dysfunction. Aseptic meningitis can occur, especially in patients with migraine, and there is an increased risk of thromboembolic complications because of an IGIV-induced increase in serum viscosity.

The mechanism of action of IGIV is not fully understood. Experimental evidence suggests that high-dose immunoglobulin may attenuate complement-dependent immune damage (Basta et al., 1989), which may explain its benefit in DM. In addition, IGIV may inhibit complement deposition, neutralize cytokines, interfere with Fc-receptor–mediated phagocytosis, downregulate autoantibody production, and/or provide other immunomodulatory effects through the presence of anti-idiotypic antibodies (Dalakas, 1997). The specific action of IGIV responsible for its effectiveness in human inflammatory myopathies has yet to be convincingly documented.

Cyclophosphamide and cyclosporine have also been employed in DM and PM, but their side effects, long-term consequences, and limited risk-benefit profiles limit their use to those patients with aggressive, steroid-unresponsive disease with increasing systemic involvement. The absence of well-controlled studies with these compounds, either individually or in combination, also limits their usefulness. Oral doses of cyclophosphamide are 1 to 2.5 mg/kg per day, keeping the leukocyte count above 2500/μL. The side effects of hemorrhagic cystitis, alopecia, infertility, bone marrow suppression, and an increased future incidence of malignant tumors, however, make this a treatment of last resort. Even under these circumstances, cyclophosphamide should be employed as it is used in patients with necrotizing vasculitis, namely, as intravenous therapy, with a dose of 3 g administered over 5 to 6 days, carefully monitoring the leukocyte and granulocyte counts, and with several monthly boosters of 750 to 1000 mg/m².

Cyclosporine, which inhibits the interleukin-2 activation of T cells and other reactions involved in T-cell activation, exerts its effects by binding to a specific immunophilin (Walsh et al., 1992), and can cause nephrotoxicity, hypertension, and hepatotoxicity. Although several limited reports suggest that cyclosporine may be of benefit in DM and PM (Heckmatt et al., 1989; Mehregan and Su, 1993), the high cost of this medication and its potential side effects limit its usefulness. Oral doses can be started at 6 mg/kg per day with reduction to 4 mg/kg per day to limit renal side effects. Monitoring trough serum levels of the drug is helpful in this regard, aiming for 100 to 150 μg/mL.

Plasmapheresis should theoretically be of benefit in the inflammatory myopathies, especially DM, because it can decrease levels of circulating immune complexes and immunoglobulins. In a double-blind placebo-controlled trial in 39 patients with steroid-resistant PM and DM, however, plasmapheresis was devoid of therapeutic benefit (Miller et al., 1991).

The most prominent feature distinguishing IBM from DM and PM is the lack of responsiveness to immunosuppressive therapy. In fact, in cases of steroid-resistant PM, repeat biopsy has often confirmed the pathologic hallmarks of IBM (Amato et al., 1996). However, because a small percentage of patients with IBM do respond to steroids, a 3-month trial of oral prednisone is warranted (Fig. 10-6). If no clinical benefit is achieved, then a trial of IGIV should be

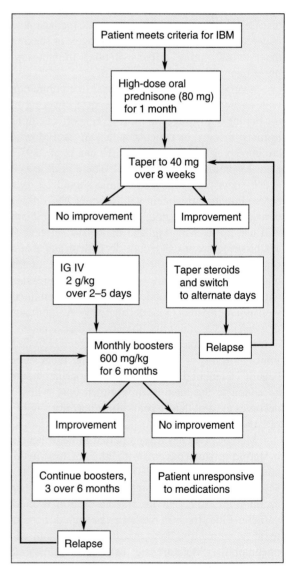

Figure 10–6.   Treating inclusion body myositis (IBM)

instituted. In a double-blind, placebo-controlled trial of IGIV in 19 patients with IBM, "functionally important" improvement was demonstrated in 6 (28%) (Dalakas et al., 1997A). The gains were modest at best, however, and the small sample size may have prevented a more robust demonstration of the efficacy of IGIV in IBM. Clearly, more specific therapy for IBM awaits the identification and clarification of the mechanisms responsible for its pathogenesis

For additional information on the drugs discussed in this chapter see chapters 8, 51, 52, 59, 60, and 64 in *Goodman and Gilman's The Pharmacological Basis of Therapeutics* (Ninth Edition), McGraw-Hill, New York, 1996.

REFERENCES

Amato AA, Gronseth GS, Jackson CE et al.: Inclusion body myositis: clinical and pathological boundaries. *Ann Neurol* 1996;40:581–586.

Arahata K, Engel AG: Monoclonal antibody analysis of mononuclear cells in myopathies. I: Quantitation of subsets according to diagnosis and sites of accumulation and demonstration and counts of muscle fibers invaded by T cells. *Ann Neurol* 1984;16:193–208.

Arahata K, Engel AG: Monoclonal antibody analysis of mononuclear cells in myopathies. III: Immunoelectron microscopy aspects of cell-mediated muscle fiber injury. *Ann Neurol* 1986;19:112–125.

Arahata K, Engel AG: Monoclonal antibody analysis of mononuclear cells in myopathies. IV: Cell-mediated cytotoxicity and muscle fiber necrosis. *Ann Neurol* 1988A;23:168–173.

Arahata K, Engel AG: Monoclonal antibody analysis of mononuclear cells in myopathies. V: Identification and quantitation of T8+ cytotoxic and T8+ suppressor cells. *Ann Neurol* 1988B;23:493–499.

Argov Z, Tiram E, Eisenberg I et al.: Various types of hereditary inclusion body myopathies map to chromosome 9p1-q1. *Ann Neurol* 1997;41:548–551.

Arsura E, Brunner NG, Namba T, Grob D: High-dose intravenous methylprednisolone in myasthenia gravis. *Arch Neurol* 1985;42:1149–1153.

Asbury AK, Arnason BG, Adams RD: The inflammatory lesion in idiopathic polyneuritis: its role in pathogenesis. *Medicine* 1969;48:173–215.

Askanas V, Engel WK: New advances in the understanding of sporadic inclusion-body myositis and hereditary inclusion-body myopathies. *Curr Opin Rheumatol* 1995;7:486–496.

Askanas V, Engel WK, Alvarez RB: Light and electron microscopic localization of beta-amyloid protein in muscle biopsies of patients with inclusion-body myositis. *Am J Pathol* 1992;41:31–36.

Askanas V, McFerrin J, Alvarez RB et al.: Beta APP gene transfer into cultured human muscle induces inclusion-body myositis aspects. *Neuroreport* 1997;8:2155–2158.

Askari AD: The heart in polymyositis and dermatomyositis. *Mt Sinai J Med* 1988;55:479–482.

Bain PG, Motomura M, Newsom-Davis J et al.: Effects of intravenous immunoglobulin on muscle weakness and calcium-channel autoantibodies in the Lambert-Eaton myasthenic syndrome. *Neurology* 1996;47:678–683.

Barnes BE, Mawr B: Dermatomyositis and malignancy: a review of the literature. *Ann Intern Med* 1976;84:68–76.

Basta M, Kirshbom P, Frank MM, Fries LF: Mechanism of therapeutic effect of high-dose intravenous immunoglobulin: attenuation of acute, complement-dependent immune damage in a guinea pig model. *J Clin Invest* 1989;84:1974–1981.

Behrens L, Bender A, Johnson MA, Hohlfeld R: Cytotoxic mechanisms in inflammatory myopathies: co-expression of Fas and protective Bcl-2 in muscle fibres and inflammatory cells. *Brain* 1997;120:929–938.

Ben-Smith A, Goodall JC, Gaston JS, Winer JB: Stimulation of peripheral blood lymphocytes with *Campylobacter jejuni* generates a gamma/delta T cell response in patients with Guillain-Barré syndrome. *Clin Exp Immunol* 1997;109:121–126.

Bohan A, Peter JB, Bowman RL, Pearson CM: Computer-assisted analysis of 153 patients with polymyositis and dermatomyositis. *Medicine* 1977;56:255–286.

Callen JP: Malignancy in polymyositis/dermatomyositis. *Clin Dermatol* 1988;6:55–63.

Carpenter S, Karpati G, Heller I, Eisen A: Inclusion body myositis: a distinct variety of idiopathic inflammatory myopathy. *Neurology* 1978;28:8–17.

Castleman B: The pathology of the thymus gland in myasthenia gravis. *Ann NY Acad Sci* 1966;135:496–503.

Chiba A, Kusunoki S, Obata H et al.: Serum anti-GQ-1b IgG antibody is associated with ophthalmoplegia in Miller Fisher syndrome and Guillain-Barré syndrome: clinical and immunohistochemical studies. *Neurology* 1993;43:1911–1918.

Chiba A, Kusunoki S, Shimizu T, Kanazawa I: Serum IgG antibody to ganglioside GQ1b is a possible marker of Miller Fisher syndrome. *Ann Neurol* 1992;31:677–679.

Chou SM: Myxovirus-like structures in a case of human chronic polymyositis. *Science* 1967;158:1453–1455.

Connolly AM, Pestronk A, Mehta S et al.: Serum IgM monoclonal autoantibody binding to the 301 to 314 amino acid epitope of beta-tubulin: clinical association with slowly progressive demyelinating polyneuropathy. *Neurology* 1997;48:243–248.

Dalakas MC: Intravenous immune globulin therapy for neurologic diseases. *Ann Intern Med* 1997;126:721–730.

Dalakas MC, Illa I, Dambrosia JM et al.: A controlled trial of high-dose intravenous immune globulin infusions as treatment for dermatomyositis. *N Engl J Med* 1993;329:1993–2000.

Dalakas MC, Illa I, Gallardo E, Juarez C: Inclusion body myositis and paraproteinemia: incidence and immunopathologic correlations. *Ann Neurol* 1997A;41:100–104.

Dalakas MC, Sonies B, Dambrosia J et al.: Treatment of inclusion-body myositis with IVIg: a double-blind, placebo-controlled study. *Neurology* 1997B;48:712–716.

de Carvalho M, Luis ML: Relapsing chronic low-dose corticosteroid-responsive multifocal motor neuropathy with conduction block. *Electromyogr Clin Neurophysiol* 1997;37:95–97.

DeVere R, Bradley WG: Polymyositis: its presentation, morbidity and mortality. *Brain* 1975;98:637–666.

Dyck PJ, Daube J, O'Brien P et al.: Plasma exchange in chronic inflammatory demyelinating polyradiculoneuropathy. *N Engl J Med* 1986;314:461–465.

Dyck PJ, Lais AC, Ohta M et al.: Chronic inflammatory polyradiculoneuropathy. *Mayo Clin Proc* 1975;50:621–637.

Dyck PJ, Litchy WJ, Kratz KM et al.: A plasma exchange versus immune globulin infusion trial in chronic inflammatory demyelinating polyradiculoneuropathy. *Ann Neurol* 1994;36:838–845.

Dyck PJ, O'Brien PC, Oviatt KF et al.: Prednisone improves chronic inflammatory demyelinating polyradiculoneuropathy more than no treatment. *Ann Neurol* 1982;11:136–141.

Eaton LM, Lambert EH: Electromyography and electrical stimulation of nerves in diseases of motor units: observations on myasthenic syndrome associated with malignant tumors. *JAMA* 1957;163:1117.

Elmqvist D, Lambert EH: Detailed analysis of neuromuscular transmission in a patient with the myasthenic syndrome sometimes associated with bronchogenic carcinoma. *Mayo Clin Proc* 1968;43:689–713.

Emslie-Smith AM, Engel AG: Microvascular changes in early and advanced dermatomyositis: a quantitative study. *Ann Neurol* 1990;27:343–356.

Enders U, Karch H, Toyka KV et al.: The spectrum of immune responses to *Campylobacter jejuni* and glycoconjugates in Guillain-Barré syndrome and in other neuroimmunological disorders. *Ann Neurol* 1993;34:136–144.

Engel AG: Myasthenic syndromes, in Engel AG, Franzini-Armstrong C (eds): *Myology*. New York, McGraw-Hill, 1994, pp 1806–1835.

Engel AG, Arahata K: Monoclonal antibody analysis of mononuclear cells in myopathies. II: Phenotypes of autoinvasive cells in polymyositis and inclusion body myositis. *Ann Neurol* 1984;16:209–215.

Engel AG, Hohlfeld R, Banker BQ: Inflammatory myopathies, in Engel AG, Franzini-Armstrong C (eds): *Myology*. New York, McGraw-Hill, 1994, pp 1335–1383.

Engel AG, Lambert EH, Howard FM: Immune complexes (IgG and C3) at the motor end-plate in myasthenia gravis: ultrastructural and light microscopic localization and electrophysiologic correlations. *Mayo Clin Proc* 1977;52:267–280.

Engel AG, Nagel A, Fukuoka T et al.: Motor nerve terminal calcium channels in Lambert-Eaton myasthenic syndrome: morphologic evidence for depletion and that the depletion is mediated by autoantibodies. *Ann NY Acad Sci* 1989;560:278–290.

Engel AG, Sahashi K, Fumagilli G: The immunopathology of acquired myasthenia gravis. *Ann NY Acad Sci* 1981;377:158–174.

Epstein MA, Sladky JT: The role of plasmapheresis in childhood Guillain-Barré syndrome. *Ann Neurol* 1990;28:65–69.

Euwer RL, Sontheimer RD: Amyopathic dermatomyositis: a review. *J Invest Dermatol* 1993;100:124S–127S.

Fambrough DM, Drachman DB, Satyamurti S: Neuromuscular junction in myasthenia gravis: decreased acetylcholine receptors. *Science* 1973;182:293-295.

Feasby TE, Gilbert JJ, Brown WF et al.: An acute axonal form of Guillain-Barré polyneuropathy. *Brain* 1986;109:1115–1126.

Flachenecker P, Wermuth P, Hartung HP, Reiners K: Quantitative assessment of cardiovascular autonomic function in Guillain-Barré syndrome. *Ann Neurol* 1997;42:171–179.

French Cooperative Group on Plasma Exchange in Guillain-Barré Syndrome: Appropriate number of plasma exchanges in Guillain-Barré syndrome. *Ann Neurol* 1997;41:298–306.

French Cooperative Group on Plasma Exchange in Guillain-Barré Syndrome: Efficiency of plasma exchange in Guillain-Barré syndrome: role of replacement fluids. *Ann Neurol* 1987;22:753–761.

French Cooperative Group on Plasma Exchange in Guillain-Barré Syndrome: Plasma exchange in Guillain-Barré syndrome: one-year follow-up. *Ann Neurol* 1992;32:94–97.

Fukunaga H, Engel AG, Lang B et al.: Passive transfer of Lambert-Eaton myasthenic syndrome with IgG from man to mouse depletes the presynaptic membrane active zones. *Proc Natl Acad Sci USA* 1983;80:7636–7640.

Fumagalli G, Engel AG, Lindstrom J: Ultrastructural aspects of acetylcholine receptor turnover at the normal end-plate and in autoimmune myasthenia gravis. *J Neuropathol Exp Neurol* 1982;41:567–579.

Fyhr IM, Moslemi AR, Tarkowski A et al.: Limited T-cell receptor V gene usage in inclusion body myositis. *Scand J Immunol* 1996;43:109–114.

Gajdos P, Chevret S, Clair B et al.: Clinical trial of plasma exchange and high-dose intravenous immunoglobulin in myasthenia gravis. Myasthenia Gravis Clinical Study Group. *Ann Neurol* 1997;41:789–796.

Goebels N, Michaelis D, Engelhardt M et al.: Differential expression of perforin in muscle-infiltrating T cells in polymyositis and dermatomyositis. *J Clin Invest* 1996;97:2905–2910.

Gorson KC, Allam G, Ropper AH: Chronic inflammatory demyelinating polyneuropathy: clinical features and response to treatment in 67 consecutive patients with and without a monoclonal gammopathy. *Neurology* 1997;48:321–328.

Gottdiener JS, Sherber HS, Hawley RJ, Engel WK: Cardiac manifestations in polymyositis. *Am J Cardiol* 1978;41:1141–1149.

Grob D, Brunner NG, Namba T: The natural course of myasthenia gravis and effect of therapeutic measures. *Ann NY Acad Sci* 1981;377:652–669.

Guillain-Barré Syndrome Steroid Trial Group: Double-blind trial of intravenous methylprednisolone in Guillain-Barré syndrome. *Lancet* 1993;341:586–590.

Guillain-Barré Syndrome Study Group: Plasmapheresis and acute Guillain-Barré syndrome. *Neurology* 1985;35:1096–1104.

Gutmann L, Crosby TW, Takamori M, Martin JD: The Eaton-Lambert syndrome and autoimmune disorders. *Am J Med* 1972;53:354–356.

Hafer-Macko C, Hsieh ST, Li CY et al.: Acute motor axonal neuropathy: an antibody-mediated attack on axolemma. *Ann Neurol* 1996;40:635–644.

Hafer-Macko CE, Sheikh KA, Li CY et al.: Immune attack on the Schwann cell surface in acute inflammatory demyelinating polyneuropathy. *Ann Neurol* 1996;39:625–635.

Hahn AF: Experimental allergic neuritis (EAN) as a model for the immune-mediated demyelinating neuropathies. *Rev Neurol* 1996;152:328–332.

Hahn AF, Bolton CF, Pillay N et al.: Plasma-exchange therapy in chronic inflammatory demyelinating polyneuropathy: a double-blind, sham-controlled, cross-over study. *Brain* 1996;119:1055–1066.

Hahn AF, Bolton CF, Zochodne D, Feasby TE: Intravenous immunoglobulin treatment in chronic inflammatory demyelinating polyneuropathy: a double-blind, placebo-controlled, cross-over study. *Brain* 1996;119:1067–1077.

Hall SM, Hughes RAC, Atkinson PF et al.: Motor nerve biopsy in severe Guillain-Barré syndrome. *Ann Neurol* 1992;31:441–444.

Hartung HP, Pollard JD, Harvey GK, Toyka KV: Immunopathogenesis and treatment of the Guillain-Barré syndrome—Part 1. *Muscle Nerve* 1995;18:137–153.

Hartung, HP, Pollard JD, Harvey GK, Toyka KV: Immunopathogenesis and treatment of the Guillain-Barré syndrome—Part 2. *Muscle Nerve* 1995;18:137–153.

Harvey GK, Gold R, Hartung HP, Toyka KV: Non-neural-specific T lymphocytes can orchestrate inflammatory peripheral neuropathy. *Brain* 1995;118:1263–1272.

Heckmatt J, Hasson N, Saunders C et al.: Cyclosporin in juvenile dermatomysositis. *Lancet* 1989;13:1063–1066.

Henriksson KG, Lindvall B: Polymyositis and dermatomyositis—diagnosis, treatment and prognosis. *Prog Neurobiol* 1990;35:181–193.

Ho TW, Hsieh ST, Nachamkin I et al.: Motor nerve terminal degeneration provides a potential mechanism for rapid recovery in acute motor axonal neuropathy after *Campylobacter* infection. *Neurology* 1997;48:717–724.

Hohlfeld R, Kalies I, Kohleisen B et al.: Myasthenia gravis: stimulation of antireceptor autoantibodies by autoreactive T cell lines. *Neurology* 1986;36:618–621.

Illa I, Gallardo E, Gimeno R et al.: Signal transducer and activator of transcription 1 in human muscle: implications in inflammatory myopathies. *Am J Pathol* 1997;151:81–88.

Jahnke U, Fischer EH, Alvord EC: Sequence homology between certain viral proteins and proteins related to encephalomyelitis and neuritis. *J Immunol* 1992;148:2446–2451.

Jenkyn LR, Brooks PL, Forcier RJ et al.: Remission of the Lambert-Eaton syndrome and small cell anaplastic carcinoma of the lung induced by chemotherapy and radiotherapy. *Cancer* 1980;46:1123–1127.

Joffe MM, Love LA, Leff RL et al.: Drug therapy of the idiopathic inflammatory myopathies: predictors of response to prednisone, azathioprine, and methotrexate and a comparison of their efficacy. *Am J Med* 1993;94:379–387.

Kissel JT, Levy RJ, Mendell JR, Griggs RC: Azathioprine toxicity in neuromuscular disease. *Neurology* 1986;36:35–39.

Kissel JT, Mendell JR, Rammohen KN: Microvascular deposition of complement membrane attacks complex in dermatomyositis. *N Engl J Med* 1986;314:329–334.

Kuwabara S, Nakajima M, Matsuda S, Hattori T: Magnetic resonance imaging at the demyelinative foci in chronic inflammatory demyelinating polyneuropathy. *Neurology* 1997;48:874–877.

Lang B, Johnston I, Leys K et al: Autoantibody specificities in Lambert-Eaton myasthenic syndrome. *Ann NY Acad Sci* 1993;681:382–393.

Lang B, Newsom-Davis J, Wray D et al.: Autoimmune aetiology for myasthenic (Eaton-Lambert) syndrome. *Lancet* 1981;2:224–226.

Lang B, Vincent A, Murray NM, Newsom-Davis J: Lambert-Eaton myasthenic syndrome: immunoglobulin G inhibition of Ca2 + flux in tumor cells correlates with disease severity. *Ann Neurol* 1989;25:265–271.

Lanska DJ: Indications for thymectomy in myasthenia gravis. *Neurology* 1990;40:1828–1829.

Lennon VA, Lindstrom JM, Seybold ME: Experimental autoimmune myasthenia gravis: cellular and humoral immune responses. *Ann NY Acad Sci* 1976;274:283–299.

Limburg PC, The TH, Hummel-Tappel E, Oosterhuis HJ: Anti-acetylcholine receptor antibodies in myasthenic gravis. *J Neurol Sci* 1983;58:357–370.

Lindberg C, Borg K, Edstrom L et al.: Inclusion body myositis and Welander distal myopathy: a clinical, neurophysiological and morphological comparison. *J Neurol Sci* 1991;103:76–81.

Maier H, Schmidbauer M, Pfausler B et al.: Central nervous system pathology in patients with the Guillain-Barré syndrome. *Brain* 1997;120:451–464.

Manfredini E, Nobile-Orazio E, Allaria S, Scarlato G: Anti-alpha- and beta-tubulin IgM antibodies in dysimmune neuropathies. *J Neurol Sci* 1995;133:79–84.

Mantegazza R, Andreetta F, Bernasconi P et al.: Analysis of T cell receptor repertoire of muscle-infiltrating T lymphocytes in polymyositis: restricted V alpha/beta rearrangements may indicate antigen-driven selection. *J Clin Invest* 1993;91:2880–2886.

Mantegazza R, Antozzi C, Peluchetti D et al.: Azathioprine as a single drug or in combination with steroids in the treatment of myasthenia gravis. *J Neurol* 1988;235:449–453.

Massa R, Weller B, Karpati G et al.: Familial inclusion body myositis among Kurdish-Iranian Jews. *Arch Neurol* 1991;48:519–522.

McEvoy KM, Windebank AJ, Daube JR, Low PA: 3,4-Diaminopyridine in the treatment of Lambert-Eaton myasthenic syndrome. *N Engl J Med* 1989;321:1567–1571.

Mehregan DR, Su WP: Cyclosporine treatment for dermatomyositis/polymyositis. *Cutis* 1993;51:59–61.

Melendez-Vasquez C, Redford J, Choudhary PP et al.: Immunological investigation of chronic inflammatory demyelinating polyradiculoneuropathy. *J Neuroimmunol* 1997;73:124–134.

Mendell JR, Sahenk Z, Gales T, Paul L: Amyloid filaments in inclusion body myositis: novel findings provide insight into nature of filaments. *Arch Neurol* 1991;48:1229–1234.

Meriney SD, Hulsizer SC, Lennon VA, Grinnell AD: Lambert-Eaton myasthenic syndrome immunoglobulins react with multiple types of calcium channels in small-cell lung carcinoma. *Ann Neurol* 1996;40:739–749.

Metzger AL, Bohan A, Goldberg LS et al.: Polymyositis and dermatomyositis: combined methotrexate and corticosteroid therapy. *Ann Intern Med* 1974;81:182–189.

Miller FW, Leitman SF, Cronin ME et al.: Controlled trial of plasma exchange and leukapheresis in polymyositis and dermatomyositis. *N Engl J Med* 1992;326:1380–1384.

Miller RG, Parry GJ, Pfaeffl W et al.: The spectrum of peripheral neuropathy associated with ARC and AIDS. *Muscle Nerve* 1988;11:857–863.

Milner P, Lovelidge CA, Taylor WA, Hughes RA: PO myelin protein produces experimental allergic neuritis in Lewis rats. *J Neurol Sci* 1987;79:275–285.

Mimori T: Structures targeted by the immune system in myositis. *Curr Opin Rheumatol* 1996;8:521–527.

Mirabella M, Alvarez RB, Bilak M et al.: Difference in expression of phosphorylated tau epitopes between sporadic inclusion-body myositis and hereditary inclusion-body myopathies. *J Neuropathol Exp Neurol* 1996;55:774–786.

Mirabella M, Alvarez RB, Engel WK et al.: Apolipoprotein E and apolipoprotein E messenger RNA in muscle of inclusion body myositis and myopathies. *Ann Neurol* 1996;40:864–872.

Morgenthaler TI, Brown LR, Colby TV et al.: Thymoma. *Mayo Clin Proc* 1993;68:1110–1123.

Motomura M, Lang B, Johnston I et al.: Incidence of serum anti-P/O-type and anti-N-type calcium channel autoantibodies in the Lambert-Eaton myasthenic syndrome. *J Neurol Sci* 1997;147:35–42.

Moulin DE, Hagen N, Feasby TE et al.: Pain in Guillain-Barré syndrome. *Neurology* 1997;48:328–331.

Muchnik S, Losavio AS, Vidal A et al.: Long-term follow-up of Lambert-Eaton syndrome treated with intravenous immunoglobulin. *Muscle Nerve* 1997;20:674–678.

Murakami N, Ihara Y, Nonaka I: Muscle fiber degeneration in distal myopathy with rimmed vacuole formation. *Acta Neuropathol* 1995;89:29–34.

Myasthenia Gravis Clinical Study Group: A randomized clinical trial comparing prednisone and azathioprine in myasthenia gravis: results of the second interim analysis. *J Neurol Neurosurg Psychiat* 1993;56:1157–1163.

Nagel A, Engel AG, Lange B et al.: Lambert-Eaton myasthenic syndrome IgG depletes presynaptic membrane active zone particles by antigenic modulation. *Ann Neurol* 1988;24:552–558.

Namba T, Brown SB, Grob D: Neonatal myasthenia gravis: report of two cases and review of the literature. *Pediatrics* 1970;45:488–504.

Nevo Y, Pestronk A, Kornberg AJ et al.: Childhood chronic inflammatory demyelinating neuropathies: clinical course and long-term follow-up. *Neurology* 1996;47:98–102.

Newsom-Davis J, Leys K, Vincent A et al.: Immunological evidence for the co-existence of the Lambert-Eaton myasthenic syndrome and myasthenia gravis in two patients. *J Neurol Neurosurg Psychiat* 1991;54:452–453.

Newsom-Davis J, Murray NM: Plasma exchange and immunosuppressive drug treatment in the Lambert-Eaton myasthenic syndrome. *Neurology* 1984;34:480–485.

Nicolle MW, Stewart DJ, Remtulla H et al.: Lambert-Eatom myasthenic syndrome presenting with severe respiratory failure. *Muscle Nerve* 1996;19:1328–1333.

Oddis CV, Medsger TA: Current management of polymyositis and dermatomyositis. *Drugs* 1989;37:382–390.

Oh SJ, Kim DS, Head TC, Claussen GC: Low-dose guanidine and pyridostigmine: relatively safe and effective long-term symptomatic therapy in Lambert-Eaton myasthenic syndrome. *Muscle Nerve* 1997;20:1146–1152.

O'Neill JH, Murray NM, Newsom-Davis J: The Lambert-Eaton myasthenic syndrome: a review of 50 cases. *Brain* 1988;111:577–596.

Oosterhuis HJ: The natural course of myasthenia gravis: a long-term follow up study. *J Neurol Neurosurg Psychiat* 1989;52:1121–1127.

Oosterhuis HJ, Limburg PC, Hummel-Tappel E, The TH: Anti-acetylcholine receptor antibodies in myasthenia gravis. Part 2. Clinical and serological follow-up of individual patients. *J Neurol Sci* 1983;58:371–385.

Ozdemir C, Young RR: The results to be expected from electrical testing in the diagnosis of myasthenia gravis. *Ann NY Acad Sci* 1976;274:203–222.

Pachman LM: Juvenile dermatomyositis. *Mt Sinai J Med* 1988;55:465–470.

Papatestas AE, Genkins G, Kornfeld P et al.: Effects of thymectomy in myasthenia gravis. *Ann Surg* 1987;206:79–88.

Penn AS, Jaretzki A 3d, Wolff M et al.: Thymic abnormalities: antigen or antibody? Response to thymectomy in myasthenia gravis. *Ann NY Acad Sci* 1981;377:786–804.

Plasma Exchange/Sandoglobulin Guillain-Barré Syndrome Trial Group: Randomized trial of plasma exchange, intravenous immunoglobulin, and combined treatments in Guillain-Barré syndrome. *Lancet* 1997;349:225–230.

Plotz PH, Dalakas M, Leff RL et al.: Current concepts in the idiopathic inflammatory myopathies: polymyositis, dermatomyositis, and related disorders. *Ann Intern Med* 1989;111:143–157.

Prevots DR, Sutter RW: Assessment of Guillain-Barré syndrome mortality and morbidity in the United States: implications for acute flaccid paralysis surveillance. *J Infect Dis* 1997;175:S151–S155.

Pruitt JN 2nd, Showalter CJ, Engel AG: Sporadic inclusion body myositis: counts of different types of abnormal fibers. *Ann Neurol* 1996;39:139–143.

Roberts M, Willison H, Vincent A, Newsom-Davis J: Serum factor in Miller Fisher variant of Guillain-Barré syndrome and neurotransmitter release. *Lancet* 1994;343:454–455.

Roscelli JD, Bass JW, Pang L: Guillain-Barré syndrome and influenza vaccination in the U.S. Army, 1980-1988. *Am J Epidemiol* 1991;133:952–955.

Rostami A, Gregorian SK: Peptide 53-78 of myelin P2 protein is a T cell epitope for the induction of experimental autoimmune neuritis. *Cell Immunol* 1991;132:433–441.

Rostami A, Gregorian SK, Brown MJ, Pleasure DE: Induction of severe experimental autoimmune neuritis with a synthetic peptide corresponding to the 53-78 amino acid sequence of the myelin P2 protein. *J Neuroimmunol* 1990;30:145–151.

Rubenstein AE, Horowitz SH, Bender AN: Cholinergic dysautonomia and Eaton-Lambert syndrome. *Neurology* 1979;29:720–723.

Sahashi K, Engel AG, Lambert EH, Howard FM Jr: Ultrastructural localization of the terminal and lytic ninth complement component (C9) at the motor end-plate in myasthenia gravis. *J Neuropathol Exp Neurol* 1980;39:160–172.

Said G, Lacroix C, Chemouilli P et al: Cytomegalovirus neuropathy in acquired immunodeficiency syndrome: a clinical and pathological study. *Ann Neurol* 1991;29:139–146.

Sanders DB, Howard JF Jr, Massey JM: 3,4-Diaminopyridine in Lambert-Eaton myasthenic syndrome and myasthenia gravis. *Ann NY Acad Sci* 1993;681:588–590.

Santorelli FM, Sciacco M, Tanji K et al.: Multiple mitochondrial DNA deletions in sporadic inclusion body myositis: a study of 56 patients. *Ann Neurol* 1996;39:789–795.

Schady W, Goulding PJ, Lecky BR et al.: Massive nerve root enlargement in chronic inflammatory demyelinating polyneuropathy. *J Neurol Neurosurg Psychiat* 1996;61:636–640.

Schlesinger I, Soffer D, Lossos A et al.: Inclusion body myositis: atypical clinical presentations. *Eur Neurol* 1996;36:89–93.

Schmidt B, Toyka KV, Keifer R et al.: Inflammatory infiltrates in sural nerve biopsies in Guillain-Barré syndrome and chronic inflammatory demyelinating neuropathy. *Muscle Nerve* 1996;19:474–487.

Schneider C, Gold R, Dalakas MC et al.: MHC class I-mediated cytotoxicity does not induce apoptosis in muscle fibers nor in inflammatory T cells: studies in patients with polymyositis, dermatomyositis, and inclusion body myositis. *J Neuropathol Exp Neurol* 1996;55:1205–1209.

Schonberger LB, Bregman DJ, Sullivan-Bolyai JZ et al.: Guillain-Barré syndrome following vaccination in the National Influenza Immunization Program, United States, 1976–1977. *Am J Epidemiol* 1979;110:105–123.

Schumacher HR, Schimmer B, Gordon GV et al.: Articular manifestations of polymyositis and dermatomyositis. *Am J Med* 1979;67:287–292.

Schwimmbeck PL, Dyrberg T, Drachman DB, Oldstone MB: Molecular mimicry and myasthenia gravis: an autoantigenic site of the acetylcholine receptor alpha-subunit that has biologic activity and reacts immunochemically with herpes simplex virus. *J Clin Invest* 1989;84:1174–1180.

Sekul EA, Chow C, Dalakas MC: Magnetic resonance imaging of the forearm as a diagnostic aid in patients with sporadic inclusion body myositis. *Neurology* 1997;48:863–866.

Sghirlanzoni A, Peluchetti D, Mantegazza R et al.: Myasthenia gravis: prolonged treatment with steroids. *Neurology* 1984;34:170–174.

Shahar E, Shorer Z, Roifman CM et al.: Immune globulins are effective in severe pediatric Guillain-Barré syndrome. *Pediatr Neurol* 1997;16:32–36.

Sharief MK, Ingram DA, Swash M: Circulating tumor necrosis factor-alpha correlates with electrodiagnostic abnormalities in Guillain-Barré syndrome. *Ann Neurol* 1997;42:68–73.

Simmons Z, Wald JJ, Alberts JW: Chronic inflammatory demyelinating polyradiculoneuropathy in children: I. Presentation, electrodiagnostic studies, and initial clinical course, with comparison to adults. *Muscle Nerve* 1997;20:1008–1015.

Sivakumar K, Semino-Mora C, Dalakas MC: An inflammatory, familial, inclusion body myositis with autoimmune features and a phenotype identical to sporadic inclusion body myositis: studies in three families. *Brain* 1997;120:653–661.

Sivieri S, Ferrarini AM, Lolli F et al.: Cytokine pattern in the cerebrospinal fluid from patients with GBS and CIDP. *J Neurol Sci* 1997;147:93–95.

Sorensen TT, Holm EB: Myasthenia gravis in the county of Viborg, Denmark. *Eur Neurol* 1989;29:177–179.

Stanley EF, Drachman DB: Effect of myasthenic immunoglobulin on acetylcholine receptors of intact mammalian neuromuscular junctions. *Science* 1978;200:1285–1287.

Stefansson K, Dieperink ME, Richman DP et al.: Sharing of antigenic determinants between the nicotinic acetylcholine receptor and proteins in *Escherichia coli, Proteus vulgaris,* and *Klebsiella pneumoniae*: possible role in the pathogenesis of myasthenia gravis. *N Engl J Med* 1985;312:221–225.

Stewart JD, McKelvey R, Durcan L et al.: Chronic inflammatory demyelinating polyneuropathy (CIDP) in diabetics. *J Neurol Sci* 1996;142:59–64.

Sullivan DB, Cassidy JT, Petty RE: Dermatomyositis in the pediatric patient. *Arthritis Rheum* 1977;20:327–331.

Sunohara N, Nonaka I, Kamei N, Satoyoshi E: Distal myopathy with rimmed vacuole formation: a follow-up study. *Brain* 1989;112:65–83.

Takamori M, Hamada T, Komai K et al.: Synaptotagmin can cause an immune-mediated model of Lambert-Eaton myasthenic syndrome in rats. *Ann Neurol* 1994;35:74–80.

Takamori M, Iwasa K, Komai K: Antibodies to synthetic peptides of the alpha1A subunit of the voltage-gated calcium channel in Lambert-Eaton myasthenic syndrome. *Neurology* 1997;58:1261–1265.

Targoff IN: Humoral immunity in polymyositis/dermatomyositis. *J Invest Dermatol* 1993;100:116S–123S.

The Dutch Guillain-Barré Study Group: Treatment of the Guillain-Barré syndrome with high-dose immune globulins combined with methylprednisolone: a pilot study. *Ann Neurol* 1994;35:749–752.

Thornton CA, Ballow M: Safety of intravenous immunoglobulin. *Arch Neurol* 1993;50:135.

Tindall RS: Humoral immunity in myasthenia gravis: biochemical characterization of acquired antireceptor antibodies and clinical correlations. *Ann Neurol* 1981;10:437–447.

Tindall RS, Rollins JA, Phillips JT et al.: Preliminary results of a double-blind, randomized, placebo-controlled trial of cyclosporine in myasthenia gravis. *N Engl J Med* 1987;316:719–724.

Toyka KV, Drachman DB, Griffin DE et al.: Myasthenia gravis: study of humoral immune mechanisms by passive transfer to mice. *N Engl J Med* 1977;296:125–131.

Tymms KE, Webb J: Dermatopolymyositis and other connective tissue diseases: a review of 105 cases. *J Rheumatol* 1985;12:1140–1148.

Tzartos SJ, Kokla A, Walgrave SL, Conti-Tronconi BM: Localization of the main immunogenic region of human muscle acetylcholine receptor to residues 67-76 of the alpha subunit. *Proc Natl Acad Sci USA* 1988;85:2899–2903.

Tzartos SJ, Seybold ME, Lindstrom JM: Specificities of antibodies to acetylcholine receptors in sera from myasthenia gravis patients measured by monoclonal antibodies. *Proc Natl Acad Sci USA* 1982;79:188–192.

Uchitel OD, Protti DA, Sanchez V et al.: P-type voltage-dependent calcium channel mediates presynaptic calcium influx and transmitter release in mammalian synapses. *Proc Natl Acad Sci USA* 1992;89:3330–3333.

van der Meche FGA, Schmitz PIM, Dutch Guillain-Barré Syndrome Study Group: High-dose intravenous immunoglobulin versus plasma exchange in Guillain-Barré syndrome. *N Engl J Med* 1992;326:1123–1129.

Van Es HW, Van den Berg LH, Franssen H et al.: Magnetic resonance imaging of the brachial plexus in patients with multifocal motor neuropathy. *Neurology* 1997;48:1218–1224.

Viglione MP, O'Shaughnessy TJ, Kim YI: Inhibition of calcium currents and exocytosis by Lambert-Eaton syndrome antibodies in human lung cancer cells. *J Physiol* 1995;488:303–317.

Villanova M, Kawai M, Lubke U et al.: Rimmed vacuoles of inclusion body myositis and oculopharyngeal muscular dystrophy contain amyloid precursor protein and lysosomal markers. *Brain Res* 1993;603:343–347.

Vriesendorp FJ, Mishu B, Blaser MJ, Koski CL: Serum antibodies to GM1, GD1b, peripheral nerve myelin, and *Campylobacter jejuni* in patients with Guillain-Barré syndrome and controls: correlation and prognosis. *Ann Neurol* 1993;34:130–135.

Walsh CT, Zydowsky LD, McKeon FD: Cyclosporin A, the cyclophilin class of peptidylprolyl isomerases, and blockade of T cell signal transduction. *J Biol Chem* 1992;267:13115–13118.

Waterman SA, Lang B, Newsom-Davis J: Effect of Lambert-Eaton myasthenic syndrome antibodies on autonomic neurons in the mouse. *Ann Neurol* 1997;42:147–156.

Wiedemann HP, Matthay RA: Pulmonary manifestations of the collagen vascular diseases. *Clin Chest Med* 1989;10:677–22.

Willison HJ, Veitch J, Paterson G, Kennedy PG: Miller Fisher syndrome is associated with serum antibodies to GQ1b ganglioside. *J Neurol Neurosurg Psychiat* 1993;56:204–206.

Yang CC, Alvarez RB, Engel WK, Askanas V: Increase of nitric oxide synthases and nitrotyrosine in inclusion body myositis. *Neuroreport* 1996;8:153–158.

Yuki N, Takahashi M, Tagawa Y et al.: Association of *Campylobacter jejuni* serotype with antiganglioside antibody in Guillain-Barré syndrome and Fisher's syndrome. *Ann Neurol* 1997;42:28–33.

Yunis EJ, Samaha FJ: Inclusion body myositis. *Lab Invest* 1971;25:240–248.

EXTRAPYRAMIDAL DISORDERS

John B. Penney, Jr., and Anne B. Young

The term extrapyramidal disorder is used to refer to conditions in which the quality and quantity of spontaneous skeletal muscle movements are abnormal. Abnormalities in tone (the resistance of the muscles to passive stretch) are common, but actual muscle weakness or paralysis is not considered part of a pure extrapyramidal disorder. Of the classic extrapyramidal disorders, several, such as Parkinson's disease, Huntington disease, and hemiballismus, are associated with specific pathologies in the basal ganglia and its connections. Other extrapyramidal disorders, such as tics and idiopathic torsion dystonia, are suspected to be caused by basal ganglia dysfunction, although standard neuropathologic examinations have revealed no abnormalities in this brain region. Although tremor is usually considered an extrapyramidal disorder, only certain types are likely to involve the basal ganglia, with the rest arising from dysfunctions in cerebellar, thalamic, brain stem, or even peripheral neural circuits. Spasticity is an abnormality of tone resulting from lesions of the pyramidal system and descending brain stem to spinal cord pathways.

Detailed in this chapter are the common presenting symptoms and diseases associated with disorders of the extrapyramidal system. To appreciate the pathophysiology of each it is important to understand the anatomy and neurochemistry of the basal ganglia and related pathways.

FUNCTIONAL AND NEUROCHEMICAL ANATOMY OF THE BASAL GANGLIA

Basal Ganglia Structures

The deep forebrain structures comprising the basal ganglia include the caudate nucleus and the putamen, the medial and lateral globus pallidus, the subthalamic nucleus, the substantia nigra pars compacta, and substantia nigra pars reticulata (Albin et al., 1989). The cerebral cortex and brain stem project to the caudate nucleus and putamen which, in turn, project through the globus pallidus and substantia nigra pars reticulata to the thalamus and brain stem and from there to other regions of the cerebral cortex and spinal cord (Figure 11-1).

Corpus striatum. The caudate nucleus, the putamen, the nucleus accumbens, and the olfactory tubercle have similar histologic features and are collectively referred to as the corpus striatum (Graybiel and Ragsdale, 1983). The caudate nucleus is important for integrating cognitive function and the putamen for coordinating movement. These two regions receive major excitatory, glutamatergic inputs from the cerebral cortex. The caudate nucleus receives input from the association cortices, whereas afferents to the putamen emanate mainly from the primary motor and sensory cortices (Graybiel, 1995). The caudate/putamen also receives excitatory projections from the intralaminar nuclei of thalamus. A major dopaminergic pathway to the corpus striatum arises from the substantia nigra pars compacta and ventral tegmental area. Serotoninergic and noradren-

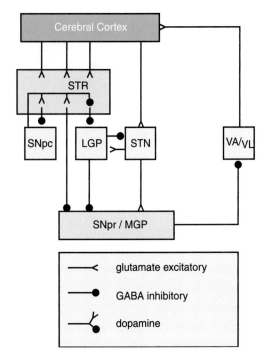

Figure 11–1. Neuroanatomic organization of the extrapyramidal system. Abbreviations: STR, corpus striatum; SNpc, substantia nigra pars compacta; STN, subthalamic nucleus; LGP, lateral globus pallidus; SNpr, substantia nigra pars reticulata; MGP, medial globus pallidus; VA/VL, ventroanterior and ventrolateral nuclei of the thalamus.

ergic projections to the caudate/putamen originated in raphe nuclei and locus ceruleus, respectively, which are found in the brain stem.

The corpus striatum is comprised of two organizational compartments—the matrix and the striosomes (Graybiel, 1995). The striosomes are interconnected patches embedded in the matrix and were first discovered because of lower levels of acetylcholinesterase staining on striatal sections (Graybiel and Ragsdale, 1983). The two compartments have different connections. Motor and sensory cortex project principally to the matrix of the putamen, whereas association and cingulate cortices project to the matrix of the caudate nucleus. These projections are discretely organized in a somatotopic and functionally specific fashion. The matrix not only receives

major projections from layers III and V of the cerebral cortex, but also from the thalamus, the ventral tegmental area, and the dorsal pars compacta of the substantia nigra. The striosomes receive projections from deep layers of the medial prefrontal cortex, insulotemporal cortex, and basolateral amygdala, as well as from the ventral pars compacta.

These differential projections to striosome and matrix provide a substrate for the basal ganglia modulation of limbic and motorsensory tasks (Mink and Thach, 1993; Graybiel, 1995). Although the exact roles these two circuits play in different basal ganglia disorders is still under investigation, striosomal circuits may be more involved in tics, obsessive-compulsive, and attention deficit disorders, whereas the matrix circuits may be more involved in motor/sensory disorders.

Most (90%) striatal neurons are medium spiny projection neurons, with the remainder being aspiny interneurons (Albin, et al., 1989). The interneurons include somatostatin/neuropeptide Y/nitric oxide synthase-positive neurons, which are exclusively confined to the matrix, and large aspiny acetylcholine neurons, which exist in both matrix and striosome compartments and which send their processes from one region to the other. All other striatal neurons appear to confine their dendritic processes to the compartment in which their somata resides. The vast majority of the matrix and striosome spiny projection neurons appear to use γ-aminobutyric acid (GABA) as a neurotransmitter along with a neuropeptide such as enkephalin, substance P, or dynorphin (Penney and Young, 1986). While many GABA/enkephalin neurons project to the lateral portion of the globus pallidus (Albin, et al., 1989, 1992), GABA/substance P/dynorphin neurons innervate the medial segment of the globus pallidus and the substantia nigra pars reticulata. Striosomal efferent neurons are comprised of GABA/substance P/dynorphin neurons, with fewer GABA/enkepahlin neurons. Striosomes project primarily to the pars compacta of the substantia nigra (Gerfen, 1984; Gerfen et al., 1987; Graybiel, 1995). GABA/benzodiazepine, dopamine D1 and D2 and cholinergic muscarinic receptors are highly concentrated in the corpus striatum.

The medial globus pallidus and the substantia nigra pars reticulata. The medial globus pallidus and the substantia nigra pars reticulata are comprised of large multipolar GABAergic neurons similar to those in the lateral globus pallidus. The medial globus pallidus receives the majority of its striatal projections from the putamen and, in turn, projects to the pars oralis of the ventral lateral thalamic nucleus, which in turn projects to the supplementary motor cortex (Schell and Strick, 1984; Albin et al., 1989). This pathway joining the putamen, medial globus pallidus, thalamus, and supplementary motor cortex may be the primary route whereby the basal ganglia influence spontaneous movements.

The substantia nigra pars reticulata receives the majority of its striatal afferents from the caudate nucleus and projects to the ventral anterior and medial dorsal nuclei of the thalamus, which in turn project to the prefrontal cortex. There is another major output that travels from the pars reticulata to the superior colliculus (Albin et al., 1989). This pathway influences eye movements. Both the medial globus pallidus and the substantia nigra pars reticulata project to the brain stem reticular formation, influencing gait and posture.

The lateral globus pallidus and subthalamic nucleus. Like the medial globus pallidus, the lateral globus pallidus consists of large GABAergic neurons. The lateral pallidal neurons send their axons to the subthalamic nucleus, the medial globus pallidus, and the substantia nigra pars reticulata (Albin et al., 1989). The subthalamic nucleus also receives excitatory, presumably glutamatergic, projections from the cerebral cortex, particularly the motor regions. The subthalamic nucleus neurons are also thought to be excitatory, utilizing glutamic acid as a neurotransmitter. The subthalamic nucleus projects to the lateral pallidum and corpus striatum, and to the medial segment of the globus pallidus and the pars reticulata of the substantia nigra.

Thus, information from the GABA/enkephalin striatal matrix neurons goes to the lateral globus pallidus from whence it is relayed by way of the subthalamic nucleus to the medial segment of the globus pallidus and the substantia nigra pars reticulata. The lateral globus pallidus also projects directly to the medial globus pallidus and the substantia nigra pars reticulata. Here the information is processed along with that derived from the matrix substance P/dynorphin direct projections to the substantia nigra and medial pallidum.

Direct and indirect pathways. The "direct" pathway from the cerebral cortex to the corpus striatum to the medial globus pallidus/substantia nigra pars reticulata to the thalamus to the cerebral cortex is a positive or reinforcing feedback loop that helps maintain and execute ongoing motor programs (Albin et al., 1989; DeLong, 1990). The "indirect" pathway travels from the cerebral cortex to the corpus striatum to the lateral globus pallidus, the subthalamic nucleus, the medial globus pallidus/substantia nigra pars reticulata, the thalamus, and the cerebral cortex. This represents a negative feedback circuit that may be involved in suppressing unwanted motor programs.

The substantia nigra pars compacta. The dopaminergic pathway from the substantia nigra pars compacta to the corpus striatum is a critical pathway in extrapyramidal motor function. It provides a dense innervation to all areas of the caudate/putamen and, to a lesser extent, certain regions of the cerebral cortex and subthalamic nucleus (Graybiel and Ragsdale, 1983; Gerfen et al., 1987). Striosomes are innervated by dopamine

afferents earlier in development than matrix. Specific pars compacta regions project preferentially to striosome rather than matrix. The ventral-caudal densocellular portion as well as the substantia nigra pars lateralis project primarily to striosomes. The more dorsal region of the pars compacta and the ventral tegmental area project primarily to matrix.

Clinical Implications

Although the complex circuitry of the basal ganglia is not yet precisely defined, some generalizations can be made that allow for the interpretion of clinical symptomatology in terms of neuronal circuitry (Albin et al., 1989; DeLong, 1990; Mink and Thach, 1993; Graybiel, 1995).

A limbic circuit, which is relatively self-contained and includes the medial prefrontal, orbitofrontal, insulotemporal cortices, the basolateral amygdala, the striosomes, the ventral pallidum, and the densocellular area of the substantia nigra pars compacta is likely to modulate emotional and motivational aspects of motor function and behavior. A motor and sensory circuit, which includes association, motor, and sensory cortices, striatal matrix, dorsal medial and lateral pallidum, subthalamic nucleus, substantia nigra pars reticulata, thalamus, superior colliculus, and the brain stem modulates motor behavior and associative learning. This latter circuit can be divided into two separate, but interconnecting, circuits, the so-called "direct" and "indirect" pathways. The direct pathway travels from the cerebral cortex to the matrix to the medial pallidum and pars reticulata and thence to the thalamus and cerebral cortex. Dopaminergic input from the substantia nigra pars compacta stimulates this circuit through activation of D1 dopamine receptors. The indirect pathway courses from the cerebral cortex to the matrix to the lateral pallidum to the subthalamic nucleus to the medial pallidum/pars reticulata and thence to the thalamus and the cerebral cortex. This circuit is inhibited by dopaminergic inputs through activation of dopamine D2 receptors.

Accordingly, dopamine affects the direct and indirect pathways differently, causing distinct alterations in motor function. The various disorders of the basal ganglia, as well as rational pharmacotherapy, can generally be understood within the framework of these circuits.

PARKINSON'S DISEASE

Clinical Description

Presenting symptoms. Typically, Parkinson's disease is unilateral in onset and can begin either with an intermittent resting tremor of the limb, usually the hand, or a slowness of movement (Stacy and Jankovic, 1992; Gelb et al, 1998). The tremor is coarse, about 46 Hz, and might be first noted while walking or holding a book or newspaper. Moreover, the tremor dampens with action and worsens with stress. Accompanying symptoms are slowness of movement of the limb, decreased arm swing, dragging of the foot, stooped posture, and a shuffling gait. Writing may become smaller and manipulation of objects more difficult. Spontaneous movements, particularly of the face, may diminish. A year or two after the onset of symptoms, movements become stiffer, both sides become involved, and balance is affected. Persons may feel dizzy or unsteady, particularly when in a crowded area where a bump or a jolt may knock them off balance.

Diagnostic criteria. In the absence of an alternative diagnosis, the diagnosis of Parkinson's disease depends on the presence of at least three of the four cardinal features of the disorder: a resting tremor, rigidity (increased resistance throughout the range of passive manipulation of a limb about a joint) that is usually of the cogwheel type, bradykinesia, and postural instability. Accompanying signs are a loss of facial expression (masked faces), micrographia, poor fine motor coordination, a stooped flexed posture and the "freeze" phenomenon, which is a tendency to suddenly cease moving when startled by a new sensory input.

Decision trees. The disease must be distinguished from other parkinsonian syndromes (Table 11-1), including drug-induced parkinsonism, progressive supranuclear palsy, striatonigral degeneration (Shy-Drager syndrome), diffuse Lewy body disease, and corticobasal ganglionic degeneration (Stacy and Jankovic, 1992; Gelb et al., 1998). With every patient it is critical to determine whether medications are being taken that block dopamine function. These include antipsychotics, such as chlorpromazine and haloperidol, as well as drugs used for treating nausea or gastric immotility, such as prochlorperazine or metaclopramide. Reserpine may also cause parkinsonism.

Other parkinsonian syndromes must be considered if the patient presents without a tremor (Fig. 11-2). Progressive supranuclear palsy (PSP) usually affects postural reflexes early, with patients often

Table 11-1
Symptoms in Parkinsonian Syndromes

	PD	PSP	MSA	CBGD
Bradykinesia/rigidity	+ +	+ +	+ +	+ +
Postural instability	+	+ + +	+	+
Resting tremor	+ +	+/−	+/−	+/−
Asymmetry	+ +	+/−	+/−	+ +
Response to L-dopa	+ +	+/−	+	+/−
Abnormal saccades	−	+ +	−	+
Orthostatic hypotension	+/−	+/−	+ +	−
Pyramidal tract findings	−	−	+	+
Ataxia	−	−	+	−
"Alien-limb"	−	−	−	+

Abbreviations: PD, Parkinson's disease; PSP, progressive supranuclear palsy; MSA, multisystem atrophy; CBGD, corticobasal ganglionic degeneration.

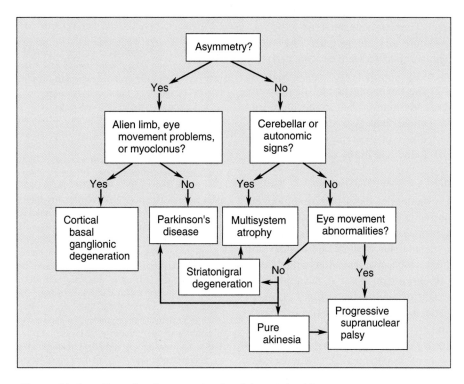

Figure 11–2. *Algorithm for assessing bradykinesia/rigidity symptoms in movement disorders. Dementia is not considered in this chart.*

presenting with unexplained frequent falls (Stacy and Jankovic, 1992; Jankovic and Tolosa, 1998). Abnormalities of voluntary saccades, particularly in the vertical direction, as well as neck and truncal rigidity out of proportion to limb rigidity, should raise the suspicion of PSP. The Shy-Drager syndrome and striatonigral degeneration may be subsets of a broader clinical syndrome, multisystem atrophy (MSA), which has a characteristic pathology but can present with several syndromes. Although these patients may have some tremor, they frequently have spasticity in the legs, extensor plantar responses, orthostatic hypotension, and, occasionally, ataxia. Patients with cortical basal ganglionic degeneration often display the "alien limb" phenomenon in which the arm or leg spontaneously, and involuntarily, assumes unusual postures. Typically, diffuse Lewy body disease presents as a dementia with a tendency for visual hallucinations, although it may sometimes

present as parkinsonism that responds poorly to levodopa. While a complete lack of tremor is often an indication the patient is suffering from one of these other conditions, the most powerful diagnostic tool for Parkinson's disease is a good response to dopamine agonists.

Although idiopathic Parkinson's disease responds remarkably well to symptomatic therapy in its early stages, the underlying pathologic loss of substantia nigra neurons progresses inexorably (Burton and Calne, 1984). Certain late complications associated with the progression of the disease may, in fact, be provoked by therapy. These include drug-induced dyskinesias and the "on-off" phenomenon, characterized by an oscillation between a severe parkinsonian state and a more mobile state accompanied by dyskinesia (Marsden et al., 1982; Fahn and Bressman, 1984; Marsden, 1994). Two types of dyskinesias are seen, the most common of which is "peak dose" dyskinesia. These movements tend to be choreoathetoid in nature and are increased by stress, although patients rarely perceive them as a problem. The other type of dyskinesia is biphasic dyskinesia which occurs at the beginning or end of a dosing interval. Biphasic dyskinesias are much more distressing to the patient than peak dose dyskinesias and tend to be ballistic or dystonic in nature. Often they become disabling late in the day.

Pathophysiology.   The major pathology in Parkinson's disease is the loss of the dopamine-producing cells of the substantia nigra and, to a lesser extent, of the ventral tegmental area (Hornykiewicz and Kish, 1987). Prior to death many of these neurons develop eosinophilic intracytoplasmic inclusions called Lewy bodies. Loss of more than 80% of the pigmented dopaminergic cells of the substantia nigra results in a significant reduction in the number of presynaptic dopamine terminals and dopamine uptake sites, a loss of tyrosine hydroxylase activity, and a decrease in the dopamine content of the putamen (Hornykiewicz and Kish, 1987). The loss of dopaminergic innervation is less severe in the caudate nucleus, the nucleus accumbens, and the frontal cerebral cortex, which receive innervation primarily from the ventral tegmental area. Levels of dopamine metabolites, such as homovanillic acid and DOPAC, do not decrease as much as dopamine itself, presumably because of an increase in the activity of the remaining dopamine terminals. Studies of postmortem material suggest that the number of dopamine D1 and D2 receptors are increased in untreated Parkinson's patients (Lee et al., 1978; Palacios et al., 1993). Treated patients, on the other hand, tend not to demonstrate such changes in receptor numbers, either because of the long-term stimulation of these receptors with drugs, or because of secondary changes in postsynaptic striatal neurons.

The loss of dopamine input to the corpus striatum diminishes the dopamine D2 receptor–mediated inhibition of the corpus striatum, resulting in an overactivity of the indirect pathway and a reduction in dopamine D1 receptor–mediated excitation of the striatum which leads to an underactivity of the direct pathway. In this model, patients have difficulty executing and maintaining a sequenced motor task because of diminished direct pathway function and have excessive inhibition of non-task-related movements, resulting in akinesia and bradykinesia, because of excessive indirect pathway activity.

Norepinephrine-containing cells in the locus ceruleus, and consequently norepinephrine terminals in the forebrain, are also lost in Parkinson's disease (Hornykiewicz and Kish, 1987). Animals with experimental parkinsonism show evidence of increased acetylcholine turnover in brain (Mao et al., 1977), although these changes have not been confirmed in parkinsonian patients. Parkinson's disease patients respond favorably to cholinergic muscarinic receptor antagonists, especially with regard to tremor.

GABA receptors are decreased in the lateral globus pallidus and increased in the medial globus pallidus and substantia nigra in untreated laboratory animals with experimental parkinsonism (Pan et al., 1985; Robertson et al., 1989). These data are consistent with the notion that the indirect pathway is overactive and the direct pathway underactive in patients with Parkinson's disease. GABAergic agonists are of benefit in patients with Parkinson's disease by relieving stress-related increases in symptoms. A decrease in the concentration of serotonin has been reported from studies of brains of patients with Parkinson's disease, although there is little evidence for an actual loss of raphe nucleus neurons (Hornykiewicz and Kish, 1987). Cerebrospinal fluid serotoninergic markers appear to be reduced in depressed, as opposed to nondepressed, patients with this condition (Mayeux et al., 1984). Accordingly, antidepressants aimed at manipulating the serotonin system are commonly used to treat the affective illness associated with Parkinson's disease.

Enkephalin and dynorphin are present in high concentrations in the corpus striatum, the former being primarily expressed in the indirect pathway GABAergic neurons and the latter in the direct pathway GABAergic cells. Although both opioid and cannabinoid receptors are highly expressed in the output areas of the striatum, there have been few studies of the effects of opioids or cannabinoids on parkinsonian symptoms (Maneuf et al., 1994, 1996).

Although glutamate, substance P, neurotensin, somatostatin, and cholecystokinin might all be involved in Parkinson's disease, no drugs have yet been approved that selectively manipulate these systems. Because inhibition of glutamatic acid neurotransmission, either of the corticostriatal pathway or the subthalamopallidal pathway, should, theoretically, be of benefit, clinical trials are now under way to test this hypothesis (Klockgether and Turski, 1992).

Selective vulnerability.   The pathogenesis of the dopamine cell loss in Parkinson's disease is likely due to several factors, the first of which is age-related loss of dopamine cells. Both postmortem and positron emission tomography (PET) data suggest that humans naturally lose dopamine neurons and dopamine terminals with age (Brooks, 1994). This phenomenon, combined with genetic and environmental factors, contributes to the increased incidence of Parkinson's disease with age (Rajput et al., 1984). Moreover, some may be born with a smaller than average number of dopamine neurons and therefore, with normal aging, lose a sufficient number to become symptomatic. Others may possess genetic risk factors that accelerate the rate of loss with aging. A documented phenomenon is early environmental exposure to certain toxins or infectious agents that deplete the number of dopamine neurons. With these individuals the superimposed loss of neurons with age precipitates symptoms.

In a minority of patients there is a clear family history of Parkinson's disease, with both dominantly inherited and mitochondrially inherited factors appearing to play a role in some. In one family with dominantly inherited parkinsonism, a mutation in the α-synuclein gene has been documented (Polymeropoulos et al., 1997). α-Synuclein was subsequently found to be a major component of Lewy bodies (Spillantini et al., 1997). Mitochondrial dysfunction increases free radicals as by-products of inefficient energy metabolism. Inasmuch as the substantia nigra expresses large amounts of free radical scavenging systems such as glutathione and catalase, which are markedly depleted in parkinsonian brains, it is possible that free radical dysregulation may play an important role in the pathophysiology of this disorder.

Exogenous or environmental factors. The influenza pandemic following World War I was accompanied by rare cases of von Economo encephalitis. These patients often developed an acute parkinsonian syndrome (Poskanzer and Schwab, 1963) frequently accompanied by additional signs such as oculogyric crises. Others who suffered from the influenza developed similar syndromes months to years later. Pathologic studies of postencephalitic brains revealed the presence of neurofibrillary tangles in the substantia nigra, rather than the characteristic Lewy bodies found in idiopathic parkinsonism. The virus apparently infected and destroyed substantia nigra neurons, producing parkinsonism immediately, or as a late complication. This influenza virus was responsible for many cases of parkinsonism until the 1930s. Since then individuals with other types of encephalitis have ocassionally developed parkinsonism. Several toxins have been associated with the development of parkinsonism:

1. Manganese. Experimental animals and miners exposed to high levels of manganese develop a parkinsonian syndrome (Barbeau, 1985). The pathology is characterized by loss of pallidal and substantia nigra neurons presumably as a direct effect of the metal.

2. Carbon Monoxide. Acute exposure to high levels of carbon monoxide produces a parkinsonian syndrome (Richter, 1945), which generally does not respond to L-dopa. It too is characterized by a loss of striatal and globus pallidus neurons. The lack of response to L-dopa indicates this syndrome differs from idiopathic Parkinson's disease.

3. MPTP. Persons injected wih a meperidine preparation contaminated with MPTP develop an acute parkinsonism syndrome (Langston, et al., 1984a, 1984b), as do experimental animals given MPTP alone. It is believed that MPTP is converted by MAO type B to an active metabolite, MPP+, which is accumulated in dopamine terminals by way of the dopamine high-affinity transport system. The MPP+ stored in dopamine neurons binds to neuro-

melanin and is slowly released and inhibits complex I of the mitochondrial electron transport chain, thereby producing excess free radicals which kill the neurons. Although MPP+ inhibits complex I in other cells as well, it is more rapidly cleared than from the dopamine cell.

PET scans of several asymptomatic persons who took MPTP showed reduced numbers of dopamine terminals (Calne et al., 1985). Because several of these individuals have since developed symptomatic disease, the notion that loss of neurons during aging contributes to the development of the condition is reinforced.

Rationale for therapy

Symptomatic therapy. Parkinson's disease can be treated by replacing, or substituting for, the dopamine depletion in brain (Fig. 11-3). In the early stages of Parkinson's disease virtually complete symptomatic relief can be achieved with intermittent use of dopamine receptor agonists or the dopamine precursor, levodopa (L-dopa).

Regular and time-release preparations of levodopa are available that dissolve in the stomach at different rates (Yeh et al., 1989). Because the drug is absorbed only from the duodenum, opening of the pyloric valve governs the rate of its delivery to the intestine. The facilitated transfer system responsible for the transport of neutral and aromatic amino acids transports levodopa into the bloodstream. Thus, a protein-rich meal may interfere with the absorption of levodopa from the intestine (Nutt et al., 1984). The blood-brain barrier has a similar facilitated-transport mechanism to transfer levodopa into the brain. Thus, neutral amino acids in either the intestine or blood can alter the accumulation of levodopa in brain (Nutt et al., 1984).

In early Parkinson's disease the therapeutic response to levodopa varies little with the rate of levodopa delivery to brain because, presumably, the administered levodopa is stored in the remaining dopamine terminals until use. With more advanced disease, patients experience fluctuations in symptomatic relief such as a noticeable onset to drug effect and a deterioration at the end of dose. These fluctuations correlate closely with levodopa and plasma amino acid blood levels (Nutt et al., 1984). Thus, the "off" state correlates with insufficient drug levels, while

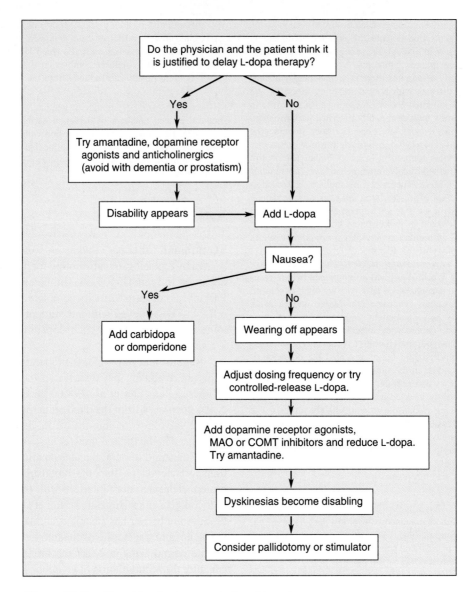

Figure 11–3. *Algorithm for treatment of parkinsonism.*

the "on" state correlates with sufficient or excessive blood levels of the drug. The different responses of early and late disease probably result from a progressive loss of presynaptic dopamine terminals. In early Parkinson's disease there are probably sufficient surviving dopamine terminals to store levodopa until there is neuronal demand. As the disease progresses, however, there are no terminals available for dopamine storage and therefore the clinical response reflects only the immediately available levodopa. A "wearing-off" phenomenon develops in which the therapeutic response does not last until the next dose. Dyskinesias develop suggesting an overdose of levodopa when there are insufficient dopamine terminals to remove excess dopamine from the synaptic cleft (Nutt, 1990). As the disease advances, synaptic levels of dopamine become more and more dependent on the moment to moment levels of levodopa in brain, making fluctuations even more prominent. Added to this may be an increase in the sensitivity of postsynaptic responses to dopamine (Nutt and Holford, 1996).

Therapy with levodopa raises dopamine availability in the brain. Because the dopamine is metabolized by MAO, there is an increase in free radicals produced. Some hypothesize those free radicals may accelerate the rate of disease progression (Spina and Cohen, 1989), although clinical data are conflicting. Some argue that levodopa therapy should be postponed as long as possible to minimize potential free radical damage (Fahn and Bressman, 1984), whereas others recommend that levodopa therapy should be instituted as soon as possible to reduce morbidity and mortality (Markham and Diamond, 1986). This issue is now being examined prospectively in a controlled clinical study.

Both dopamine D1 and D2 receptors play key roles in Parkinson's disease (Palacios et al., 1993), with optimal relief of parkinsonian symptoms requiring stimulation of both. Most currently available dopamine agonists, such as bromocriptine, pergolide, ropinerole, and pramipexole act predominantly at the D2 receptor site (Jankovic and Marsden, 1993; Parkinson Study Group, 1997). Although all these dopamine receptor agonists may be effective as monotherapy in early Parkinson's disease, evidence suggests that some D1 stimulation is necessary for a maximal reponse.

Although dopamine D2 receptor agonists aggravate dyskinesias in those who have already developed it and the "on/off" phenomenon as a result of levodopa therapy, dyskinesias and "on/off" have not been reported in patients receiving D2 receptor agonists alone. Whether dopamine D1 receptor stimulation is necessary for production of dyskinesias is unclear. It is also possible patients who tolerate dopamine D2 receptor agonist monotherapy simply do not have sufficiently advanced disease to display dyskinesias.

Rarely, patients lose the ability to respond to levodopa. The mechanism of this response failure is unclear since levodopa can be converted to dopamine independent of dopamine terminals. More commonly, therapy is limited by the disabling side effects of levodopa.

Drugs that increase the release of dopamine, block its reuptake, or prevent its metabolism are also helpful in Parkinson's disease. Even amphetamines have been used in some cases. In addition, tricyclic antidepressants are useful adjunctive therapy and monoamine oxidase B and catechol-O-methyl transferase inhibitors are sometimes employed to enhance the effects of levodopa.

Manipulation of neurotransmitter systems other than dopamine may be of benefit in Parkinson's disease. For many years, muscarinic cholinergic receptor antagonists were the mainstay of antiparkinsonian therapy, with trihexyphenidyl and benztropine being the most commonly used agents of this class, although others are available as well. Use of these drugs is usually limited by side effects such as confusion, dry mouth, and urinary retention.

Enhancement of GABAergic receptor activity with benzodiazepines can be helpful for those who experience panic or anxiety attacks when their medications wear off. Another approach currently being investigated is the use of glutamic acid receptor antagonists. Since glutamate is the neurotransmitter of the corticostriatal, corticosubthalamic, and subthalamofugal pathways, glutamate receptor antagonists could reduce some symptoms of this disorder by toning down these overactive circuits.

Preventive therapy. Preventive therapies are aimed at halting or delaying further loss of dopamine terminals in symptomatic and presymptomatic Parkinson's patients. Several different approaches along these lines have been pursued experimentally. One has been to block MAO because it has been hypothesized to metabolize environmental agents into toxic metabolites, whereas another is to reduce free radicals in brain. A third strategy has been to limit potential glutamate-induced excitotoxicity by blocking NMDA receptors. Trials of selegiline or eldepryl, selective MAO inhibitors, and α-tocopherol, a free radical scavenger, have so far not suggested these approaches delay progression of the disease. Other free-radical scavengers are now being tested since vitamin E does penetrate the brain efficiently. By slowing the loss of dopamine terminals through preventive therapy it would be possible to maintain patients in a state in which they respond to symptomatic therapy for a much longer period of time.

CHOREA

Clinical Manifestations

Chorea is a term used to describe brief, involuntary, random, elemental movements of the limbs. The movements are simple, quick, and can resemble normal restless movements and yet are not part of any planned behavior. The movements can be bilateral or unilateral, although when both sides of the body are involved they are not synchronous. More prolonged choreoathetotic movements involve a degree of dystonia that superimposes a more prolonged contraction of agonists and antagonists on the quick choreic movements and leads to a writhing type of movement. Depending on the etiology, chorea may develop insidiously or suddenly. Sudden or subacute onset usually indicates a vascular, structural, autoimmune, or metabolic disorder, whereas insidious, progressive onset usually suggests a neurodegenerative disorder.

Differential Diagnosis

Drug-induced choreas. Drug-induced chorea is most commonly seen following the long-term use of dopamine D2 receptor antagonists (Tolosa et al., 1993). The chorea is usually noted months or years after the onset of drug treatment with the movements manifesting as chorea, dyskinesia, or dystonia. Because their onset occurs after prolonged drug therapy, the disorders are termed tardive chorea, tardive dyskinesia, or tardive dystonia. If drug treatment is halted at the first sign of involuntary movements, they are usually, but not always, reversible. If the drug therapy is continued, a permanent, lifelong movement disorder usually results that does not improve after terminating the use of the offending

agent. Although the elderly are more susceptible to the development of tardive dyskinesia, all age groups are vulnerable. While tardive movement disorders are most commonly encountered with the use of neuroleptics for the treatment of psychiatric illness, they can occur in patients receiving antipsychotics or dopamine antagonists for nausea or gastric immotility.

Chorea is also induced in parkinsonian patients treated with levodopa (Nutt, 1990). Muscarinic cholinergic receptor antagonists can also induce chorea and dystonia, particularly in individuals with a preexisting basal ganglia disease (Tolosa et al., 1993). Levodopa- and anticholinergic-induced chorea is reversible with lowering or discontinuation of the medication.

Metabolic disorders. A host of acquired and inherited metabolic disorders can induce chorea (Shoulson, 1986). The most common metabolic abnormalities that cause chorea are pregnancy (or estrogen therapy) or hyperthyroidism. Completion of pregnancy, termination of estrogen therapy, or treatment of hyperthyroidism usually results in complete reversal of the symptoms.

Autoimmune disorders. Autoimmune disorders can produce chorea presumably secondary to the production of anticaudate antibodies (Shoulson, 1986; Kiessling et al., 1993; Giedd et al., 1995). Sydenham chorea usually begins 2 to 3 weeks after a streptococcal A infection and worsens over several days. The movements can be severe and accompanied by tics and personality changes. The disorder usually improves gradually over weeks. Some individuals who develop chorea sporadically in later life have a prior history of Sydenham chorea. Likewise, individuals with estrogen-induced and hyperthyroid-induced chorea sometimes have had a prior history of Sydenham chorea.

Patients with systemic lupus erythematosis or other collagen vascular diseases can experience chorea either as a presenting symptom or in the context of an established disease. Chorea has also been seen as a remote effect of systemic carcinoma. This syndrome apparently results from the production of antitumor antibodies that cross-react with the corpus striatum.

Vascular or structural disorders. Hemiballismus or hemichorea usually results from a structural abnormality in the subthalamic nucleus caused by ischemic damage, tumor, or infection (Buruma and Lakke, 1986). The disorder is manifested by large-amplitude, choreic and ballistic movements of the limbs on one side of the body and frequently involves dyskinesias of the face. The movements can be of such large amplitude that they are physically exhausting to the patient. Fortunately, if the acute period can be survived, the movements abate over time and eventually are manifested only by unilateral chorea.

Although the abnormal subthalamic nucleus is downstream from the dopamine system, dopamine receptor angagonists have some beneficial effects in the treatment of ballistic movements. In addition, benzodiazepines, valproate and barbiturates are sometimes used to reduce the magnitude of the movements. No specific therapy exists for this condition.

Genetic disorders. *Recessive, childhood onset.* There are many inherited disorders of amino acid metabolism, lipid metabolism, and mitochondrial disorders that cause chorea and dystonia. While rare, these are readily diagnosed with metabolic tests. Many are accompanied by other neurological and systemic signs and symptoms (Shoulson, 1986; Lyon et al., 1996).

Dominant, adult onset: Huntington disease. Clinical manifestations. Huntington disease (HD) is an autosomal dominant neurodegenerative disorder characterized by midlife onset of progressive cognitive decline, motor incoordination, and involuntary movements (Harper, 1996). George Huntington first described the condition in 1872 while studying a familial disorder among residents on Long Island. Huntington disease has a prevalence of approximately 10/100,000 and, because of its late age of onset, about 30/100,000 are at 50% risk at any given time. Although the average age of onset for HD is 35 to 40 years, the range is very broad with cases occurring as young as age 3 years and as late as 90

years. Although the disease was originally thought to display full penetrance, is is now appreciated this is not always the case. Interestingly, those who inherit the gene from their father have a statistical chance of an age of onset 3 years earlier than those who inherit it from their mother, with approximately 80% of those who become symptomatic before their twentieth birthday having inherited the disease from their father. This phenomenon is called anticipation.

Age of onset is difficult to define because HD begins insidiously, with personality and behavioral changes and minor motor incoordination occurring many years before overt symptoms became apparent. At diagnosis, most display abnormal choreic movements, impaired fine motor coordination, and latency in generating voluntary saccades (Young et al., 1986; Penney et al., 1990). As the disease progresses, organizational abilities and memory become impaired, speech becomes abnormal, the eye movement disorder worsens, and motor coordination is increasingly compromised. Although muscle tone and posture are often normal early in the disease, dystonic posturing becomes more prominent as the condition worsens, eventually becoming the predominant symptom. In advanced stages, speech becomes unintelligible, swallowing is severely impaired, and walking ceases. The disease typically progresses over 15 to 20 years, with the patient requiring full-time care at the end stage. Death is not caused by the primary illness but occurs from secondary causes such as pneumonia.

Genetic studies. Despite considerable interest in the genetics and biochemistry of HD there was little progress in identifying the gene until the late 1970s (Young, 1994). At this time Nancy Wexler and Allan Tobin organized a workshop sponsored by the Hereditary Disease Foundation to discuss strategies for finding the HD gene. David Housman, David Botstein, and Ray White attended the workshop and suggested that the recently described recombinant DNA techniques could be exploited for this purpose. A key element in the proposed project was to identify a large multigenerational HD family for the collection of DNA samples. In 1979, a collaborative project between scientists in Venezuela and the United States was initiated to examine what appeared to be a very large family with HD living on the shores of Lake Maracaibo, Venezuela. By 1983, the HD gene was localized to the end of the short arm of chromosome 4 (Gusella et al., 1983) and, a decade later, the mutation in the HD gene was identified as a (CAG)n trinucleotide repeat disorder (Huntington's Disease Collaborative Research Group, 1993). Methodologies established by this group of scientists are now considered standard for positional cloning of novel genes (Young, 1994).

While the wild-type gene has a stretch of 10–28 CAGs, in the HD mutant form, the stretch is increased from 39 to more than 100 CAGs (Huntington's Disease Collaborative Research Group, 1993; Rubinsztein, 1996). The discovery of the CAG expansion provides an explanation for many of the features of this disorder. Thus, there is an inverse correlation between age of onset and the length of the CAG repeat (Gusella et al., 1997). Anticipation with paternal descent can be explained by the finding that repeat expansion most frequently occurs in males apparently during spermatogenesis (MacDonald, 1993). New mutations were identified when the parent, usually the father, has a CAG repeat greater than 28 that apparently expands further in the next generation (Goldberg et al., 1993); Myers et al., 1993; Davis et al., 1994; Durr et al., 1995). It has now been determined that repeat numbers of less than 28 are stably transmitted from generation to generation, whereas the repeat numbers of 29 to 35 are often not stably transmitted and yet are not associated with HD (Rubinsztein, 1996). Repeat numbers of 36 to 39 are also unstably transmitted but may or may not be associated with the disease (incomplete penetrance). Repeat numbers greater than 40 are associated with disease and are not stably transmitted.

The factors responsible for expansion of the repeat number are unknown.

Anatomic pathology. Huntington disease is characterized by a loss of neurons predominantly in the caudate nucleus and putamen, with some loss in the cerebral cortex and other areas as well. Overall brain weight is decreased in HD owing in part to a decrease in white matter as well as to the loss of neurons. In the cerebral cortex, the cells in layers V and VI appear to be most affected, with the degree of gross and microscopic degeneration, corrected for age at death, correlating with the CAG repeat number (Furtado et al., 1996; Penney, 1997). Detailed pathologic analysis of several hundred HD cases suggests that the striatal degeneration begins in the dorsal medial caudate nucleus and dorsolateral putamen and progresses ventrally (Vonsattel, 1985). All caudate nucleus and putamen neurons are not affected equally (Aronin et al., 1983; Dawburn et al., 1985; Ferrante et al., 1985, 1987; Reiner et al., 1988), with a selective sparing of the interneurons in the corpus striatum and a selective vulnerability of certain projection neurons from this brain region. In juvenile onset HD, the striatal pathology is severe and is more widespread in the cerebral cortex, cerebellum, thalamus, and globus pallidus (Albin et al., 1990; Myers et al., 1991).

Neurochemical pathology. GABA. Neurochemical studies of HD brains found a significant decrease in the striatal concentration of GABA (Perry et al., 1973). Subsequent studies confirmed the loss of GABAergic neurons and demonstrated that GABA levels are also decreased in striatal projection regions, the lateral and medial globus pallidus, and the substantia nigra.

GABA receptors, as measured by binding studies and in situ hybridization of mRNA expression, are also found to be abnormal in HD brain. GABA receptor number is moderately reduced in the caudate nucleus and putamen, and increased in the substantia nigra pars reticulata and lateral segment of the globus pallidus (Albin et al., 1989) in HD brain, consistent with up-regulation in striatal projection areas after denervation.

ACETYLCHOLINE. Acetylcholine is the neurotransmitter utilized by large aspiny interneurons in the corpus striatum. In initial postmortem studies, choline acetyltransferase (ChAT) activity was found to be decreased in the corpus striatum of HD brain, suggesting a loss of cholinergic neurons (Spokes, 1980). However, relative to the loss of GABAergic neurons, cholinergic interneurons are spared (Ferrante et al., 1987). Thus, the density of ChAT and acetylcholinesterase-positive neurons is in fact relatively increased in corpus striatum of HD brain compared to age-matched controls.

SUBSTANCE P. Substance P is contained in many of the medium spiny neurons of the corpus striatum, which project predominantly to the medial globus pallidus and substantia nigra, and is usually co-localized with dynorphin and GABA. Substance P levels decline in the corpus striatum and substantia nigra pars reticulata of the HD brains. In end-stage disease, immunohistochemical studies of substance P immunoreactivity indicate a significant loss of substance P neurons. At earlier stages of the illness, there appears to be a selective sparing of substance P neurons that project to the medial globus pallidus as compared to those projecting to the substantia nigra pars reticulata (Reiner et al., 1988; Albin et al., 1989).

OPIOID PEPTIDES. Enkephalin is contained in the medium spiny projection neurons of the indirect pathway that projects to the lateral globus pallidus. Enkephalin is colocalized with GABA in cells that also contain a predominance of dopamine D2 receptors. Immunohistochemical studies of enkephalin-like immunoreactivity in brains of early-stage HD patients indicate a loss of enkephalin neurons projecting to the lateral globus pallidus (Reiner et al., 1988; Albin et al., 1989). These cells appear to be lost prior to the substance P cells that project to the medial globus pallidus.

CATECHOLAMINES. Biogenic amine (dopamine and serotonin) containing neurons project to the corpus striatum from the substantia nigra pars compacta, the ventral tegmental area and the raphe nucleus. While norepinephrine projections to human corpus striatum are minimal, the serotonin and dopamine levels, on a per-gram basis, are actually increased in this brain area in HD, reflecting the sparing of these afferent projections in the face of a loss of intrinsic striatal neurons (Albin et al., 1989). Dopamine neurons in the substantia nigra are spared in both adult and juvenile onset forms of the disorder.

SOMATOSTATIN/NEUROPEPTIDE Y AND NITRIC OXIDE SYNTHASE. Measurements of somatostatin and neuropeptide Y levels in HD corpus striatum indicate four- to five-fold increases above those found in normal tissues. Immunohistochemical studies reveal absolute sparing of neuropeptide Y/somatostatin/nitric oxide synthase-positive interneurons in the HD corpus striatum (Aronin et al., 1983; Dawburn et al., 1985; Ferrante et al., 1985; Beal et al., 1986). These neurons appear resistant to the disease process.

EXCITATORY AMINO ACIDS. Glutamate-induced neurotoxicity has been proposed as an explanation for the selective cell death ovserved in HD. Levels of glutamate and quinolinic acid (an endogenous neurotoxin that is synthesized as a by-product of serotonin metabolism) are little changed in HD corpus striatum, although recent MRI spectroscopy studies suggest increased glutamate levels *in vivo*. The glial enzyme responsible for quinolinic acid synthesis is increased approximately five-fold in HD corpus striatum as compared to normal brain tissue (Foster et al., 1985), whereas the enzyme responsible for quinolinate degradation is increased only 20 to 50% in HD. Thus, quinolinic acid synthesis may be increased in HD.

Studies of excitatory amino-acid (EAA) receptors in HD brain indicate major losses of NMDA, AMPA, kainate, and metabotropic glutamate receptors in the corpus striatum and AMPA and kainate receptors in the cerebral cortex (Young et al., 1988; Albin et al., 1990; Dure IV et al., 1991; Wagster et al., 1994). Indeed, NMDA receptors are virtually absent in advanced HD, with significant declines in NMDA receptor numbers reported in several presymptomatic and early-stage cases.

Selective vulnerability. Certain striatal cell types are selectively lost in HD. Medium spiny neurons that project to the lateral globus pallidus and which contain GABA and enkephalin are affected very early in the disease, as are GABA and substance P-containing neurons that project to the substantia nigra pars reticulata (Albin et al., 1989). Loss of the GABA/enkephalin neurons projecting to the lateral globus pallidus disinhibits the lateral pallidum, which, in turn, more actively inhibits the subthalamic nucleus. The decreased activity of the subthalamic nucleus is likely to be responsible for the choreiform movements seen in HD; lesions of the subthalamic nucleus have long been recognized as a cause of chorea. Loss of GABA/substance P neurons projecting to the substantia nigra pars reticulata is likely to be responsible for the abnormal eye movements observed in HD. This pathway normally inhibits substantia nigra pars reticulata neurons projecting to the superior colliculus which, in turn, regulates saccades. In juvenile onset cases, the pathways described previously are even more severely affected and, in addition, striatal projections to the medial globus pallidus are lost early.

The protein encoded by the HD gene, huntingtin, is expressed throughout the brain and other tissues (DiFiglia, 1995; Gutekunst et al., 1995; Sharp, 1995; Trottier, 1995). In brains of unaffected individuals, the protein is primarily neuronal and cytoplasmic. Most neurons in brain express the protein, although recent work suggests it is more intensely expressed in matrix neurons than in striosomal neurons and in projection neurons more so than in interneurons (Ferrante et

al., 1997; Kosinski et al., 1997). Thus, selective neuronal vulnerability appears to correlate with the amount of huntingtin normally expressed in certain neuronal populations.

As is the case in HD brain, in mice transgenic for the N-terminal fragment of the HD gene with expanded repeats, the huntingtin protein forms dense aggregates in the nucleus of neurons (Mangiarini et al., 1996; Davies et al., 1997). Indeed, striatal projection neurons, but not interneurons, develop these neuronal intranuclear inclusions. The transgenic mice develop the inclusions weeks before the onset of symptoms. These findings suggest that the huntingtin protein with the expanded repeats, or a fragment thereof, is abnormally targeted to the nucleus where it might alter nuclear control of cell function.

Rationale for therapy

Symptomatic therapy. There is as yet no effective, preventive therapy for HD. Many types of medications, however, have been tried, with none demonstrating any significant beneficial effect (Folstein, 1989; Harper, 1996). Dopamine receptor antagonists and antipsychotics are used extensively to control the psychiatric symptoms and involuntary movements characteristic of HD. The involuntary movements reflect an imbalance between dopaminergic and GABAergic neurons, with antipsychotics used to combat the excessive dopaminergic activity. These medications themselves cause significant cognitive and extrapyramidal side effects, however, and unless the patient is psychotic or very irritable, there is little evidence they provide any benefit. Antipsychotics often induce or worsen dysphagia or motor symptoms. The newer antipsychotics, risperidone, clozepine, and olanzepine, seem to be particularly useful in the treatment of HD since they produce fewer extrapyramidal side effects and yet reduce paranoia and irritability.

Tetrabenazine and reserpine, both of which reduce brain dopaminergic function, help alleviate the abnormal involuntary movements encountered early in the disease. These agents, however, can induce depression. Because depression is a common feature of the condition itself, this side effect limits the use of reserpine and tetrabenazine. In late disease, dopamine receptor-containing cells are lost and therefore dopamine receptor antagonists have little or no therapeutic efficacy.

Antipsychotic, antidepressant, and antianxiety agents can be useful for the treatment of psychosis, depression, and irritability (Shoulson, 1986), but their administration should be limited to periods when the patient is experiencing symptoms. Indeed, medications that are useful at one stage of the illness may be ineffective or even detrimental at another stage because of the disease progression.

GABA receptor agonists have been tested in HD because of the profound decrease in striatal GABA levels and the GABA receptor supersensitivity in striatal projection areas (Shoulson, 1986). Benzodiazepines have been found of benefit for treating those whose movements and cognitive functioning worsen with stress and anxiety. Low doses of these drugs should be used to avoid sedation. In general, most HD patients do well with no medication.

For those with early-onset HD and parkinsonian symptoms, dopamine receptor agonists may be tried (Shoulson, 1986), although they are of limited benefit. Furthermore, L-dopa can induce or worsen myoclonus in those patients, whereas baclofen may be helpful in reducing the increased muscle tone in rigid HD patients.

PREVENTIVE THERAPY. Although the genetic defect in HD is known, it is not yet clear how it leads to selective neuronal degeneration. Preventive therapies aimed at reducing oxidative stress and excitotoxicity may ultimately prove useful in slowing or arresting progress of the disease (Shoulson and Kieburtz, 1997). Just as in Wilson's disease, where the genetic defect was unknown for years, preventive treatment of the secondary effects of copper accumulation resulted in a "cure." In this regard, the hypothesis that HD is related to abnormal energy metabolism and excitotoxic-induced cell death deserves attention (Beal, 1992). The disorder itself may cause cell death by provoking the intranuclear aggregation of N-terminal fragments of the huntingtin protein which may, in turn, affect cellular and metabolic function (Davies et al., 1997; DiFiglia et al., 1997). Such defects may affect certain neurons more than others because of a greater susceptibility to excitotoxic-induced injury. If this is the case, preventive therapy with excitatory amino acid receptor antagonists, or by rescue from free radical damage, might prevent or delay the onset

and progression of the disorder (Beal, 1995). Indeed, in animal models of amyotrophic lateral sclerosis, free radical scavengers and excitatory amino acid receptor antagonists delay the progression of disease (Beal, 1995). Similar strategies may work in HD (Shoulson and Kieburtz, 1997). Clinical trials of glutamate receptor antagonists and enhancers of complex II of the mitochondrial electron transport chain are now in progress.

DYSTONIA

Clinical Manifestations

There are both primary and secondary causes of dystonia, with their clinical symptomatology varying with the cause (Fahn, 1988; Fahn et al., 1988). Dystonia as a symptom is defined as distorted movements and posture resulting from the simultaneous, involuntary contraction of agonist and antagonist muscles. In the foot, dystonia may be extension and inversion of the foot and marked flexion of the toes. In the hand, the wrist may be flexed but the fingers extended. The neck or trunk may be twisted, and the face may develop a range of movements from forced closure or opening of the jaw, contraction of the lids, or pursing of the lips. Dystonic postures are often bizarre and disabling but always disappear during sleep and sometimes during relaxation. Dystonia can involve any part of the body and is usually described according to the parts affected, such as segmental (extremity, axial, or cranial) or generalized. Patients may use "sensory tricks" to control the movements such as touching the chin to relieve torticollis.

Secondary dystonias are numerous and can result from inherited metabolic disorders such as the amino acidoses and lipidoses, carbon monoxide poisoning, or traumatic events, such as stroke, truama, or subdural hematoma (Calne and Lang, 1988; Jankovic and Fahn, 1993). The age of onset and clinical manifestations of the secondary dystonias are variable depending on the etiology.

Primary dystonias are inherited disorders, with several of the responsible genes already identified (Segawa et al., 1976; Fahn, 1988; Kramer et al., 1990; Lee et al., 1991; Waters et al., 1993; Bressman et al., 1994; Ichinose et al., 1994; Knappskog et al., 1995; Ludecke et al., 1995) (Fig. 11-4). These conditions can be inherited as autosomal dominant, autosomal recessive, or x-linked and can be associated with other disorders such as myoclonus, tremor, and/or parkinsonism. In many families the penetrance is variable, with some individuals manifesting dystonia in childhood and others in adulthood.

Although each type of inherited dystonia is different, in general dystonia that begins in childhood usually involves the legs first, followed by the trunk, neck, and upper extremities. Childhood-onset dystonia usually generalizes and causes significant physical, but never cognitive, impairment. In contrast, dystonia that begins in adulthood rarely generalizes, being typically segmental (trunk, neck, or upper extremities) or cranial (eyes or mouth). Onset of segmental and axial dystonias is usually between the ages of 20 and 50, with the cranial dystonias most commonly seen between 50 and 70 years of age.

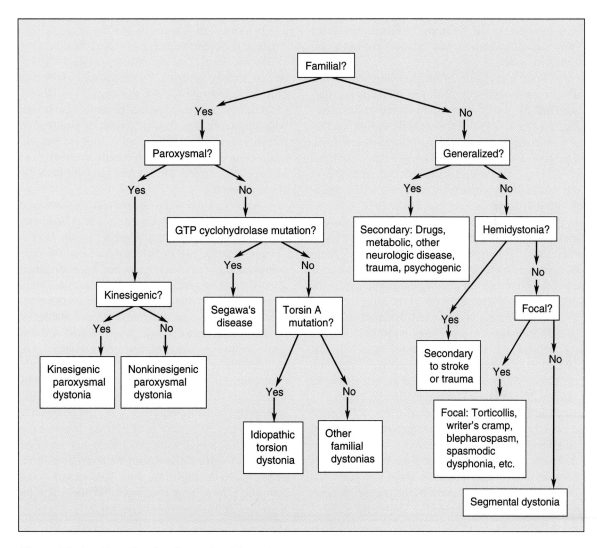

Figure 11-4. Algorithm for diagnosis of dystonia.

Neurochemical Pathology

Few data are available on the neurochemical changes associated with the various forms of dystonia (Hornykiewicz et al., 1986, 1988; Chase et al., 1988; Lang et al., 1988; Leenders et al., 1988; Otsuka et al., 1992; Eidelberg et al., 1993, 1995; Perlmutter et al., 1997). In none of the primary dystonias is there any evidence of focal neuronal degeneration in brain. Studies of monoamine systems have generally been negative, although studies of brains from individual dystonia pedigrees are lacking. Since individuals with dystonia do not die from the illness, but rather from secondary causes, few brains have been collected for study.

The main exception to the preceding is Segawa's disease, an autosomal recessive dystonia that is characterized by diurnal fluctuations (better in the morning and worse in the afternoon and evening) and by dramatic improvement with low doses of levodopa. The gene for Segawa's disease has been identified as GTP-cyclohydrolase I, an enzyme involved in the synthesis of biopterin, a necessary cofactor for tyrosine hydroxylase (Segawa et al., 1976; Ichinose et al., 1994). In these individuals tyrosine hydroxylase activity is reduced and synaptic dopamine levels decreased. It is hypothesized that during sleep synaptic dopamine levels are partially replenished but upon awakening they are rapidly depleted, resulting in the development of dystonia later in the day.

Lubag disease, an x-linked dystonia observed in the Philippines, is associated with parkinsonism (Wilhelmsen et al., 1991; Waters et al., 1993a, 1993b). Symptomatic individuals display a decrease in ^{11}C-fluorodopa uptake on PET scan, suggesting an abnormality of dopamine metabolism in brain.

The loss of the GAG codon in the DYT1 gene causes most cases of autosomal dominantly inherited childhood-onset dystonia (Ozelius et al., 1997). This mutation has a high frequency in Ashkenazi Jews because of a founder mutation about 300 years ago in Lithuania. This gene encodes the protein torsin A which is intensely expressed in dopamine cells of the substantia nigra, granule cells of the cerebellum, and dentate granule cells and pyramidal cells of the hippocampus (Penney et al., 1997). The function of this protein is unknown as are its effects on dopamin-

ergic function, although the failure of these patients to respond to levodopa suggests that dopaminergic activity is unaffected.

Approach to Therapy

The usual approach for treating any dystonia is to first determine whether it is responsive to levodopa or dopamine receptor agonists (Calne and Lang, 1988; Fahn et al., 1988). If not, muscarinic cholinergic receptor antagonists, baclofen, tegretol, and long-acting benzodiazepines may be attempted (Fahn, 1983; Calne and Lang, 1988; Fahn et al., 1988). Trials of different medications should be conducted systematically so that the efficacy, or lack thereof, can be clearly assessed. Often patients experience only limited benefit to these therapies. In childhood-onset dystonias, some appear to improve significantly with long-term, high-dose treatment with muscarinic receptor antagonists (Fahn, 1983). In these patients, medication trials of at least 6 months are suggested, as beneficial effects often takes some time to become apparent.

Surgery, particularly stereotaxic thalamotomy and, more recently, pallidotomy, has been attempted as treatments for dystonia (Cooper, 1976). Despite the considerable risk of severe dysarthria and other complications that accompany the bilateral procedures needed for generalized dystonia and spasmodic torticollis, the advent of sophisticated imaging and recording techniques have made this a viable approach for the most severe cases. Pallidal and thalamic microstimulation on one side, combined with pallidotomy or thalamotomy on the other, may be investigated as an option. The local injection of botulinum toxin every 2 to 4 months has proved effective in treating focal dystonia (Brin et al., 1987); Jankovic and Orman, 1987; Lew et al., 1994). Injections of the affected muscles causes limited but sufficient weakness to afford relief from the dystonic contractions. While the injections must be repeated, so far few side effects have been noted. While a few patients develop excessive weakness acutely, this wears off within a week or so, with subsequent doses adjusted to eliminate this problem. Occasionally, patients develop antibodies to the toxin that diminishes long-term effectiveness.

TREMORS

Clinical Manifestations

A tremor is the involuntary rhythmic movement of a limb, a portion of a limb, the head, jaw, tongue, or vocal cords. They are usually divided into resting, kinetic, and postural subtypes (Hallett, 1986; Findley, 1992). Resting tremors are most commonly observed in Parkinson's disease, although they can occur in isolation. Kinetic and postural tremors occur in isolation, as part of another neurological disorder, or as a result of a metabolic imbalance or medication (Fig. 11-5).

The most common type of kinetic tremor is the exaggerated physiologic tremor that is usually of low amplitude and high frequency (12 cycles/sec). The tremor is worsened by exercise, hyperthyroidism, and various drugs, including caffeine, adrenergic receptor agonists, lithium, and valproic acid.

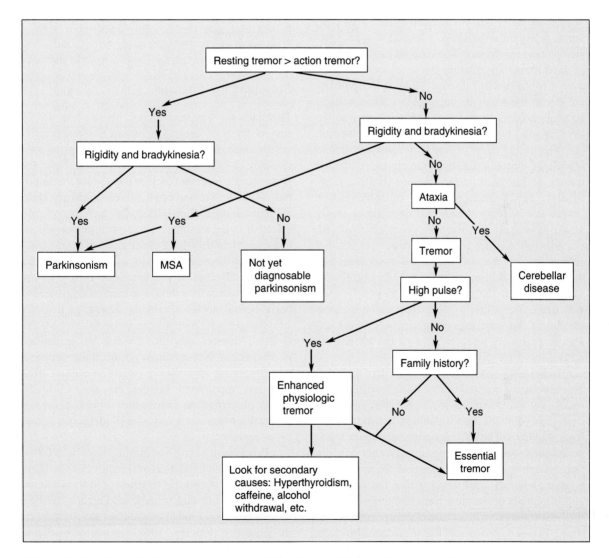

Figure 11–5. Algorithm for assessing tremor. Abbreviations: MSA, multisystem atrophy.

The next most common tremor is the so-called essential or familial tremor, which is somewhat slower than exaggerated physiologic tremor. Essential tremor can involve the extremities as well as the head, tongue, lips, and voice. The tremor worsens with stress and, when severe, can be quite disabling. Persons with this tremor frequently have an affected first-degree relative, with the location and severity of the tremor varying considerably within a family. The limbs may be affected asymmetrically, with a purely unilateral tremor usually suggesting another cause. The tremor frequently improves after an alcoholic drink and commonly is made worse by caffeine, stress, or hyperthyroidism as is the case with exaggerated physiologic tremor. The tremor is asynchronous in the different limbs unlike the synchronous resting tremor of Parkinson's disease. Holding a cup of liquid in one hand may be impossible without spilling it, while holding it with two hands is better as the asynchronous movements tend to cancel each other.

Tremor can occur with several disorders such as myoclonic dystonia with lightening jerks, orthostatic tremor, and isolated postural tremor (Hallett, 1986; Findley, 1992). The genetics of inherited kinetic tremor are currently being examined (Durr et al., 1993). It is likely that multiple genes are involved. Families often differ in their tendency for alcohol responsiveness, the association with myoclonus and dystonia and parkinsonism. It is likely that the genetic identification of the disorders in different families will make it possible to determine which nuances in clinical characteristics are genetically based and which are simply representative of the phenotypic variability of the disorder.

Individuals with cerebellar disorders also display kinetic and postural tremors. The low-frequency oscillating tremor results from proximal instability of the limb, with the tremor abating when the extremity is stabilized. The differentiation between cerebellar tremor and essential tremor is usually not difficult. Cerebellar tremor worsens when the limb approaches a target, whereas in essential tremor the amplitude and magnitude of the movement remains essentially the same throughout the course of a purposeful movement. Persons with cerebellar disorders also have marked impairment of fine motor coordination in addition to the tremor, whereas those with essential tremor usually have relatively intact fine motor coordination.

Neurochemical Pathology

Examination of the brains of patients dying with familial tremor revealed no specific pathology and no particular biochemical defects. While lesions of cerebellar afferents or efferents can result in a tremor, the specific chemical abnormalities responsible for the tremor remain unknown. Imaging studies have helped elucidate the circuitry involved in tremor (Jenkins et al., 1993; Wills et al., 1994).

Rationale for Therapy

Therapies for essential tremor involve the use of several types of agents, including β-adrenergic receptor antagonists, benzodiazepines, and primidone (Findley, 1992). The most useful have been the β-adrenergic receptor blockers that reduce the amplitude of the tremor and often induce significant clinical improvement. Benzodiazepines have been found effective in the treatment of essential tremor and, in low doses, can be helpful either alone or in combination with β-adrenergic receptor antagonists. Because tolerance develops to the beneficial effects of the benzodiazepines they should be used on an as-needed basis before social events or during particularly stressful periods. Alcohol can be useful in the treatment of tremor, although the risk of alcoholism is of concern. Nevertheless, an alcoholic beverage prior to a meal may allow a patient to eat and drink with less impairment. Finally, low doses (25–250 mg/d) of primidone can reduce essential tremor, especially when combined with β-adrenergic receptor antagonists.

Few pharmacologic treatments have been found effective for cerebellar tremor (Findley, 1992). There are reports of successful treatment of this condition with clonazepam and primidone. Perhaps the best approaches for cerebellar tremor are stereotaxic thalamotomy (Findley, 1992) or microstimulation (Hubble et al., 1996).

TICS

Clinical Manifestations

Tics are repetitive, stereotyped movements resulting from sequential or co-contraction of several muscles groups which are either rapid or slightly sustained (dystonic). Most frequently, the face, neck, and upper extremity are involved, although the trunk and the leg can also be involved. Sometimes vocalizations or involuntary sniffing or grunting are manifestations of tics. Tic movements are usually preceded by a sensation of discomfort or a need to move. Unlike choreic or myoclonic disorders or tremor, tics can be voluntarily suppressed for brief periods of time. Tics do not affect intellect and are not accompanied by any additonal pyramidal or extrapyramidal signs or symptoms. Obsessive-compulsive disorder may be a comorbid condition in many cases.

Tic disorders have been divided into three syndromes (Lees, 1985; Kurlan, 1989; Jankovic, 1992). Transient tic of childhood occurs in up to 10% of those below 15 years of age and lasts less than 1 year and does not recur. Chronic motor tic is manifest as a single repetitive motor tic that usually begins within the first three decades of life and remains thereafter. The third type of tic disorder is Tourette's syndrome. Tourette's syndrome is characterized by an onset younger than 15 years of age and by both vocal and motor tics that wax and wane in severity and character but are present for life. The tics can be severe and can become physically and socially disabling. Usually, however, they are mild and primarily a social nuisance. It is estimated that as many as 1/1000 individuals has this disorder. The syndrome appears to be dominantly inherited, although with incomplete penetrance. Other family members may manifest the disorder as either simple tics or obsessive-compulsive disorder (Cath et al., 1992). The gene or genes for Tourette's syndrome have not yet been identified.

Neurochemical Pathology

The brains of only a few persons who suffered from Tourette's syndrome have been examined, with no clear neuropathological or neurochemical abnormality emerging (Anderson et al., 1992; Haber and Wolfer, 1992; Singer, 1992). The few neurochemical studies on postmortem brain suggest abnormalities in the dopamine system. Indeed, recent studies in living twins with Tourette's syndrome suggest a greater number of dopamine D2 receptors in the twin with the worst clinical manifestations (Wolff et al., 1996). MRI studies of persons with Tourette's suggest that the normal left-right caudate asymmetry is lost (Singer et al., 1993; Hyde et al., 1995). Functional MRI and PET activation studies suggest an imbalance in the orbitofrontal-caudate circuitry (Singer et al., 1993; Hyde et al., 1995).

Recently, several individuals with poststreptococcal Sydenham chorea have been noted to manifest tics and OCD in addition to chorea (Kiessling et al., 1993). This has led to investigations of the possibility that some patients with tic disorders may have an autoimmune disorder with anticaudate nucleus antibodies after streptococcal infections.

Rationale for Therapy

Although the chemical pathology of tics is unknown, it was noted sometime ago that tic disorders are very responsive to low doses of dopamine D2 receptor antagonists or drugs that block vesicular dopamine accumulation, such as reserpine and tetrabenazine (Lees, 1985). Tics may also be responsive to the α-adrenergic receptor agonist, clonidine, and the benzodiazepine clonazepam. In all cases, therapy is symptomatic and does not affect the overall course of the illness. Many patients do quite well on no medication at all. Therapy should be reserved for those whose tics are significantly disrupting schooling, social relationships, or employment. The drugs rarely eliminate totally the tics and the potential side effects are considerable. Education of the family, teachers, and employers may be sufficient to alleviate many problems. Only if these measures do not suffice should medications be prescribed.

Since there are always concerns about long-term side effects with dopamine receptor antagonists, it is reasonable to begin with other drugs even though their success rate may not be as good. For this reason, clonidine is often the drug of choice. Although there is some controversy as to the effectiveness of this agent (Cohen et al., 1979; Goetz et al., 1987) it has no known long-term side effects. The therapy should be started at a low dose (0.05 mg bid) which is gradually increased over weeks until side effects appear or symptom relief is obtained. Care must be taken that the patient does not abruptly terminate the therapy because headache and hypertension can result.

If clonidine is ineffective, a trial of tetrabenazine is possible since tardive dyskinesia has not been described with this drug and it is often quite effective. Doses of 25 mg qd building to 25 mg tid is the usual strategy. Reserpine is rarely used because of hypotension and depression. Almost all dopamine receptor antagonists are effective in the treatment of tic disorders, with the most popular agents being pimozide, haloperidol, and fluphenazine. Pimozide appears to have fewer cognitive side effects than haloperidol and antipsychotics with significant anticholinergic actions (Regeur et al., 1986). Risperidone and clozepine do not appear to be particularly effective in this condition. The general strategy for treatment is to begin with as low a dose as possible for 2 to 3 weeks, gradually increasing the dose until symptom relief is achieved or side effects occur. For those who do require medication, the development of drug-induced tardive dyskinesias is always of concern. The patient should be informed of this possibility and be followed closely for any indication of this long-term side effect.

Treatment for the obsessive-compulsive disorder that often accompanies Tourette's syndrome includes fluoxetine, clomipramine, or other serotonin selective reuptake inhibitors. This class of drug has been found to be quite helpful for the behavioral problems associated with Tourette's syndrome (Kurlan, 1989).

WILSON'S DISEASE

Clinical Manifestations

Wilson's disease is an autosomal recessively inherited disorder that results in copper accumulation in many organs and tissues, including brain, liver, kidney, and cornea (Wilson, 1912). It was first described by S.A. Kinnier Wilson in 1912 as "a definite symptom-complex whose chief features are generalized tremor, dysarthria and dysphagia, muscular rigidity and hypertonicity, emaciation, spasmodic contractions, contractures, and emotionalism. Mental symptoms may be transient, such as that seen with toxic psychosis, but not severe, or more chronic, including a general restriction of the mental horizon, and a certain facility or docilility without delusions or hallucinations. These may not be as progressive as the somatic symptoms. In some cases of Wilson's disease the mental symptoms may be very slight or absent" (Wilson, 1912). Although Wilson described most of the clinical manifestations of the disease he did not appreciate that the liver was involved and did not note abnormal pigmentation around the cornea. The latter, which is due to the deposition of copper in the cornea, is called Kayser-Fleischer (KF) rings (Schienberg and Stenlieb, 1984; Brewer et al., 1988; Brewer, 1995).

Wilson's disease is caused by a mutation in a copper transporter gene localized on chromosome 13 (Bull et al., 1993; Tanzi et al., 1993; Cox, 1995; DiDonato and Sarkar, 1997). Patients usually present in the second or third decade with predominant neurologic, hepatic, or psychiatric symptoms (about one-third in each group) (Starosta-Rubinstein et al., 1987; Brewer et al., 1988; Akil and Brewer, 1995). Occasionally, patients present in the first decade or as late as the sixth decade.

Neurological presentations are most commonly characterized by dysarthria, dysphagia, poor fine motor coordination, tremor, and rigidity. Less frequently, patients present with chorea, dystonia, or cerebellar ataxia. If diagnosis is not prompt, deterioration is rapid with progressive liver disease and progressive dysarthria or anarthria, dystonia, wing-beating tremor, and death. As initially described, behavioral and personality changes, depression, and emotional lability are common. Siblings are often identified with unexplained hepatitis, hemolytic anemia, or renal dysfunction. The diagnosis must be considered in all patients with movement disorders and/or dysarthria with or without psychiatric complaints since the condition is readily treatable.

Clinical Diagnosis

The KF rings are readily detected either at the bedside (70%) or by slit-lamp examination (97%) (Scheinberg and Sternlieb, 1984; Brewer et al., 1988), with their presence assuring diagnosis of Wilson's disease in more than 99% of cases.

The most accurate test for the diagnosis in the absence of cholestatic liver disease, which can lead to copper accumulation, is measurement of hepatic copper from liver biopsy (Brewer et al., 1988). In untreated patients, values of greater than 200 μg/g dry weight of liver are diagnostic. Normal values are <50 mg/g dry weight of liver.

Measurement of 24 h urine copper is a simple test that usually distinguishes unaffected individuals from those with Wilson's disease. Whereas normal urinary copper excretion in the absence of therapy is 20 to 45 μg/24 h, in Wilson's disease excretion is almost always greater than 80 μg/24 h. A 24 h urine copper excretion of greater than 125 μg is virtually diagnostic. If the value ranges between 45 and 125 μg/24 h, the patient might be either a heterozygote or a homozygote. A 48 h measurement of copper excretion may improve the accuracy of the test.

Quantification of serum ceruloplasmin is the most commonly employed diagnostic test for Wilson's disease. In 10% of patients, however, the ceruloplasmin level is normal (>20 mg/dL). Even in those whose ceruloplasmin levels are low (<20 mg/dL) at one point in the illness, the level can rise because of liver disease, pregnancy, or estrogen administration. Decreased serum ceruloplasmin levels also occur in other conditions, such as protein loss, copper deficiency, Menkes syndrome, and fulminant hepatitis, and in individuals who are heterozygous for Wilson's disease.

Thus, if a patient presents with a suspicious neurologic or psychiatric disorder, a slit-lamp examination should be performed. If positive, the diagnosis is almost certain. Serum ceruloplasmin, serum copper, and 24 h urine copper excretion should be measured to substantiate the diagnosis and to provide a baseline for monitoring therapy. If the tests are ambiguous, liver biopsy should be performed. An MRI scan can also be helpful as no patients manifesting neurological symptoms have been identified with a normal MRI. Although the gene for Wilson's disease has been identified, most cases involve unique mutations within each family and, at the current time, sequencing each of the cases is impractical. As chip technology develops, improved genetic testing and molecular diagnosis should become available.

Rationale for Therapy

Once a diagnosis is established, the patient should be started on a decoppering agent (Scheinberg and Sternlieb, 1984; Brewer et al., 1988; Brewer, 1995) and cautioned to avoid foods with high copper content such as red meat, liver, chocolate, nuts, mushrooms, and shellfish. The patient's main water source should be checked for copper content. Patients should be monitored frequently for the first 2 months or so of therapy to assess medication side effects and worsening of symptoms. Although an initial dose of 250 mg D-penicillamine four times per day 30 to 60 min before meals is recommended, about 10 to 30% of neurologically ill patients worsen during the first few months of therapy. A possible reason for this deterioration is that free serum copper levels rise initially because of mobilization of copper stores in liver and peripheral tissues which, in turn, damage the brain. Initial treatment with 250 mg D-penicillamine two or three times per day with monitoring of free serum and urine copper to effect an excretion of 125 μg/24 h may be a better strategy. The D-penicillamine dose can then be increased to 1 g/d once the free serum copper levels and urinary excretion of copper begin to fall. Frequent monitoring should include measurements of serum copper, serum ceruloplasmin, and 24 h urine copper levels to assess compliance. Yearly slit-lamp exams should be performed to monitor the completeness of the decoppering.

Since D-penicillamine has a high frequency of toxic side effects, CBC, including reticulocyte counts, differential, and platelet counts should be monitored two to three times a week and urinalysis performed once a week during the first month. Lupus-like syndromes, dermatitis, stomatitis, lymphadenopathy, thrombocytopenia, agranulocytosis, and other problems are associated with D-penicillamine therapy.

Additional decoppering agents include British antilewisite, triethylene-tetramine dihydrochloride (Trien, Trientine), and zinc (Brewer, 1995). The dose of Trien is usually 1 to 1.5 g/d, and therapy should be monitored as with D-penicillamine. Renal, bone marrow, and dermatologic toxicity are most common with this agent.

Zinc acetate (150 mg/d) has been found to maintain the decoppered state in patients intolerant to D-penicillamine and/or Trien (Brewer, 1995). Zinc acetate is well-tolerated with very few side effects and can be used effectively for maintenance therapy but is not recommended for initial therapy. In some cases patients are unable to tolerate the gastric irritation associated with this substance. Its mechanism of action is thought to be due to induction of metallothionein in the intestine that, in turn, chelates dietary and biliary copper, enhancing copper excretion in the feces, thereby reducing its absorption.

Despite optimal treatment, many patients continue to have neurologic problems such as dysarthria, dystonia, parkinsonism, chorea, tremor, or combinations thereof. Symptomatic therapy in these cases is the same as that used for the primary movement disorders discussed previously.

For additional information on the drugs discussed in this chapter see chapters 10, 18, 19, and 22 in *Goodman & Gilman's The Pharmacological Basis of Therapeutics* (Ninth Edition), McGraw-Hill, New York, 1996.

REFERENCES

Akil M, Brewer GJ: Psychiatric and behavioral abnormalities in Wilson's disease. *Adv Neurol* 1995;65:171–178.

Albin RL, Reiner A, Anderson KD, et al.: Striatal and nigral neuron subpopulations in rigid Huntington's disease: implications for the functional anatomy of chorea and rigidity akinesia. *Ann Neurol* 1990;27:357–365.

Albin RL, Reiner A, Anderson KD, et al.: Preferential loss of striatoexternal pallidal projection neurons in presymptomatic Huntington's disease. *Ann Neurol* 1992;31:425–430.

Albin RL, Young AB, Penney JB: The functional anatomy of basal ganglia disorders. *Trends Neurosci* 1989;12:366–375.

Albin RL, Young AB, Penney JB, et al.: Abnormalities of striatal projection neurons and N-methyl-D-aspartate receptors in presymptomatic Huntington's Disease. *New Engl J Med* 1990;322:1293–1298.

Anderson GM, Pollak ES, Chatterjee D, et al.: Postmortem analysis of subcortical monoamines and amino acids in Tourette syndrome. *Adv Neurol* 1992;58:123–133.

Aronin N, Cooper P, Lorenz L, et al.: Somatostatin is increased in the basal ganglia in Huntington's disease. *Ann Neurol* 1983;13:519–526.

Augood SJ, Penney JB, Friberg IK, et al.: Expression of early onset dystonia gene (DYT1) in human brain. *Ann Neurol* 1998, in press.

Barbeau A: Manganese and extrapyramidal disorders. *Neurotoxicology* 1985;5:13–36.

Beal MF, Kowall NW, Ellison DW, et al.: Replication of the neurochemical characteristics of Huntington's disease by quinolinic acid. *Nature* 1986;321:168–172.

Beal MF: Does impairment of energy metabolism result in excitotoxic neuronal death in neurodegenerative illnesses? *Ann Neurol* 1992;31:119–130.

Beal MF: *Mitochondrial Dysfunction and Oxidative Damage in Neurodegenerative Diseases.* Austin: RG Landes Co., 1995.

Bressman SB, de Leon D, Kramer PL, et al.: Dystonia in Ashkenazi Jews: clinical characterization of a founder mutation. *Ann Neurol* 1994;36:771–777.

Brewer G, Yuzbasiyan-Gurkham V, Young A: The treatment and diagnosis of Wilson's disease. *Curr Opin Neurol Neurosurg* 1988;1:302–306.

Brewer GJ: Practical recommendations and new therapies for Wilson's disease. *Drugs* 1995;50:240–249.

Brin M, Fahn S, Moskowitz C, et al.: Localized injections of botulinum toxin for the treatment of focal dystonia and hemifacial spasm. *Movement Dis* 1987;2:237–254.

Brooks DJ: Functional imaging of movement disorders, in Marsden, CD Fahn S (eds): *Movement Disorders,* 3rd ed. Oxford: Butterworth-Heinemann, 1994, pp 65–87.

Bull PC, Thomas GR, Rommens JM, et al.: The Wilson's disease gene is a putative copper transporting P-type ATPase similar to the Menkes gene. *Nat Genet* 1993;5:327–337.

Burton K, Calne D: Pharmacology of Parkinson disease. *Neurol Clin* 1984;2:461–472.

Buruma O, Lakke J: *Ballism.* Amsterdam: Elsevier, 1986.

Calne D, Langston J, Martin W, et al.: Positron emission tomography after MPTP: Observations relating to the cause of Parkinson disease. *Nature* 1985;317:246–248.

Calne DB, Lang AE: Secondary dystonia. *Adv Neurol* 1988;50:933.

Cath DC, Hoogduin CAL, van de Wetering BJM, et al.: Tourette syndrome and obsessive-compulsive disorder: an analysis of associated phenomena. *Adv Neurol* 1992;58:33–42.

Chase TN, Tamminga CA, Burrows H: Positron emission tomographic studies of regional cerebral glucose metabolism in idiopathic dystonia. *Adv Neurol* 1988; 50:237–241.

Cohen D, Young J, Nathanson A, Shaywitz B: Clonidine in Tourette's syndrome. *Lancet* 1979;2:551–552.

Cooper I: *Dystonia: Surgical Approaches to Treatment and Physiological Implications.* New York: Raven Press, 1976.

Cox DW: Genes of the copper pathway. *Am J Hum Genet* 1995;56:828–834.

Davies SW, Turmaine M, Cozens B, et al.: Formation of neuronal intranuclear inclusions underlies the neurological dysfunction in mice transgenic for the HD mutation. *Cell* 1997;90:537–548.

Davis MB, Bateman D, Quinn NP, et al.: Mutation analysis in patients with possible but apparently sporatic Huntington's disease. *Lancet* 1994;344:714.

Dawburn D, Dequidt ME, Emson PC: Survival of basal ganglia neuropeptide Y-somatostatin neurones in Huntington's disease. *Brain Res* 1985;340:251–260.

DeLong MR: Primate models of movement disorders of basal ganglia origin. *Trends Neurosci* 1990;13:281–289.

DiDonato M, Sarkar B: Copper transport and its alterations in Menkes and Wilson diseases. *Biochimica Biophysica Acta* 1997;1360:316.

DiFiglia M, Sapp E, Chase O, et al.: Huntingtin is a cytoplasmic protein associated with vesicles in human and rat brain neurons. *Neuron* 1995;14:1075–1081.

DiFiglia M, Sapp E, Chase KO, et al. Aggregations of huntingtin in neuronal intranuclear inclusions and dystrophic neurites in brain. *Science* 1997;277:1990–1993.

Dure IV LS, Young AB, Penney JB: Excitatory amino acid binding sites in the caudate nucleus and frontal cortex of Huntington's disease. *Ann Neurol* 1991;30:785–793.

Durr A, Dode C, Hahn V, et al.: Diagnosis of "sporadic" Huntington's disease. *Neurol Sci* 1995;129:51.

Durr A, Stevanin G, Jedynak CP, et al.: Familial essential tremor and idiopathic torsion dystonia are different genetic entities. *Neurology* 1993;43:2212–2214.

Eidelberg D, Moeller JR, Ishikawa T, et al.: The metabolic topography of idiopathic torsion dystonia. *Brain* 1995;118:1473–1484.

Eidelberg D, Takikawa S, Wilhelmsen K, et al.: Positron emission tomographic findings in Filipino X-linked dystonia parkinsonism. *Ann Neurol* 1993;34:185–191.

Fahn S: High dosage anticholinergic therapy in dystonia. *Neurology* 1983;33:1255–1261.

Fahn S: Concept and classification of dystonia. *Adv Neurol* 1988;50:18.

Fahn S, Bressman S: Should levodopa therapy for parkinsonism be started early or late? Evidence against early treatment. *Can J Neurol Sci* 1984;11:200–206.

Fahn S, Marsden C, Calne D: *Dystonia.* New York: Raven Press, 1988.

Ferrante R, Beal M, Kowall N, et al.: Sparing of acetylcholinesterase-containing striatal neurons in Huntington's disease. *Brain Res* 1987;411:162–166.

Ferrante R, Kowall N, Beal M, et al.: Selective sparing of a class of striatal neurons in Huntington's disease. *Science* 1985;230:561–564.

Ferrante RJ, et al: Heterogeneous topographic and cellular distribution of huntingtin expression in the normal human striatum, *J Neurosci* 1997;17:3052.

Findley LJ: Tremors: Differential diagnosis and pharmacology, in Jankovic J, Tolosa E (eds): *Parkinson Disease and Movement Disorders.* Urban and Schwarzenberger, Baltimore–Munich, 1988 pp243–261.

Folstein SE: *Huntington's Disease: A Disorder of Families.* Baltimore: Johns Hopkins University Press, 1989.

Foster A, Whetsell W, Bird E, Schwarcz R: Quinolinic acid phosphoribosyltransferase in human and rat brain: activity in Huntington's disease and in quinolinate-lesioned rat striatum. *Brain Res* 1985;336:207–214.

Furtado S, Sucherowsky O, Rewsasle NB, et al.: Relationship between trinucleotide repeats and neuropathological changes in Huntington's disease, *Ann Neurol* 1996;39:132–136.

Gelb DJ, Oliver E, Gilman S: NINDS diagnostic criteria for Parkinson disease, in preparation, 1998.

Gerfen C: The neostriatal mosaic: Compartmentalization of corticostriatal input and striatonigral output systems. *Nature* 1984;311:461–464.

Gerfen C, Herkenham M, Thibauld J: The neostriatal mosaic 2. Patch-directed and matrix-directed mesostriatal dopaminergic and nondopaminergic system. *J Neurosci* 1987;7:3915–3934.

Giedd JN, Rapoport JL, Kruesi MJP, et al.: Sydenham's chorea: magnetic resonance imaging of the basal ganglia. *Neurology* 1995;45:2199–2202.

Goetz C, Tanner C, Wilson R, et al.: Clonidine and Gilles de la Tourette's syndrome: double-blind study using objective rating methods. *Ann Neurol* 1987;21:307–310.

Goldberg YP, Kremer B, Andrew SE, et al.: Molecular analysis of new mutations for Huntington's disease, intermediate alleles and sex of origin effects. *Nat Genet* 1993;5:174–179.

Graybiel A, Ragsdale C: *Biochemical Anatomy of the Striatum.* New York: Raven Press, 1983.

Graybiel AM: Building action repertoires: memory and learning functions of the basal ganglia. *Curr Opin Neurobiol* 1995;5:733–741.

Gusella J, Persichetti F, MacDonald ME: The genetic defect causing Huntington's disease: repeated in other contexts? *Mol Med* 1997;3:238–246.

Gusella J, Wexler N, Conneally P, et al.: A polymorphic DNA marker genetically linked to Huntington's disease. *Nature* 1983;306:234–238.

Gutekunst CA, Levey AI, Heilman DJ, et al.: Identification and localization of huntingtin in brain and human lymphoblastoid cell lines with antifusion protein antibodies. *Proc Natl Acad Sci USA* 1995;92:8710.

Haber SN, Wolfer D: Basal ganglia peptidergic staining in Tourette syndrome: a follow-up study. *Adv Neurol* 1992;58:145–150.

Hallett M: *Differential Diagnosis of Tremor.* New York: Elsevier Science, 1986.

Harper PS: Huntington's Disease: Major Problems in Neurology. 1996;31:438.

Hornykiewicz O, Kish S: Biochemical Pathophysiology of Parkinson Disease. *Adv Neurol* 1987;45:19–34.

Hornykiewicz O, Kish S, Becker L, et al.: Biochemical Evidence for Brain Neurotransmitter Changes in Idiopathic Torsion Dystonia (Dystonia Musculoram Deformans). *Adv Neurol* 1987;50:157–165.

Hornykiewicz O, Kish SJ, Becker LE, et al.: Brain neurotransmitters in dystonia musculorum deformans. *N Engl J Med* 1986;315:347–353.

Hubble JP, Busenbark KL, Wilkinson S, et al.: Deep brain stimulation for essential tremor. *Neurology* 1996;46:1150–1153.

Huntington's Disease Collaborative Research Group: A novel gene containing a trinucleotide repeat that is expanded and unstable on Huntington's disease chromosomes. *Cell* 1993;72:971–983.

Hyde TM, Stacey ME, Coppola R, et al.: Cerebral morphometric abnormalities in Tourette's syndrome: A quantitative MRI study of monozygotic twins. *Neurology* 1995;45:1176–1182.

Ichinose H, Ohye T, Takahashi E, et al: Hereditary progressive dystonia with marked diurnal fluctuation caused by mutations in the GTP cyclohydrolase I gene. *Nat Genet* 1994;8:236–242.

Jankovic J: Diagnosis and classification of tics and Tourette syndrome. *Adv Neurol* 1992;58:714.

Jankovic J, Fahn S: Dystonic disorders, in Jankovic J, Tolosa E (eds): *Parkinson Disease and Movement Disorders.* Baltimore: Williams & Wilkins, 1993, pp 337–374.

Jankovic J, Marsden CD: Therapeutic strategies in Parkinson disease, in Jankovic J, Tolosa E (eds): *Parkinson Disease and Movement Disorders.* Baltimore: Williams & Wilkins, 1993, pp. 115–144.

Jankovic J, Orman J: Botulinum A toxin for cranialcervical dystonia: a double-blind placebo-controlled study. *Neurology* 1987;37:616–623.

Jankovic J, Tolosa E: *Parkinson Disease and Movement Disorders.* Baltimore: Williams & Wilkins, 1988.

Jenkins IH, Bain PG, Colebatch JG, et al.: A positron emission tomography study of essential tremor: evidence for overactivity of cerebellar connections. *Ann Neurol* 1993;34:82–90.

Kiessling LS, Marcotte AC, Culpepper L: Antineuronal antibodies in movement disorders. *Pediatrics* 1993;92:39–43.

Klockgether T, Turski L: Toward an understanding of the role of glutamate in experimental parkinsonism: agonist-sensitive sites in basal ganglia. *Ann Neurol* 1992;34:585–593.

Knappskog P, Flatmark T, Mallet J, et al.: Recessively inherited L-dopa-responsive dystonia caused by a point mutation (Q381K) in the tyrosine hydroxylase gene. *Hum Mol Genet* 1995;4:1209–1212.

Kosinski CM, Cha JJ, Young AB, et al.: Huntingtin immunoreactivity in the rat neostriatum: differential accumulation in projection and interneurons. *Exp Neurol* 1997;144:239–247.

Kramer PL, De Leon D, Ozelius L, et al.: Dystonia gene in Ashkenazi Jewish population is located on chromosome 9q32-34. *Ann Neurol* 1990;27:114–120.

Kurlan R: Tourette's syndrome. *Neurology* 1989;39:1625–1630.

Lang AE, Garnett ES, Firnau G, et al.: Positron tomography in dystonia. *Adv Neurol* 1988;50:249–253.

Langston J, Forno L, Rebert C, Irwin I: Selective nigral toxicity after systemic administration of 1-methyl-4-phenyl-1,2,3,6-tetrahydropyridine (MPTP) in the squirrel monkey. *Brain Res* 1984a;292:390–394.

Langston J, Langston E, Irwin I: MPTP-induced parkinsonism in human and nonhuman primates: clinical and experimental aspects. *Acta Neruol Scand* 1984b;70(Suppl 100):49–54.

Lee L, Kupke K, Caballargonzaga F, et al.: The phenotype of the x-linked dystonia-parkinsonism syndrome: an assessment of 42 cases in the Philippines. *Medicine* 1991;70:179–187.

Lee T, Seeman P, Tajpu A, et al.: Receptor basis for dopaminergic supersensitivity in Parkinson disease. *Nature* 1978;273:59–61.

Leenders KL, Quinn N, Frackowiak RS, Marsden CD: Brain dopaminergic system studied in patients with dystonia using positron emission tomography. *Adv Neurol* 1988;50:243–247.

Lees A: *Tics and Related Disorders.* New York: Churchill Livingstone, 1985.

Lew MF, Shindo M, Moskowitz CB, et al.: Adductor laryngeal breathing dystonia in a patient with lubag (x-linked dystonia-Parkinsonism syndrome). *Mov Disord* 1994;9:318–320.

Ludecke B, Dworniczak B, Bartholome K: A point mutation in the tyrosine hydroxylase gene associated with Segawa's syndrome. *Hum Genet* 1995;95:123–127.

Lyon G, Adams RD, Kolodny EH: *Neurology of Hereditary Metabolic Diseases of Children.* New York: McGraw-Hill, 1996.

MacDonald ME, Barnew G, Srinidhi J, et al.: Gametic but not somatic instability of CAG repeat length in Huntington's disease. *J Med Genet* 1993;30:982–986.

Maneuf YP, Crossman AR, Brotchie JM: Modulation of GABAergic transmission in the globus pallidus by the synthetic cannabinoid WIN 55,2122. *Synapse* 1996;22:382–385.

Maneuf YP, Mitchell IJ, Crossman AC, Brotchie JM: On the role of enkephalin cotransmission in the GABAergic striatal efferents to the globus pallidus. *Exp Neurol* 1994;125:65–71.

Mangiarini L, Sathasivam K, Seller M, et al.: Exon 1 on the HD gene with an expanded CAG repeat is sufficient to cause a progressive neurological phenotype in transgenic mice. *Cell* 1996;87:493–506.

Mao C, Cheney D, Marco E, et al.: Turnover times of gamma-aminobutyric acid and acetylcholine in nucleus caudatus, nucleus accumbens, globus pallidus, and substantia nigra: effects of repeated administration of haloperidol. *Brain Res* 1977;132:375–379.

Markham C, Diamond S: Modification of Parkinson disease by longterm levodopa treatment. *Arch Neurol* 1986;43:405–407.

Marsden C, Parkes J, Quinn N: Fluctuations of Disability in Parkinson Disease: Clinical Aspects. in Marsden, CD, Fahn, S, *Movement Disorder*. London: Butterworths Scientific, 1982 pp. 96–122.

Marsden CD: Problems with longterm levodopa therapy for Parkinson disease. *Clin Neuropharmacol* 1994;17(Suppl 2):S32–S44.

Mayeux R, Stern Y, Cote L, Williams B: Altered serotonin metabolism in depressed patients with Parkinson disease. Neurology 1984;34:642–646.

Mink JW, Thach WT: Basal ganglia intrinsic circuits and their role in behavior. *Curr Opin Neurobiol* 1993;3:950–957.

Myers RH, Vonsattel JP, Stevens TJ, et al.: Clinical and neuropathological assessment of severity in Huntington's disease. *Neurology* 1991;38:341–347.

Myers RH, MacDonald ME, Koroshetz WJ, et al.: De novo expansion of a (CAG)n repeat in sporadic Huntington's disease. *Nat Genet* 1993;5:168–173.

Nutt J: Levodopa-induced dyskinesias: review, observations and speculations. *Neurology* 1990;40:340–345.

Nutt J, Woodward W, Hammerstad J, et al.: The on-off phenomenon in Parkinson disease: relation to levodopa absorption and transport. *N Engl J Med* 1984;310:483–488.

Nutt JG, Holford NHG: The response to levodopa in Parkinson disease: imposing pharmacological law and order. *Ann Neurol* 1996;39:561–573.

Nutt JG: Levodopa-induced dyskinesia: review, observations and speculations. *Neurology* 1990;40:340–345.

Otsuka M, Ichiya Y, Shima F, et al.: Increased striatal ^{18}F-Dopa uptake and normal glucose metabolism in idiopathic dystonia syndrome. *J Neurol Sci* 1992;111:195–199.

Ozelius L, Hewett JW, Page CE, et al.: The early onset torsion dystonia gene (DYT1) encodes an ATP-binding protein. *Nat Genet* 1997;17:40–48.

Palacios JM, Landwehrmeyer B, Mengod G: Brain dopamine receptors: characterization, distribution, and alteration in disease, in Jankovic J, Tolosa E (eds): *Parkinson Disease and Movement Disorders*. Baltimore: William & Wilkins, 1993, pp 35–54.

Pan H, Penney J, Young A: GABA and benzodiazepine receptor changes induced by unilateral 6-hydroxydopamine lesions of the medial forebrain bundle. *J Neurochem* 1985;45:1396–1404.

Parkinson Study Group: Safety and efficacy of pramipexole in early Parkinson disease: a randomized dose-ranging study. *JAMA* 1997;278:125–130.

Penney J, Young A: Striatal inhomogeneities and basal ganglia function. *Movement Dis* 1986;1:3–15.

Penney JB: CAG repeat number governs the development rate of pathology in Huntington's disease. *Ann Neurol* 1997, 41:689–692

Penney JB, Young AB, Shoulson I, et al.: Huntington's disease in Venezuela: seven years of follow-up on symptomatic and asymptomatic individuals. *Movement Dis* 1990;5:93–99.

Perlmutter JS, Stambuk MK, Markham J, et al.: Decreased [18F]Spiperone binding in putamen in idiopathic focal dystonia. *J Neurosci* 1997;17:843–850.

Perry T, Hanson S, Kloster M: Deficiency of gamma-aminobutyric acid in brain. *N Engl J Med* 1973;288:337–342.

Polymeropoulos MH, Lavedan C, Leroy E, et al.: Mutation in the alphasynuclein gene identified in families with Parkinson disease. *Science* 1997;276:2045–2048.

Poskanzer D, Schuab R: Evidence for a single etiology related to subclinical infection about 1920. *J Chronic Dis* 1963;16:961–973.

Rajput AH, Offord KP, Beard CM, Kurland LT: Epidemiology of parkinsonism: incidence classification and mortality. *Ann Neurol* 1984;16:278–282.

Regeur L, Pakkenberg B, Fog R, Pakkenberg H: Clinical features and longterm treatment with pimozide in 65 patients with Gilles de la Tourette's syndrome. *J Neurol Neurosurg Psychiatry* 1986;49:791–795.

Reiner A, Albin R, Anderson K, et al.: Differential loss of striatal projections neurons in Huntington's disease. *Proc Natl Acad Sci USA* 1988;85:5733–5737.

Richter R: Degeneration of the basal ganglia in monkeys from chronic carbon disulfide poisoning. *J Neuropathol Exp Neurol* 1945;4:324–353.

Robertson RG, Clarke CE, Boyce S, et al.: GABA/benzodiazepine receptors in the primate basal ganglia following treatment with MPTP: evidence for the differential regulation of striatal output by dopamine? In Crossman AC, Sambrook MA (eds): *Neural Mechanisms in Disorders of Movement*. London: John Libbey, 1989, pp. 165–173.

Rubinsztein DC, Leggo J, Coles R, et al.: Phenotypic characterization of individuals with 3040 CAG repeats in the Huntington's disease (HD) gene reveals HD cases with 36 repeats and apparently normal elderly individuals with 3639 repeats. *Am J Hum Genet* 1996;59:16–22.

Schell G, Strick P: The origin of thalamic inputs to the arcuate premotor and supplementary motor areas. *J Neurosci* 1984;4:539–560.

Scheinberg I, Sternlieb I: *Wilson's Disease*. Philadelphia: WB Saunders, 1984.

Segawa M, Hosaka A, Miyagawa F, et al.: Hereditary progressive dystonia with marked diurnal fluctuation. *Adv Neurol* 1976;14:215–233.

Sharp AH: Widespread expression of Huntington's disease gene (IT15) protein product. *Neuron* 1995;14:1065–1074.

Shoulson I: *Huntington's Disease*. Philadelphia: WB Saunders, 1986.

Shoulson I: On chorea. *Clin Neurophamacol* 1986;9(Suppl 2):S84–S99.

Shoulson I, Kieburtz K: Neuroprotective therapy for Huntington's disease, in Bar PR, Beal MF (eds): *Neuroprotection in CNS Diseases*. New York: Marcel Dekker, 1997, pp. 457.

Singer HS: Neurochemical analysis of postmortem cortical and striatal brain tissue in patients with Tourette syndrome. *Adv Neurol* 1992;58:135–144.

Singer HS, Reiss AL, Brown JE et al.: Volumetric MRI changes in basal ganglia of children with Tourette's syndrome. *Neurology* 1993;43:950–956.

Spillantini MG, Schmidt ML, Lee VMY, et al.: α-Synuclein in Lewy bodies. *Nature* 1997;388:839–840.

Spina M, Cohen G: Dopamine turnover and glutathione oxidation: implications for Parkinson disease. *Proc Natl Acad Sci USA* 1989;85:1398–1400.

Spokes E: Neurochemical alterations in Huntington's disease. *Brain* 1980;103:179–210.

Stacy M, Jankovic J: Differential diagnosis of Parkinson disease and the parkinsonism plus syndromes. *Neurol Clin* 1992;10:341–359.

Starosta-Rubinstein S, Young AB, Kluin K, et al.: Clinical assessment of 31 Wilson's patients: correlations with structural changes on MRI. *Arch Neurol* 1987;44:365–370.

Tanzi RE, Petrukhin K, Chernov I, et al.: The Wilson's disease gene is a copper transporting ATPase with homology to the Menkes disease gene. *Nat Genet* 1993;5:344–350.

Tolosa E, Alom J, Marti MJ: Drug-induced dyskinesias, in Jankovic J, Tolosa E (eds): *Parkinson Disease and Movement Disorders.* Baltimore: Williams & Wilkins, 1993, pp. 375–397.

Trottier Y, Devys D, Imbert G, et al.: Cellular localization of the Huntington's disease protein and discrimination of the normal and mutated form. *Nat Genet* 1995;10:104–110.

Vonsattel JP, Myers RH, Stevens TJ, et al.: Neuropathological classification of Huntington's disease. *Neuropathol Exp Neurol* 1985;44:559–577.

Wagster MV, Hedreen JC, Peyser CE, et al.: Selective loss of [³H]kainic acid and [³H]AMPA binding in layer VI of frontal cortex in Huntington's disease. *Exp Neurol* 1994;127:70–75.

Waters CH, Faust PL, Powers J, et al.: Neuropathology of lubag (x-linked dystonia parkinsonism). *Movement Disord* 1993;8:387–390.

Waters CH, Takahashi H, Wilhelmsen KC, et al.: Phenotypic expression of x-linked dystonia-parkinsonism (lubag) into two women. *Neurology* 1993;43:1555–1558.

Wilhelmsen KC, Weeks DE, Nygaard TG, et al.: Genetic mapping of "Lubag" (x-linked dystonia-parkinsonism) in a Filipino kindred to the pericentromeric region of the X chromosome. *Ann Neurol* 1991;29:124–131.

Wills AJ, Jenkins IH, Thompson PD, et al.: Red nuclear and cerebellar but no olivary activation associated with essential tremor: a positron emission tomography study. *Ann Neurol* 1994;36:636–642.

Wilson S: Progressive lenticular degeneration: a familial nervous disease associated with cirrhosis of the liver. *Brain* 1912;34:295–509.

Wolff SS, Jones DW, Knable MB, et al.: Tourette syndrome: prediction of phenotypic variation in monozygotic twins by caudate nucleus D-2 receptor binding. *Science* 1996;273:1225.

Yeh K, August T, Bush D, et al.: Pharmacokinetics and bioavailability of Sinemet CR: a summary of human studies. *Neurology* 1989;38(Suppl 2):25–38.

Young A, Greenamyre J, Hollingworth Z, et al.: NMDA receptor losses in putamen from patients with Huntington's disease. *Science* 1988;241:981–983.

Young AB: Huntington's disease: lessons from and for molecular neuroscience. *Neuroscientist* 1994, preview issue: 30–37.

Young AB, Shoulson I, Penney JB, et al.: Huntington's disease in Venezuela: neurological features and functional decline. *Neurology* 1986;36:244–249.

C H A P T E R   1 2

MULTIPLE SCLEROSIS

Joseph B. Guarnaccia, Timothy L. Vollmer, and Stephen G. Waxman

Multiple sclerosis (MS) is the most common cause of acquired demyelination of the central nervous system, which, in essence, appears to be an inflammatory process directed at brain and spinal cord myelin. Relatively prevalent in the Western Hemisphere and Europe, MS is a major cause of chronic neurologic disability in adults. It imposes various degrees of physical, emotional, economic, and social hardship for most, if not all, afflicted persons. Estimates range from 300,000 to 400,000 individuals affected in the United States. Although its precise cause remains unknown, and a cure remains elusive, disease-modifying drug therapies are available to treat the underlying pathophysiology and to enhance the quality of life. The purpose of this chapter is to review the current understanding of the epidemiology, pathophysiology, and clinical features of MS and to detail its pharmacologic management.

CLINICAL FEATURES

Epidemiology

Since the 1920s, numerous epidemiologic investigations have attempted to define the worldwide incidence and prevalence of multiple sclerosis (MS). Both geographic variation and temporal fluctuations have been found. Many of these studies support the hypothesis that exposure to a transmissible factor, such as a virus, or some other environmental agent influences the risk of acquiring the disease. This hypothesis is based on three types of epidemiologic evidence: 1) population surveys, 2) migration studies, and 3) clusters.

Studies of death rates and the prevalence of MS have demonstrated a pattern of increasing incidence with distance from the equator. This south-north (north-south in the southern hemisphere) risk gradient has led epidemiologists to divide the world into high ($\geq$30 in 100,000), medium (5 to 29 in 100,000), and low (<5 in 100,000) prevalence zones (Kurtzke, 1975a, b) (Fig. 12-1). High-risk zones are located in

North America and Europe, above 40 degrees latitude north of the equator, and in Australia and New Zealand, in the Southern Hemisphere.

Prevalence estimates of MS. Although repeated surveys of the same regions have frequently suggested greater prevalence rates, the relationship between MS risk and latitude continues to hold in many areas, particularly in North America, Australia, and New Zealand. In some European countries, changes in ascertainment methods probably contributed to revised estimates of higher prevalence rates. For instance, Spain, Italy, Sardinia, and Cyprus, all of which were considered to be in low-risk zones, were recently identified as having prevalence rates of greater than 40 in 100,000. Curiously, there is also unexplained geographic variation among these regions. For instance, the island of Malta has a much lower rate of MS than the island of Sicily, which is 100 miles away. Israel, a country of immigrants, has a higher rate of MS than would be expected on the basis of its latitude. In parts of the British Isles, MS reaches almost epidemic proportions, with the highest rates in the world

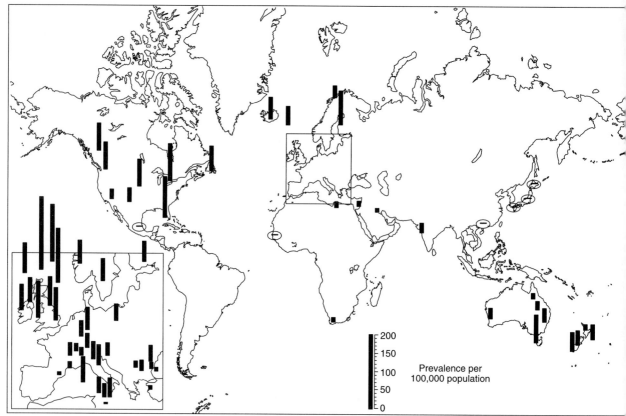

Figure 12–1. *Prevalence of multiple sclerosis throughout the world. (Bars represent estimates of prevalence obtained from population-based surveys. Where areas have been studied repeatedly, only estimates from surveys in which case-ascertainment was judged to be most complete and which were carried out most recently have been shown). Reprinted with permission from Martyn C, 1991.*

found in the Orkney and Shetland Islands off the coast of Scotland, with prevalence rates of 309 in 100,000 and 184 in 100,000, respectively (Poskanzer et al., 1980). Similarly, MS is also relatively prevalent in Norway, Sweden, Finland, and Denmark. By contrast, except for English-speaking whites of South Africa, MS is extremely rare in native Africans and has a very low prevalence among the Japanese.

Migration studies.   Several migration studies have also supported the concept of geographically based incidence. The disease risk changes in groups of individuals who move be-

tween localities, suggesting that risk can be altered by different environments. A case-controlled study of the U.S. veteran population from World War II showed that the risk of MS in subgroups of recruits from different prevalence zones was related to birthplace, but modified by residences at entry into the armed forces (Kurtzke et al., 1985) (Table 12-1). This phenomenon was also noted in black veterans, whose overall prevalence of MS was half that of whites. Migrant studies in Israel showed that both place of origin and age at immigration influenced the rate of disease in different ethnic groups. Thus, the prevalence was higher for immigrants of Ashkenazi origin from the higher-prevalence areas of northern Europe than for those of Sephardic origin from the lower-prevalence areas of Asia and Africa. These differences depended on age at migra-

Table 12-1

The effect of migration in the time between birth and entry to military service on the risk of multiple sclerosis in U.S. veterans. Numbers are case/control ratios.

Residence at birth (by tier of latitude)	Residence at entry to military service (by tier of latitude)			
	North	Middle	South	Total
North	1.41	1.26	0.70	1.38
Middle	1.30	1.04	0.72	1.04
South	0.73	0.62	0.56	0.57
Total	1.39	1.04	0.58	1.04

With permission from Martyn, C, 1991.

tion for the Ashkenazi immigrants, with those who migrated before puberty tending to have a very low risk of MS compared with those who migrated later in life. This suggests that the risk of acquiring MS depends on exposure to some environmental factor before the age of 15. These differences in risk of MS based on age of immigration are also noted in multigenerational studies of immigrants to London from Africa and Asia and to South Africa from Europe. Whether these differences are better explained by the genetic background of migrant groups or indigenous populations continues to be debated, although most believe in some contribution from the environment.

Clusters of MS. The Faeroe Islands, which are located in the North Atlantic between Iceland and Norway, did not report any cases of MS before 1943. After 1945 there was an increase to 10 cases of MS per 100,000 population, followed by a decline in prevalence over the next several years. This change in prevalence has been linked to the 1940–1945 occupation of the islands by British troops. Kurtzke has speculated that the British harbored a "primary MS affectation" (PMSA), an asymptomatic condition that could cause disease in individuals at risk. Following a latent period of at least 2 years after exposure, those aged 11 to 45 were susceptible to developing MS. Some 46 cases of MS were subsequently identified between 1943 and 1982. Kurtzke later described a second epidemic in Iceland around the same period, which also coincided with the presence of foreign troops. Similar epidemics, however, have not been seen in other geographic areas with historically low incidence after occupation by British or American troops.

A number of other geographic clusters of MS have been analyzed, with most dismissed as chance occurrences. One in Key West, Florida, involved 37 patients with definite or probable MS, 34 of whom developed the disease while living on the island, and nine of whom were community nurses.

Genetics

Confounders of race and ethnicity have made it extremely difficult to isolate completely the environmental factors that contribute to susceptibility to MS. Descendants of settlers from comparably high-risk areas of Scandinavia and western Europe settled Canada and the northern and western United States, which also have relatively high prevalence rates (Fig. 12-2). Although Japan is located a similar distance north of the equator, however, the incidence of MS is low in that country. Furthermore, a number of studies show that different ethnic groups living in the same area have different risks for the disorder. Thus, the disease is rare in black Africans and unknown in ethnically pure native populations, including Eskimos, Inuits, Native Americans, Australian aborigines, New Zealand Maoris, Pacific Islanders, and Lapps.

Determinants of genetic susceptibility to MS come from studies of twins and multiply affected family members. In Western countries, first-degree relatives of patients have an estimated lifetime risk 20 to 50 times that of the general population. Concordance rates in monozygotic twins are approximately

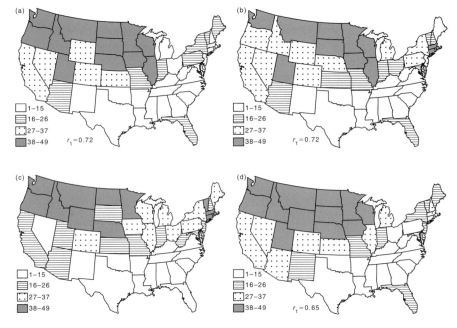

Figure 12–2. *The relative prevalence of MS in the United States using Kurtzke's control ratios for the U.S. World War II veteran MS population (c) compared with the distribution of foreign-born Scandinavians in 1930 (a), for "foreign white stock" (1930) in (b), and for Scandinavian ancestry (1980) in (d). Reprinted with permission from Compston A, Ebers G, 1990.*

30% according to several studies, in contrast with less than 5% in dizygotic twins and siblings. Furthermore, there is an indication that some discordant twins, or asymptomatic family members, may harbor a similar susceptibility to demyelinating disease as determined by the finding of asymptomatic lesions on magnetic resonance imaging (MRI) in some of these individuals. These studies have not, however, found a consistent correlation between disease pattern or severity and familial incidence. Specific genes linked to MS have not been identified, and the pattern of inheritability is consistent with a polygenic trait (see the following).

Genome screening. Multi-institutional, collaborative studies are being conducted to identify candidate genes for MS through whole genome screening. These studies have excluded approximately 90% of the human genome as major genetic determinants

for MS. The most consistent genetic link is to the HLA region on chromosome 6p21, which is compatible with the finding of the increased susceptibility to MS of individuals who carry certain HLA alleles. Although American and British investigators have demonstrated a modest linkage to the HLA region (The Multiple Sclerosis Study Group, 1996; Sawcer et al., 1996), Canadian scientists found no such linkage, but rather a strong genetic effect from a location on chromosome 5p, similar to that reported by Finnish scientists (Ebers et al., 1996). Certain HLA alleles are known to be associated with a greater risk of MS, particularly the HLA-DR2 (subtype Drw15) haplotype. Although there is a four-fold increased risk of MS for white Europeans and North Americans carrying the DR2 allele, the predictive value of this is limited because 30 to 50% of patients are DR2 negative, and DR2 is present in 20% of the general population.

Other Risk Factors

Women have about double the risk as men for developing MS at a younger age. The gender ratio equalizes with MS onset after age 40. The period of greatest risk is between the second and the sixth decades, although MS has been described in young children and older adults. Childhood MS does not differ significantly from the adult form in presentation and clinical course, according to several studies. The onset of MS after age 60 is rare and comprises less than 1% of some series.

Higher socioeconomic status has been identified consistently as a risk factor and antecedent viral infections have been associated with disease relapses. Physical trauma has been suggested as a cause of MS, but this is controversial because neither retrospective nor prospective studies have definitely demonstrated a relationship. Pregnancy studies tend to show that although women are at reduced risk for disease activity during gestation, risk increases during the first 6 months of the postpartum period.

Pathology and Pathogenesis

The cause of MS is unknown, with no conclusive evidence that a virus, or any other infectious agent, is the sole cause of the disorder. Viruses have been proposed, however, as the most likely etiologic candidates based on interpretations of the epidemiologic data and some of their well-described properties. Particular infectious viruses may alter immunity, exist in latent forms in the CNS and cause demyelination in the CNS (Table 12-2). Furthermore, there is some evidence that MS patients have altered immune responses to common viruses, including a heightened reactivity to measles virus. A model of persistent viral infection of the CNS is subacute sclerosing panencephalitis, a rare sequela of measles infections occurring years after an apparently uncomplicated illness. Several viruses, and some bacteria, are associated with acute disseminated encephalomyelitis (ADEM). This is usually a monophasic, demyelinating illness, histopathologically similar, although not identical, to MS. Canine distemper virus, which is closely related to measles, has been postulated to be

Table 12-2

Possible Mechanisms of Virus-Induced Demyelination

Direct viral effects

  Viral infection of oligodendrocytes or Schwann cells causing demyelination through cell lysis or an alteration of cell metabolism

  Myelin membrane destruction by the virus or viral products

Virus-induced immune-mediated reactions

  Antibody and/or cell-mediated reactions to viral antigens on cell membrane

  Sensitization of host to myelin antigens

    Breakdown of myelin by infection with introduction into the circulation

    Incorporation of myelin antigens into the virus envelope

    Modification of antigenicity of myelin membranes

  Cross-reacting antigens between virus and myelin proteins

  Bystander demyelination

Viral disruption of regulatory mechanisms of the immune system

With permission from RA Shubin, Weiner LP, 1989.

the "primary MS affectation" factor of Kurtzke that spread to the native Faeroe Islanders from dogs brought to the island by British troops. Theiler's murine encephalomyelitis virus, a picornavirus, is an experimental model for CNS demyelination in rodents, its natural hosts.

A disease similar to myelopathic (spinal) forms of MS is caused by the retrovirus, human T-cell lymphotropic virus type I (HTLV-I). The condition is known in different geographic locations as tropical spastic paraparesis (TSP) or HIV-associated myelopathy (HAM). Both TSP and HAM are slowly progressive myelopathies, characterized by vasculopathy and demyelination. Evidence that MS is caused by

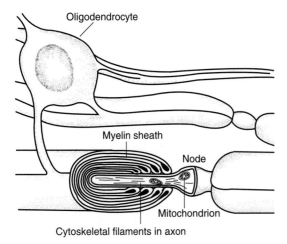

Oligodendrocyte

Myelin sheath

Node

Mitochondrion

Cytoskeletal filaments in axon

Figure 12–3. *The myelin-oligodendrocyte unit.*

a retrovirus remains inconclusive, however, despite the fact that nucleic acid sequences of HTLV-I have been reported in some patients. Extensive CNS demyelination associated with subacute infection by herpes simplex virus type 6 (HSV6) has also been described.

The myelin-oligodendrocyte unit.   Myelin is a complex, metabolically active laminated sheath surrounding large-diameter axons. It is formed by apposing extensions of the membrane bilayers of oligodendrocytes in the CNS and by Schwann cells in the peripheral nervous system (PNS) (Fig. 12-3). The internal surfaces of the sheath are continuous with the cytoplasm of their respective myelin-forming cells. Although the myelin sheath is susceptible to direct damage, it also fails if its parent cell is destroyed. The CNS and PNS myelin systems have quite different vulnerabilities to inflammatory insults, with PNS myelin rarely affected in CNS demyelinating disease processes, and vice versa. Differences also exist between PNS and CNS myelin in structural protein composition, antigenicity, and the functional relationships with their respective component cells. Within CNS myelin, the most abundant structural protein is proteolipid protein (50%), which is exposed to the extracellular environment (Fig. 12-4). Next in relative abundance is myelin basic protein (30%), which is located on the internal side of the membrane bilayer. Other proteins, although present in small quantities, may be important as autoantigens in the immunopathogenesis of MS, including myelin-associated glycoprotein (1%) and myelin-oligodendrocyte glycoprotein (<1%.)

Because the CNS myelin-oligodendrocyte unit covers more axons than the PNS myelin-oligodendrocyte unit, it is probably more vulnerable to injury. Thus, as many as 35 CNS axons can be myelinated by one oligodendrocyte, compared with one axon per Schwann cell in the PNS.

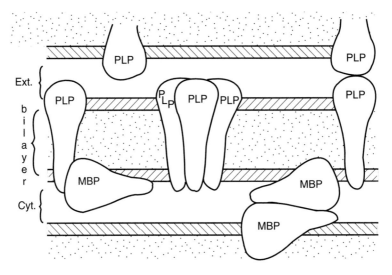

Figure 12–4.   *The molecular organization of the CNS myelin bilayer. Cyt—cytoplasmic apposition; Ext—extracellular apposition; MBP— myelin basic protein; PLP—proteolipid protein. With permission from Kamholtz J, 1989.*

Myelin is a high-resistance, low-capacitance substance that, along with a nonuniform distribution of sodium channels, confines the production of the action potentials to the exposed, specialized regions of the axon (Waxman, 1982). These nodes of Ranvier are formed at the discontinuous edges of adjacent myelin sheaths. Depolarization of the axonal membrane proceeds along the nodes of Ranvier and jumps in a discontinuous, energy-efficient manner from node to node in a rapid process termed saltatory conduction (Fig. 12-5).

Because the myelin-oligodendrocyte unit is susceptible to damage from a host of metabolic, infectious, ischemic/anoxic, and inflammatory processes, demyelination is a prominent feature of numerous disorders. Demyelinating diseases share the characteristics of destruction of the myelin sheath with relative sparing of axons and other supporting elements. A number of these insults, including carbon monoxide poisoning, other toxic exposures, hepatic dysfunction, vitamin B_{12} deficiency, and viral or postviral infections, have been eliminated as contributing causes of MS. Primary inflammatory demyelination caused by processes such as those associated with MS and ADEM is characterized by perivascular infiltrates of inflammatory cells and a multifocal distribution of lesions in the subcortical white matter, which may have a symmetrical or confluent pattern.

Pathology. The study of MS has benefited greatly from the histologic examination of demyelinating lesions (MS plaques) of apparently different ages in the same patient and from comparisons between patients who differed in clinical characteristics and temporal profiles. Some have died from fulminant MS of recent onset and others from unrelated causes or medical complications of end-stage disease.

Postmortem findings in MS brain and spinal cord are usually unremarkable. There may be mild atrophy of the cortex with ventricular enlargement of the brain stem and spinal cord. The exposed surfaces of the ventral pons, medulla, corpus callosum, optic nerves, and spinal cord may contain firm, pinkish gray depressions, indicating underlying demyelinating plaques. Plaques are found throughout the white matter and occasionally gray matter. There is a propensity for plaques to occur in certain white-matter areas, however, especially those near small veins and postcapillary venules. These include areas bordering the lateral ventricles in places where subependymal veins course along the inner walls and in the brain stem and spinal cord, where pial veins lie next to white matter. Individual plaques in periventricular locations frequently enlarge and become confluent,

particularly along the posterior horns of the lateral ventricles. Discrete plaques with an ovoid appearance that extend perpendicularly from the ventricle into white matter are called Dawson's fingers. Histologically, these are circumscribed areas of inflammation, with or without demyelination, encircling parenchymal veins and following their radial extension into the deep white matter. Both clinically and pathologically, the optic nerves and cervical spinal cord are frequently involved in demyelinating disease. Their propensity for plaque formation is attributed to the slight mechanical stretching to which these areas are subjected during eye movement or flexion of the neck, although this remains an unproven theory. Other areas of the brain commonly involved are the floor of the fourth ventricle, periaqueduct, corpus callosum, brain stem, and cerebellar tracts. The corticomedullary junction may also show some involvement, although subcortical U fibers are usually spared.

Multifocal demyelination is the rule with MS. In an autopsy series of 70 MS patients (Ikuta and Zimmerman, 1976), only 7% had brain lesions (excluding the optic nerves), without spinal cord lesions, and 13% had spinal cord, without brain lesions (Table 12-3).

Histopathology. Although the earliest changes preceding demyelination are debated, perivascular infiltrates of lymphocytes, plasma cells, and macrophages have been observed both in demyelinated and normally myelinated white matter in the brains of MS patients. These cells may collect in the perivenular Virchow-Robin spaces—potential spaces between blood vessels and the brain parenchyma that are continuous with the cerebrospinal fluid system. This is taken as evidence for a primary pathogenic role of the immune system in MS (Prineas, 1990). Indirect evidence that this inflammatory reaction does not occur solely as a consequence of changes in myelin comes from the presence of similar perivascular cuffs of lymphocytes in the retina of MS patients, which lacks myelinated fibers. Similarly, sheathing around the retinal vessels, and focal disruptions in the blood-retinal vascular interface have been observed in MS patients.

There are differing interpretations about the mechanism of myelin breakdown in MS plaques. Some suggest the monocytes are simply scavengers of myelin sheaths damaged by some other process; others believe that monocytes actively participate in the demyelination. Macrophage membranes contain clathrin-coated pits that have been observed to be contiguous with the myelin sheath. This is postulated to be the site

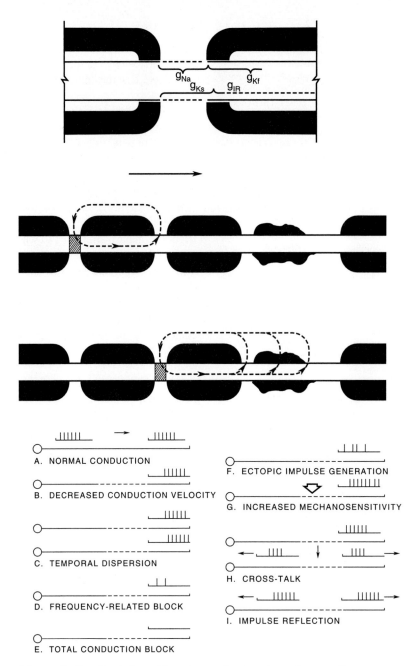

Figure 12–5. *Depiction of impulse conduction through normally myelinated and demyelinated axons (top). Working model of ion channel organization of the myelinated fiber: gNa = Na channels; gkf = fast K channels; gks = slow K channels; gIR = inward rectifier; (middle) conduction through normally myelinated (upper) and demyelinated (lower) regions; (bottom) conduction abnormalities in demyelinated fibers. B-E would lead to negative and F-I to positive neurological signs. With permission from Waxman SG, 1990.*

Table 12-3

Extent and regional distribution of plaques in 70 autopsied cases of MS in the United States

	Optic nerve	Cerebrum	Cerebellum	Midbrain	Pons	Medulla	Spinal cord
Extensive plaques	32 cases (46%)	36 (51%)	13 (19%)	17 (27%)	27 (39%)	17 (25%)	37 (53%)
Large plaques	23 cases (33%)	18 (26%)	30 (43%)	24 (38%)	24 (34%)	26 (39%)	18 (26%)
Small plaques	13 cases (19%)	14 (20%)	18 (26%)	12 (19%)	14 (20%)	16 (24%)	14 (20%)
No plaques	1 case (1%)	2 (3%)	9 (13%)	10 (16%)	5 (7%)	8 (12%)	1 (1%)

In a few cases microscopic preparations were unavailable for the optic nerve, midbrain, and medulla, and these cases were omitted.

With permission from Ikuta F, Zimmerman HM, 1976.

of Fc-dependent antibody-receptor interactions that lead to the opsonization of myelin by monocytes. Macrophages have also been observed to invade directly the myelin sheath, causing vesicular eruptions within the myelin.

Myelin degradation products within the cytoplasm of macrophages are markers for acute demyelination. These internalized myelin fragments have a composition and ultrastructure similar to normal myelin. With degradation, the ultrastructural features are lost, neutral lipid droplets are formed, and the macrophages develop a "foamy" appearance. These macrophages are cleared much more slowly from the lesion area and have been found up to 6 months to 1 year following acute demyelination.

Freshly demyelinated areas are characterized by hypercellularity, with B cells, plasma cells, CD4+ and CD8+ T cells, and early reactive macrophages found within the plaque and at the plaque margin. Acute axonal changes may be detected morphologically in the form of beading. Remyelination, or abortive remyelination, is frequently observed at the plaque border, and sometimes recurrent demyelination is noted within or contiguous to these areas. Occasionally, entire plaques are remyelinated. These are described as shadow plaques because they appear both grossly and radiographically to blend with the surrounding, normally appearing white matter. The remyelinating cell population is unknown. The source of remyelinating oligodendrocytes could be mature cells escaping destruction within the lesion, those migrating in from plaque borders, or young oligodendrocytes that have regenerated from precursor cells. It has been suggested that the degree of destruction of mature oligodendrocytes determines the remyelin-

ation potential within a given lesion, which may vary among patients. Schwann cells are also reported to migrate into the spinal cord and remyelinate axons. As compared with normal neurons, remyelinated axons have thinner myelin sheaths with shortened myelin segments and wider internodes. Experimentally, demyelinated axons can reestablish electrophysiologic function, but the extent to which this accounts for functional recovery in MS is unknown. Following remyelination of experimentally demyelinated axons by transplanted glial cells, relatively normal conduction properties are restored (Honmou et al., 1996), suggesting that cell transplantation may be a useful therapeutic strategy for this condition.

Chronic plaques with inactive central areas typically have low numbers of macrophages and other inflammatory cells, although an actively demyelinating margin displays an inflammatory infiltrate. Chronically demyelinated axons are embedded in a matrix of fibrous astroglial processes, hence the term "sclerosis." Blood vessel walls may be thickened with hyalinization. Remyelination potential is perhaps reduced in older lesions, rather than acute lesions, because they contain fewer surviving oligodendrocytes.

Magnetic resonance imaging (MRI) is a very sensitive procedure for indirectly visualizing plaque morphology (Figs. 12-6 to 12-10). Although conventional MRI signal changes do not reliably distinguish edema from demyelination, gliosis, or axonal loss, these lesions frequently are referred to as demyelinat-

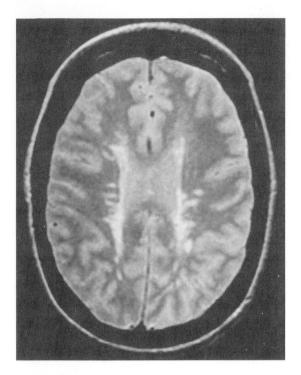

Figure 12–6. *Proton density MRI of the brain in a patient with MS. Note the typical periventricular distribution of hyperintense signal abnormalities.*

ing plaques. Sagittal, coronal, and axial MRI views of the brain and spine provide a topographic depiction of disease-involved areas in individual patients. Sagittal views of the brain are best for showing plaques in the corpus callosum and their extensions upward through the corona radiata toward the cortex. Coronal sections show the pattern of white-matter disease along the ventricular walls; axial sections are best for general topographic location and quantification of lesions. The MS lesions are visualized as increased intensities (white) on T2-weighted (spin echo) images, which provide good contrast with the darker normal white matter, but insufficient contrast with ventricular cerebrospinal fluid (CSF). On proton density images, lesions are brighter than CSF, which is dark, and the normal-appearing white matter. Fluid-attenuated inversion recovery (FLAIR) images enhance the light–dark contrast between lesions and the surrounding white matter.

MRI, MRS, and the evolution of pathology. Serial MRI provides dynamic information about lesion pathology. The integrity of the blood-brain barrier is visualized by an enhancing agent, gadolinium-diethyenetriaminepentaacetic acid (Gd-DPTA), a paramagnetic substance that increases the T1 relaxation time of adjacent mobile water protons, making lesions appear bright on T1-weighted images. Blood-brain barrier permeability is associated with the presence of vesicles within endothelial cells that contain Gd. It has been demonstrated in laboratory animals and humans that enhancement with Gd-DPTA reflects perivascular inflammation. Serial MRI scanning with Gd-DPTA shows enhancement in early lesions that lasts from 2 weeks to 3 months. As enhancement resolves, lesions disappear completely or leave a hyperintense T2-weighted signal. The ap-

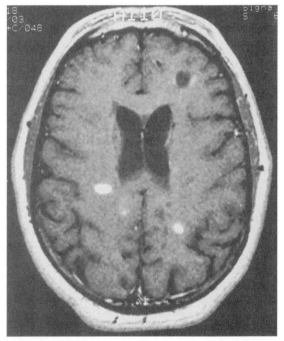

Figure 12–7. *T1 image with gadolinium. Note the enhancing lesions in the subcortices of both hemispheres. In the upper left, in the frontal cortex, there is a hypointense signal abnormality that demonstrates slight enhancement at the margin.*

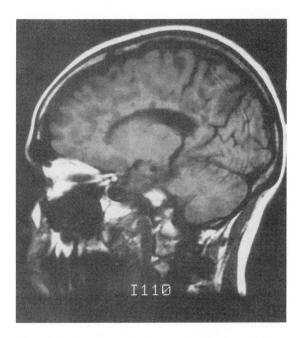

Figure 12–8. *Sagittal T1 view showing hypointense signal in the corpus callosum, indicating plaque involvement.*

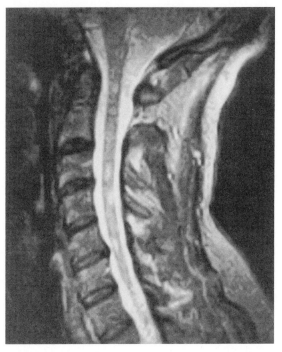

Figure 12–10. *Sagittal view of the cervical spinal cord, showing multiple lesions on T2-weighted images.*

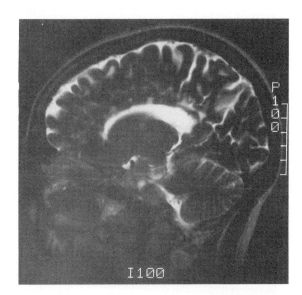

Figure 12–9. *Same view as in Figure 12-8. T2-weighted image showing corresponding signal changes.*

pearance of lesions is often not accompanied by clinical symptoms, although lesion activity has some association with the clinical course of MS. For instance, new lesions are much more likely to enhance in patients with secondary rather than primary progressive MS. The changes noted on T2 and contrast-enhanced T1 are indicative of vasogenic edema and expansion of the extracellular water. Detection of active lesions may be increased with higher doses of Gd-DPTA.

Magnetic resonance spectroscopy (MRS), which quantifies brain metabolites in vivo, provides indications of axonal integrity through the proton resonance of N-acetylaspartate (NAA), a neuronal constituent. Larger plaque volumes on conventional MRI and a more disabling or progressive clinical course have been associated with lower levels of N-acetylaspartate (NAA) within plaques.

Pathologic variants of MS. There are variants of MS with distinctive clinical and pathologic features. Schilder's myeloclastic diffuse sclerosis is characterized by large, bilateral symmetrical areas of demyelination of the centrum semiovale (the area of white matter above the ventricles), with or without smaller isolated plaques. Children comprise a high proportion of these cases. The clinical picture may consist of dementia, relapses and remissions, pseudotumor cerebri with increased intracranial pressure, or psychiatric symptoms. Histopathologically there are sharply delineated foci of demyelination with fibrillary gliosis, giant multinucleated or swollen astrocytes, and perivascular cuffing of inflammatory cells with some axonal damage.

Marburg's disease is an acute fulminant form of MS characterized by a large hemispheric lesion as well as brainstem involvement, and CSF pleocytosis and oligoclonal bands. Edema is prominent in the early stages of this disease, with myelin destruction being extensive and axonal loss severe.

Bálo's concentric sclerosis is another fulminant, but usually monophasic, variant in which there are concentric laminated zones of alternating myelinated and demyelinated areas.

Two other variants of MS, acute disseminated encephalomyelitis (ADEM) and neuromyelitis optica (Devic's disease), are more common and therefore described in more detail in the following.

Experimental allergic encephalomyelitis. Although there is no natural counterpart to MS in other mammals, a demyelinating condition, experimental allergic encephalomyelitis (EAE), can be induced (Fig. 12-11). This animal model is important not only in understanding the pathophysiology of the immune process in MS but also in designing and testing potential pharmacologic treatments. The histopathology of EAE is similar to MS, with perivenous inflammatory infiltrates and variable degrees of demyelination. Experimental allergic encephalomyelitis is induced by immunization with myelin antigen-containing preparations, including crude brain-spinal cord homogenates and whole or parts of myelin proteins, with or without the addition of adjuvant and pertussis toxin, depending on the preparation and method. The disease may also be adoptively transferred by T cells sensitized to myelin antigens between syngeneic mouse strains. In this case, there is an additional requirement for antibodies directed against myelin constituents to produce significant demyelination. Typically, EAE is a monophasic illness with complete or nearly

complete recovery, but relapsing EAE has been induced in guinea pigs and common marmosets. It has also been studied in a murine model with a transgenic T-cell receptor to a specific amino acid sequence of myelin basic protein. Although EAE is an imperfect model of MS, insights gained from its study have contributed to the understanding of the T-cell receptor and MHC biology, autoantigens and autoantibodies of potential relevance in MS, regulation of the immune response, and the genetics of CNS demyelination.

Immunopathogenesis. The prevailing view of MS is that it is a disorder of cell-mediated immunity directed against one or more myelin antigens in the CNS (Fig. 12-12). The histopathology of the early demyelinated MS plaque strongly implicates a key role for T lymphocytes (Raine, 1991). The CD4 helper T-cell subset is prominent early in lesion pathogenesis and is thought to initiate the inflammatory cascade. Moreover, CD8 suppressor/cytotoxic T cells found at the lesion perimeter and perivascular spaces, may have a counterregulatory effect on pro-inflammatory processes. In addition, there is localized upregulation (increased sensitivity) of the immune response with the expression of major histocompatibility complex (MHC) class I and class II on both immune and nonimmune cells, including astrocytes and blood vessel endothelial cells. Thus, these cells may potentially participate in the immune response by presenting myelin autoantigens to CD8 and CD4 cells. Notably, oligodendrocytes do not appear to express class I or II MHC antigens, suggesting that they do not have a primary role in immunopathogenesis. Macrophages within the lesions are recruited to the CNS from the periphery and/or are derived from resident microglial cells.

Although a specific autoantigen has not been identified in MS, the working hypothesis is that there is a T-cell proliferative response to one or more myelin antigens. The early T-cell receptor specificities to myelin antigens may not reflect the T-cell receptor repertoire in established disease however, because of the phenomenon of epitope spreading, by which later in situ T cells acquire affinities for a greater range of autoantigens. Peripheral T cells from MS patients are reactive to multiple CNS myelin antigens, including myelin basic protein (MBP), proteolipid protein (PLP), myelin-associated glycoprotein (MAG), and myelin oligodendrocyte glycoprotein (MOG). However, normal individuals also harbor T cells reactive to MBP and PLP.

If MS is caused by activated, myelin-autoreactive T cells, it implies a breakdown of the mechanisms of immune tolerance. Central immune tolerance is established in the thymus early in development and involves both positive and negative selection processes to select T cells that recognize MHC antigens and eliminate those that have an affinity for autoantigens. Peripheral immune tolerance is maintained by active suppression of potentially autoreactive cells. It is not known how tolerance to antigens is acquired in the CNS, as the latter is normally a privileged site with respect to the immune system. Evidence that T-cell exposure to MBP takes place outside the

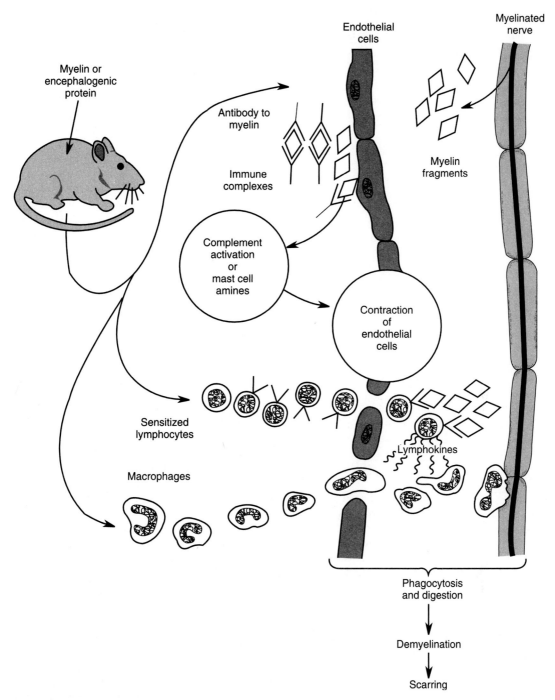

Figure 12–11. *Mouse model of inflammatory demyelination: experimental allergic encephalomyelitis (EAE).*

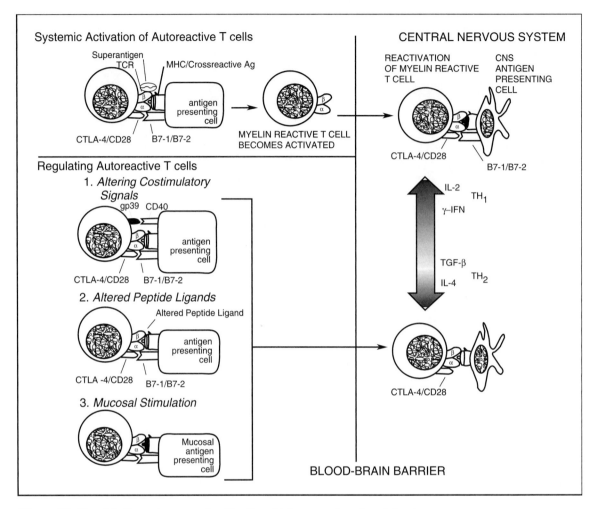

Figure 12–12. *Myelin antigen-reactive T cells, which are activated and develop into Th₁ cells, can traffic to the CNS, and cause inflammation and demyelination. Under different activating conditions (altered costimulatory signals, altered peptide ligans, mucosal presentation) antigen-specific cells of a Th₂ phenotype develop, and these can regulate the proinflammatory action of Th₁ cells. With permission from Windhagen et al., 1996.*

CNS, however, comes from the discovery of the Golli-MBP gene (for gene expressed in the oligodendrocyte lineage). This gene, which is expressed in the fetal thymus, spleen, and white blood cells, may provide a mechanism for the positive or negative selection of MBP-reactive T cells in the thymus.

Studies are being conducted to determine whether there are limited sets of pathogenic T-cell clones in MS patients. Much of this work has focused on T-cell alpha-beta chain receptor specificities, as determined by gene rearrangements and antigen-induced proliferation studies. Brain tissue, cerebrospinal fluid, and peripheral blood from patients all serve as sources of T cells for these studies. In some cases of MS, and in rodent EAE, activated T cells are found with a limited repertoire of variable region alpha-beta receptors, which may or may not be specifically reactive to particular peptide fragments of MBP. When comparing different patients and animal strains, MBP-reactive T cells show wide variability in receptor gene expression and MHC specificity. The fact that individuals who are HLA DR2+ have a greater risk of MS implies that specific T-cell receptor interactions are important. Steinman and collaborators have shown that persons who are HLA DR2+ have major B-cell and T-cell responses to peptide fragments of MBP within the 84 to 103 peptide region (Steinman et al., 1995).

Such work has therapeutic implications for the design of peptides that may block or stimulate protective responses by altering disease-causing T-cell receptor–antigen-MHC interactions. This approach, using a number of different peptides, has experimental validation in EAE and is in the early stages of clinical trials.

Other subtypes of T cells may also have pathogenic roles in MS. Thus, T cells bearing receptors with gamma-delta chains (versus alpha-beta chains for CD4 and CD8 cells) are also found in plaques.

A number of pathophysiologic mechanisms through which the autoreactive response in MS takes place can be postulated. These include the binding of viral or bacterial antigens to T-cell receptors that are potentially autoreactive to myelin antigens (molecular mimicry) and the polyclonal activation of T cells by the binding of microbial toxins (superantigens) to common beta receptor chains.

An early step in the pathogenesis of demyelination is the diapedesis of activated lymphocytes across tight junctions of brain endothelial cells into the perivascular spaces. As indicated previously, endothelial cells may play a role in presenting antigen to T cells through induced MHC class I and II receptors. Brain endothelial cells also facilitate T-cell transmigration, however, through the increased expression of adhesion molecules. These include ICAM-1 (intracellular adhesion molecule) and VCAM (vascular cell adhesion molecules), which attach to their corresponding ligands, LFA-1 (lymphocyte function antigen) and VLA-4 (very late activation antigen), respectively. Activated lymphocytes also express a class of enzymes called matrix metalloproteinases, which degrade type IV collagen of the extracellular matrix and facilitate migration.

A number of coreceptors and cytokines are active in the initiation, maintenance, and regulation of the local immune response. The trimolecular complex of T-cell receptor, antigen, and MHC imparts specificity to the immune response. Other receptor-mediated signals, however, are required for T-cell activation. One such signal comes from the engagement of coreceptor B7.1 on antigen-presenting cells to its corresponding ligand, CTLA-4, on lymphocytes. In the absence of this coreceptor interaction, the T cell becomes anergic to the presented antigen. Blocking this interaction using CTLA-4Ig prevents EAE and graft rejection, and may lead to another therapeutic approach for treating MS.

Other cytokine signals within the local CNS microenvironment may influence the subtypes and interactions of effector cells. Thus, CD4+ helper T cells differentiate into a TH-1 phenotype in the presence of interferon-γ (INF-γ and IL-12, and they in turn produce IL-2 and interferon-γ. The principal function of TH-1 cells is to mediate delayed type hypersensitivity responses, which leads to the activation of macrophages. The TH-1 cells are thought to mediate the pathologic effects of MS. The CD4+ helper T cells that have a TH-2 phenotype participate in antibody generation by B cells and this subset of T cells produces IL-4, -5, -6, and -10. A TH-3 phenotype, which produces transforming growth factor beta (TGF-β), has also been identified.

It is known that INF-γ stimulates macrophages to release TNF-α, and reactive nitrogen oxide metabolites and other free radical species which are toxic to myelin and oligodendrocytes. The T cells produce TNF-β (lymphotoxin) which can cause apoptosis in cultured oligodendrocytes. Moreover, interferon-γ activates and enhances the microbicidal function of macrophages and induces MHC class II expression on a variety of cells within the CNS, including endothelial cells, astrocytes, and microglia. In addition, activated macrophages express MHC class II and Fc receptors, and produce interleukin-1, and tumor necrosis factor alpha (TNF-α), all of which may contribute to pathogenesis.

Interferon-γ (type II interferon) in MS. The immune stimulatory effects of INF-γ have emerged as central to the pathophysiology of multiple sclerosis. Patients having acute attacks of MS display elevations of interferon-γ–secreting cells both in unstimulated and MBP-stimulated peripheral mononuclear cell cultures (PBMC). There is evidence of increased interferon-γ expression preceding clinical attacks in patients and increased interferon-γ in active multiple sclerosis plaques. Furthermore, interferon-γ promotes the expression of adhesion molecules on endothelial cells and increases the CD4+ T cells' proliferative response to mitogenic stimulation through a transmembrane calcium channel. This phenomenon may have some correlation to disease course as measured by clinical activity and cranial MRI. Experimental evidence that patients with chronic progressive MS have enhanced production of IL-12, may account for the increased production of interferon-γ by stimulated CD4+ cells also observed in these patients. A clinical study using interferon-γ to treat patients with relapsing-remitting MS resulted in an increase in exacerbations during the first month, halting the study (Panitch, 1987). Patients displayed INF-γ dose-dependent increases in activated monocytes (HLA-DR2+) in peripheral blood.

Immune counterregulation in MS. Counterregulatory influences on plaque pathogenesis may include CD8+ T suppressor cells. In addition, a number of cytokines have been shown to reduce inflammatory demyelination, the most important of which are interferon-β and interferon-α, the type I interferons. In active, demyelinating lesions, interferon-α and interferon-β staining is found on macrophages, lymphocytes, astrocytes, and endothelial cells, with interferon-β being the predominant cytokine found in endothelial cells in unaffected white matter. INF-β blocks some of the proinflammatory effects of INF-γ, including MHC class II antigen expression on cultured human astrocytes, and in other experimental systems it induces HLA-DR expression on cells. Additionally, INF-β blocks EAE in laboratory animals following systemic or intrathecal administration and increases suppressor cell function in vitro.

Electrophysiology of Demyelination

A number of pathophysiologic changes result in abnormal action potential conduction in demyelinated, but structurally intact, axons (Waxman, 1982). Stripped of its high-resistance, low-capacitance myelin sheath, the axon fails to carry a sufficient electrical charge to depolarize the membrane at the nodes (Fig. 12-5). The break in fast, saltatory conduction along the nodes of Ranvier is reflected in decreased conduction velocity and conduction block (Fig. 12-5). Clinically, this is best exemplified by tests of the optic nerve and chiasm. The visual evoked potential test (VEP) involves the measurement of an occipital signal (P100) by surface EEG electrodes in response to a changing visual stimulus. An increased P100 latency corresponds to demyelination and inflammation of the optic tracts in acute optic neuritis. The P100 latencies often continue to be abnormally prolonged after vision returns to normal (Fig. 12-13). It may also be prolonged in the absence of a history of visual loss, reflecting subclinical demyelination of the optic nerve. Other evoked potential tests measure, in a similar manner, conduction in myelinated afferent nerve tracts using auditory and somatic sensory stimuli. Demyelination produces other clinically measurable changes as well. Temporal dispersion of action potentials as a result of different degrees of demyelination results in different axons conducting at different speeds. Presumably this accounts for the earlier loss of vibratory sensation compared with other modalities with diseases of peripheral and central myelin (Fig. 12-5).

Destabilization of the demyelinated axonal membrane may give rise to autonomous local generation of action potentials and possibly abnormal ephaptic transmission from axon to axon. These phenomena appear to account for the "positive" symptoms of MS, including paresthesias, pain, and paroxysmal movements. These often respond to treatment with sodium channel blockers, such as carbamazepine and phenytoin. Reversible, temperature-dependent changes in the conduction properties of demyelinated axons account for the tendency for signs and symptoms in some MS patients to worsen when body temperature is elevated (Fig. 12-14).

The molecular organization of the myelinated axon. The nodal membrane of the axon is highly specialized for generation of action potentials, whereas the internodal membrane is relatively refractory to depolarization. This is primarily due to the 100-fold greater density of sodium channels at the node compared with the internode. The node also contains slow potassium channels, which modulate the prolonged depolarization that occurs with high-frequency firing. The paranodal part of the axon membrane adjacent to the node contains a relatively high density of fast potassium channels, which are rapidly activated to hyperpolarize the axon. This may serve to prevent aberrant re-excitation at the node. As a result of the low sodium channel density in the internodal portion of the axon membrane, demyelination exposes membrane that acts as a site of current loss but does not contribute to depolarization. This is a major reason for impairment of conduction in actively demyelinated axons.

Changes are observed in chronically demyelinated axons that may partially restore conduction and may account for some improvement in symptoms after an acute demyelinating attack. Continuous, but not saltatory, conduction may be restored by increases in sodium channel densities along previous internodal regions. Although the source of these channels is unknown, they could arise from the neuronal cell body or astrocytes configures to the segment of demyelinated axon.

Restoration of conduction in demyelinated fibers has been demonstrated with 4-aminopyridine (4-AP), which blocks fast potassium channels. In contrast, 4-AP has minimum effects on intact axon, presumably because myelin covers fast potassium channels, making them inaccessible to the drug. The clinical utility of 4-AP has been suggested from studies with MS patients and those with Lambert-Eaton myasthenic syndrome. In MS, the drug improves objective measures of visual function, including VEP latency, contrast sensitivity, and other aspects of neurologic function. Patients responding to the drug are more likely to have temperature-sensitive symptoms, a longer duration of disease, and more advanced disability. The ability of 4-AP to lower conduction thresholds is apparent in some of its side effects, including paresthesias, dizziness, restlessness, and confusion, and, in higher serum concentrations, generalized tonic-clonic seizures. As of this time, clinical testing of this drug in MS is continuing.

DIAGNOSIS

An attractive hypothesis, based on epidemiologic data, is that clinical MS represents the final stage of a disease process that begins prior to adulthood. According to this scheme, there is an induction phase, which occurs before the age of 15 in a genetically susceptible individual exposed to unknown immune trigger in the environment. This is followed by an asymptomatic latent period, during which there may be biological evidence of demyelination without clinical signs or symptoms. Clinical manifestations begin with an individual's first attack or subacute onset of symptoms. Estimates of the time interval from acquisition to clinical expression of the disease range from 1 to 20 years. Occasionally, MRIs performed for other purposes show typical patterns of demyelination in patients without clinical signs or symptoms of demyelinating disease. The term "latent" MS has

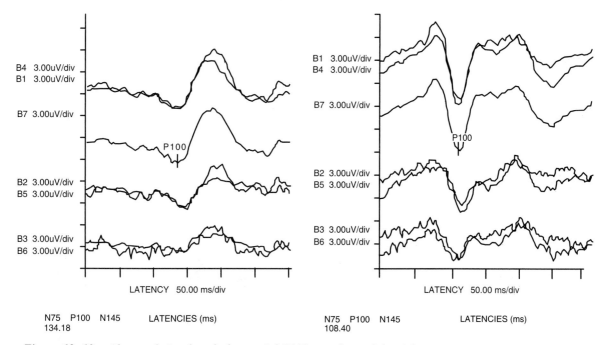

N75 P100 N145   LATENCIES (ms)
134.18

N75 P100 N145   LATENCIES (ms)
108.40

Figure 12–13. Abnormal visual evoked potential P100 waveform of the right eye (left diagram) with slowing (134 ms) compared with the left eye (108 ms) and loss of wave amplitude. Patient had optic neuritis 3 years previously and some mild visual disturbances 1 month before this test. Visual acuity was normal at testing. The technique: A black-and-white checkerboard pattern is displayed in front of a subject in a dark room. Each eye is tested separately. The pattern is alternately shifted one square horizontally to produce a pattern reversal, which is synchronized with the computer acquisition of signal by surface scalp electrodes. The waveform is a signal-averaged composite of many trials. The most characteristic abnormal response in optic neuritis is the delay of a large positive deflection at 100 ms (the P100 wave), but a variable decrease in amplitude can occur and the wave may be absent altogether.

also been used to describe individuals who have evidence of a demyelinating process without clinical expression of the disease.

A careful medical history of patients presenting with their first defined neurologic episode frequently reveals one or more past instances of transient symptoms, such as mild visual changes, numbness or tingling, or gait imbalance. These symptoms may or may not have been accorded any particular significance at the time they were experienced. In other patients, earlier episodes of extreme fatigue or difficulty concentrating may be reported (Table 12-4).

The acute episode that drives the patient to seek medical attention may not be associated with any inciting factors. Patients frequently recall, however, a temporal association with an infection, stressful period, trauma, or pregnancy. Symptoms may be fully developed when first noticed, as on awakening, or may become maximal over a variable period of time ranging from a few minutes to days. A progression of symptoms is often reported by patients, with a "stroke-like" onset being unusual. Symptoms caused by these inflammatory demyelinating events are termed attacks, exacerbations, or relapses. Individuals whose disease course is typified by these attacks are termed relapsing-remitting. The degree

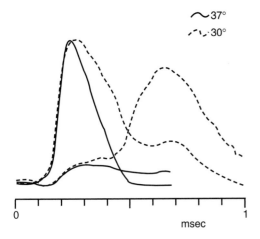

~37°
··30°

0   msec   1

Figure 12–14. Temperature-dependent characteristics of demyelinated fibers. Action potentials at two adjacent nodes of fiber demyelinated with diphtheria toxin. At 37° C (solid lines) conduction is blocked. At 30° C (dashed lines) action potential at first node is prolonged, and second node is excited more than 300 ms later. With permission from Sears, Bostock, 1981.

of remission from attacks is highly variable but, commonly in the early stages of the disease, it may begin soon after symptoms peak and be complete or well underway within 6 to 8 weeks. Those whose MS begins with an insidious onset of neurological symptoms are termed chronic progressive and are less likely to experience resolution, but their symptoms may appear to stabilize for periods of time. At the time of the first attack it is important to consider the possibility of acute demyelinating encephalomyelitis (ADEM), a nonrecurrent attack of demyelination.

A relationship between age and type of presenting symptom was noted in a study of 1096 patients (Weinshenker et al., 1989). The results revealed a greater likelihood of patients developing chronic motor weakness and hence a progressive course, after age 40 (Table 12-5).

Diagnostic Criteria

There are several classification schemes for MS. All have in common the definition of clinically definite

Table 12-4
Frequency of initial symptoms (left) and symptoms during the course of illness (right).

Symptom	Incidence	Symptom	Incidence
Sensory disturbance of limbs	33%	Balance abnormalities	78%
Disturbance of gait and balance	18%	Impaired sensation	71%
Visual loss in one eye	17%	Fatigue	65%
Double vision	13%	Paraparesis	62%
Progressive weakness	10%	Urinary disturbance	62%
Acute myelitis syndrome	6%	Sexual disturbance	60%
Sensory disturbance of face	3%	Visual loss in one eye	55%
L'hermitte's symptom	3%	Weakness of one limb	52%
Pain	2%	Incoordination of limbs	45%
		Double vision	43%
		Abnormal sensory experiences	40%
		Pain	25%
		Facial paralysis	15%
		Epilepsy	5%
		Hearing loss	4%
		Facial pain (tic douloreux)	2%

With permission from Scheinberg LC, Smith CR, 1987.

Table 12-5

Initial presentation in a total clinic population

Age at onset (yrs)	n	Percentage with initial presentation					
		Optic neuritis	Sensory	Motor (acute)	Motor (insidious)	Diplopia and/or vertigo	Limb ataxia and/or impairment of balance
<20	131	22.9	46.5	6.1	3.8	17.6	13.7
20–29	435	22.8	52.2	7.3	6.2	12.4	11.3
30–39	310	13.2	44.2	6.8	14.5	11.0	14.8
40–49	173	9.2	33.5	2.9	30.6	16.8	12.7
>49	47	6.3	31.9	4.2	46.8	12.8	10.6
Total	1096	17.2	45.4	6.2	13.9	12.9	13.2

With permission from Weinshenker et al., 1989.

MS (Table 12-6) which, by history and examination, requires two or more attacks in the CNS white matter separated by time and location, establishing both temporal and spatial dissemination of lesions. The episodes must be separated by at least 1 month with-

Table 12-6

The Schumacher criteria for the diagnosis of "clinically definite" MS

1. Age of onset between 10 and 50 years
2. Objective neurologic signs present on examination
3. Neurologic symptoms and signs indicative of CNS white-matter disease
4. Dissemination in time: (a) two or more attacks (lasting at least 24 h) and separated by at least 1 month (an attack is defined as the appearance of new symptoms or signs or worsening of previous ones); or (b) progression of symptoms and signs for at least 6 months
5. Dissemination in space: two or more noncontiguous anatomical areas involved
6. No alternative clinical explanation

Adapted with permission from Miller AE, 1990.

out interval continuous worsening, and must not be due to a single anatomical lesion of the neuroaxis. For example, ocular symptoms with unilateral somatic motor findings or crossed sensory loss of the face and body, may be caused by single brain-stem lesions. This definition does not include recurrent optic neuritis in the same eye as a separate lesion.

To account for purely progressive forms of the disease, a pattern of progressive neurologic dysfunction for at least 6 months in the absence of another cause also meets the criteria (Schumacher et al., 1965). As there is no specific diagnostic test for MS, the constellation of clinical signs and symptoms and radiographic and laboratory results provide the basis for the diagnosis. The terms "probable" or "possible" MS have been incorporated into classifications when evidence exists for only one attack or one lesion, or when attacks cannot be corroborated by physical evidence.

Since the publication of these classifications, several diagnostic tests have enhanced the sensitivity and specificity of the diagnosis of MS (Table 12-7). The importance of MRI and evoked potentials is discussed in the preceding. The most characteristic CSF finding is the presence of intrathecally produced immunoglobulin. This is usually determined by an index comparing CSF to serum IgG, corrected for albumin levels (Table 12-8). A qualitative measure is the presence of oligoclonal protein banding in the

Table 12-7

Evaluations that may be useful in the diagnosis and management of MS in individual patients

Test	Remarks
MRI scans of the brain and/or spine	T1, T2, proton density, gadolinium-enhanced, FLAIR images
Cerebrospinal fluid exam	Protein, cells, glucose, lyme testing, IgG index, oligoclonal bands, VDRL
Evoked potentials	Visual, brain-stem auditory, somatosensory
Neuropsychological testing	
Urodynamic studies	
Serologies	ANA with extractable nuclear antigens (rho, la, rnp); anticardiolipin antibodies, angiotensin converting enzyme levels, serum lyme titers, B_{12} level.

γ-globulin spectrum measured by immunofixation or isoelectric focusing. The presence of two or more oligoclonal bands in CSF that are not detected in serum constitutes a positive test. Other CSF parameters common in MS are shown in Table 12-9. These and other tests have been incorporated into the most recent diagnostic criteria for MS (Poser et al., 1983). The Poser criteria allow "paraclinical" evidence provided by diagnostic testing to fulfill the requirement for a second, spatially separate lesion (Table

Table 12-8

Calculation of CSF IgG Index

$$\text{CSF IgG Index} = \frac{\text{CSF IgG/CSF albumin}}{\text{serum IgG/serum albumin}}$$

12-10). Furthermore, the term "laboratory-supported" definite MS applies to patients who do not meet the criteria for "clinically definite" MS but have elevated CSF IgG or oligoclonal bands.

The diagnostic value of ancillary tests. More than 90% of patients with clinically definite MS have an abnormal MRI scan and more than two-thirds have elevated CSF γ-globulins or oligoclonal bands. Although an MRI is not required to confirm the diagnosis of clinically definite MS, imaging is more sensitive than a CSF exam or evoked potentials (EPs) in identifying patients with suspected multiple sclerosis. Certain MRI criteria for the diagnosis of MS are both sensitive and specific: 1) the presence of three or four abnormal signal intensities on proton density

Table 12-9

CSF parameters in MS

Total protein
   Normal in 60% of MS patients
   >110 mg/dL very rare
Leukocytes
   Normal in 66%
   >5 lymphocytes/mm³ in 33%
   Irregularly correlated with exacerbation
   Lymphocyte subsets:
      >80% CD3 +
      2:1 ratio of CD4 + : CD8 +
      16–18% B lymphocytes
      Plasma cells rarely found
Glucose
   Normal
Immunoglobulin (IgG)
   Increased in amount
   Increased IgG index (>0.7)
   Increased IgG synthetic rate (>3.3 mg/day)
   Oligoclonal IgG bands
   Increased ratio kappa/lambda light chains
   Free kappa light chains
Tissue markers
   Increased MBP-like material in active phases

With permission from Whitaker JN, Benveniste EN, Zhou S, 1990.

Table 12-10

Diagnostic criteria for multiple sclerosis

I. Clinically definite multiple sclerosis
   A. Two attacks and clinical evidence of two separate lesions
   B. Two attacks: clinical evidence for one lesion and paraclinical (CT, MRI, EP) evidence of another, separate lesion

II. Laboratory-supported definite multiple sclerosis
   The laboratory support is the demonstration in CSF of oligoclonal bands (OB) or increased synthesis of IgG. The serum banding pattern and IgG should be normal. Other causes of CSF changes, such as syphilis, subacute sclerosing panencephalitis, sarcoidosis, collagen vascular disease, and similar disorders, should be excluded.
   A. Two attacks; either clinical or paraclinical evidence of one lesion; and CSF OB/IgG
   B. One attack; clinical evidence of two separate lesions, and CSF OB/IgG
   C. One attack; clinical evidence of one lesion and paraclinical evidence of another, separate lesion; and CSF OB/IgG

III. Clinically probable multiple sclerosis
   A. Two attacks and clinical evidence of one lesion
   B. One attack and clinical evidence of two separate lesions
   C. One attack; clinical evidence of one lesion and paraclinical evidence of another, separate lesion

IV. Laboratory-supported probable multiple sclerosis
   A. Two attacks and CSF OB/IgG

With permission from Brass LM, Stys PK, 1991.

or T2-weighted images; 2) lesions in a periventricular location; 3) lesion size greater than 5 mm, and 4) infratentorial lesions. These criteria were 96% specific and 81% sensitive in correctly classifying 1500 consecutive cranial MRI scans on patients with clinical evidence of MS (Offenbacher et al., 1993). Other characteristic MRI lesions include elliptical lesions located adjacent to the lateral ventricles perpendicular to the anteroposterior axis of the brain, corresponding to Dawson's fingers, and are lesions originating along the inferior aspect of the corpus callosum.

Brain MRI scanning also gives prognostic information on an individual's risk of developing MS after a clinically isolated attack consistent with a demyelinating event with both the presence and number of lesions in the cerebral white matter being predictive (Morrissey, 1993) (Table 12-10).

Although brain and spinal cord imaging is a necessary adjunct to the clinical diagnosis of MS, sole reliance or inaccurate interpretation of MRI findings can lead to an erroneous diagnosis because a number of other disorders have a similar radiographic appearance. Moreover, nonspecific T2-weighted signal abnormalities increase beyond 40 years of age.

Cardinal Signs and Symptoms by Region

Visual pathways. Inflammation and demyelination of the optic nerve and chiasm are common in MS, with optic neuritis occurring in nearly 20% of patients as their first symptom, and in 70% of patients during the course of the illness. A high percentage of patients who present with isolated optic neuritis later develop MS. One prospective study found a conversion rate to MS in 74% of women and 34% of men by 15 years following a first episode of optic neuritis. Others found rates of conversion of 20 to 30% over a shorter time span. In these studies, the risk of conversion to MS after optic neuritis has also been found to be higher in women.

Optic neuritis is commonly reported as an acute loss of vision developing over several days to a week. Often, mild discomfort or pain on movement of the affected eye, or in the periorbital area, precedes or accompanies the visual loss. Unilateral optic nerve involvement is far more common than bilateral or sequential presentations. The visual loss usually involves a decrease in both light sensitivity and color saturation alone or in combination with an altitudinal field deficit or enlarged central scotoma. In acute optic neuritis, direct ophthalmoscopic examination of the affected eye may reveal a pale or swollen optic disk depending on the proximity of the involved segment to the optic nerve head. Other abnormalities can be demonstrated by dilated indirect ophthalmoscopic examination. These abnormalities include paleness around the peripheral retinal venules (perivenous sheathing), focal leakage of fluid demonstrated by fluorescein angiogram, and cells in the vitreous. These modifications occur in the absence of myelinated fibers in the retina and suggest that changes in vascular permeability may be a primary event in MS and not just secondary to demyelination.

Abnormal visual evoked responses are highly sensitive in the diagnosis of acute optic neuritis and in detecting past episodes in which there is no noticeable optic atrophy and vision has returned to normal. The main utility of visual evoked potentials in the diagnosis of MS is in the detection of subclinical involvement of the optic pathways to establish the presence of multiple lesions in the central nervous system, particularly in the differential diagnosis of spinal cord disease or in cases of possible or probable MS.

A useful symptom associated with subclinical optic neuropathy is Uhtoff's phenomenon. Although it has many causes, Uhtoff's phenomenon is most frequently encountered in connection with demyelinating lesions of the optic tracts. Uhtoff's phenomenon is characterized by deterioration of vision in one or both eyes associated with an elevation of body temperature due to fever, exercise, hot weather, etc. It may be brought on by other circumstances as well, such as exposure to bright lights, emotional stress, or fatigue. When the precipitant associated with visual loss is removed, the vision returns to normal.

A bedside test for acute, chronic, or subclinical optic neuropathy relies on Marcus Gunn's phenomenon. This is the tendency of both eyes to redilate when the affected eye is subjected to continuous, direct light stimulation. A positive test demonstrates the effects of interruption of the afferent light pathway in the affected eye on the pupillary reflexes of both the affected (direct response) and unaffected eye (consensual response). It can best be demonstrated by the swinging flashlight test in a darkened room with each eye alternately exposed to direct light. With direct light stimulation on the unaffected side, both the ipsilateral and affected contralateral pupils constrict normally because of a normal direct and consensual response. Direct light stimulation of the affected side, however, affects constriction in both eyes because both the consensual and direct pupillary reflex require an intact afferent arc. Like visual evoked potentials, Marcus Gunn's phenomenon may remain persistently abnormal despite the return of full vision following an episode of optic neuritis, or may be abnormal with subclinical involvement of the optic nerve. Although optic neuritis may be idiopathic, or associated with demyelinating disease, it may also occur with infection (syphilis, lyme, tuberculosus, contiguous sinusitis, several viruses, some of which occur with immunodeficiency associated with AIDS) or other systemic inflammatory diseases (sarcoid, Behçet's, lupus erythematosus). Severe bilateral visual loss, either concurrently or in succession due to optic neuropathy, occurs in Leber's hereditary optic neuropathy, a mitochondrial disease predominantly affecting males. Interestingly, although the Leber's mitochondrial DNA mutation has been found in a small group of patients with otherwise typical MS and severe visual loss, it does not appear to determine genetic susceptibility to MS.

The prognosis is generally favorable for recovery from an initial attack of optic neuritis, with the period of recovery being 4 to 6 weeks. For milder degrees of visual loss, there is a 70% chance of recovering normal vision within 6 months. This result does not appear to be influenced by treatment with corticotropin or corticosteroids. The chance for visual recovery when acute visual loss is moderate or severe, however, is favorably influenced by such treatments. The timing of corticosteroid therapy may be relevant to the degree of recovery, with early use thought to be more effective than delayed treatment.

Spinal cord.   The spinal cord is frequently affected in MS patients with either acute or long-standing disease. Cord involvement is likely to be responsible for symptoms such as sensory loss, paresthesias, and motor weakness, especially when they begin bilaterally. Incoordination of gait, bladder and bowel dysfunction, erectile sexual dysfunction, and pain are also symptoms commonly associated with spinal cord lesions. Dystonias or myoclonus are reported, although they may occur with brain-stem involvement as well.

Spinal cord dysfunction can occur acutely, as in transverse myelitis, subacutely, or insidiously. The cervical spinal cord is affected about-two thirds of the time, followed by the thoracic spinal cord. Altered sensation resulting from incomplete transverse myelitis may occur in nearly half of patients as their initial symptom of MS. Sensory symptoms typically begin in the distal extremities and travel proximally. They build to a maximum over a few days to a week or two, and resolve over a similar period in the reverse order in which they appeared. A tingling pins-and-needles sensation, or numbness, ascends from the distal lower extremities to the trunk or involves the arm and leg of the same side. Sensory deficits are rarely complete and usually produce few objective findings on examination. Paresthesias are almost invariant. There may or may not be complaints of urinary hesitancy or urgency and upper motor neuron signs (i.e. deep tendon reflexes) may be increased, normal, or, rarely, diminished, with a Babinski sign present or absent. Loss of superficial abdominal reflexes (if not caused by abdominal surgery) is a sensitive sign of spinal cord disease.

Patients may complain that head movements precipitate sharp pain or paresthesias that radiate from the neck down the back, or to the arms or the legs. This is the L'hermitte's sign which indicates the presence of a lesion in the cervical spinal cord that is stimulated by slight stretching of the cord when the neck is flexed. Although suggestive of MS, L'hermitte's sign is not pathognomonic and can occur in other disorders, including spinal cord trauma, vitamin B_{12} deficiency, radiation myelitis, herpes zoster infection, and spinal cord compression.

Other symptoms include the acute or insidious onset of spastic monoparesis, paraparesis, or hemiparesis, which, like the sensory deficits, are rarely complete at onset. Mixed motor and sensory involvement, usually loss of vibration or position sense, is the rule. Upper motor neuron signs are, more often than not, bilaterally present even when weakness is noticed in only one limb.

MRI is the procedure of choice for evaluating the spinal cord for intramedullary lesions, vascular malformations, developmental anomalies, or extramedullary compression. The MRI appearance of demyelinating plaques on sagittal section of the cord generally reveals a distinct hyperintense area on T2 or proton density images, with its long axis parallel to that of the cord. The area may span one or more cord segments, or be multifocal in different segments. Axial views may show lesions in the central cord involving both gray and white matter, or in the posterior, anterior, or lateral funiculi. Plaques frequently appear patchy on cross-sectional views of the cord.

Acute plaques that enhance with gadolinium and cause mild swelling of the cord may be mistaken for a tumor if they are solitary. Spinal cord atrophy, presumably due to axonal loss within demyelinated plaques, has been correlated with the degree of physical disability. As with optic neuritis and brainstem syndromes, the risk of progression to MS after a clinically isolated spinal cord syndrome is also increased dramatically by the presence of cerebral white matter lesions (Morrissey et al., 1993) (Table 12-11).

An attack of transverse myelitis that is incomplete, and therefore does not cause paraplegia, is more likely to lead to MS than complete transverse myelitis. The presence of oligoclonal bands in cerebrospinal fluid can distinguish patients with a first presentation of MS from those with postinfections. Viral infections of the spinal cord are accompanied by higher CSF cell counts and protein levels than are usually encountered in demyelinating disease. Disease localized to the spinal cord is more likely to lead to a progressive rather than a relapsing remitting course. Often the diagnosis of MS is complicated by the fact that brain MRI may be normal or show nondiagnostic white-matter abnormalities of a pattern that is commonly seen in older patients.

Brain stem and cerebellum. Demyelinating plaques in the posterior fossa (e.g. the brain stem and cerebellum) often cause disabling symptoms out of proportion to their size or number in comparison with other regions of the neuraxis. Indeed, disease in this location accounts for the classic Charcot's triad of symptoms in MS: nystagmus, intention tremor, and scanning speech. In the autopsy series of Ikuta and Zimmerman (1976), the proportion of cases in which the posterior fossa structures were free of any disease were, in descending order: midbrain (16%), cerebellum (13%), medulla (12%), pons (7%). These findings compare with disease-free areas of the optic nerve, cerebrum, and spinal cord of 1%, 3%, and 1% respectively. Although brain-stem involvement may cause symptoms that are seen in disease affecting other regions, such as hemiparesis or paraparesis and sensory deficits, specialized functions subserved in that region may also be affected, including conjugate eye movements, articulation, swallowing, and respiration. Plaques in the cerebellar subcortex and tracts cause limb and truncal ataxia, nystagmus, vertigo, and scanning dysarthric speech. Some patients who have intact motor strength are totally disabled because of severe ataxia in the trunk and limbs.

Table 12-11

Prognosis of clinically isolated syndromes related to presence of an abnormal MRI (top chart) and the number of lesions on MRI (lower chart)

Brain MRI at presentation and relationship to clinical outcome		
	MRI abnormal	MRI normal
Number of patients	57	32
Mean follow-up time (months)	64	63
Progression to multiple sclerosis		
All cases	41 (72%)	2 (6%)
Optic neuritis	23/28 (82%)	1/16 (6%)
Brainstem	8/12 (67%)	0/5
Spinal cord	10/17 (59%)	1/11 (9%)
Cases seen within 2 months of onset of symptoms	34/45 (76%)	1/29 (4%)

Number of brain lesions detected by MRI at presentation and relationship to clinical outcome				
	Number of lesions detected by MRI			
	0	1	2–3	4–10	>10
Number of patients	32	6	18	13	20
Progression to multiple sclerosis	2 (6%)	1 (17%)	12 (67%)	12 (92%)	16 (80%)
EDSS ≥3 at follow-up	0	0	3 (17%)	4 (30%)	11 (56%)
Mean number of new lesions detected by MRI at follow-up (range)	1.3 (0–12)	5 (0–11)	7.2 (0–26)	10.5 (0–26)	15.4 (0–38)

With permission from Morrissey et al., 1993.

Eye movement abnormalities. Although not specific to multiple sclerosis, a number of eye movement abnormalities are associated with this condition. The most characteristic is the uncoupling of eye movements on lateral gaze, known as intranuclear ophthalmoplegia (Fig. 12-15). This sign may be unilateral or bilateral, complete or incomplete. It occurs with lesions of the medial longitudinal fasciculus (MLF), a tract that connects the third nerve nucleus of one side (controls adduction of ipsilateral eye) with the sixth nerve nucleus of the opposite side (controls abduction of the ipsilateral eye). The eye ipsilateral to the lesion either cannot adduct or slowly adducts past the midline on gaze to the opposite side. The contralateral eye abducts fully in the same direction but overshoots with a coarse beating nystagmus. Although isolated ocular motor abnormalities are rare, when they occur the third and sixth cranial nerves are most commonly involved.

Other signs and symptoms. Trigeminal neuralgia may be present at the onset or during the course of MS. The prevalence of this condition was nearly 2%

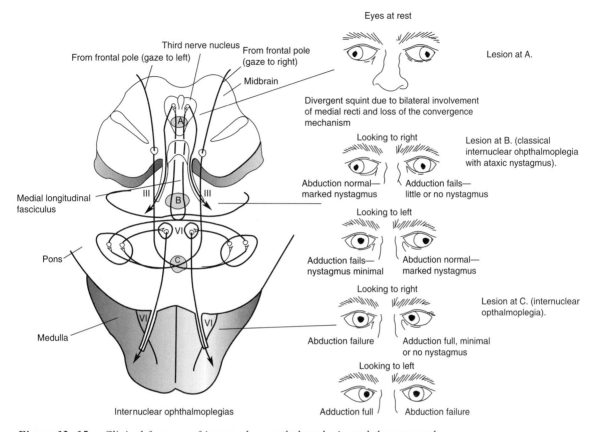

Figure 12–15. *Clinical features of internuclear opthalmoplegia and the neuronal connections responsible for conjugate eye movements. With permission from Patten, 1996.*

in a survey of a large MS population. A mild facial palsy with lower motor neuron features is present in some patients. A rare symptom that has been associated with MS and other disorders is facial myokymia, an undulating, wavelike, fascicular twitching of facial muscles. Involvement of the brain-stem respiratory centers leading to complications is usually a feature of advanced disease, but may also occur in acute relapses.

Cerebrum. Many plaques visualized in the subcortical white matter occur in "silent" areas of the brain and consequently are asymptomatic. Cerebral plaques may, however, uncommonly cause hemiparesis similar to that seen with stroke, hemisensory loss, cortical blindness, and aphasia. Cognitive deficits in MS are associated not only with total plaque burden but also with lesions in the corpus callosum. Cognitive deficits most commonly found in MS include reductions in short-term memory, abstract and conceptual reasoning, verbal fluency, and visuospatial reasoning. Extrapyramidal movement disorders are rare, but may be caused by plaques located in subcortical gray-matter structures, such as the basal ganglia, caudate nucleus, and subthalamic nuclei.

Some elements of the differential diagnosis. Issues relating to the differential diagnosis of MS are listed on Table 12-12. The most important clinical and pathologic variants of CNS demyelinating dis-

Table 12-12

Some conditions that could be mistaken for multiple sclerosis

Multifocal lesions, often with relapsing/remitting course	Remarks
Vasculitides	
Systemic lupus erythematosus	Clinical criteria for SLE. May cause neuromyelitis optica (see text). CSF oligoclonal bands may be positive.
Anticardiolipin antibody syndrome	Livido reticularis, hypercoagulable state (spontaneous abortion, deep vein thrombosis). Anticardiolipin antibodies, lupus anti-coagulant, false + VDRL. Gray as well as white matter affected, stroke and hemorrhages.
Sjögren's syndrome	Sicca syndrome. Anti-Ro (SS-A), La (SSB) antibodies.
Behçet's syndrome	Relapsing iridocyclitis, uveitis, oral and genital ulcerations. Meningoencephalitis. Abducens nerve palsy. More prevalent Japan, Near East, Mediterranean area, and men more than women.
Sarcoidosis	Cranial nerve palsies. Encephalopathy, mass lesions, hydrocephalus, menigitis, hypophyseal/hypothalamic involvement, seizures, uveitis. Peripheral nerve, muscle. Pulmonary involvement, fevers, weight loss, positive CSF oligoclonal bands. Angiotensin converting enzyme levels, calcium; polyclonal gammopathy.
Cerebrovascular occlusive disease	
Moyamoya disease, other intracranial vascular disease	Lesions following vascular distribution. Gray matter dysfunction (e.g., aphasia, visual field deficits) stroke-like onset. New onset hypertension, cardiovascular disease risk factors (e.g., diabetes, hypertension, smoking).
Spirochete infections	
Meningovascular syphilis	Meningitis, cranial nerve palsies, dementia, autonomic dysfunction, tabes dorsalis. Positive VDRL, FTA antibodies. Risk factors (e.g. HIV positivity)
Neuroborrelioses	Meningitis, cranial and peripheral neuropathies, dementia. Hx. erythema chronica migrans, migratory arthritis. Positive oligoclonal bands. Positive tests in serum and CSF for Borrelia burgdorferi (i.e. culture, ELISA, Western blot, PCR).
Other	
Paraneoplastic effects of malignant diseases	
Migrant sensory neuritis of Wartenberg	
Systemic histiocytosis X	

(*continued*)

Table 12-12

Some conditions that could be mistaken for multiple sclerosis (*continued*)

Symmetrical signs and symptoms, progressive course	*Remarks*

Multisystem atrophies
   Hereditary spinocerebellar ataxia, olivopontine
   cerebellar degeneration, Machado-Joseph disease.
   Familial spastic paraplegia
	Autosomal dominant or recessive. Pyramidal tract signs, cerebellar ataxia. Dystonias, spinal, brainstem, cerebellar atrophy. CSF without elevated IgG or oligoclonal bands.

Subacute combined degeneration of the cord (B$_{12}$ deficiency)	*Ataxic or spastic paraparesis with/without loss of patellar, achilles reflexes. Paresthesias in extremities. Mental signs, visual impairment. Low serum B$_{12}$, gastric achlorhdria, macrocytic anemia. Schilling test for B$_{12}$ absorption.*
Myelopathies due to infections *(myelitis-CMV, VZV, HSV; TSP&HAM-HTLV-1)*	*Meningoencephalitis. CSF pleocytosis. Follows acute viral illness. Edematous changes to necrotizing myelitis. Acute and convalescent viral titers, positive HTLV-1 antibodies in serum and CSF-oligoclonal bands present.*
Primary lateral sclerosis Dysmyelinating diseases (adult-onset metachromatic leukodystrophy (MLD), adrenoleukodystrophy (ALD), adrenomyeloneuropathy)	*Spastic quadriparesis, pseudobulbar affect, dysarthria, intact sensation. Onset fifth to sixth decade.* *Peripheral nerve involvement. Recessive or X-linked recessive (carrier state may be symptomatic).* *MLD: personality changes, dementia may be initial findings. arylsulfatase A.* *ALD: adrenal failure, spastic paraparesis. Very long chain fatty acids.*
Spondylytic myelopathy	

Single lesions, often a relapsing-remitting course	*Remarks*
Spinal cord tumors	*Meningioma (foramen magnum), Schwannomas (extradural dumbbell shape), lipomas (ass. with spinal dysraphic states), chordomas (basisphenoid, sacrococcygeal area), astrocytomas (fusiform enlargement), metastases, ependymomas (filum terminatle, cauda equina). Signs and symptoms vary: local pain, L'hermitte's sign, bony involvement, long tract signs, sensory level.*
Primary CNS lymphoma	*Cerebrum, cerebellum, brainstem. Periventricular location common. Unifocal or multifocal. Behavioral, personality changes, increased intracranial pressure. Immunodeficiency (HIV, Wiskott-Aldrich syndrome, ataxia-telangiectasia) or immunosuppressed states (e.g. renal transplantation).*

(*continued*)

Table 12-12

Some conditions that could be mistaken for multiple sclerosis (*continued*)

Single lesions, often a relapsing-remitting course	Remarks
Arteriovenous malformations of the spinal cord (spinal dural AV fistulas, cavernous malformations)	*Dural fistulas occur in lower thoracic and lumbar cord, occasionally intracranial. Onset middle age and older, in men more commonly than women. Symptoms exacerbate with exercise or due to venous thrombosis. Pain and progressive spastic paraparesis. Dx: MRI, myelogram, spinal arteriography.*
Arnold Chiari malformations Spinal cord syrinx Arachnoid cyst	*Suspended or "cape-like" distribution of disassociated sensory loss (impairment pain, temp). May exhibit periodic worsening with improvement.*

Modified from Brass LM, Stys PK, 1991.

ease are ADEM and Devic's neuromyelitis optica, both of which differ from MS in their prognoses and treatment.

Acute disseminated encephalomyelitis. Acute disseminated encephalomyelitis has clinical and pathologic features indistinguishable from early MS. It enters the differential when a patient presents with a clinically isolated episode of demyelination following an acute illness or vaccination, or it may occur without an antecedent event. Measles is the most common antecedent infection, followed by varicella, rubella, mumps, scarlet fever, and pertussis. The condition is most common in children and young adults. Acute optic neuritis is often bilateral when it occurs in connection with ADEM. Cerebrospinal fluid typically shows greater inflammatory changes, including blood cell counts with neutrophilic pleocytoses and elevated protein. The CSF oligoclonal bands are typically negative, or only transiently positive, during the acute phase. Although ADEM is usually monophasic and responds to corticosteroids or corticotrophin, multiphasic and recurrent variants have been described. Multiphasic ADEM is defined by one or more clinically distinct attacks following the original acute episode, and the recurrent variant by subsequent episodes that are clinically identical to the original attack. In ADEM and its variants, MRI may show small, multifocal T2-weighted signal abnormalities indicative of large, lobar masslike areas that may involve gray matter. Furthermore, features common in MS, namely, plaques in the periventricular white matter and corpus callosum, are not generally observed in ADEM.

Although a number of systemic inflammatory disorders can cause white-matter disease, CNS manifestations are seldom the sole or presenting feature. These diseases are usually distinguished by their extra-CNS signs and symptoms. The CNS systemic lupus erythematosus (SLE) causes infarcts or hemorrhages as a result of thrombosis or vasculitis. Psychosis, seizures, confusion, or somnolence may occur primary or secondary to infection or other organ failure. A myelitis or myelopathic picture, with or without a Devic's-like optic neuritis, may be associated with SLE, as may oligoclonal banding in the CNS. Other inflammatory diseases that may be associated with CSF oligoclonal banding include sarcoidosis and Behçet's disease; conversely, antinuclear antibodies may be found in as many as one third of MS patients.

Neuroborreliosis. Neuroborreliosis due to *Borrelia burgdorferi* infection may cause meningitis, encephalomyelitis, or peripheral neuropathy (CNS lyme disease). Encephalomyelitis is a rare complication of *Borrelia burgdorferi* infection (lyme borreliosis), occurring in less than 0.1% of all cases (Halperin et al., 1996). Where lyme disease is endemic, occasional patients who have otherwise typical signs, symptoms, and laboratory findings of MS, and no objective evidence for CNS lyme infection, may be inappropriately treated by some physicians with prolonged courses of intravenous antibiotics (personal observation). Typical CNS symptoms of lyme encephalomyelitis are memory impairment and cognitive dysfunction, although multifocal disease primarily involving CNS white matter is reported, and oligoclonal banding may be present in CSF. Objective evidence for CNS neuroborreliosis includes intrathecal production of specific antibody, positive CSF cultures or detection of *B. burgdorferi DNA* by polymerase chain reaction.

Tropical spastic paraparesis and HIV-associated myelopathy. Tropical spastic paraparesis (TSP) and HIV-associated myelopathy (HAM) are terms describing a chronic demyelinating inflammatory disease of the spinal cord caused by a retrovirus, human T-cell lymphotrophic virus type I (HTLV-I). This virus is endemic to areas of Japan, the West Indies, and South America. Features of TSP and HAM that are similar to MS include CSF oligoclonal bands and elevated IgG, the presence of white-matter abnormalities on cranial MRI, and a partial response to immunotherapies. However, TSP and HAM may be distinguished from MS by a finding of HTLV-1 antibodies or detection of HTLV-1 DNA by PCR, peripheral nerve involvement, serum oligoclonal banding, multilobed lymphocytes in CSF or blood, a positive serologic test for syphilis, a sicca syndrome, and pulmonary lymphocytic alveolitis.

Neuromyelitis optica. Neuromyelitis optica, also known as Devic's disease, is a variant of MS with distinct clinical and pathologic features. The clinical picture is that of an acute or subacute optic neuropathy and severe transverse myelopathy. The interval between the visual loss and myelopathy is usually less than 2 years but may be longer. Pathologic findings are limited to demyelination in the optic nerves and severe necrosis that may involve most of the spinal cord. Outside of the optic nerves and chiasm the brain appears normal. The CSF findings include a normal opening pressure, variable pleocytosis up to a few hundred white cells per mm with increased numbers of neutrophils and elevated protein. Oligoclonal banding and abnormal IgG synthesis in the CSF are typically absent. The disease may be monophasic or multiphasic and is reported in association with acute disseminated encephalomyelitis (ADEM), systemic lupus erythematosus, mixed connective tissue disease, and tuberculosis. The Devic's clinical picture is more common in Japan and it appears to have distinct immunogenetic characteristics. The prognosis for neurologic recovery is poor. Various treatments have been used with variable success, including alkylating agents such as cyclophosphamide, corticotropin, corticosteroids, and plasmapheresis.

Clinical Course and Natural History

There are a few well-recognized clinical patterns associated with MS that are used for classifying the condition into subtypes (Fig. 12-16). The clinical spectrum is dominated at one end by relapses followed by complete or nearly complete remissions and on the other end by insidious, nonremitting neurologic progression. These two forms are referred to as relapsing-remitting and primary progressive, respectively. The latter is distinguished from progression after a relapsing-remitting course, which is called secondary chronic progressive, or progression with infrequent relapses, which is progressive relapsing. The term "benign MS" has been abandoned in the new classification.

The clinical characteristics of MS may be associated with both age at presentation and initial symptoms. A relapsing-remitting course has a greater association with females and an earlier age presentation with sensory symptoms and optic neuritis. A progressive course is more likely in males and those who present in their fifth and sixth decades with insidious onset of motor weakness (Weinshenker et al., 1989).

Prognosis. In a survey of 1099 clinic patients, 51% were able to walk without assistance (Weinshenker et al., 1989). In this study, 66% of patients were relapsing-remitting at the onset of their disease versus 34% with some progressive features. The conversion rate from relapsing-remitting to chronic progressive was 12% within 5 years of diagnosis, 41% within 10 years, and 66% within 25 years.

In other studies, steady, although slow, rates of disease progression have been noted, with the proportion of patients with mild disease decreasing over time. The Weinshenker study found that, on average, the time from diagnosis to disability requiring some assistance to walk was 15 years for all patients, and 4.5 years for patients with progressive disease. These data on prognosis for relapsing-remitting patients are consistent with a study of 308 patients who were observed for 25 years (Runmarker and Anderson, 1993) (Fig. 12-17). Both studies found that being female and having a younger age of onset had a favorable prognosis, as did sensory attacks (including optic neuritis) with complete recovery, low frequency of attacks in the early years of the disease, and minimal disability after the first 5 years (Runmarker and Anderson, 1993; Weinshenker et al., 1991).

The biological factors underlying the variability in MS at the onset of the disease, and those that influence the conversion to a progressive course, are centrally important for scientific inquiry and designing a rational treatment plan for individual patients.

MRI studies. Insights have been gained in understanding the pathophysiology of MS and how it relates to the clinical course through serial MRI studies. Although the association between MRI-measured plaque volume and disability is variable in cross-sectional studies, increases in lesion area correspond to increases in disability in longitudinal studies (The INFB Multiple Sclerosis Study Group, 1995). Likewise, clinical disease activity accompanies new lesion activity as measured by gadolinium enhancement on T1. Lesions typically enlarge over a period of 2 to 4 weeks and then decrease in size at 6 weeks. Lesions that are hyperintense on T2 and hypointense on T1-weighted images may have clinical significance. These lesions may correspond to areas of gliosis, more severe demyelination, or greater axonal loss.

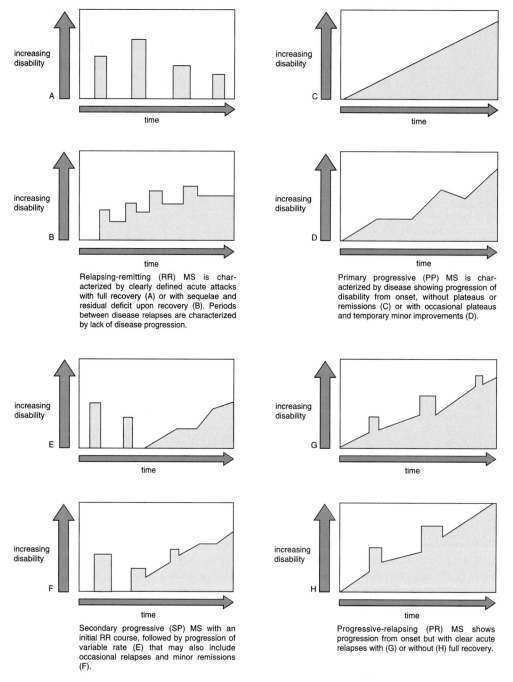

Relapsing-remitting (RR) MS is characterized by clearly defined acute attacks
with full recovery (A) or with sequelae and
residual deficit upon recovery (B). Periods
between disease relapses are characterized
by lack of disease progression.

Primary progressive (PP) MS is characterized by disease showing progression of
disability from onset, without plateaus or
remissions (C) or with occasional plateaus
and temporary minor improvements (D).

Secondary progressive (SP) MS with an
initial RR course, followed by progression of
variable rate (E) that may also include
occasional relapses and minor remissions
(F).

Progressive-relapsing (PR) MS shows
progression from onset but with clear acute
relapses with (G) or without (H) full recovery.

Figure 12–16.   *Four clinical patterns of MS. Reproduced with permission from
Lublin, Reingold, 1996.*

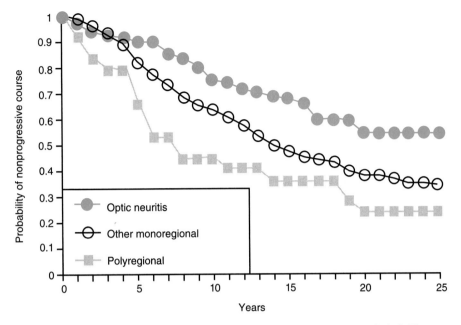

Figure 12–17. *Prognosis in patients with bout onset, possible MS included. The graph shows life-table analysis with the start of a progressive course as the endpoint. Onset symptoms from optic nerves compared with other monoregional symptoms and polyregional symptoms. With permission from Runmarker B, Anderson O, 1993.*

Serial MRI studies of patients with mild relapsing-remitting disease show new lesion activity from month to month and an increase in affected white matter over time, even in the absence of clinical signs of progression. It has been suggested that change in disease course from relapsing-remitting to chronic-progressive reflects this accumulation of demyelinating plaques.

Another variable is the degree of spinal cord involvement, which tends to be associated with more disability than cerebral disease. Serial MRI studies of patients with relapsing-remitting disease and secondary progressive disease show comparable increases in lesion activity over time. The MRI plaque volume of patients with primary progressive disease, however, is generally less than in patients with secondary progressive disease, with the lesions of the former being less likely to enhance after gadolinium administration.

PHARMACOTHERAPY

Drugs with anti-inflammatory and immunosuppressive actions are used to treat multiple sclerosis.

The goals of immunotherapy in MS are to improve the outcome from relapses, minimize the risk of future relapses, and delay or prevent neurologic progression of the disease. Glucocorticoids and corticotropin have had the longest and most widespread use in the treatment of MS. High-dose, intravenous methylprednisolone, the preferred glucocorticoid at this time, accelerates recovery and improves function over the short term during acute relapse. Neither this treatment nor the chronic use of oral steroids, however, appears to improve function over the long term, although a small minority of patients seem to become dependent on steroids to prevent relapse.

The past few years have witnessed the introduction of new immunomodulating drugs. Nonselective agents include the antiviral cytokine, interferon-β. There are two preparations of interferon-β approved for use in multiple sclerosis, interferon beta-1b and interferon beta-1a. A therapy purported to be a selective approach to therapy is glatiramer acetate.

The efficacy measurement for drugs used to treat MS relies primarily on neurologic examination, supplemented by quantitative MRI to measure plaque formation and activity. The most commonly used disability scale in these studies are the Kurtzke Functional Status Scale (FSS) and the Kurtzke Extended Disability Status Scale (EDSS), developed more than 30 years ago (Table 12-13). Both scales are ordinally based and rank neurologic functions commonly affected by MS.

Treatment of Acute Relapses

Glucocorticosteroids and corticotropin. In 1949, Dr. Phillip Hench reported that 14 patients with rheumatoid arthritis benefited from compound E (cortisone) and cortico-

Table 12-13

Milestones in the Kurtzke Disability Status Scale (EDSS)

0—normal neurologic examination

1 to 2.5—minimal disability in one or more functional systems (e.g. pyramidal, brain stem, sensory, cerebral/mental, cerebellar, bowel and bladder, visual, other)

3 to 4.5—moderate to marked disability in one or more functional systems, but able to walk at least 300 m at the upper range

5 to 5.5—marked disability in one or more functional systems. Able to walk without aid at least 100 m at the upper range

6—requires unilateral assistance (e.g. cane or crutch to walk at least 100 m)

6.5—requires bilateral assistance (e.g. walker, or two canes or crutches to walk at least 20 m)

7 to 7.5—wheelchair bound

8 to 8.5—restricted to bed

10—death due to MS

tropin treatment. The discovery of the clinically important anti-inflammatory effects of steroids won Dr. Hench and two chemists, E.C. Kendall and T. Reichstein, the Nobel Prize in Medicine or Physiology, and resulted in the wide application of these drugs for the treatment of autoimmune diseases and inflammatory states. The first use of these agents in multiple sclerosis was reported in 1950 when small groups of patients were treated in unblinded fashion with adrenocorticotropin hormone (ACTH). Although the studies could not prove ACTH was efficacious, patients seemed to improve with therapy. Although other uncontrolled studies of ACTH tended to show little or no effect on the chronic course of the disease, it appeared to be of some benefit in ameliorating relapses. Similarly, studies of ACTH in optic neuritis demonstrated significant improvements in the rate and extent of visual function within the first month of therapy, but with no differences between groups after 1 year (Myers, 1992). Although several studies using oral prednisone similarly reported improvement in function after relapses, chronic use of oral steroids for up to 2 years had no impact on neurologic progression.

In the early 1980s published reports of both open and blinded studies indicated that intravenous methylprednisolone improved short-term outcome in relapsing MS patients. Randomized studies comparing ACTH with intravenous methylprednisolone showed the latter was as effective as ACTH but had fewer side effects. Initial doses of intravenous methylprednisolone ranged from 20 mg/kg per day for 3 days to 1 g for 7 days. As a result of these findings, interest in corticotropin therapy has become largely historical since a short course of intravenous methylprednisolone is more convenient for patients and has fewer side effects than ACTH treatment.

Dose recommendations for intravenous methylprednisolone vary. The doses and duration of treatment in studies range from 500 to 1500 mg per day, in bolus or divided doses, for 3 to 10 days (Myers, 1992). The duration of therapy may be shortened if there is a rapid response, or lengthened if there is no improvement.

The risk with short courses of intravenous methylprednisolone therapy is small. Rarely, cardiac arrhythmias, anaphylactic reactions, and seizures are reported. These effects are minimized by infusing the drug over 2 to 3 h. It is best to administer the drug in a supervised medical setting when the patient is receiving it for the first time. Other adverse reactions to this agent when used in MS patients include minor infections (urinary tract infections, oral or vaginal candidiasis), hyperglycemia, gastrointestinal complaints (dyspepsia, gastritis, aggravation of a preexisting ulcer, acute pancreatitis), psychiatric symptoms (depression, euphoria, emotional lability), facial flushing, disturbance of taste, insomnia, mild weight gain, paresthesias, and exacerbation of acne. There is also a well-defined steroid withdrawal syndrome after abrupt discontinuation of high-dose therapy that consists of myalgias, arthralgias, fatigue, and fever. This can be minimized by a tapering course of oral prednisone, beginning at 1 mg/kg per day. Alternatively, nonsteroidal anti-inflammatory agents, such as ibuprofen, may be used in place of prednisone.

High-dose glucocorticosteroid therapy consistently reduces the number of gadolinium-enhancing lesions in MS as detected on MRI, presumably by restoring the integrity of the blood-brain barrier. A number of actions of glucocorticosteroids may contribute to these effects. Thus, glucocorticosteroids counter vasodilation by inhibiting the production of its mediators, including nitric oxide. The immunosuppressive actions of glucocorticosteroids may reduce the trafficking of inflammatory cells into the perivenular spaces of the brain. These actions include inhibition of proinflammatory cytokine production, reduction of activation markers on immune and endothelial cells, and a reduction in antibody production. Glucocorticosteroids inhibit the actions of T lymphocytes and macrophages and reduce the expression of IL-1, -2, -3, -4, -6, and -10; TNF-α; and interferon-γ. Glucocorticosteroids also inhibit expression of the IL-2 receptor and signal transduction, and MHC Class II expression on macrophages. In addition, CD4 T cells are affected to a greater extent than CD8 T cells by this treatment. Glucocorticosteroids have not shown consistent effects on other immune markers in MS. Oligoclonal bands are not changed in most patients on this therapy, and temporary reductions in the CSF Ig synthesis rate do not correlate with clinical improvement.

Although it has been difficult to distinguish the immunosuppressive effects from the immediate anti-inflammatory effects of glucocorticosteroids in MS, a landmark study of optic neuritis (Beck et al., 1992) indicated that patients receiving high-dose intravenous methylprednisolone had a reduced risk of a second attack of demyelination for 2 years compared to the placebo and oral prednisone groups.

The Beck study randomized 457 patients in three treatment groups: intravenous methylprednisolone 1 g per day for 3 days, followed by oral prednisone 1 mg/kg per day for 11 days; oral prednisone alone at 1 mg/kg per day for 14 days; oral placebo for 14 days. By day 15 the rate of return of visual function, as measured by visual fields and contrast sensitivity, but not visual acuity, was significantly greater in the intravenous group than with placebo or prednisone alone. By 6 months posttreatment there continued to be a mild but significant treatment effect on these measures. After 2 years, however, the rate of recurrent optic neuritis in either eye was significantly greater in the oral prednisone group (27%) than either the intravenous (13%) or placebo groups (15%). Of those who did not have definite or probable MS at entry, 13% (50 of 389) had a second attack within 2 years, satisfying the criteria for the disorder. The risk was greatest in those whose MRI scan at baseline had at least two lesions of a typical size and location for multiple sclerosis. Among this group the risk of a second attack was significantly reduced in the intravenous methylprednisolone group (16%) as compared with the prednisone (32%) and placebo (36%) groups. The effect of intravenous methylprednisolone in delaying the development of clinically definite MS did not extend into the third and fourth years of therapy.

Based on these results, high-dose intravenous methylprednisolone is warranted for treating acute attacks of optic neuritis in patients with abnormal MRI scans, if not for the more rapid return of vision, then to forestall the development of clinically definite MS.

More recent studies have compared oral administration of corticosteroids, either with prednisone or methylprednisolone, with standard doses of intravenous methylprednisolone therapy in treating acute relapses. These studies have not shown a therapeutic advantage for high dose intravenous therapy. However, the conclusions that may be drawn from these results are limited by the lack of comparable doses, the lack of control groups and the lack of demonstration of efficacy from intravenous therapies that had been demonstrated in other studies. Furthermore, the studies have not employed MRI as an outcome measure. Therefore, more definitive clinical studies, which should incorporate assessments of blood-brain barrier integrity as measured by MRI, are needed to provide a rationale for abandoning intravenous glucocorticosteroids.

Chronic Immunosuppression

Immunosuppression with cyclophosphamide. Cytotoxic drugs have been used to induce long-term remissions in patients with rapidly progressive MS.

The most well studied immunosuppressant in this regard is cyclophosphamide, an alkylating agent developed 40 years ago to treat malignancies. Cyclophosphamide has a dose-dependent, cytotoxic effect on white blood cells and other rapidly dividing cells. Initially, lymphocyte counts are reduced more than granulocyte counts, with higher doses affecting both. At doses less than 600 mg/m^2, B cells are affected more than T cells, and CD8 T cells more so than CD4 T cells. Higher doses affect CD8 and CD4 T cells equally. Temporary stabilization of rapidly progressive patients for up to 1 year has been achieved with high-dose intravenous cyclophosphamide (400 to 500 mg per day for 10 to 14 days), inducing a leukopenic nadir of 900 to 2000 cells per cubic millimeter. Blinding to therapy could not be achieved in these studies because of the inevitable development of alopecia in treated patients. Reprogression after the first year occurs in as many as two thirds of the intensively treated patients, requiring the need for either a second induction with high-dose cyclophosphamide or monthly booster doses of 1 mg. Responders to this therapy tend to be younger, with shorter disease durations. Another randomized, placebo-controlled study reported no benefit from induction cyclophosphamide treatments (The Canadian Cooperative Multiple Sclerosis Study Group, 1991).

Other studies have confirmed the efficacy of maintenance protocols using cyclophosphamide with or without induction in stabilizing chronic progressive patients and relapsing-remitting patients. Booster therapy with cyclophosphamide, after an induction dose, significantly delayed, for up to 2.5 years, treatment failure in patients younger than 40 years old with secondary progressive multiple sclerosis (Weiner et al., 1993). Its endorsement as a standard treatment, however, is limited by the side effects experienced by some patients, including nausea and vomiting.

Immunosuppression with cladribine.   Cladribine (2-chlorodeoxyadenosine) is a purine analogue resistant to deamination by adenosine deaminase. Cladribine is selectively toxic to dividing and resting lymphocytes because of a shunt pathway preferentially used in those cells. A single course of treatment can induce a lymphopenia that may persist for 1 year. While the drug was demonstrated to stabilize rapidly progressive patients in a double-blinded, cross-over study, these clinical benefits were not duplicated in a multicenter study of patients with primary and secondary chronic progressive MS. The hematologic effects of cladribine include bone marrow suppression of all blood-forming elements. Significant declines in white blood cell subsets with CD3, CD4, CD8, and CD25 markers persist for up to 1 year after a course of treatment.

Other Immunosuppressive Treatments

The requirement for long-term therapy of multiple sclerosis has led to the study and use of other commonly used immunosuppressants that pose less risk when used chronically. Because studies have demonstrated these drugs may be partially beneficial in slowing the disease process they are still used in selected patients.

Azathioprine.   Azathioprine is a purine antagonist that is converted to its active analogue, 6-mercaptopurine, in the intestinal wall, liver, and red blood cells. Its major use is in prevention of allograft rejection in organ transplantation, management of graft versus host disease, and treatment of refractory rheumatoid arthritis. Metabolites of 6-mercaptopurine inhibit enzymes involved in the purine salvage pathway, resulting in the depletion of cellular purine stores and suppression of DNA and RNA synthesis. In white blood cells, it causes a delayed cytotoxicity that is relatively selective for replicating antigen-responsive cells. In neurologic diseases, azathioprine is used most extensively in myasthenia gravis and in MS in doses ranging from 2.0 to 3.0 mg/kg per day. Only partial therapeutic efficacy in MS has been demonstrated, however, with this treatment. The British and Dutch Multiple Sclerosis Azathioprine Trial Group (1988) included 354 patients over 3 years in a double-blind, randomized study. The mean decline in the treated group versus the control group was 0.62 versus 0.80 Kurtzke disability points. A mild decrease in average relapse frequency from 2.5 to 2.2 was not statistically significant. Another study showed a modest effect in decreasing exacerbation frequency, which was greater in the second year of treatment. A large meta-analysis of azathioprine treatment in both double-blind and single-blind studies confirmed a small difference in favor of treated patients after the second and third years of therapy.

There are minimal long-term risks from azathioprine therapy in MS patients, with slight increased risk of malignancy found only for treatment durations of 5 years or greater

(Confavreux et al., 1996). Gastrointestinal upset may be caused by a mucositis that, if minor, can be treated by lowering the dose or by taking the medication with food.

Cyclosporine. Cyclosporine A, an isolate from the soil fungus *Tolypocladium inflatum,* inhibits the proliferation of autoreactive T lymphocytes by inhibiting signal transduction pathways. It is effective in the prevention of graft rejection in organ transplantation and has improved the outcome of allogeneic bone marrow transplantation. Cyclosporine binds to an intracellular immunophilin receptor, with the complex acting on calcineurin, a serine-threonine phosphatase. Treatment of patients with rapidly progressing MS with cyclosporine in doses sufficient to maintain trough levels of 310 to 430 ng/mL for 2 years resulted in a significant but modest reduction of the increase in disability scores and delayed the time to becoming wheelchair bound (The Multiple Sclerosis Study Group, 1990). A large withdrawal rate was observed for both cyclosporine (44%) and placebo (33%) treated groups. The dose was initiated at 6 mg/kg per day, with serum levels later adjusted to maintain a serum creatinine level within 1.5 times baseline. Nephrotoxicity and hypertension were the most common reasons for withdrawal of the drug. Another 2-year, randomized, double-blind study showed a beneficial effect on progression, relapse rate, and severity. The general use of cyclosporine in MS is limited, however, because of its low therapeutic index, nephrotoxicity, and other cumulative risks from chronic therapy.

Methotrexate. Low-dose oral methotrexate therapy has emerged as an effective, relatively nontoxic treatment for various inflammatory diseases, notably rheumatoid arthritis and psoriasis. A folic acid antagonist, methotrexate inhibits a variety of biochemical reactions, with effects on protein, DNA, and RNA synthesis. Although it is not known which effects of methotrexate are relevant in the treatment of MS, methotrexate inhibits IL-6 activity, decreases IL-2 and TNF-α-receptor levels, and exerts an antiproliferative effect on mononuclear cells. In relapsing-remitting MS patients a significant reduction in exacerbation frequency has been found with treatment. One study showed no effect on the number of chronic progressive patients who worsened at 18 months of treatment. A larger, randomized, double-blind study of 60 patients with chronic progressive disease using low-dose (7.5 mg per week) methotrexate, however, found no effect in the decline in ambulation but a significant effect in preserving upper extremity function (Goodkin et al., 1995). Thus, methotrexate is a relatively safe treatment option for patients with chronic progressive disease, particularly those who are nonambulatory.

Other Nonspecific Immunosuppressive Therapies

Total lymph node irradiation. Total lymph node irradiation has been used to treat both malignant and autoimmune diseases, including Hodgkin's lymphoma and refractory rheumatoid arthritis. It also prolongs graft survival in organ transplants and induces a prolonged immunosuppression with decreases in absolute blood lymphocyte counts. In placebo-controlled studies using sham irradiation, total lymph node irradiation in doses of 1980 cGy given over 2 weeks resulted in delayed time to progression in two double-blind studies. The effectiveness of the treatment correlates with the degree of lymphopenia, which is extended by the use of low-dose corticosteroids.

Plasma exchange. Plasma exchange has been reported to stabilize patients with fulminant forms of CNS demyelinating disease, including acute disseminated encephalomyelitis. In studies of MS it has been combined with ACTH and cyclophosphamide and shown to shorten the time to recovery in relapsing patients without demonstrating a significant clinical advantage at 1 year. A small, randomized, single-blind crossover study in patients with secondary progressive disease that compared plasma exchange and azathioprine did not show significant differences in plaque activity as measured by MRI.

Intravenous γ-globulin. Intravenous γ-globulin has shown some benefit in reducing exacerbation frequency and disability over 2 years in patients with relapsing-remitting MS. As with plasma exchange, it has been used to stabilize patients with ADEM and fulminant forms of MS. Currently it is being studied as a treatment for refractory optic neuritis and chronic progressive MS.

Mitoxantrone. Mitoxantrone, an anthracenedione antineoplastic drug that inhibits both DNA and RNA synthesis, has been used in some European MS centers to treat patients with chronic progressive disease. In the United States, investigators who studied mitoxantrone in an open-label fashion in a small group of progressive MS patients concluded it had no benefit. A recent, unblinded study, however, suggested an effect of mitoxantrone in reducing clinical relapses and active MRI lesions.

Interferon

Preliminary studies of interferon (IFN) therapy in multiple sclerosis began in the early 1980s. First described by Isaacs and Lindenmann in 1957 as a soluble substance that protected cells from viral infection, interferons were later found to have potent antiproliferative and immunomodulatory properties as well. Subsequent research was spurred by the possibility that interferons might be effective anticancer therapies. These substances are classified as type I, which includes interferon-α (15 subtypes) and interferon-β (1 subtype), and type II, which is interferon-γ. Two other types of IFNs are interferon-τ

and interferon-ω. Type I interferons have similar structural and functional characteristics and share a common receptor; type II interferons are structurally different from the others and interact with a different receptor. Both, however, have biologically similar actions. Interferons bind to cell surface receptors and activate a family of transcriptional agents called STAT proteins (Signal Transducers and Activators of Transcription), which form a complex with a DNA binding protein that translocates to the nucleus and directs transcription of IFN-stimulated genes (ISGs) (Pfeffer, 1997) (Fig. 12-18). Type I and type II interferons differentially activate proteins involved in the tyrosine-dependent phosphorylation of STAT proteins, which may impart some of their specificity in cytokine signaling.

Type I interferons. Both interferon-α and interferon-β are composed of 166 amino acid glycoproteins that share 34% sequence homology. Genes for

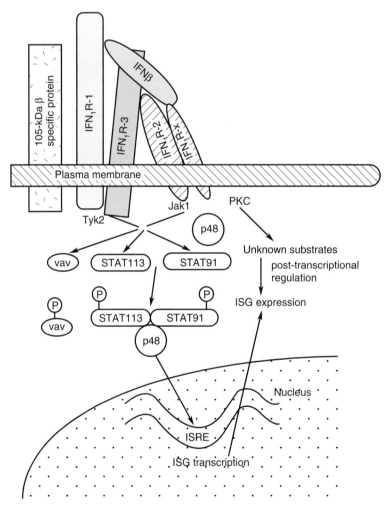

Figure 12–18. *Schematic representation of the type I interferon system. Both INF-β and INF-α bind to the same cell surface receptor. With permission from Pfeffer LM, Constantinescu SN, 1997.*

both are located on chromosome 9, with interferon-α primarily produced by leukocytes and interferon-β by fibroblasts. A variety of cells, however, produce both. The production of these interferons is induced by double-stranded viral RNA, IFN-α, and IFN-γ. The antiviral effects come from the selective induction of certain enzymes, including 2'5' oligoadenylate, which is a marker for interferon activity. The type I interferons are also antiproliferative and promote the differentiation of cells. A list of the immune modulating effects of type I and type II interferons is displayed in Table 12-14.

An important first step in the chronic treatment of multiple sclerosis was taken with the release of interferon beta-1b in 1993 as this was the first approved noncytotoxic drug that demonstrated a significant impact on the course of the disease. The drug received an expedited review based on the results of a multicenter phase III study showing a significant dose-related effect on relapse frequency, time to first relapse, severity of relapses, and reduction of lesions as measured by MRI (The IFNB Multiple Sclerosis Study Group, 1993). There was also a trend toward a reduction of disability in the interferon-treated groups as compared with the placebo group. The MRI was a critical surrogate marker for biological efficacy, showing that patients given interferon-β had stabilization of T2-weighted lesion volumes in contrast with the increase in lesion frequency and volume in the placebo group.

A second interferon-β (interferon beta-1a) was approved for use in patients with MS in April 1996, based on the results of a phase III study showing a modest effect in reducing disability over 2 years. Reduction of disease activity, as measured by gadolinium-enhancing lesions on MRI scan, was also demonstrated with this drug.

Interferon beta-1b. Interferon beta-1b is a nonglycosylated protein produced in *Escherichia coli* from a recombinant interferon-β gene. Interferon beta-1b has a serine substituted for cysteine at position 17 which provides its stability. The dose used in MS patients is 8 million international units (MIU), or 0.25 mg, injected subcutaneously every other day. Serum levels after a 0.25-mg dose peak within 8 to 24 h and decline to pretreatment levels by 48 h. The biological activity of interferon beta-1b is determined by measurements of serum levels of beta$_2$-microglobulin, neopterin, and 2',5' oligoadenylate synthetase activity in peripheral blood mononuclear cells. In healthy subjects a single injection of 8 MIU causes a rise in these biological markers, which peak in 48 to 72 h and remain elevated after 1 week of injections every other day (Fig. 12-19). The beta$_2$-microglobulin peaks at 2 mg/mL after a single injection and remains elevated after 1 week of injections.

Phase III pivotal study. The clinical efficacy of interferon beta-1b as a treatment for MS was demonstrated in a double-blind, placebo-controlled clinical trial of 372 subjects with relapsing-remitting MS (The IFNB Multiple Sclerosis Study Group, 1993). Subjects were 66% female and 95% white. Their average age was 36 and their average duration of MS was 4 years. The patients had a mean of 3.5 exacerbations of disease in the 2 years before the study. The three treatment groups included a high-dose group receiving 8 MIU, a low-dose group receiving 1.6 MIU, and controls. After 2 years, annual exacerbation rates were significantly lower for those on high-dose interferon therapy compared with placebo, with an intermediate effect shown for the low-dose group (annual exacerbation rates: 1.27 for controls; 1.17 for 1.6 MIU, and .84 for 8 MIU). There was a twofold reduction in moderate and severe exacerbations with the 8 MIU dose. A significantly greater proportion of subjects in the high-dose interferon group were exacerbation-free at 2 years: 36 (8 MIU) compared with 18 (placebo) (p = 0.007). Furthermore, MRI findings supported the clinical response to interferon treatment. The MRI scans were performed annually on all patients, and, on a subset of 52 patients, every 6 weeks for 1 year. Both studies demonstrated significant reductions in active lesions, the appearance of new lesions, and the total disease burden in the high-dose group (Paty et al., 1993). Despite these findings, disability scores as measured by the EDSS did not change significantly in either treatment or placebo groups after 3 years. Nonetheless, there was a trend toward reduced disability in the high-dose group. However, the study was not powered adequately to detect a moderate effect on disability.

Adverse effects from treatment or placebo caused 16 patients to withdraw from the study, 10 of whom were taking 8 MIU of interferon and 5 of whom were taking 1.6 MIU. Reasons for withdrawal included abnormalities in liver function tests, injection site pain, fatigue, cardiac arrhythmia, allergic reactions, nausea, headache, "flu syndrome," confusion, and "felt sick" (Table 12-15). There was also one suicide and four attempted suicides among patients given interferon beta-1b. Overall, side effects were most common in the 8-MIU group, including injection site reactions (69%), fever (58%), and myalgias (41%). These side effects tended to lessen in severity after 3 months of treatment, approaching the frequency reported by placebo-treated subjects at 1 year.

Based on the results of this study interferon beta-1b was approved for patients with relapsing-remitting multiple sclerosis who are still ambulatory. In a 5-year follow-up on the original cohorts it was found that while the decrease in exacerbation frequency persisted, it became nonsignificant by

Table 12-14

IFN Effects on Immune Function

	Immunoactivating effects	*Immunoinhibiting effects*
Type I IFNs (IFN-α and IFN-β)	Increase of MHC class I molecule expression	Inhibition of the abnormal IFN-γ–induced MHC class II expression on many cell types (astrocytes included)
	Slight to moderate increase of MHC class II molecule expression on antigen-presenting cells only	Inhibition of mitogen-induced T-lymphocyte proliferation
	Increase of activity of differentiated T cytotoxic cells	Increase of T suppressor cell function (particularly if reduced, as in active MS)
	Increase of IgG production	Inhibition of mitogen-induced IgG and of IL-4–induced IgG1 and IgE production
		Reduction of IFN-γ production by T cells
Type II IFN (IFN-γ)	Increase of MHC class I molecule expression	
	Increase of MHC class II molecule expression on APC and other cell types	
	Induction of Th$_1$ lymphocyte differentiation (potentially encephalitogenic lymphocytes)	
	Activation of T cytotoxic and NK lymphocyte maturation and function	
	Activation of B-cell maturation, Ig production, and Ig class switching	
	Enhancement of macrophage function (with release of potentially CNS-damaging products)	
	Enhancement of TNF-α (a potentially demyelinating cytokine)	
	Inhibition of T suppressor lymphocyte maturation and function	
	Inhibition of maturation and function of Th$_2$ lymphocytes (which may counteract encephalitogenic Th$_1$ lymphocyte activity)	

With permission from Durelli L, 1997.

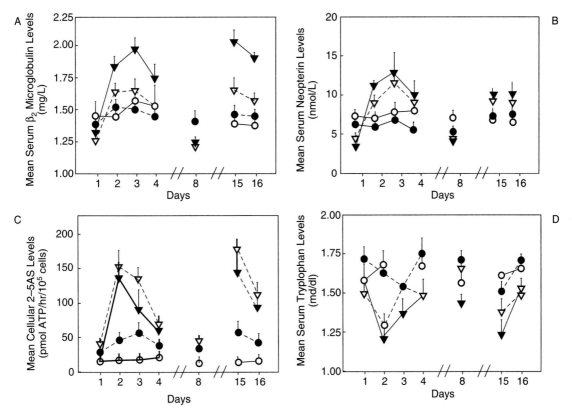

Figure 12–19. *The mean and SE values for serum B₂-microglobulin (A), serum 2,5-OAS activity in PBMC (C), and serum tryptophan (D) are shown, for eight healthy subjects per dose group receiving 0.09 (○); 0.9 (●), 9.0 (▽); or 45.0 (▼) MU INF-β-1b (old units, which are one fifth current international units) s.c. The day 1 sample was taken before the first injection; samples on days 2, 3, 4, and 8 follow that single injection. Subjects received further injections on days 8, 10, 12, and 14; samples were assayed on days 15 and 16 following these every-other-day injections. With permission from Witt, 1997.*

Table 12-15

IFN Beta-1b Side Effects

Injection site reactions	85%	Neutropenia	18%
Flu-like symptoms complex	76%	Menstrual disorder	17%
Fever	59%	Leukopenia	16%
Asthenia	49%	Malaise	15%
Chills	46%	Palpitations	8%
Myalgia	44%	Dyspnea	8%
Sweating	23%	Injection site necrosis	2%

With permission from The IFNB Multiple Sclerosis Study Group, 1993.

year 3. It was noted that the dropouts in all groups tended to have higher exacerbation rates and progression of disease as measured by MRI than those who completed the study (The INFB Multiple Sclerosis Study Group and the University of British Columbia MS/MRI Analysis Group, 1995).

A number of investigators have sought to define the mechanism of action of interferon-β in MS. It has been found to inhibit gelatinase secretion by activated T lymphocytes in vitro, impeding migration through an artificial basement membrane. Other studies have demonstrated a decline in the number of adhesion molecules, enhancement of IL-10 secretion, inhibition of T-cell activation, reduction of tumor necrosis factor, and stimulation of IL-6 production in response to interferon-β.

Interferon beta-1a. Interferon beta-1a is a full-sequence, glycosylated recombinant interferon produced in Chinese hamster ovary cells. It is administered by intramuscular injection at a dose of 6 MIU per week. A single injection at this dose increases serum β_2-microglobulin levels in healthy patients which peaks by 48 h and remains elevated at a lower level for 4 days. This dose was chosen for study because, although it induced biological markers, side effects could be suppressed with acetaminophen, preserving the blind.

The clinical trial examining the efficacy of interferon beta-1a used time to sustained progression of 1 EDSS point as a primary outcome measure, and relapse frequency as a secondary outcome measure to examine whether it slowed progression of neurologic disability (Jacobs et al., 1996). The study demonstrated that by the end of 2 years, 34.9% of patients in the placebo group and 21.9% of patients in the treatment group met the defined endpoint (p = 0.02). Exacerbations were also significantly decreased by 30% in patients who completed 2 years, and by 18% in all patients. The number and volume of gadolinium-enhanced lesions, but not T2-weighted lesion volume, showed a significant decrease in treated patients. Side effects to interferon beta-1a were similar to those reported for interferon beta-1b, including headache (not significantly different between treated and controls), flu-like symptoms, muscle aches, fever, asthenia, and chills.

Other interferons. Although *interferon*-α has also been tested both in relapsing-remitting and chronic progressive MS, it is not currently approved for this indication in the United States. The results of a small study demonstrated a significant decrease in relapse frequency and disease progression as measured by MRI.

Interferon-τ differs from type I interferons in that it is not readily induced by viruses and double-stranded DNA, it has comparatively less toxicity, and its synthesis is prolonged. It was first identified as a pregnancy identification hormone in ruminants such as sheep and cows. Interferon-τ displays immunodulatory activity like the type I interferons and blocks EAE induced by superantigen activation.

Issues in the management of patients on interferon. The approved indications for interferon-β use in MS are based on the design of the pivotal clinical trials. In the case of interferon beta-1b, it is approved for the treatment of ambulatory patients with relapsing-remitting MS to reduce the frequency of clinical exacerbations. Interferon beta-1a is approved for treatment of patients with relapsing forms of MS to slow the development of physical disability and decrease the frequency of clinical exacerbations. Neither drug is approved for patients with chronic secondary progressive or primary progressive MS. Furthermore, although these drugs differ in the frequency and degree of side effects, and in the dose and mode of administration, there is no consensus on which should be initiated in which patients (Fig. 12-20).

An expert panel was convened to assess whether patients with more severe or different subtypes of MS than those enrolled in the clinical trials should be treated with interferon beta-1b (Report of the Quality Standards Subcommittee of the American Academy of Neurology, 1994). The panel concluded that interferon beta-1b therapy might be helpful in relapsing-remitting patients older than 50 years of age and in those who were nonambulatory, provided they met criteria for frequent relapses. The panel also noted that patients with relapsing progressive disease might also benefit from interferon treatment. Criteria for terminating interferon beta-1b therapy were those used in the pivotal study. At present, the efficacy of interferon beta in treating chronic progressive disease is being tested in a clinical trial.

Side effects. Side effects of interferon therapy are dose related and tend to diminish with continued use. A list of common side effects and recommendations for management is provided in Fig. 12-20. Included are injection site reactions, flu-like symptoms, mood changes, decreases in blood cell counts, and elevation of liver functions. Gradual dose escalation, training patients or their caregivers in proper injection techniques, and monitoring patients more frequently early in the course of treatment aid in the successful management of interferon therapy. Local injection

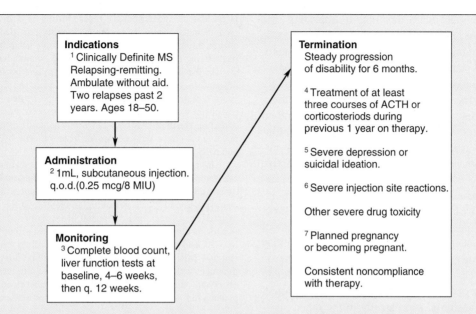

Indications
¹ Clinically Definite MS
Relapsing-remitting.
Ambulate without aid.
Two relapses past 2
years. Ages 18–50.

Administration
² 1mL, subcutaneous injection.
q.o.d.(0.25 mcg/8 MIU)

Monitoring
³ Complete blood count,
liver function tests at
baseline, 4–6 weeks,
then q. 12 weeks.

Termination
Steady progression
of disability for 6 months.

⁴ Treatment of at least
three courses of ACTH or
corticosteriods during
previous 1 year on therapy.

⁵ Severe depression or
suicidal ideation.

⁶ Severe injection site reactions.

Other severe drug toxicity

⁷ Planned pregnancy
or becoming pregnant.

Consistent noncompliance
with therapy.

¹ Expert consensus panel suggested that interferon beta-1b may be helpful for patients who ambulate with aid or are nonambulatory, those who had relapsing-progressive disease and those greater than 50 years old. (Report of the Quality Standards Subcommittee of the American Academy of Neurology, 1994)

² Recommendations for amelioratating side effects: initiate at half dose first 2 to 4 weeks. Use antipyretic/analgesic (acetaminophen, aspirin, nonsteroidal anti-inflammatory drug) 4 h prior, at the time of, and 4h after injection. Administer injection at bedtime. Patients need to be trained in proper injection techniques.

³ May temporarily discontinue drug with mild elevations of transaminases, wait until levels return to baseline and resume therapy at 25% full dose, increasing as tolerated. Persistent and high elevations of transaminases (10xs nml.) require discontinuation of drug.

⁴ Consider in patients who have been on therapy continuously for one year and having increased relapses or otherwise doing poorly, testing for neutralizing antibodies (assay done by Berlex Laboratories). Two positive titers 3 months apart indicate neutralizing antibody positivity.

⁵ More mild degrees of depression may be treated with antidepressant agents/psychotherapeutic interventions. Selective serotonin reuptake inhibitors may have an advantage in causing less fatique.

⁶ Therapy may be continued despite mild injection site reactions. Technique should be reviewed periodically by qualified health care professional. Skin necrosis at injection sites or other severe injection site reactions, (e.g., fasciitis) require temporary or permanent discontinuation of drug.

⁷ Category C. Has dose-related abortifacient activity in animals given in 2.8 to 40 times recommended human dose. Spontaneous abortions (4) reported.

Figure 12–20.   *The use of interferon beta-1b (Betaseron).*

site reactions are often the most troublesome side effect. They range from mild erythema to necrosis at the site of injection. Biopsies have revealed leukocytoclastic infiltrates and vascular thrombosis. Warming the solution and injecting the drug slowly minimizes the discomfort related to the injection. Flu-like symptoms may be reduced by concomitant use of acetaminophen or other nonsteroidal antiinflammatory agents and by scheduling injections during times when patients are less likely to be active (e.g. during the evening before bedtime). Mild degrees of depression may be managed pharmacologically. The treating physician must be vigilant, however, for persistent or more severe forms of depression or emotional lability. A short drug holiday may help determine the contribution of interferon therapy to changes in mood states. Patients who do not tolerate one interferon-β preparation may sometimes be transferred successfully to the other.

Neutralizing antibodies to interferon-β. Neutralizing antibodies occur with IFNβ-1b and IFNβ-1a therapy. In clinical trials neutralizing antibodies were detected in 38% of patients receiving interferon-1b (INFβ Multiple Sclerosis Study Group, 1996). Exacerbation rates in antibody-positive patients equaled or exceeded those in placebo-treated controls. The percentage of neutralizing antibody positive patients did not differ between the 1.6-MIU and the 8-MIU groups, and side effects were as common in the antibody-negative as in the antibody-positive group. It is recommended that patients given interferon beta-1b be tested for neutralizing antibodies if they have been taking the drug for 1 year and continue to have multiple relapses or disease progression. If the initial test is positive or indeterminant, repeat testing in 3 months is recommended. Antibody testing is currently provided free of charge through the distributor of interferon beta-1b. Other neutralizing antibody assays are available commercially.

In the interferon-1a study neutralizing antibodies were detected in 14% of treated patients at 1 year and 22% at 2 years, compared with 4% of the placebo-treated patients (Jacobs et al., 1996). Some preliminary reports suggest that patients given interferon beta-1a who are neutralizing antibody positive also have reduced benefit from the drug by clinical and MRI measures.

It has been noted that patients beginning treatment with interferon-β may be at increased risk of exacerbations because of an initial induction of interferon-γ production. This has been suggested by data indicating an increase in the number of interferon-γ-secreting peripheral blood mononuclear cells in patients during the first 2 months of therapy with interferon beta-1b, and a study showing a higher rate of exacerbations and new MRI lesions in patients during the first 3 months of treatment with interferon beta-1a. During the interferon beta-1b pivotal study, a reduction in attack frequency in treated patients did not occur until after 2 months of treatment.

Glatiramer Acetate (formerly Copolymer 1)

Glatiramer acetate was approved for use in relapsing-remitting multiple sclerosis in 1996. It is administered subcutaneously daily at a dose of 20 mg which does not produce detectable serum levels. The drug is a mixture of synthetic polypeptides composed of the acetate salts of four L amino acids: glutamic acid, alanine, tyrosine, and lysine (Table 12-16). Following injection glatiramer acetate is rapidly degraded

Table 12-16
Composition of Glatiramer acetate*

Amino acid	N-Carboxyanhydride used for reaction	Amount used in the reaction (mM)		Molar ratio of amino acid in copolymer
Alanine	Alanine	8.6	75	6.0
Glutamic acid	Benzyl glutamate	6.0	23	1.9
Lysine	N-Trifluoroacetyl-lysine	14.0	52	4.7
Tyrosine	Tyrosine	3.0	14	1.0

* molecular weight 23,000
With permission from Bornstein et al., 1990.

into smaller molecular weight fragments. The drug is indicated for reducing the frequency of relapses in patients with relapsing-remitting MS. In its pivotal phase III study, glatiramer acetate reduced exacerbation rates by one third (Johnson et al., 1995). The decrease in exacerbations was more significant in patients with minimal to mild disability. Mild skin reactions may occur at the injection site, including erythema and swelling. Although the drug rarely produces ongoing systemic side effects, its use may be limited in patients who experience a "vasogenic" reaction immediately after injection. The drug is classified in Category C with respect to pregnancy, indicating that no adverse effects were noted in animal reproduction studies. In contrast, interferons are in Category B. Therefore, the risk of MS patients becoming pregnant on immunomodulation therapy might influence the choice of glatiramer acetate.

Glatiramer acetate was one of a series of treatments developed by the Weizmann Institute in the early 1970s in a study of experimental allergic encephalomyelitis. It contains amino acids found in high abundance in myelin basic protein, but instead of inducing EAE the compound suppresses the disease in a variety of laboratory animals challenged with either whole white matter or myelin basic protein in complete Freund's adjuvant. Although the mechanism of action is unknown, there is evidence that it binds directly to MHC class II complexes, either displacing or inhibiting myelin basic protein binding. Alternatively, it may induce MBP-specific suppressor cells (Fig. 12-21).

The results of the pivotal study replicated those of an earlier placebo-controlled trial that showed both a significant reduction in exacerbation frequency and a higher proportion of exacerbation-free patients. A significant effect on slowing disability in secondary progressive MS was not demonstrated in a two-center study, although one center demonstrated a mild, statistically significant effect.

The phase III study involved 251 patients at 11 centers and revealed a significant reduction of relapse rates, increase in relapse-free patients, and prolonged time to first relapse in treated patients (Johnson et al., 1995). A suggestion of delayed neurologic progression with therapy was indicated by a greater proportion of placebo patients who worsened by 1 EDSS point or more and a higher proportion of treated patients who improved by 1 EDSS point. The percentage of progression-free patients, however, was the same in both groups. General side effects of glatiramer acetate were minimal compared with interferon treatment. However, 15% of treated patients experienced a transient reaction, characterized by flushing, chest tightness with palpitations, anxiety, or dyspnea, which also occurred in 3.2% of placebo-treated patients. This reaction, the cause of which is unknown, lasts from 30 s to 30 min and is not associated with ECG changes.

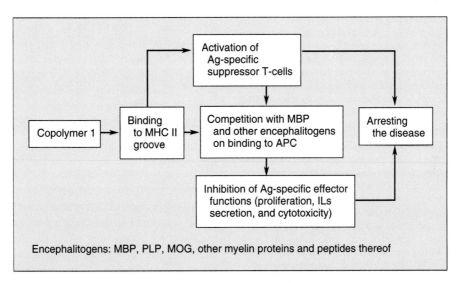

Figure 12–21. *Proposed mechanism of action of Glatiramer acetate (formerly copolymer 1). From Arnon, 1996.*

Other Treatment Issues

Early treatment.   At the present time, these therapies are approved only for patients with clinically definite MS who have evidence of active disease. They are not indicated for those who have probable MS based on a single attack. There is some debate, however, as to how early to intervene with long-term therapy. The present cost of treatment is high (about $10,000 per year), but is potentially balanced against the costs of treating the attacks and other disease complications, and of preservation of economic productivity. The issue of whether early administration of IFNB-1a in patients presenting with their first attack of demyelinating disease could delay a subsequent second attack is currently under study. The flow chart shown in Fig. 12-22 is based on recommendations by an expert panel, with some modifications since the panel originally addressed only interferon beta-1b treatment.

Combination drug therapy.   Another issue that may be increasingly studied is combination treatment with drugs that have different mechanisms of action. For instance, the in vitro combination of glatiramer acetate and interferon beta-1b has an additive effect in reducing proliferation of interferon-γ of myelin basic protein reactive cell lines from healthy volunteers. As of this date, the clinical use of interferon-β and glatiramer acetate in combination has not been reported. Some centers have experimented with bolus cyclophosphamide and methylprednisolone as induction therapy, followed by interferon-β maintenance treatment to stabilize progressive patients. At this time, however, any evidence that combination therapies in MS may be beneficial must be regarded as preliminary since neither the safety nor efficacy of such treatment protocols have been tested in adequately controlled clinical trials.

New treatment strategies.   There are a number of potential immunologic interventions that may be beneficial in the treatment of MS (Table 12-17). This number is likely to increase further with a greater understanding of the immune pathogenesis of the disease. Some therapies that are being tested in preliminary clinical studies include TGF-β, T-cell vaccination, anti-α_4 integrin antibodies, phosphodiesterase inhibitors, anti-CD4 antibodies, and T cell antagonist peptides. Sometimes the results of these preliminary studies are at variance with expectations, reflecting the as-yet incomplete understanding of the pathogenesis of MS. For instance, treatment with antitumor necrosis factor antibodies in two rapidly progressive MS patients had no affect on clinical status but did cause a transient increase in gadolinium-enhancing lesions as measured by MRI (van Oosten et al., 1996).

SYMPTOMATIC THERAPY

Common symptoms of MS and their pharmacologic management are briefly outlined in this section. Patients with fever of any cause may experience pseudoexacerbations, due in part to reversible temperature-dependent changes in the conduction properties of demyelinated axons. Methylprednisolone therapy should not be administered when there is an untreated infection, particularly if it may be causing a worsening of symptoms. Many patients with advanced disability take multiple combinations of drugs for symptoms. It is important to remember that the potential for side effects (e.g. cognitive dysfunction secondary to anticholinergics) is increased as more drugs are used to control other symptoms, including drugs for bladder control, GABA agonists for spasticity, and tricyclics and antiepileptics for pain and depression (Fig. 12-23). It is often difficult to determine in such patients whether new symptoms, such as fatigue or muscle weakness, are due to the effects of drugs or the disease.

In general medical care, patients with MS may require special measures to compensate for motor disability (e.g. special tables for gynecologic examinations). MS is seldom, however, a contraindication with respect to procedures or treatments for other medical conditions. It is also not by itself a contraindication for general or regional anesthesia, pregnancy, normal childbirth, or immunizations. Carefully conducted studies have shown no detrimental effects from influenza immunizations on either exacerbation rates or the course of the disease.

Spasticity

Spasticity results from an upper motor neuron pattern of weakness due to interruption of inhibitory inputs to the segmental spinal cord reflex arcs. Spasticity is caused by lesions that affect the descending pyramidal tracts. This is the most common pattern of motor involvement in MS and results in symptoms of weakness, muscle stiffness, cramps, and spasms of the upper or lower extremities, with the latter being most common. In moderately severe spasticity,

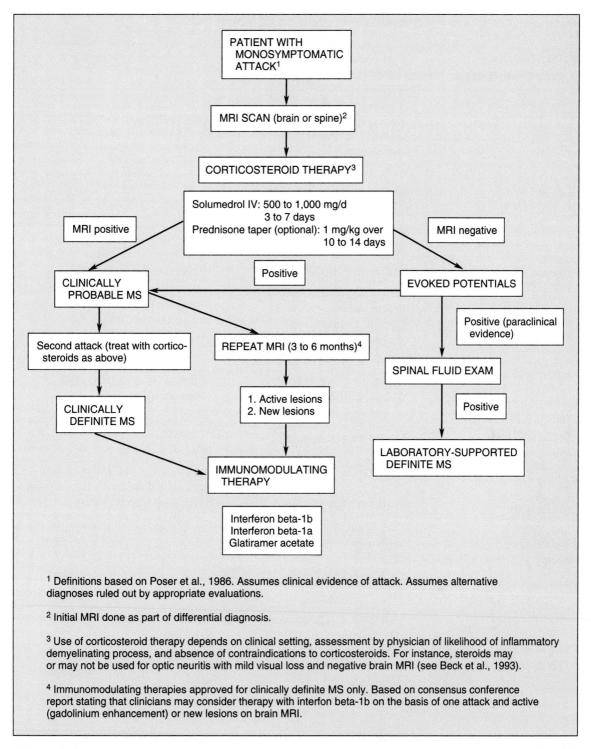

Figure 12–22. *Algorithm for clinical decision-making (applies to relapsing MS patients only, not primary progressive).*

Table 12-17

Accepted and emerging disease-modifying therapies for MS

Therapeutic strategy	Treatment options	Major putative mechanism of action
Non-specific immunosuppression	Cyclophosphamide[1] Azathioprine[1] Methotrexate[1] Total lymphoid irradiation[2] Cladribine[2] Mitoxantrone Glucocorticosteroids[1]	Global reduction of T-cell population
Reduce T-lymphocyte trafficking across vascular endothelial cells into the central nervous system	Glucocorticosteroids[1] Antibodies to adhesion molecules:[3] VLA-4, ICAM-I, L-selectin and integrins TGFβ,[3] IFNβ[4]	Decrease the expression of adhesion molecules on T-lymphocytes and vascular endothelial cells
	Matrix metalloproteinase inhibitors,[3] IFNβ[4]	Inhibit proteases that facilitate T-cell trafficking
Inhibit T-cell receptor-peptide/MHC-II interaction	Copolymer I[4] Altered peptide ligands[3]	Block or compete with the binding of encephalitogenic peptides to the MHC-II molecule
	TCR peptide vaccination	Generation of antibodies against peptides within the TCR
	IL-10,[5] TGFβ,[3] IFNβ[4]	Reduce MHC-II molecule expression
Induction of T-cell anergy	Antibodies to B7 and CD28 molecules[5] Soluble MHC-II/peptide complexes[3]	T-cells are anergised when TCR/peptide/MHC-II interaction occurs in the absence of co-signalling
Alter the balance of proinflammatory (Th-1) and immunomodulatory (Th-2) cytokines	Antibodies to TNFα,[3] IL-1, and soluble IL-2; TNF receptors,[3] and antagonists to IL-1R[5]	Reduce proinflammatory (Th-1) cytokine activity
	IFNβ,[4] IFNα[3]	Antagonise production of proinflammatory cytokines induced by IFNγ
	IFNβ,[4] TGFβ,[3] IL-10[5]	Increase immunomodulatory (Th-2) cytokine activity

(continued)

Table 12-17

Accepted and emerging disease-modifying therapies for MS (*continued*)

Therapeutic strategy	Treatment options	Major putative mechanism of action
	Glucocorticosteroids[1]	Reduce Th-1 cytokine secretion and macrophage function
	Matrix metalloproteinase inhibitors	Block cleavage of pro-TNFα to TNFα
	Methotrexate	Reduces level of soluble IL-2 receptor
	Intravenous immunoglobulin	Reduction of proinflammatory cytokines
Promote remyelination	Insulin-like growth factor-1[3]	Enhance oligodendrocyte survival in vitro and may promote maturation of oligodendrocyte precursors

[1] Unlabelled use in the USA and Europe.
[2] Unlabelled use in the USA.
[3] Phase I-II clinical trials.
[4] Approved for use in relapsing forms of MS in the USA and Europe.
[5] Preclinical testing.
VLA = very late antigen; ICAM = intercellular adhesion molecule; TGF = transforming growth factor; IFN = interferon; TCR = T-cell receptor; TNF = tumor-necrosis factor; IL = interleukin
From Andersson PB, Waubant E, Goodkin D, 1997.

joint movement is difficult. Extensor spasms are more commonly encountered and involve the quadriceps, which extend the knee. Flexor spasms involving the knee joints are usually painful and harder to treat. Where movement of an extremity is seriously impaired, joint contractures may develop. Symptoms may increase, however, with fever, urinary tract infections, and, in some patients, interferon-β therapy (Shapiro, 1994).

Baclofen. Baclofen is an analogue of γ-aminobutyric acid (GABA), which is an inhibitory neurotransmitter in the spinal cord and brain. Baclofen inhibits both monosynaptic and polysynaptic spinal cord reflexes and may exert some effects at supraspinal sites. Its main dose limitation is its CNS depressant effects, typified by sedation or confusion. Constipation and urinary retention are other possible dose-limiting ef-

fects. Peak levels after oral administration of baclofen are achieved in 2 to 3 h, and the serum half-life is 2.5 to 4 h. Between 70 and 80% of baclofen is excreted in the urine unchanged. The drug may be started at 5–10 mg administered at bedtime and increased gradually to a t.i.d. or q.i.d. dosing. Some patients require total doses of 100 to 120 mg per day or more. Intrathecal baclofen, delivered by a rate-controlled, implanted pump, is an alternative to patients who continue to have severe spasticity despite maximum oral doses.

Other GABA agonists. Diazepam or clonazepam may be used to augment the effects of baclofen, particularly to control nighttime muscle spasms, although they tend to have more CNS depressant effects than baclofen. Clonazepam is longer acting than the others, up to 12 h, and may be used in

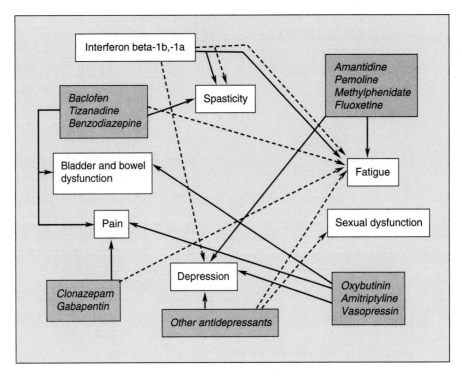

Figure 12–23. *Treatment of multiple sclerosis emphasizing drug effects on various symptoms. Solid arrows indicate beneficial effect of drug on symptoms. Broken arrows indicate possible negative effect. Both types of arrows indicate positive or negative effect.*

doses of 0.5 to 1 mg once or twice each day. Diazepam is given in 2- to 10-mg doses up to three times a day.

Tizanadine.   Tizanadine is an α_2-adrenergic receptor agonist used in Europe to treat spasticity and recently (1997) approved for use in the United States. It is thought to act on spinal motor neurons through polysynaptic, as opposed to monosynaptic, pathways. Following oral administration, peak plasma levels are achieved in 1.5 h, and the serum half-life is 2.5 h. Oral bioavailability is 40% owing to first-pass metabolism in the liver. Although the drug has one tenth to one fiftieth the potency of clonidine in lowering blood pressure, symptomatic hypotension may occur after an 8-mg dose. Because of a risk of hepatocellular injury, it is recommended that amino-

transferase levels be monitored after 1, 3, and 6 months and periodically thereafter. Tizanadine should also be used with caution in elderly patients and those with impaired renal function owing to decreased clearance of the drug. Initial doses are 2 to 4 mg and are increased up to 24 mg per day.

Other drugs used to treat spasticity.   Dantrolene sodium is an option for patients with severe spasticity who do not respond to other agents. The risk of severe hepatocellular injury and side effects limit its general use in MS. Paroxysmal spasms of the arms or legs may respond to antiepileptic agents, including carbamazepine, phenytoin, or valproic acid. These may also be effective in treating paroxysmal symptoms of any kind, including pain, as in trigeminal neuralgia, myoclonus, or dysphonia.

Detailed information on the doses and routes of administration for the more common drugs used to treat MS is provided in Table 12-18.

Bladder and Bowel Dysfunction

Bladder dysfunction is one of the most common symptoms in MS and can be prominent even in those with otherwise mild symptoms. A spastic bladder is characterized by a limited storage capacity for urine due to disinhibited detrusor contractions. It is managed primarily by anticholinergic smooth muscle relaxants such as oxybutynin chloride or tricyclic antidepressants with anticholinergic effects, such as imipramine or amitriptyline. Oxybutynin may be taken in doses ranging from 5 to 10 mg b.i.d. to q.i.d., or the tricyclic antidepressants started at 25 to 50 mg at bedtime, being increased as needed.

Hyoscyamine sulfate is a belladonna alkaloid with anticholinergic properties. It may be taken 0.125 mg every 4 h. An extended release form delivers 0.375 mg every 12 h.

Vasopressin is a useful alternative or adjunctive agent to reduce urination. It is administered as a nasal spray once a day, either in the evening or in the morning. Other agents include propantheline bromide and dicyclomine hydrochloride.

Failure to empty the bladder may result from weak detruser contractions or detruser contractions against a closed external sphincter (detruser–external sphincter dyssynergia). The former is perhaps best managed by intermittent catheterization to reduce postvoid urine residuals, but cholinergic drugs, such as bethanechol, have also been used. α-Adrenergic receptor blocking agents that relax the sphincter may also be used to treat the latter, including terazosin and phenoxybenzamine. Clonidine, an α$_2$-agonist, may also be used.

Bowel dysfunction may include constipation, diarrhea, or incontinence. Anticholinergic drugs used to treat spasticity, bladder dysfunction, or depression may aggravate a preexisting tendency to constipation. A bowel regimen that includes regular fiber in the diet, a bulk agent, stool softeners, and laxatives, if needed, may be advised.

Fatigue

The physiologic basis for fatigue in MS is poorly understood. Some fatigue is probably related to the greater energy required to overcome muscle spasticity in order to conduct activities of daily living. Fatigue in MS, however, can also be a very prominent, or the most prominent, symptom in some patients with minimal or no disability. Clinical depression should also be excluded as a cause for lack of energy. The two drugs commonly used to treat fatigue are amantadine, an indirect acting dopamine receptor stimulant, and pemoline, an amphetamine-like drug. Amantadine, prescribed at 100 mg b.i.d., is generally well tolerated and has a mild effect on fatigue. It may rarely cause livido reticularis of the skin. Pemoline is prescribed at doses of 18.75 to 37.5 mg once per day. Because tachyphylaxis may occur to the antifatigue effect of pemoline, it is advisable patients interrupt therapy 1 or 2 days a week.

Pain

Pain sometimes occurs in patients with spinal cord involvement. It usually parallels sensory symptoms in its distribution and is described as burning and paresthesialike or, alternatively, as a deep pain. Agents used to control this pain include tricyclic antidepressants and antiepileptic drugs, including those with GABA-agonist properties such as gabapentin, diazepam, or clonazepam. Baclofen, the muscle relaxant, also may display some activity in this regard.

ACKNOWLEDGMENTS

JBG acknowledges the generous support of Mr. Tommy Hilfiger, his wife Susan, and his sister Suzie Clapp for the Yale Neuroimmunology Fellowship. JBG and TLV also acknowledge the support of the Nancy Davis Foundation for MS and Center Without Walls. SGW acknowledges the support of the National MS Society and the Veterans Administration. We also thank John Booss, M.D. for his thoughtful review of this manuscript and Justin Hayes for editorial assistance.

Table 12-18

**List of Selected Medications and Available Doses
(and route of administration if not oral)**

Drug	Trade name	Dosage (Route)
IMMUNOMODULATING THERAPIES		
Approved Agents		
Glatiramer acetate	Copaxone	20 mg (SC)
Interferon beta-1a	Avonex	6 MIU (IM)
Interferon beta-1b	Betaseron	8 MIU (SC)
Others		
Azathioprine	Imuran	50 mg
Cladribine	Leustatin	0.07 mg/kg (SC or IV)
Cyclophosphamide	Cytoxan	400–800 mg/m^2 (IV)
Methotrexate		2.5 mg
Methylprednisolone	Solumedrol	500–1000 mg (IV)
SYMPTOMATIC THERAPIES		
Spasticity		
Dantrolene	Dantrium	25, 50 mg
Diazepam	Valium	2, 5, 10 mg
Baclofen	Lioresal	10, 20 mg; 25–300 µg (IT)
Tizanidine	Zanaflex	2, 4, 6 mg
Bladder management		
Bethanechol	Urecholine	5, 10, 25, 50 mg
Clonidine	Catapres	0.1, 0.2, 0.3 mg
Desmopressin	DDAVP Nasal Spray	10 mcg
Dicyclomine	Bentyl	10, 20 mg
Flavoxate	Urispas	100 mg
Hyoscyamine	Levsin, Levsinex	0.125, 0.375 mg
Imipramine	Tofranil	10, 25, 50 mg
Oxybutynin	Ditropan	5 mg
Phenoxybenzamine	Dibenzyline	10 mg
Propantheline	Pro-Banthine	7.5, 15 mg
Terazosin	Hytrin	1, 2, 5, 10 mg
Fatigue		
Amantadine	Symmetrel	100 mg
Fluoxetine	Prozac	10, 20 mg
Methylphenidate	Ritalin	5, 10, 20, 20 mg
Pemoline	Cylert	18.75, 37.5 mg
Pain, spasms, and other paroxysmal symptoms		
Carbamazepine	Tegretol	100, 200 mg
Clonazepam	Klonopin	0.5, 1, 2 mg
Gabapentin	Neurontin	100, 300, 400 mg
Phenytoin	Dilantin	30, 100 mg
Divalproex	Depakote	125, 250, 500 mg

Abbreviations: IM, intramuscular; IT, intrathecal; IV, intravenous; SC, subcutaneous.

For additional information on the drugs discussed in this chapter see chapters 7, 9, 10, 18, 19, 20, 30, 50, 51, and 59 in *Goodman & Gilman's The Pharmacological Basis of Therapeutics* (Ninth Edition), McGraw-Hill, New York, 1996.

REFERENCES

Anderson PB, Waubant E, Goodkin D: How should we proceed with modifying treatments for multiple sclerosis? *Lancet* 1997;349:586–587.

Arnon R: The development of cop 1 (Copakone®), an innovative drug for treatment of multiple sclerosis: personal reflections. *Immunology Letters* 1996;50:1–15.

Beck RW, Cleary PA, Anderson MM Jr et al.: A randomized, controlled trial of corticosteroids in the treatment of acute optic neuritis. *N Engl J Med* 1992;326:581–588.

Bornstein MB, Miller AE, Slogle S, et al.: Clinical trials of cop 1 in multiple sclerosis in Cook SD (ed): *Handbook of Multiple Sclerosis.* New York, Marcel Dekker, 1990, pp 469–480.

Brass LM, Stys PK: *Handbook of Multiple Sclerosis.* New York, Churchill Livingstone, 1991, p 299. Originally from Poser CM et al.: New diagnostic criteria for multiple sclerosis: guidelines for research protocols. *Ann Neurol* 1983;13:227–231.

British and Dutch Multiple Sclerosis Azathioprine Trial Group: Double-masked trial of azathioprine in multiple sclerosis. *Lancet* 1988;23:179–183.

Compston A, Ebers GC: The genetics of multiple sclerosis, in Cook SD (ed): *Handbook of Multiple Sclerosis.* New York, Marcel Dekker, 1990, pp 25–39.

Confavreux C, Saddier P, Grimaud J, et al.: Risk of cancer from azathiprine therapy in multiple sclerosis: a case controlled study. *Neurology* 1996;46:1607–1612.

Durelli L: Recombinant interferon-α in the treatment of multiple sclerosis: effects on exacerbation rate, magnetic resonance imaging of lesion activity, and cytokines, in Reder AT (ed): *Interferon Therapy of Multiple Sclerosis.* New York, Marcel Dekker, 1997, pp 307–342.

Ebers GC, Kukay K, Bulman DE et al.: A full genome search in multiple sclerosis. *Nature Genetics* 1996;13:472–476.

Goodkin DE, Rudick RA, Medendorp SV et al.: Low-dose (7.5 mg) oral methotrexate reduces the rate of progression in chronic progressive multiple sclerosis. *Ann Neurol* 1995;37:30–40.

Halperin JJ, Logigian EL, Finkel MF, Pearl RA: Practice parameters for the diagnosis of patients with nervous system Lyme borreliosis (Lyme disease). *Neurology* 1996;46:619–627.

Honmou O, Felts PA, Waxman SG, Kocsis J: Restoration of normal conduction properties in demyelinated spinal cord axons in the adult rat by transplanation of exogenous Schwann cells. *J Neurosci* 1996;16:3199–3208.

Ikuta F, Zimmerman HM: Distribution of plaques in seventy autopsy cases of multiple sclerosis in the United States. *Neurology* 1976;26:26–28.

Jacobs LD, Cookfair DL, Ruckick RA et al.: Intramuscular interferon beta-1a for disease progression in relapsing multiple sclerosis. *Ann Neurol* 1996;39:285–294.

Johnson KP, Brooks BR, Cohen JA et al.: Copolymer 1 reduces relapse rate and improves disability in relapsing-remitting multiple sclerosis: results of a phase III multicenter, double-blind, placebo-controlled trial. *Neurology* 1995;45:1268–1276.

Kamholtz J: Molecular genetics of myelin basic protein in mouse and humans, in Kim SU (ed): *Myelination and Demyelination: Implications for Multiple Sclerosis.* New York, Plenum Press, 1989, pp 49–59.

Kurtzke JF: A reassessment of the distribution of multiple sclerosis. Part one. *Acta Neurol Scand* 1975a;51:110–136.

Kurtzke JF: A reassessment of the distribution of multiple sclerosis. Part two. *Acta Neurol Scand* 1975b;51:137–157.

Kurtzke JF, Beebe GW, Norman JE Jr.: Epidemiology of multiple sclerosis in US veterans. III. Migration and the risk of MS. *Neurology* 1985;35:672–678.

Lublin FD, Reingold SC, for the National Multiple Sclerosis Society (USA) Advisory Committee on Clinical Trials of New Agents in Multiple Sclerosis: Defining the clinical course of multiple sclerosis: results of an international survey. *Neurology* 1996;46:907–911.

Martyn, CN: The epidemiology of multiple sclerosis, in Matthews WB, Allen IV, Martyn CN (eds): *McAlpine's Multiple Sclerosis.* New York, Churchill Livingstone, 1991, pp 3–40.

Miller AE: Clinical features, in Cook SD (ed): *Handbook of Multiple Sclerosis.* New York, Marcel Dekker, 1990, pp 169–186.

Morrissey SP, Miller DH, Kendall BE et al.: The significance of brain magnetic resonance imaging abnormalities at presentation with clinically isolated syndromes suggestive of multiple sclerosis: a 5-year follow-up study. *Brain* 1993;116:135–146.

Myers LW: Treatment of multiple sclerosis with ACTH and corticosteroids, in Rudick RA, Goodkin DE (eds): *Treatment of Multiple Sclerosis: Trial Design, Results and Future Perspectives.* New York, Springer-Verlag, 1992, pp 135–156.

Offenbacher H, Fazekas F, Schmidt R et al.: Assessment of MRI criteria for a diagnosis of MS. *Neurology* 1993;43:905–909.

Panitch HS, Haley AS, Hirch RL, Johnson KP: Exacerbations of multiple sclerosis in patients treated with gamma interferon. *Lancet* 1987;8538:893–895.

Patten J: *Neurological Differential Diagnosis,* 2d ed. London, Springer-Verlag, 1996 p 98.

Paty DW, Li DKB et al.: Interferon beta-1b is effective in relapsing-remitting multiple sclerosis. II. MRI analysis results of a multicenter, randomized, double-blind, placebo-controlled trial. *Neurology* 1993;43:662–667.

Pfeffer LM, Constantinescu SN: The molecular biology of interferon-β from receptor binding to transmembrane signaling, in Reder AT (ed): *Interferon Therapy of Multiple Sclerosis*. New York, Marcel Dekker, 1997, pp 1–39.

Poser CM, Paty DW, Scheinberg L et al.: New diagnostic criteria for multiple sclerosis: guidelines for research protocols. *Ann Neurol* 1983;13:227–231.

Poskanzer DC, Prenney LB, Sheridan JL, Kondy JV: Multiple sclerosis in the Orkney and Shetland Islands. I: Epidemiology, clinical factors and methodology. *J Epidem Comm Hlth* 1980;34:229–239.

Prineas JW: Pathology of multiple sclerosis, in Cook S (ed): *Handbook of Multiple Sclerosis*. New York, Marcel Dekker, 1990, pp 187–218.

Raine CS: Multiple sclerosis: a pivotal role for the T cell in lesion development. *Neuropath App Neurobiol* 1991;17:265–274.

Report of the Quality Standards Subcommittee of the American Academy of Neurology: Practice advisory on selection of patients with multiple sclerosis for treatment with Betaseron. *Neurology* 1994;44:1537–1540.

Runmarker B, Anderson O: Prognostic factors in a multiple sclerosis incidence cohort with twenty-five years of follow-up. *Brain* 1993;116:117–134.

Sadovnick AD, Ebers GC: Epidemiology of multiple sclerosis: a critical overview. *Can J Neurol Sci* 1993;20:17–29.

Sawcer S, Jones HB, Feakes R et al.: A genome screen in multiple sclerosis reveals susceptibility loci on chromosome 6p21 and 17q22. *Nature Genetics* 1996;13:464–468.

Scheinberg LC, Smith CR: Signs and symptoms of multiple sclerosis, in Scheinberg LC, Holland NJ (eds): *A Guide for Patients and Their Families,* 2d ed. New York, Raven Press, 1987, pp 45.

Schumacher GA, Beebe G, Kibler RF et al.: Problems of experimental trials of therapy in multiple sclerosis: report by the panel on the evaluation of experimental trials of therapy in multiple sclerosis. *Ann NY Acad Sci* 1965;122:552–568.

Sears TA, Bostock H: Conduction failure in demyelination: Is it inevitable?, in Waxman SG and Richie JM (eds): *Demyelinating Disease: Basic and Clinical Electrophysiology*. Raven Press, New York, 1981, pp 357–375.

Shapiro RT: Symptom management in multiple sclerosis. *Ann Neurol* 1994;36:S123–S129.

Shubin RA, Weiner LP: Viruses and demyelinzation, in Kim SU (ed): *Myelination and Demyelination: Implications for Multiple Sclerosis*. New York, Plenum Press, 1989, 129–143. Originally from Weiner LP, Johnson RT, Herndon RM: Viral infections and demyelinating disease. *N Engl J Med* 1973;288:1103.

Steinman L, Waisman A, Altmann A: Major T cell responses in multiple sclerosis. *Mol Med Today* 1995;1:79–83.

The Canadian Cooperative Multiple Sclerosis Study Group: The Canadian cooperative trial of cyclophosphamide and plasma exchange in progressive multiple sclerosis. *Lancet* 1991;337:441–446.

The IFNB Multiple Sclerosis Study Group: Interferon beta-1b is effective in relapsing-remitting multiple sclerosis. I. Clinical results of a multicenter, randomized, double-blind, placebo-controlled trial. *Neurology* 1993;43:655–661.

The INFB Multiple Sclerosis Study Group, the University of British Columbia MS/MRI Analysis Group: Interferon beta-1b in the treatment of multiple sclerosis: final outcome of the randomized controlled trial. *Neurology* 1995;45:1277–1285.

The IFNB Multiple Sclerosis Study Group, the University of British Columbia MS/MRI Analysis Group: Neutralizing antibodies during treatment of multiple sclerosis with interferon beta-1b: experience during the first three years. *Neurology* 1996;47:889–894.

The Multiple Sclerosis Study Group: Efficacy and toxicity of cyclosporine in chronic progressive multiple sclerosis: a randomized, double-blinded, placebo-controlled clinical trial. *Ann Neurol* 1990;27:591–605.

The Multiple Sclerosis Study Group: A complete genomic screen for multiple sclerosis underscores a role for the major histocompatibility complex. *Nature Genetics* 1996;13:469–471.

van Oosten BW, Barkoff F, Truyen L et al.: Increased MRI activity and immune activation in two multiple sclerosis patients treated with the monoclonal anti-tumor necrosis factor antibody cA2. *Neurology* 1996;47:1531–1534.

Waxman SG: Current concepts in neurology: membranes, myelin and the pathophysiology of multiple sclerosis. *N Engl J Med* 1982;306:1529–1532.

Waxman SG: Pathophysiology of multiple sclerosis, in Cook SD (ed): *Handbook of Multiple Sclerosis*. New York, Marcel Dekker, 1990 pp 219–249.

Weiner HL, Mackin GA, Orav EJ et al.: Intermittent cyclophosphamide pulse therapy in progressive multiple sclerosis: final report of the northeast cooperative multiple sclerosis treatment group. *Neurology* 1993;43:910–918.

Weinshenker BG, Bass B, Rice GP et al.: The natural history of multiple sclerosis: a geographically based study. *Brain* 1989;112:133–146.

Weinshenker BG, Rice GP, Noseworthy JH et al.: The natural history of multiple sclerosis: a geographically based study. *Brain* 1991;114:1045–1056.

Whitaker JN, Benveniste EN, Zhou S: Cerebrospinal fluid, in Cook SD (ed): *Handbook of Multiple Sclerosis*. New York, Marcel Dekker, 1990, pp 251–270.

Windhagen A, Nicholson LB, Weiner HL, et al.: Role of Th1 and Th2 cells in neurologic disorders, in Romasnani S (ed): *Th1 and Th2 Cells in Heart Valve Disease*. Chem. Immunol., Krajec, Basal, vol. 63, 1996, pp 171–186.

Witt P: Pharmacokinetics of interferon-β and the biological markers it induces, in Reder AT (ed): *Interferon Therapy of Multiple Sclerosis*. New York, Marcel Dekker, 1997, pp 77–93. Originally reported in Witt PL et al.: Pharmacokinetics of biological responses in vivo after single and multiple doses of interferon-B. *J Immunother* 1993;13:191–200.

PAIN

Richard Payne and Gavril W. Pasternak

Pain is a more terrible lord of mankind than even death itself.
— Albert Schweitzer

Current pharmacotherapies make adequate pain control a realistic and achievable goal for virtually all patients, especially those with chronic pain-complicating medical illness. A thorough assessment of the pain and an accurate diagnosis is the key to successful management. Special attention should be paid to those pain syndromes caused by pathology that can be treated directly, such as metastatic disease. Individualization of therapy is the cornerstone of pain management. The vast majority of patients can be managed with systematically administered analgesics, but when this fails interventional approaches should be considered and addressed by physicians experienced in their use. Many factors other than simple nociceptive input affect the perception of pain. Conversely, uncontrolled pain may have a disastrous impact on all aspects of function and quality of life. Adequate pain management, ideally in a multidisciplinary setting, should therefore be viewed as a high priority for all patients.

Pain, defined by the International Association of Pain as "a sensory or emotional process associated with tissue damage or described in those terms . . ." (Mersky, 1986), is the most common reason for patients to seek out a physician, with 40 million visits per year for evaluation of new pain complaints (Foley, 1996). Society pays a high price to treat chronic pain, $4 billion in direct and indirect medical costs and 515 million lost workdays (Bonica, 1985), which represents an estimated loss of as much as $65 million per year in diminished work productivity.

Unrelieved acute and chronic pain can be considered a public health emergency. Nearly 64 million people suffer from trauma-related pain each year, and another 20 million in the United States are exposed annually to pain associated with surgical procedures, many of whom experience uncontrolled postoperative pain (Jacox et al., 1992). Surveys suggest that approximately 35 million people suffer from chronic headaches and another 16 million people have chronic back pain (Harris, 1985). Burns are yet another source of severe pain, affecting as many as 2 million people per year, and half of all cancer patients, and 90% of those with advanced disease, require treatment for pain. Of these cancer patients, almost half are not managed adequately with the available analgesics (Jacox et al., 1994; Cleeland et al., 1994). Pain is also a common problem associated with acquired immunodeficiency syndrome (AIDS), occurring in over 80% of these patients (Breitbart et al., 1996). Although statistics cannot provide a full understanding of the suffering that needs to be addressed, they do give an indication of the extent of the problem faced by society.

Pain is a subjective sensation that is often difficult for the patient to describe and an observer to assess. It is further complicated by the wide variations in sensitivity among individuals. Even within a particular patient the response to a nociceptive insult can vary dramatically depending on the context in which it is perceived. The meaning of pain can markedly influence the suffering it induces and the ability of a patient to tolerate it. For example, excruciating low back pain in a patient with a remote history of cancer may suddenly diminish with assurances it does not imply metastatic disease from recurrent cancer.

NOCICEPTIVE AND ANTINOCICEPTIVE PHYSIOLOGY

One important aspect of the sensory nervous system is that it makes it possible to focus attention without distractions. Without the ability to sublimate stimuli, humans would be overwhelmed by the simultaneous presentation of the wide range of available sensory input. Focusing requires the ability to filter unneeded input, putting it on hold where it can be accessed when needed. The same types of systems are important in the appreciation of pain. For example, pain is often less troublesome when a patient is distracted. Conversely, in the absence of distractions, such as when a patient is going to sleep, pain may be more problematic. Stress can also modify the perception of pain. In a classic study Beecher found that severely wounded soldiers required far fewer painkillers than civilians undergoing elective surgery (Beecher, 1946). Many people have had similar experiences in a less dramatic context. Oftentimes it is difficult to remember the bump during a game that later becomes a large bruise. Conversely, minimal injuries can provoke severe pain in other situations. Thus, the perception of pain is dependent both on pathways presenting the nociceptive stimuli to the central nervous system and on antinociceptive systems that modulate these sensations. Pain can be treated by targeting either, or both, systems.

To understand pain it is important to appreciate its physiology (Payne and Fasternak, 1992). Nociception can be dissected into fast and slow pain. Fast pain is rapidly transmitted through the neospinothalamic pathway to the thalamus and is readily identified and localized. Slow pain, on the other hand, is responsible for the emotional "hurting." This is the pain compo-

nent that is associated with suffering and is relieved by opioids, such as morphine. Indeed, many patients receiving morphine have observed that the pain no longer hurts even though it is still present. Slow pain is transmitted rostrally through a multisynaptic circuit that includes a variety of limbic structures, which explains its emotional aspects.

The localization of pain perception within the brain is still unsettled. Many areas of the central nervous system are important in processing and interpreting nociceptive stimuli. Peripheral and spinal systems have been well studied, and their ability to respond to nociceptive stimuli through reflex withdrawal well established, even in the presence of spinal transections, but is this pain? Brainstem and limbic systems play a prominent role in the perception of pain (Rainville et al., 1997), as do descending modulatory and spinal pathways. The conscious perception of pain, therefore, is dependent on a complex interaction of a wide range of central pathways.

Periphery

Nociceptors, sensory receptors that respond to noxious or tissue-damaging stimuli, are widely distributed in skin and subcutaneous tissues, muscles, joints, and viscera, and have been defined by both their morphology and physiologic responses to noxious chemical, mechanical, or thermal stimuli (Willis, 1985; Perl, 1984). Two types of fibers are central in the perception of pain: the myelinated A delta fiber (6 μ; 35 m/s) and the unmyelinated C fiber (1 to 2 μ; 1 m/s). The A delta fibers are activated primarily by mechanical stimuli through a receptor ensheathed within an axon–Schwann cell–keterinocyte complex. C fibers, on the other hand, are polymodal and respond to chemical, mechanical, or thermal stimuli. Unlike the A delta fiber, there is no well-defined "receptor," and it has been suggested that this may simply be a "free nerve ending." In microneurography studies, activation of these unmyelinated fibers at frequencies greater than 1.5 m/s have been reported to induce dull, aching, or burning pain, whereas stimulation of the myelinated nociceptor induces a sharp or stinging pain (Torebjork and Hallin, 1979).

Under normal circumstances, cutaneous nociceptors are not spontaneously active. They can be sensitized, however, which decreases their thresholds and increases the intensity of nociceptive stimuli. Moreover, sensitized nociceptors may also show spontaneous activity. Although the mechanisms of nociceptor sensitization have not been defined, prostaglandins, especially PGE_1, bradykinin, and other mediators have been implicated (Steranka et al., 1987; Goldstein et al., 1983; Pela et al., 1996; Dray et al., 1992). The clinical importance of these factors is well illustrated by the analgesic efficacy of nonsteroidal anti-inflammatory agents and bradykinin receptor antagonists.

Spinal Cord and Ascending Pathways

Nociceptive afferents, which comprise as many as 25% of unmyelinated ventral root fibers in humans, make their first synapse in the substantia gelatinosa (lamina II) of the dorsal horn, with additional polysynaptic relays into lamina V. Neurons in laminae I and II are predominately "nociceptive-specific," whereas those in lamina V receive both nociceptive and nonnociceptive inputs, leading to their designation as wide dynamic range cells. Both neuronal types are important in pain perception. Substantia gelatinosa neurons exert minor excitatory and major inhibitory effects segmentally in the cord, providing an important modulation of nociceptive input.

Nociceptive signaling then ascends to higher structures via the spinothalamic tract, predominantly with fibers originating from neurons within laminae I and V. The spinothalamic tract can be divided physiologically and anatomically into the neospinothalamic and paleospinothalamic tracts, which are responsible for conducing "first and second pain," respectively (Willis, 1985). For example, pricking the skin with a pin produces a nociceptive stimulus that is quickly conducted by A delta fibers to the neospinothalamic pathway, which is responsible for transmitting the well-localized pricking sensation. This is then followed by a less pleasant "second pain," which is conveyed by the paleospinothalamic system from C fiber input. The neospinothalamic tract conducts "fast" pain monosynaptically from the dorsal horn to the ventroposterolateral nucleus of the thalamus and then to the somatosensory cortex. Its input is predominantly from A delta and C fibers and it conveys information concerning the quality, intensity, and location of the nociceptive input. The paleospinothalamic tract differs in a number of respects. Unlike the neospinothalamic tract, the paleospinothalamic tract is not topographically organized and projects to the medial and posterior thalamic nuclei through multisynaptic pathways, with extensive interactions with the reticular system. From the thalamus, this system projects diffusely to limbic areas of the brain, explaining its conduction of the poorly localized "suffering," or the affective component of pain.

Anatomically and physiologically, the spinal trigeminal nucleus and adjacent reticular formation are a direct extension of the dorsal horn and serve as the first relay in the transmission of facial pain. Taking this into consideration, the processing of facial pain is analogous to spinal mechanisms.

The Cerebral Cortex and Pain

Although many of the physiologic systems associated with the conduction of pain are well established, the localization of its conscious perception remains somewhat controversial. While nociceptive-specific neurons have been localized in the primate cerebral cortex, cortical lesions are typically not very effective in relieving pain. As noted earlier, the paleospinothalamic pathway is presumed to mediate the affective, "suffering" component of pain. Sectioning this pathway is difficult owing to its diffuse nature with extensive synapses in the reticular and limbic systems. Recent work suggests, however, that the anterior cingulate cortex may play a particularly important role in pain perception (Rainville et al., 1997).

Descending Modulatory Pathways

Descending systems play a major role in the modulation of nociceptive input at the level of the dorsal horn (Fields and Basbaum, 1978; Sherry, 1976; Maciewicz, 1992). Stimulation of the periaqueductal gray provokes a profound analgesia (Reynolds, 1969) that is mediated, at least in part, by descending pathways acting at the spinal level (Fields and Basbaum, 1978; Basbaum and Fields, 1984). The neurons in the periaqueductal gray project to the rostral ventral medulla, including the nucleus raphe magnus. This area, in turn, projects to the spinal cord. A second descending pain-inhibiting pathway originates in the locus coeruleus.

PHARMACOLOGY OF ANTINOCICEPTIVE OPIOID SYSTEMS

Although many neurotransmitters have been implicated in the modulation of pain perception, the opioid systems are most important owing to their effectiveness in attenuating severe pain. Thus, the most potent, clinically useful analgesics are opioids. Although first envisioned as a single system, a number of distinct opioid systems have been identified (Pasternak, 1993). All are capable of modulating severe pain and have clinical significance.

The filtering of sensory input is an important property of the nervous system. Being able to focus attention on specific inputs without extraneous distractions is essential for survival. The opioid system provides an important filtering approach toward the relief of pain. Electrical stimulation studies (Reynolds, 1969) provided the first experimental evidence for an active antinociceptive system within the brain. Subsequent studies revealed that the electrical stimulation of selected brain regions produces a profound analgesic response that could be antagonized by the opioid antagonist naloxone, implying the existence of endogenous opioid systems (Akil et al., 1976). It has now been established that this endogenous opioid system comprises a number of opioid peptides (Table 13-1), which act through a family of opioid receptors (Table 13-2). The complexity of this system has progressively increased over the years, with the addition of a number of additional opioid peptides and receptor subclasses. Each opioid receptor system is quite distinct pharmacologically and can modulate pain independently of the others. These systems often work in concert, however, producing actions far more effective than is possible with one alone. Thus, the endogenous opioid system represents a redundant pain modulatory system with many potential targets for the relief of pain.

The Opioid Peptides

Three major classes of opioid peptides have been identified, each with its own gene and peptide precursor (Table 13-1) (Evans et al., 1988). The enkephalins, first discovered using bioassays (Hughes, 1975; Hughes et al., 1975) and receptor binding assays (Pasternak et al., 1975), are pentapeptides with the structures Tyr-Gly-Gly-Phe-Met or Tyr-Gly-Gly-Phe-Leu. Both [Met^5]enkephalin and [Leu^5]enkephalin are generated from a larger precursor peptide through complex processing (Evans et al., 1988). Additional peptides containing the requisite Tyr-Gly-

Table 13-1

Endogenous and synthetic opioid peptides

Endogenous opioids	
[Leu^5]enkephalin	**Tyr-Gly-Gly-Phe-Leu**
[Met^5]enkephalin	**Tyr-Gly-Gly-Phe-Met**
Dynorphin A	**Tyr-Gly-Gly-Phe-Leu-**Arg-Arg-Ile-Arg-Pro-Lys-Leu-Lys-Trp-Asp-Asn-Gln
Dynorphin B	**Tyr-Gly-Gly-Phe-Leu-**Arg-Arg-Gln-Phe-Lys-Val-Val-Thr
α-Neoendorphin	**Try-Gly-Gly-Phe-Leu-**Arg-Lys-Tyr-Pro-Lys
β-Neoendorphin	**Tyr-Gly-Gly-Phe-Leu-**Arg-Lys-Tyr-Pro
β$_h$-Endorphin	**Tyr-Gly-Gly-Phe-Met-**Thr-Ser-Glu-Lys-Ser-Gln-Thr-Pro-Leu-Val-Thr-Leu-Phe-Lys-Asn-Ala-Ile-Ile-Lys-Asn-Ala-Try-Lys-Lys-Gly-Glu
Endomorphin 1	Try-Pro-Trp-Phe-NH$_2$
Endomorphin 2	Try-Pro-Phe-Phe-NH$_2$
Orphanin FQ/Nociceptin	Phe-Gly-Gly-Phe-Thr-Gly-Ala-Arg-Lys-Ser-Ala-Arg-Lys-Leu-Ala-Asp-Gln
Synthetic	
DAMGO	[D-Ala^2,MePhe^4,Gly(ol)^5]enkephalin
DPDPE	[D-Pen^2,D-Pen^5]enkephalin
DSLET	[D-Ser^2,Leu^5]enkephalin-Thr^6
DADL	[D-Ala^2,D-Leu^5]enkephalin
CTOP	D-Phe-Cys-Tyr-D-Trp-Orn-Thr-Pen-Thr-NH$_2$
[D-Ala^2,Glu^4]Deltorphin	Tyr-D-Ala-Phe-Glu-Val-Val-Gly-NH$_2$
Morphiceptin	Tyr-Pro-Phe-Pro-NH$_2$
PL-017	Tyr-Pro-MePhe-D-Pro-NH$_2$

Table 13-2

Opioid receptor classification and localization of analgesic actions

Receptor		Analgesia	Other
Mu			
	Mu$_1$	Supraspinal	Prolactin release
			Acetylcholine release in the hippocampus
			Feeding
	Mu$_2$	Spinal	Respiratory depression
			Gastrointestinal transit
			Dopamine release by nigrostriatal neurons
			Guinea pig ileum bioassay
			Feeding
	M6G	Supraspinal/spinal	
Kappa			Psychotomimesis
			Sedation
	Kappa$_1$	Spinal/supraspinal	Diuresis
			Feeding
	Kappa$_2$	Unknown	Unknown
	Kappa$_3$	Supraspinal	
Delta			Mouse vas deferens bioassay
			Dopamine turnover in the striatum
			Feeding
	Delta$_1$	Supraspinal	
	Delta$_2$	Spinal and supraspinal	

Some of the actions attributed to a general family of receptor have not yet been associated with a specific subtype. All the correlations in this table are based upon animal studies, which can show species differences.

Gly-Phe motif are present within the preproenkephalin sequence, but their physiologic and pharmacologic relevance has not yet been established.

The discovery of the dynorphin family followed soon after the enkephalins (Chavkin et al., 1982; Chavkin and Goldstein, 1981). Dynorphin A is a heptadecapeptide (Table 13-1) with potent opioid activity. Structurally, the sequence of [Leu^5]enkephalin is present at the NH$_2$-terminus, leading many to prematurely assume that [Leu^5]enkephalin was a breakdown product of dynorphin A. Preprodynorphin and preproenkephalin are, however, distinct gene products (Evans et al., 1988). Additional Tyr-Gly-Gly-Phe-Leu- sequences were identified within preprodynorphin, leading to the identification of sev-

eral additional potential opioid peptides, including dynorphin B and α-neoendorphin (Table 13-1). As with the extended enkephalin peptides present within preproenkephalin, the physiologic significance of these dynorphins has not yet been fully established.

β-Endorphin is the third member of opioid peptides (Evans et al., 1988; Li and Chung, 1976). Containing the same first five amino acids as [Met^5]enkephalin, β-endorphin is by far the largest of the opioid peptides. As with the other families, β-endorphin is generated from a larger precursor peptide, prepro-opiomelanocortin (Fig. 13-1) (Li and Chung, 1976). This single precursor also yields the important stress hormone adrenocorticotrophin hormone (ACTH), as well as melanocyte stimulatory hormone

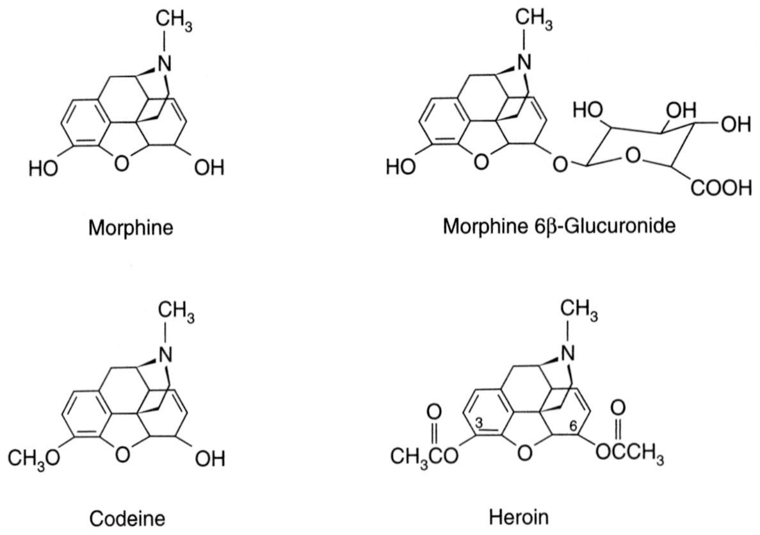

Figure 13–1. *Structure of morphine and related opioids.*

(MSH). Physiologically, β-endorphin is released by the same stimuli as ACTH, leading to the interesting suggestion that it may be responsible for the diminished responses to pain seen in people experiencing stress.

These peptides have a number of similarities beyond sharing a conserved NH$_2$-terminus. All are analgesics and interact with the various opioid receptor classes, albeit with varying affinities and selectivities and all are quite labile physiologically owing to the presence of highly efficient peptidases. Major synthetic efforts have now led to agents with far greater stability, many of which contain D-alanine at the second position (Evans et al., 1988). Furthermore, it has been possible to develop very highly selective peptides for all of the various opioid receptor subtypes. These have proven extremely valuable in defining the various opioid receptor systems. Some of these agents are presented in Table 13-1.

A major question in the area of opioid pharmacology has been the endogenous ligand for the mu receptors. Although peptides such as β-endorphin label mu receptors with reasonably high affinities, the evidence implicating them as the endogenous mu ligand has not been particularly strong. Recently, a new class of opioid peptide, the endomorphins, have been identified (Table 13-1) (Zadina et al., 1997). Unlike the other opioid peptides, endomorphins have both high affinity and selectivity for the mu receptors. Their pharmacology is only now being established and additional work is needed to firmly establish their pharmacologic significance.

Several groups have identified yet another peptide related to the opioid family, orphanin FQ (Reinscheid et al., 1995) or nociceptin (OFQ/N) (Meunier et al., 1995). Originally identified as a ligand for a cloned member of the opioid receptor family (Pan et al., 1994, 1995, 1996a–b; Bunzow et al., 1994; Lachowicz et al., 1995; Mollereau et al., 1994; Wang et al., 1994; Wick et al., 1994; Uhl et al., 1994; Keith Jr. et al., 1994; Chen et al., 1994; Fukuda et al., 1994), OFQ/N is a heptadecapeptide with a great deal of homology to dynorphin A. Although the presence of phenylalanine as the first amino acid distinguishes it from the traditional opioid peptides, its pharmacology is even more unique. Despite their different selectivities among the various opioid receptor classes, the natural opioid peptides all display at least modest affinity for the other opioid receptors. OFQ/N, on the other hand, has no appreciable affinity for any of the traditional opioid receptors (Foddi and Mennini, 1997; Ardati et al., 1997; Dooley and Houghten, 1996; Reinscheid et al., 1995; Mathis et al., 1997; Meunier et al., 1995). Furthermore, none of the traditional opioid ligands, peptides, or alkaloids label the OFQ/N receptor with affinities comparable to those seen with traditional opioid receptors.

The pharmacology of OFQ/N is quite complex. OFQ/N can clearly activate antianalgesic systems that functionally reverse opioid and nonopioid analgesia (Rossi et al., 1997; Reinscheid et al., 1995; Hara et al., 1997; Tian et al., 1997; Grisel et al., 1996; Mogil et al., 1996a; Mogil et al., 1996b; Meunier et al. 1995), while in other paradigms, OFQ/N is a potent analgesic (Xu et al., 1996; King et al., 1997; Tian et al., 1997; Rossi et al., 1996; Rossi et al., 1997). These actions have suggested the possibility of subtypes within the OFQ/N receptor family that are just beginning to be investigated. The OFQ/N system may provide future targets in the control of pain. Its ability to activate a potent antianalgesic system suggests a possible therapeutic role for OFQ/N receptor antagonists. Alternatively, it may be possible to develop analgesic OFQ/N analogues lacking the antianalgesic actions of the parent compound. Clearly, more work is needed to more fully elucidate the actions of this agent.

Opioid Receptors

The understanding of opioid receptors has been very dependent on the availability of novel agents. Before the discovery of the opioid peptides, opioid pharmacology was assessed solely with morphine and related alkaloids. Natural alkaloid derivatives, including morphine and codeine (Fig. 13-1), and thebaine, another alkaloid present in the poppy, provided the starting material for many semisynthetic agents (Reisine and Pasternak, 1996). Thousands of agents were synthesized in the hopes of obtaining a drug capable of relieving pain without the side effects characteristic of these alkaloids. Although most of these new agents retained the properties of morphine, several displayed unusual pharmacologies. Nalorphine, which is structurally similar to morphine (Fig. 13-2), was the first mu receptor antagonist and also provided the first evidence to suggest the existence of

multiple classes of opioid receptors. Clinical studies revealed that low doses of nalorphine reversed the analgesic actions of morphine. However, as the nalorphine dose increased analgesia returned, leading Martin to propose in his hypothesis of "receptor dualism" a second opioid receptor responsible for nalorphine analgesia (Martin, 1967). The nalorphine receptor has since been classified within the kappa-receptor family (Martin et al., 1976).

The concept of multiple opioid receptors (Table 13-2) has grown through extensive pharmacologic and biochemical studies, in large part owing to the availability of a wide range of novel opioid agonists and antagonists (Reisine and Pasternak, 1996; Pasternak, 1993). Using these substances the various receptors, described in the following, can be easily distinguished from one another although they share many properties. All of the opioid receptor subtypes can elicit analgesia through their own independent mechanism. This has been demonstrated by the ability of highly selective antagonists to block the actions of only a single class of opioids and by the lack of cross-tolerance among highly selective drugs. Thus, virtually all of the opioid receptor subtypes provide potential targets for the design of novel analgesics.

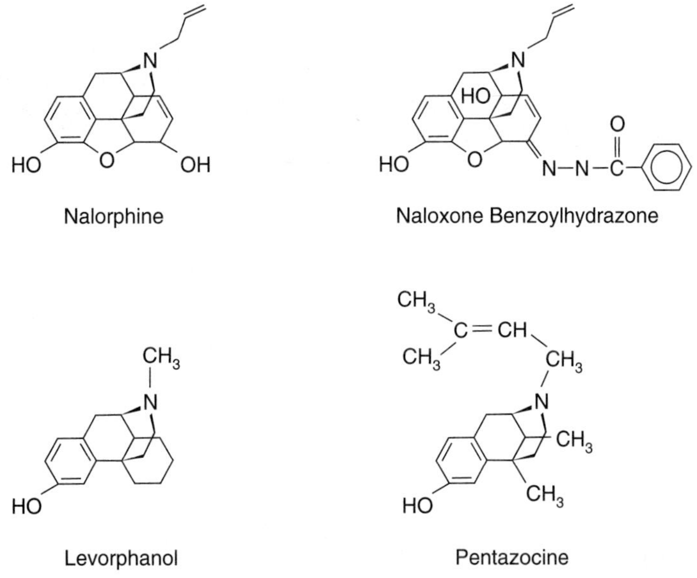

Figure 13–2.   Structure of kappa opioids.

Mu receptors.   Mu receptors were the first opioid receptors identified in receptor binding studies (Terenius, 1973; Simon et al., 1973; Pert and Snyder, 1973). Soon afterward, additional studies suggested mu-receptor subtypes (Pasternak et al., 1980a; Hahn et al., 1982a; Nishimura et al., 1984a; Rothman et al., 1987a; Lutz et al., 1985a; Lutz et al., 1984a; Toll et al., 1984a; Pasternak et al., 1980a; Pasternak and Snyder, 1975a). Although receptor binding studies played an important role in defining the existence of these two sites, the most important differences were detected in behavioral studies (Table 13-2) (Ling et al., 1986; Ling et al., 1985; Ling et al., 1983; Pasternak et al., 1980; Heyman et al., 1988; Pasternak et al., 1980; Pick et al., 1991; Paul and Pasternak, 1988; Paakkari et al., 1993; Kamei et al., 1993; Janik et al., 1992). Selective mu_1 antagonists effectively distinguished between subtypes, antagonizing systemic and supraspinal morphine without affecting gastrointestinal transit or respiratory depression. Additional studies defined the subtypes responsible for many of the other actions of morphine as well. The pharmacology of the two mu-receptor subtypes has been extensively reviewed (Reisine and Pasternak, 1996; Pasternak, 1993).

More recently, a third member of the mu-receptor family, which is responsible for the actions of an extremely potent morphine metabolite, morphine-6β-glucuronide (M6G) (Fig. 13-1) was proposed (Rossi et al., 1996a; Pasternak and Standifer, 1995a; Rossi et al., 1995a). M6G is one of the major metabolites of morphine and, with chronic morphine administration, M6G blood levels actually surpass those of morphine (Tiseo et al., 1995). Given systemically, M6G is approximately twice as potent as morphine in animal models (Paul et al., 1989; Yoshimura et al., 1973; Shimomura et al., 1971) and clinically (Lötsch et al., 1996; Thompson et al., 1995; Grace and Fee, 1996). Thus, the major analgesic activity in patients receiving chronic morphine may be due to M6G. The role of M6G may be even more important in patients with renal compromise because this is the major route for its excretion (D'Honneur et al., 1994). When the blood-brain barrier is avoided by administering the drug directly in the brains of laboratory animals, M6G is more than 100-fold more potent than morphine (Pasternak et al., 1987; Paul et al., 1989).

Evidence from a number of sources indicates that M6G analgesia is mediated through a novel receptor subtype. Antisense studies based on the MOR-1 clone revealed dramatic differences between M6G and morphine (Rossi et al., 1997a; Rossi et al., 1996a; Rossi et al., 1995a). Genetic approaches support this concept. Despite the analgesic insensitivity of the CXBK mouse to morphine, M6G is fully active (Rossi et al., 1996a). The most impressive evidence, however, is the retention of M6G analgesia in mice in which the gene encoding the mu receptor (MOR-1) has been inactivated—"knockout mouse"—making the animal insensitive to morphine. Finally, a selective M6G antagonist has been reported (Brown et al., 1997). The significance of the M6G receptor is further evident by its role in the actions of other opioids. Fentanyl is widely used in anesthesiology and pain management. Although fentanyl can act through mu receptors, it also works through M6G receptors. Foremost in the list of M6G receptor-active drugs, however, is heroin (Rossi et al., 1996a). Thus, there are three independent mu-receptor subtypes.

Delta receptors.   Delta receptors were first demonstrated in a mouse bioassay that distinguished the actions of enkephalins from those of morphine (Lord et al., 1977). This was quickly followed by the identification of highly selective delta (enkephalin-selective) binding sites in brain (Chang et al., 1980; Chang et al., 1979; Lord et al., 1977). The study of these receptors has been facilitated by the development of a large series of highly selective peptide and alkaloid agonists and antagonists, including the antagonist naltrindole (Pasternak, 1993; Reisine and Pasternak, 1996). In animal models of pain delta drugs are potent analgesics. Because they act independently from the traditional mu receptors, there is no cross-tolerance between delta drugs, morphine, or other mu agents. Delta drugs have a different side effect profile than other opioids and do not produce the typical signs of dependence in animal models. At present, no delta analgesics are clinically available, although significant effort is directed toward this objective. There now is strong evidence for two distinct delta-receptor subtypes, $delta_1$ and $delta_2$, which have been defined by a series of novel agonists and antagonists (Chakrabarti et al., 1993; Mattia et al., 1991; Jiang et al., 1991; Vanderah et al., 1994). Additional work is needed, however, to assess the full pharmacologic implications of this receptor system.

Kappa receptors.   The family of kappa receptors provided the first evidence for multiple classes of opioid receptors (Iwamoto and Martin, 1981; Martin, 1967; Martin et al., 1976). Using published results from clinical studies examining nalorphine/morphine combinations (Houde and Wallenstein, 1956; Lasagne and Beecher, 1954), Martin proposed the concept of "receptor dualism" (Martin, 1967), which he then refined into the mu/kappa classification that is widely used today (Martin et al., 1976). There are two major subdivisions within this family, although detailed binding studies have suggested as many as four (Paul et al., 1991; Cheng et al., 1992; Cheng et al., 1995; Gistrak et al., 1990; Clark et al., 1989; Paul et al., 1990). The $kappa_1$ receptors have been defined by the highly selective synthetic agonist U50,488H and the antagonist norbinaltorphimine (VonVoightlander et al., 1983; Portoghese et al., 1987). Together, these agents have defined $kappa_1$ actions. Dynorphin A is the endogenous ligand for this receptor for which it has a very high affinity (Chavkin et al., 1982; Chavkin and Goldstein, 1981). However, the selectivity of dynorphin A is somewhat limited because it also has significant affinity for other opioid receptor subtypes. The pharmacologic profile of $kappa_1$ drugs is distinct from that of other opioids. Although $kappa_1$ drugs are analgesics, they produce little gastrointestinal transit inhibition or respiratory depression. Diuresis, however, is consistently seen, which may prove to be clinically significant. Clinically, a number of agents act, at least in part, through kappa$_1$ receptors. The most widely used drug of this type is pentazocine (Fig. 13-2) (Chien and Pasternak, 1995). Several highly selective kappa$_1$ drugs have been examined clinically, but were abandoned owing to problems with dysphoric and psychotomimetic side effects. The suggestion of kappa$_1$ subtypes may be important if it is possible to dissociate these actions from their analgesic activity.

The kappa$_3$ receptor has also proven important from the clinical perspective. Formally defined using a novel opioid, naloxone benzoylhydrazone (Fig. 13-2) (Gistrak et al., 1990; Price et al., 1989; Clark et al., 1989; Paul et al., 1990), kappa$_3$ receptors are responsible for the analgesic actions of nalorphine (Paul et al., 1991) and are important for mediating the response to other clinical agents, such as nalbuphine (Pick et al., 1992) and levorphanol (Tive et al., 1992) (Fig. 13-2). As with the other opioid receptor subtypes, the binding selectivity profile of the kappa$_3$ receptor is quite distinct from the others, which has been used to define it pharmacologically.

Molecular biology of opioid receptors

Opioid receptors fall into the classification of G protein–linked seven transmembrane receptors. The delta receptor (DOR-1) was the first opioid receptor cloned (Evans et al., 1992; Kieffer et al., 1992), followed quickly by mu (MOR-1) (Bare et al., 1994; Min et al., 1994; Kozak et al., 1994; Chen et al., 1994; Uhl et al., 1994; Eppler et al., 1993; Thompson et al., 1993) and kappa$_1$ receptors (KOR-1) (Simonin et al., 1995; Knapp et al., 1995; Liu et al., 1995; Yasuda et al., 1993; Minami et al., 1993) and a novel member of the opioid family (ORL$_1$/KOR-3) (Pan et al., 1994, 1995, 1996a and 1996b; Wick et al., 1995b; Fukuda et al., 1994b; Mollereau et al., 1994b; Wang et al., 1994b; Bunzow et al., 1994b; Chen et al., 1994b; Lachowicz et al., 1995b; Wick et al., 1994b; Keith Jr. et al., 1994b; Uhl et al., 1994b; Pan et al., 1994, 1995, 1996a and 1996b). The different receptors are highly homologous, particularly in the transmembrane regions, and are clearly members of a distinct receptor family. The genes for all of these receptors contain multiple exons with a number of splice variants having been reported. However, the pharmacologic significance of these variants remains unclear. When expressed in cell lines, the various cDNA clones generate receptors with binding affinities and selectivities similar to those characterized in brain tissues.

Much effort has focused on correlating cloned receptors with opioid behavior. Initially, this was done using antisense approaches (Pasternak and Standifer, 1995). By designing cDNA probes complementary to unique regions of the mRNA's encoding the various cloned receptors, it is possible to selectively diminish the production of one opioid receptor without affecting the others. Using this approach, the importance of DOR-1 in spinal delta analgesia (Lai et al., 1994; Standifer et al., 1994), MOR-1 in morphine actions (Rossi et al., 1996a; Rossi et al., 1995a; Rossi et al., 1994a), and

KOR-1 with kappa$_1$ analgesia (Adams et al., 1994; Chien et al., 1994) was established. Mice in which the various opioid receptors have been eliminated by targeted disruption (i.e. knockout mice) also have proven helpful in examining the functional correlation between the genes and behavior. Knockout mice lacking MOR-1 are insensitive to morphine (Tian et al., 1997; Sora et al., 1997; Matthes et al., 1996).

Despite advances in the understanding of opioid pharmacology, many questions remain. Foremost is the relationship between the four clones with the numerous receptor subtypes defined pharmacologically (Pasternak, 1993). Although several splice variants have been reported for mu receptor (Zimprich et al., 1994; Bare et al., 1994), they do not explain the pharmacologically defined mu receptor subtypes. Antisense mapping of morphine, M6G, and heroin, and their activity profile in receptor knockout mice, reveals markedly different sensitivity patterns. Further studies are needed to resolve whether the pharmacologically defined subtypes represent distinct gene products or splice variants of the genes already identified. A similar situation exists for the delta receptor (Rossi et al., 1997b), which has two postulated subtypes, and for the orphan opioid receptor (Pasternak and Standifer, 1995; Pan et al., 1995; Pan et al., 1994). This fourth cloned member of the opioid receptor family, KOR-3/ORL$_1$, has high affinity for OFQ/N but not for traditional opioids. Yet a number of approaches clearly reveal a close relationship at the molecular level between KOR-3/ORL$_1$ and the kappa$_3$ receptor.

PATHOPHYSIOLOGY OF PAIN

Acute pain typically alerts someone to the presence of harmful, or potentially harmful, stimuli. On the other hand, chronic pain is not a simple extension of acute pain in time. Persistent tissue injury with activation of nociceptors, especially in the presence of inflammation, produces pharmacologic, physiologic, and anatomic changes in the central processing of nociceptive information (Wolfe, 1994). These changes involve many mechanisms, with activation of glutamic acid N-methyl-D-aspartate (NMDA) receptors being particularly important.

Some clinicians refer to the "chronic pain state" to describe patients who report pain on a long-term basis without any apparent tissue injury. Adaptation of sympathetic activity and the development of chronic vegetative signs, including a decrease in appetite, malaise, sleep disturbances, and irritability, characterize chronic pain. In fact, these psychologic counterparts to the chronic pain state are often associated with depression, anger, and other affective states, and are key in understanding the disability associated with this condition (Anonymous, 1992). Usually chronic pain does not serve to warn the patient about bodily injury and thus serves no useful function.

Clinically, several broad types of pain have been proposed: somatic, visceral, neuropathic, and complex regional pain syndromes (formerly known as sympathetically maintained pain.) (Table 13-3) (Stanton-Hicks et al., 1995; Payne, 1997).

Somatic or nociceptive pain. The most common type of pain, somatic or nociceptive, occurs as a result of activation of nociceptors in cutaneous and deep musculoskeletal tissues. It is usually well localized to the site of pathology and may be felt in superficial cutaneous or deeper musculoskeletal structures.

Visceral pain. Visceral pain results from ischemia, infiltration, compression, distention, torsion, or stretching of thoracic, abdominal, and pelvic viscera. Typically, it is poorly localized and often associated with nausea, vomiting, and diaphoresis, particularly when acute. Visceral pain is often referred to cutaneous sites that may be remote from the site of the lesion. Examples include myocardial infarctions with their associated jaw or left arm pain or deep substernal pressure, or in diaphragmatic irritation, which often produces shoulder pain. Tenderness at the referred cutaneous site may occur, occasionally making the diagnosis difficult (Cervero, 1994). Visceral pain is mediated through both the sympathetic and parasympathetic nervous systems. Recently "silent nociceptors" have been identified in visceral tissues (Gebhart, 1995). These nociceptors are not active until sensitized by inflammatory and other chemical stimuli, but once sensitized they respond with many of the same neurophysiologic characteristics as nociceptors in somatic nerves. The sensitization of silent visceral nociceptors has been implicated in the development of chronic abdominal pain associated with syndromes such as inflammatory bowel disease.

Neuropathic pain. Neuropathic pain results from injury to the peripheral and/or central nervous systems (Casey, 1991). Pain resulting from lesions to the peripheral nerves that partially or completely in-

Table 13-3
Pain Categories

Type of pain	Examples	Putative mechanisms
Nociceptive	Arthritis; fractures; bone metastasis; cellulitis	Activation of nociceptors
Visceral	Pancreatitis; peptic ulcer; myocardial infarction	Activation of nociceptors
Neuropathic	Herpes zoster; central pain; diabetic neuropathy; trigeminal neuralgia	Ectopic discharges within the nervous system; spontaneous activity in nerves; neuroma formation; others
Complex regional pain syndromes	Persistent focal pain following trauma with or without evidence of sympathetic involvement	Sensitization of spinal neurons; ephaptic transmission; others

terrupts afferent sensory transmission between the peripheral and central nervous systems has been termed "deafferentation" pain. Pain resulting from spinal cord or brain injury, such as with strokes, demyelinating disease, or traumatic injury, is termed "central pain." The recent development of animal models of neuropathic pain have provided an opportunity to examine the neurophysiologic and pharmacologic correlates of neural injury and pain (Tal and Bennet, 1993).

A complete understanding of the pathophysiology of pain in a particular patient is seldom possible, with several physiologic mechanisms frequently coexisting. Nonetheless, clinical inferences regarding pain mechanisms often have important diagnostic and therapeutic implications (Payne, 1997). For example, paroxysmal or lancinating pain should alert the physician to a neuropathic etiology, even in the absence of demonstrable sensory or motor abnormalities or reflex changes. The prescription of tricyclic antidepressant or anticonvulsant medications may successfully manage this lancinating pain when traditional analgesics such as opioids or nonsteroidal anti-inflammatory agents have failed (Swerdlow, 1984; Max, 1995).

Complex regional pain syndrome (Reflex Sympathetic Dystrophy). The sympathetic nervous system is often involved in somatic, visceral, or neuropathic pain, although its role is poorly understood and, indeed, has been challenged recently (Verdugo and Ochoa, 1994). Reflex sympathetic dystrophy, or sympathetically maintained pain, is now termed complex regional pain syndrome (CRPS) to avoid any inferences regarding the presence or absence of sympathetic involvement (Stanton-Hicks et al., 1995). Complex regional pain syndrome has been subclassified. Type I includes the traditionally recognized syndromes that do not involve primary injury to nerves. Type II corresponds to the syndromes historically termed causalgia that distinguishes patients with nerve injury. Either syndrome may present with features of regional sympathetic hyperactivity and respond to sympathetic interruption, and hence may be sympathetically mediated. These syndromes also may respond to more conventional analgesic

therapies in the absence of sympathetic nervous system interventions. Associated signs and symptoms of nerve injury or dystrophy, such as muscle atrophy, osteoporosis, or neurophysiologic and electrophysiologic signs of nerve injury, are not predictive in defining response to therapy in these syndromes (Treede et al., 1992).

Principles of Pain Assessment

Successful pain management begins with a thorough and accurate assessment of the complaint (Table 13-4). However, many physicians unfortunately remain unskilled in assessing clinical pain. In a recent large prospective study of cancer pain management, 63% of 1170 physicians surveyed indicated that inadequate pain assessment skills were the primary reason for suboptimal outcomes and patient management in their practice settings (Von Roenn et al., 1993). Several key points should be evaluated in each patient with a new or recurring pain complaint (Table 13-4).

The history should consider the location, quality, duration, intensity, temporal pattern, and aggravating or relieving factors associated with the pain. The clinician should obtain information regarding the extent of pathology or tissue damage associated with the specific disease or disorder. Although pain intensity may not always correlate with the level of pathology, especially in disorders such as cancer, AIDS, and sickle cell anemia, there is often a reasonable correlation between increasing pain and progression of disease. Psychological factors play a major role in pain management and particular attention should be paid to the patient's psychological state and coping style, and degree of family or social support. For patients with potentially life-threatening diseases, a discussion about prognosis with the primary treating physician, the patient, and the family is invaluable since it places in context the meaning of the pain.

A detailed physical examination with a focused neurologic examination is always important, but particularly so when neuropathic pain is suspected. The mental status of the patient should be evaluated because it may determine the reliability of self reports of pain.

Table 13-4
Principles of Pain Assessment

1. **Provide supportive environment for patient and family to discuss current pain problems and anticipatory fears about pain problems in future.**
2. **Ask about the pain, document its characteristics, and measure its intensity with simple tools.**
   Trust the patient's self-report.
   Measure both pain intensity and pain relief using a numerical rating scale (0–10) or visual analogue scale.
   Assess factors that exacerbate or relieve the pain, especially movement.
   Evaluate the psychological and functional impact of pain on the patient and family.
   Assess the patient for signs of depression, anxiety, and distress and treat accordingly.
   Assess prior coping style of patient and family during previously stressful periods.
   Establish any current or remote history of substance abuse in the patient or family.
3. **Determine the cause of pain.**
   Perform careful physical and neurologic examinations and any relevant laboratory or imaging studies to determine the presence and extent of somatic, visceral, and/or neurological pathology.
   Evaluate disease activity (e.g., tumor markers in cancer patients; CD4 counts in AIDs patients; hemoglobin levels and hemolysis in sickle cell anemia patients; etc.).
   Rule out additional causes of pain (e.g., infection or other disease or disorder).
   Use analgesics appropriately to facilitate the diagnostic evaluation.
   Treat the cause of pain whenever possible with disease-specific therapies.
4. **Continuously reassess the patient for analgesic needs and re-evaluate new pain complaints.**

Diagnostic testing is often necessary to determine the etiology of the pain complaint. It is important for the attending physician to personally review radiologic studies to ensure the relevant anatomy has been imaged and to assess the relevance of any abnormal findings. However, abnormalities are not always the cause of pain. For example, in a recent study of low back pain, many abnormal MRI findings that were thought to be related to the pain were not associated with pain complaints by the patient (Deyo, 1994). Documentation of disease progression may provide insights into the cause of the

pain long before objective physical signs or radiographic findings develop. Critical to a successful outcome of treatment is the need to continually reassess the patient, especially when pain is unresolved.

PRINCIPLES OF PAIN MANAGEMENT

There are several basic therapeutic strategies for pain management (Table 13-5). Although the pharmacotherapy of pain constitutes the mainstay of treatment

Table 13-5
Therapeutic Strategies in Pain Management

Type of therapy	Clinical examples	Therapeutic examples
Pharmacologic	Cornerstone of treatment for most pain syndromes	See Tables 13-6, 13-7, 13-8
Behavioral/ Psychological	Useful in almost all pain syndromes to treat coexisting anxiety and improve patient and family coping strategies	Deep breathing, relaxation exercises Cognitive-behavioral therapies
Anesthetic	Pain localized to peripheral nerve or spinal roots Midline or bilateral pain at or below thorax	Celiac plexus block for pancreatic cancer Epidural or intrathecal analgesic administration
Neurosurgical	Pain refractory to analgesic or anethestic interventions	Cordotomy or myelotomy Hypophysectomy for diffuse metastatic bone pain
Physiatric	Musculoskeletal pain and spasm	Focal application of heat, ultrasound, or cold

for most pain associated with medical disorders, experienced pain clinicians individualize and integrate additional relevant therapeutic modalities. Although the remainder of this section is concerned with the pharmacotherapy of pain, analgesic drugs should always be used with appropriate assessment of pain and the aim of balancing pain relief while maximizing the functional goals set with the patient. The analgesics most commonly used in the management of acute and chronic pain are listed in Tables 13-6, 13-7, and 13-8 and are discussed in the following section.

Mu Analgesics

Morphine. Morphine remains the most widely used opioid analgesic and is the gold standard against which all other drugs are compared. Because most opioids in clinical use are chemical derivatives of morphine, it is not surprising that most possess similar pharmacologic properties and are classified as mu receptor drugs. Morphine is particularly useful owing

to its low cost and availability. Its utility in recent years has increased with the development of slow-release formulations that enable dosing intervals to be extended to up to 24 h.

Morphine and related drugs have several sites of action within the nervous system. Animal studies reveal profound analgesic actions following microinjections of morphine into specific brain regions, such as the periaqueductal gray, nucleus raphe magnus, and locus coeruleus. Morphine also is a potent analgesic when administered at the spinal level, explaining its widespread use epidurally and intrathecally. At the spinal level, opioids act at the level of the dorsal horn, a region containing high levels of opioid receptors. Moreover, morphine and related compounds act peripherally, presumably directly on the nociceptive fibers involved with pain perception. Systemic drugs probably act through a combination of these systems. This is important because these different systems interact synergistically with each other. For example, animal studies clearly demonstrate that the dose of morphine needed to elicit

Table 13-6

Commonly Used Opioids for Cancer Pain

WHO Step II Opioids	Usual starting dose	Comment
Codeine with acetaminophen or aspirin Tylenol #2 (15 mg codeine) Tylenol #3 (30 mg codeine) Tylenol #4 (60 mg codeine)	60 mg q 3–4 h PO	Fixed combinations scheduled as DEA III; single entity as DEA II Take care not to exceed toxic doses of acetaminophen or aspirin
Hydrocodone with acetaminophen or aspirin Lorcet; Lortab: Vicodan, others	10 mg q 3–4 h PO	Same as for codeine; Vicodan-ES has 750 mg ASA/tablet
Oxycodone with acetaminophen or aspirin Percocet; Percodan; Tylox; others	5 mg q 3–4 h PO	
Tramadol	50 mg qid PO	Although a mu receptor agonist, it is not scheduled as an opioid. Nausea common. Seizures may occur at doses > 400 mg per day
WHO Step II/III Opioids		
Morphine Immediate release (MSIR)	30 mg q 3–4 h PO 10 mg q 3–4 h IV	Also available as suppository MSIR is preferred rescue analgesic for controlled-release preparations
Sustained release MS Contin; Oramorph	30 mg q 12 h PO	MS Contin and Oramorph may not be therapeutically interchangeable

Oxycodone
Sustained release
  Oxycontin
  Roxicodone
	20 mg q 12 h PO	Twice as potent as morphine; immediate-release oxycodone is recommended as rescue for Oxycontin

Hydromorphone Dilaudid; others	6 mg q 12 h PO	Sustained-release formulation in clinical development Available as a suppository

Fentanyl
  Duragesic (transdermal)
  Sublimaze; other
	25–50 μg/h
	50 μ/h i.v. infusion
		Available for transdermal administration; patches are replaced every 3 days. Potency relative to morphine close to 100:1.

Methadone Dolophine; other	20 mg q 6–8 h PO 10 mg q 6–8 h IV	Very stigmatized because used to treat heroin addiction.
Levorphanol Levodromoran	4 mg q 6–8 h PO	Relatively long-acting; may have higher incidence of psychotomimetic effects than other opioids

Table 13-7

Nonopioid Analgesics

Generic name	Trade name	Typical starting dose
Acetaminophen	Tylenol and others	650 mg q 4 h PO
Aspirin	Multiple	650 mg q 4 h PO
Ibuprofen	Motrin, Advil, and others	200–800 mg q 6 h PO
Choline-magnesium Trisalicylate	Trilisate	1000–1500 mg tid PO
Diclofenac sodium	Voltaren	50–75 mg q 8–12 PO
Diflunisal	Dolobid	500 mg q 12 PO
Etodolac	Lodine	200–400 mg q 8–12 h PO
Flurbiprofen	Ansaid	200–300 mg q 4–8 h PO
Naproxen	Naprosyn	250-750 mg q 12 h PO
Naproxen sodium	Anaprox	275 mg q 12 h PO
Oxprozin	Dayprop	600–1200 mg q daily PO
Sulindac	Clinoril	150–200 mg q 12 h PO
Piroxicam	Feldene	10–20 mg q daily PO
Nabumetone	Relafen	1000–2000 mg q daily PO
Ketoprofen	Orudis	50 mg q 6 PO
Ketorolac	Toradal	Oral: 10 mg q 4–6 h (not to exceed 10 days) Parenteral: 60 mg initially, followed by 30 mg q 6 h IV or IM (not to exceed 5 days)

analgesia can be lowered 5- to 10-fold if the dose is divided between supraspinal and spinal sites (Yeung and Rudy, 1980). Equally important, peripheral mechanisms synergize with central ones (Kolesnikov et al., 1996). Indeed, tolerance to morphine analgesia is due, in large part, to decreased peripheral sensitivity to morphine and a diminished peripheral/central synergy (Kolesnikov et al., 1996). Thus, the analgesic actions of morphine reflect a complex interaction of peripheral, spinal, and supraspinal opioid systems.

Morphine analgesia is mediated through mu receptors. Many side effects are difficult to avoid because they, too, are mediated by mu receptors. Like analgesia, these side effects can be reversed by opioid antagonists such as naloxone. One of the most common problems in the management of a patient on morphine is constipation, a result of its actions on the gastrointestinal tract. Constipation is mediated through a combination of mu opioid receptors in the central nervous system and peripherally in the myenteric plexus. While a common problem, constipation can usually be minimized with intensive bowel regimens and laxities that should be started at the same time as the medication. Addressing this issue is important because opioid use can lead to bowel obstruction. Bowel problems may remain troublesome even after prolonged use of morphine because tolerance develops more slowly to constipation than to analgesia.

Respiratory depression is another side effect that must be considered when employing morphine for pain. Although easily demonstrated in a variety of experimental and clinical settings, respiratory depression rarely becomes an issue in the clinical

Table 13-8
Adjuvant Analgesic Drugs

Drug category	Typical dose	Indications
General Purpose		
Tricyclic antidepressants	Amitriptyline 10–150 mg q HS PO Nortriptyline 25–150 mg q HS PO	Neuropathic and muscloskeletal pain
Corticosteroids	Dexamethasone 4–16 mg per day PO in divided doses Prednisone 60–80 mg per day PO in divided doses	Essential for spinal cord compression and brain herniation; also useful in malignant bone and nerve pain
Phenothiazine	Methotrimeprazine 10–15 mg IM q 6 h	Useful for opioid sparing in very tolerant patients and opioid-induced ileus
Neuropathic pain		
Anticonvulsants	Carbamazepine 200–800 mg per day PO in divided doses Valproic acid 15–60 mg/kg per day PO in divided doses Gabapentin 300–400 mg TID PO Clonazapam 0.5–1.0 mg TID PO	Useful for dysesthetic and paroxysmal lancinating pain
Antiarrhythmics and local anesthetics	Lidocaine 5 mg/kg i.v. continuous infusion in 30 min Mixelitine 450–600 mg per day in divided doses PO	Usually reserved for neuropathic pain refractory to anticonvulsants and opioids
Topical creams and ointments	Capsaicin 0.075% cream—apply to site of pain at least four times a day Eutectic mixture of local anesthetics (EMLA) cream—apply 60–90 to site before procedure	Capsaicin most often used for postherpetic neuralgia EMLA used often in children
Baclofen	5 mg BID PO—150 mg per day (divided doses)	Useful as second-line agent in neuropathic pain in combination with anticonvulsants Also used in spinal spasticity
Dissociative "anesthetics"	Ketamine 0.1–0.5 mg/kg/h i.v. or s.c.	Effects on NMDA receptors occur at lower doses than anesthetic effects; psychotomimetic effects may still occur
Dextorphan	Delsym 15 mg BID PO—1000 mg per day	Delsym is a single entity slow-release preparation; dextromethorphan also contained in common cough syrups such as Robitussin-DMO

(Continued)

Table 13-8
Adjuvant Analgesic Drugs (*Continued*)

Drug category	Typical dose	Indications
Bone pain		
Radiopharmaceuticals	Strontium-89 4 μCi/dose i.v.	Dose may be repeated if positive analgesic response and adequate marrow reserve
Bisphosphonates	Pamidronate 90 mg i.v. over 2 h, monthly	Inhibits bone resorption and improves bone pain
Osteoclast inhibitors	Calcitonin 25–150 IU i.v. BID	Also used in Paget's disease, phantom pain, and complex regional pain syndromes such as reflex sympathetic dystrophy (RSD)
Visceral pain		
Octreotide	Octreotide 100–600 μg per day vis s.c. bolus or infusion	Useful for secretory diarrhea and malignant bowel obstruction
Psychostimulants		
Over-the-counter	Caffeine 100–200 mg per day PO	One cup of coffee or 12 oz. caffeinated beverage contains 65 mg caffeine
Controlled substances	Methylphenidate 5–20 mg per day PO Dextroamphetamine sulfate 5–15 mg per day PO	Act additively with opioids for analgesia and improve alertness
Marijuana and Cannabinoids	Drabinoil 2.5–5.0 mg BID PO	Effects of smoked marijuana as analgesic reported in anecdotal reports only Possibly useful as appetite stimulant, antiemetic, and antiglaucoma agent

management of outpatients in the absence of a preexisting pulmonary disorder. Special consideration should be taken with patients with decreased pulmonary reserve and a tendency to retain carbon dioxide, such as is seen with emphysema and following lung resections for cancer. Patients may also be more sensitive to the respiratory depressant effects of morphine in the immediate postoperative period following general anesthesia, and particular care should be taken to observe them during this time. As with

analgesia, respiratory depression is mediated through mu receptors and can be readily reversed with opioid antagonists when necessary. Recent clinical reports emphasize the overuse and inappropriate use of naloxone to reverse sedation mediated by causes other than opioid overdose in patients on chronic opioid therapy (Manfreidi et al., 1996). Opioid antagonists should be used with great care because they may also reverse the analgesic actions of the drug and precipitate withdrawal in dependent patients.

Sedation is frequently seen with morphine, explaining why it is named after Morpheus, the god of sleep. Indeed, sedation is one of the most frequent dose-limiting problems in the management of severe pain. Although sedation often cannot be avoided, it can be managed with low doses of stimulants such as amphetamine or methylphenidate.

Tolerance and dependence are invariably seen with chronic morphine administration. Tolerance is characterized by the need to increase the drug dose or frequency to maintain analgesic activity. In the treatment of severe, persistent pain, such as that experienced by cancer patients, tolerance is overcome by increasing the dose or frequency of the drug (Foley, 1993). In cancer patients, for example, tolerance can be quite impressive, leading to doses over 100 times greater than those needed in opioid-naive patients. Doses may be progressively increased to regain analgesic activity, although side effects often become problematic and prevent additional increases. Most mu opioids show cross-tolerance (i.e. patients tolerant to one drug also are tolerant to another). However, cross-tolerance is often incomplete. Switching patients from one compound to another will commonly restore analgesic sensitivity.

Codeine.   Codeine is widely used for mild to moderate pain. Although structurally similar to morphine (Fig. 13-1), codeine has a low affinity for mu receptors, leading to the suggestion its analgesia is mediated primarily by morphine, the demethylated metabolite of codeine. This may also explain its lower potency despite its superior bioavailability following oral administration as compared to morphine. Pharmacologically, the actions of codeine are very similar to morphine.

Morphine-6β-glucuronide.   Morphine is converted to several metabolites. The major metabolite, morphine-3-glucuronide, is devoid of any opioid activities, in contrast with morphine-6β-glucuronide (M6G) (Fig. 13-1) which is approximately 100 times more active than morphine when given directly into the nervous system. Owing to its difficulty in penetrating the blood-brain barrier M6G is only twice as potent as morphine when administered systemically (Lötsch et al., 1996). Although both are effective analgesics, M6G and morphine differ pharmacologically. Evidence suggests that M6G acts through a unique opioid receptor that is also the site of action of heroin (Brown et al., 1997; Rossi et al., 1997; Rossi et al., 1996; Rossi et al., 1995). Although M6G is not clinically available, it is important because it accumulates during chronic administration of morphine, particularly in the presence of renal insufficiency. Indeed, in patients chronically taking morphine, serum M6G levels are typically greater than those of morphine itself. Thus, in the setting of chronic dosing with morphine, the predominent component of analgesia may be due to M6G rather than morphine.

Other morphine-related drugs.   A number of compounds structurally related to morphine are used clinically, including hydromorphone, oxymorphone, oxycodone, and hydrocodone (Fig. 13-3). Pharmacologically, these compounds are quite similar to morphine, differing primarily in their potency and duration of action. However, there are subtle differences among these agents. This is most readily demonstrated by their incomplete cross-tolerance. That is, switching a patient from one drug to another reestablishes analgesic sensitivity for reasons that are still not entirely clear. Oxycodone is now available in a sustained-release formulation, allowing twice-a-day dosing. Sustained-release hydromorphone preparations are in clinical trials.

Meperidine.   Meperidine was one of the first synthetic opioids (Fig. 13-3). Although structurally different from morphine, meperidine is also a mu receptor analgesic and has a pharmacology very similar to morphine. Meperidine is widely used despite some significant problems unique to this drug, particularly in patients with compromised renal function (Kaiko et al., 1983). Meperidine is demethylated to normeperidine, which has convulsant activity. In the presence of renal failure, normeperidine levels increase and can result in seizures. Thus, caution must be exercised when using this drug in the presence of renal failure or metabolic abnormalities. In view of the wide range of analgesics currently available, it is probably best to ignore meperidine.

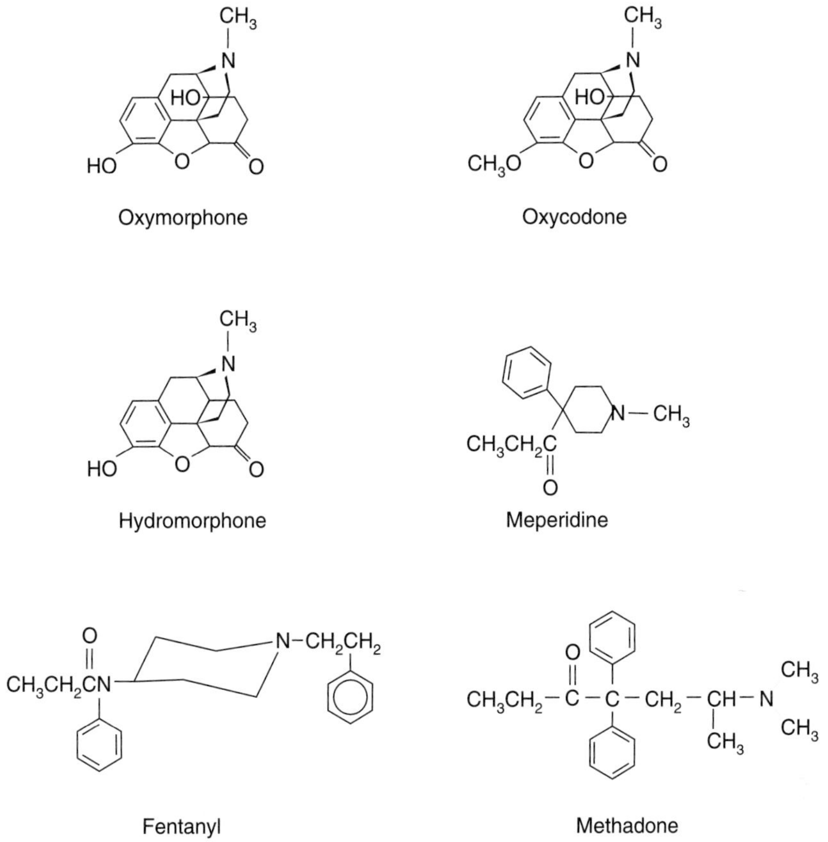

Oxymorphone

Oxycodone

Hydromorphone

Meperidine

Fentanyl

Methadone

Figure 13–3. *Structure of additional mu opioids.*

Fentanyl. Fentanyl (Fig. 13-3) and its analogues, including sufentanil and alfentanil, are exceedingly potent opioids with short durations of action, making them particularly suitable for use during anesthesia. The development of transdermal patches containing fentanyl has led to its widespread use in the management of pain. These patches release the drug at a constant rate for up to 3 days and can be readily used by patients unable to take oral medications. Pharmacokinetically, fentanyl has a very short duration of action, making it an ideal drug to be given by this route. Recently, an oral transmucosal fentanyl (OTFC) has become available for pre-anesthetic sedation of children and the treatment of acute pain complicating procedures in children and adults. In this formulation, fentanyl is embedded in a sweet-ened lozenge on a stick and can be absorbed across the oral mucosa by sucking. A similar formulation with higher doses of fentanyl is being developed to treat breakthrough pain in cancer patients (Fine et al., 1991).

Methadone. Methadone is a synthetic opioid that acts at mu receptors. Although typically associated with maintenance programs in the treatment of opioid addiction, methadone is an effective analgesic in its own right and can be very helpful in managing severe pain. Its use in opioid addiction maintenance programs should not adversely affect the decision to use methadone for pain management. Methadone has a prolonged half-life, typically about 24 h, which can be a major clinical advantage. Its utility as an analgesic is tempered, however, by its tendency to accumu-late with chronic administration because of its long half-life. Indeed, 3 to 5 days may be required to stabilize blood levels, making it difficult to titrate in patients. Structurally, propoxyphene is quite similar to methadone, but it is less potent and is typically used in conjuction with acetaminophen or aspirin to treat mild to moderate pain. Despite its low potency, propoxyphene is an active opioid analgesic. Increas-ing the dose of propoxyphene will also increase its analgesic effect.

Mixed Opioids

Over the years, many additional opioids have been developed, including a number of mixed agonist/antagonists. Most of these drugs are partial agonists or even antagonists at mu receptors, with agonist activity at kappa sites. In general, these agents should only be used in opioid-naive patients because they can reverse the actions of morphine and related drugs and even precipitate withdrawal in a dependent pa-tient. There is also a higher incidence of dysphorias and psychomimetic effects with these agents, al-though this is countered by less constipation, respira-tory depression, and dependence than is seen with pure agonists.

Pentazocine.   Pentazocine is the most widely used opioid agonist/antagonist (Fig. 13-2).   Structurally, pentazocine is a benzomorphan. It has very low af-finity for mu receptors and acts like a partial agonist. Its major analgesic actions are mediated through kappa$_1$ receptors (Chien and Pasternak, 1995). The major limitation to the use of pentazocine is its ten-dency to cause dysphoria and psychotomimetic ef-fects. Because of its potential for abuse, oral pentazo-cine is marketed in the United States in combination with naloxone to prevent its parenteral use. This increases further the chance of potential problems when the combination is given to patients who have received opioids in the past since it may precipi-tate withdrawal.

Nalorphine.   Nalorphine, a close chemical analog of morphine (Fig. 13-2), was the first opioid antago-nist and was used for many years before the develop-ment of more selective agents such as naloxone. Unfortunately, the clinical utility of nalorphine has been markedly compromised by a high incidence of psychotomimetic effects. Although nalorphine is no longer used clinically, it is important historically. Nalorphine is a potent mu receptor antagonist/kappa$_3$ receptor agonist. While low doses reverse morphine analgesia, higher doses produce analgesia through its interaction at kappa$_3$ receptors (Paul et al., 1991).

Nalbuphine.   Available for parenteral use, nal-buphine is a weak partial mu receptor agonist that elicits its analgesic actions predominently through actions at kappa$_1$ and kappa$_3$ receptors (Pick et al., 1992). Nalbuphine has less respiratory depressant and constipating effects than morphine, increasing its utility in the postoperative setting. The lack of an oral formulation, however, diminishes its clinical value.

Opioid Receptor Antagonists

There are a large number of opioid receptor antago-nists, many of which are highly selective for the various receptor subtypes. Their use is limited, how-ever, to preclinical studies, and it is not likely that they will be clinically important in the near future. Thus, their value at this time relates to the insights they provide into the various opioid systems.

Naloxone.   Clinically, naloxone (Fig. 13-4) is the most effective and popular opioid antagonist. Al-though somewhat selective for mu receptors, at suf-ficiently high doses naloxone reverses the actions of almost all opioids. Naloxone acts within seconds

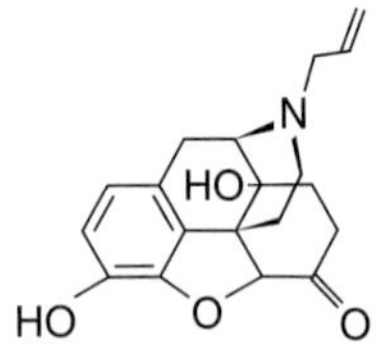

Naloxone (Narcan)

Figure 13–4.   *Structure of naloxone.*

following intravenous administration and therefore is an effective treatment for opioid overdose. It also will precipitate withdrawal in dependent patients, however, and care must be taken with this group. However, it is possible to titrate the naloxone dose to reverse respiratory depression without inducing withdrawal. For this purpose the drug is diluted and given very slowly until the patient awakens. Because naloxone has a shorter duration of action than many opioids, the physician must be alert to the possibility that the respiratory depression may recur. Given to naive subjects, naloxone has little observable activity, implying limited tonic activity of the opioid systems.

Additional Therapeutic Approaches

Intraspinal opioids. Opioid analgesics can be given epidurally or intrathecally. With these routes of administration, small doses of opioids can be used because the drugs are delivered in close proximity to the dorsal horn of the spinal cord, achieving high local concentrations in the region important in producing the pain relief. The reduced drug doses typically produce good analgesia with fewer of the side effects associated with equianalgesic doses of systemically administered opioids (Payne, 1987). Spinally administered opioids should be considered for patients whose pain is at least partially opioid-responsive, but who cannot tolerate the side effects associated with oral or parenteral opioids.

Adverse effects of spinal opioids include pruritus, urinary retention, nausea, vomiting, and respiratory depression, which is thought to reflect redistribution of the drug supraspinally (Payne, 1987). Respiratory depression may occur within the first few hours or up to 24 h later, although the risk of respiratory depression in patients who are not opioid-naive is quite low. Tolerance to the analgesic effects of spinal opioids may develop rapidly in some patients, occasionally limiting the usefulness of this route of administration.

Catheter placement is associated with a low but definite, risk of epidural infection. Nevertheless, long-term epidural analgesia is safe and effective when patients are monitored carefully and receive prompt treatment following any signs of infection. When spinal opioids are considered for the treatment of back pain in the cancer patient, magnetic resonance imaging of the spine should precede placement of an epidural catheter to ensure the absence of an epidural tumor.

Nonopioid drugs can also be administered into the epidural space. Epidural clonidine may be effective in selected patients with cancer pain, particularly for neuropathic pain, which often responds poorly to spinal opioids (Eisenach et al., 1995) Co-administration of local anesthetics, such as bupivicaine, with opioids into the epidural space may also enhance analgesia in selected cases, and may be useful when opioid tolerance develops (DuPen et al., 1992).

Adjuvant Analgesic Drugs

The adjuvant analgesics cover a broad group of drugs used as analgesics, either alone or in combination with other agents, or to counteract adverse side effects (Portenoy, 1996).

Nonsteroidal anti-inflammatory drugs (NSAIDs). The basic principles of pain assessment and management apply when using these agents, which are typically used alone for mild to moderate pain and in conjunction with opioids for more severe pain. Nonsteroidal anti-inflammatory analgesics (NSAIDs) (Table 13-7) have analgesic, anti-inflammatory, and antipyretic effects. Aspirin is the prototype of this class. Acetaminophen, which is comparable to aspirin, is included, even though it has only weak anti-inflammatory activity (Portenoy, 1996). Unlike opioids, NSAIDs and acetaminophen have limitations to their analgesic actions owing to ceiling effects. Dose increases rapidly reach maximal responses beyond which further increases yield no additional therapeutic benefits, although more side effects may be seen. This limits the use of these drugs to mild or moderate pain. Sensitivity among patients to these drugs will vary, so dose titration may be necessary to determine effective and ceiling doses. Thus, alternative drugs may be justified if side effects or ineffectiveness are encountered with a particular agent.

The NSAIDs inhibit the enzyme cyclooxygenase (Vane, 1971), thereby blocking prostaglandin synthesis. Although they have central actions as well, the primary role of prostaglandins in pain appears to be the activation and sensitization of peripheral nociceptors (Malmberg and Yaksh, 1992).

Adverse effects are commonly encountered with NSAIDs, particularly gastrointestinal toxicity. Ibuprofen at doses under 1600 mg per day has the least risk for serious gastrointestinal hemorrhage, followed by intermediate risks for aspirin, indomethacin, naproxen, and sulindac, and the highest risk with ketoprofen and piroxicam. The recent identification of two cyclooxygenase isoforms (COX-1 and COX-2) has important implications for the development of safer, and perhaps more effective, NSAIDs (Laneuville et al., 1994). The COX-1 isoenzyme is constitutively expressed in blood vessels, the gastric mucosa, and kidney, whereas COX-2 is induced in peripheral tissues by inflammation. NSAIDs which selectively inhibit COX-2 may prove to be effective analgesics with significantly less gastrointestinal and renal toxicity. Although no pure COX-2 selective drugs are clinically available at this time, meloxicam is completing clinical development.

Antidepressants. The tricyclic antidepressants are used extensively to treat neuropathic and musculoskeletal pain, as well as migraine and tension headaches. Although the analgesic actions of antidepressants have been clearly demonstrated (Spiegel et al., 1983), their additional actions are also beneficial. Thus, antidepressants effectively potentiate the analgesic actions of opioids and help relieve depression, a significant concern in many patients suffering from pain. Even the sedative actions of amitriptyline are helpful to patients with insomnia. Therapy is typically initiated at low doses (10 to 25 mg given once a day at bedtime). The dose is gradually titrated upward until the desired response is obtained. Maximal effects are usually seen, however, at doses under 150 mg per day. As with many other analgesics, patient response can vary significantly. Accordingly, if one drug is ineffective or induces limiting side effects, it is often helpful to switch to another.

Anticonvulsants. Anticonvulsants are often used for a variety of neuropathic pains, particularly those with a paroxysmal or lancinating character. Carbamazepine has proven to be one of the more effective drugs in this category, particularly for trigeminal neuralgia. Its tendency to lower blood counts can limit its utility, however, in cancer patients on chemotherapy. Phenytoin is an alternative. The recent availability of gabapentin has provided another effective agent in this class, and its use is spreading rapidly.

Additional drugs. A large number of additional drugs for the treatment of pain is available (Table 13-8). They include locally acting formulations, such as capsaicin and EMLA cream, and systemically administered lidocaine and mixelitine. Bone pain associated with cancer can be treated with radiopharmaceuticals, such as strontium-89, bisphosphonates, or calcitonin.

Alternative Approaches

When pharmacologic approaches fail, owing to either limited control of pain or the presence of unacceptable side effects, alternative approaches for the management of pain should be explored. There are a number of anesthetic and neurosurgical techniques that can be considered in specific circumstances (Fig. 13-5). In addition, simple physical and psychological interventions can be helpful.

Regional local anesthetic or neurolytic nerve blocks. Peripheral nerve blocks are most useful for the management of well-localized somatic pain. Examples include intercostal nerve block for chest wall pain, gasserian ganglion block for craniofacial pain, and paravertebral block for radicular pain (Patt, 1993). Temporary blockade of peripheral nerves may be accomplished by injection of a short-acting local anesthetic and is often performed as a screening procedure before proceeding with a more permanent block. In patients responding well to temporary block, neurolytic block using absolute alcohol or phenol may provide more sustained relief. Subarachnoid neurolytic block may be effective in patients with advanced disease and pain that is limited to a few spinal segments. Neurolytic procedures are most appropriate for individuals with a limited life expectancy because of the risk of delayed development of deafferentation pain 6 to 12 months after the procedure.

Blockade of the sympathetic nervous system may also provide effective pain relief in selected cases. Although its efficacy has been questioned, celiac plexus block can be a highly effective technique for managing pain related to pancre-

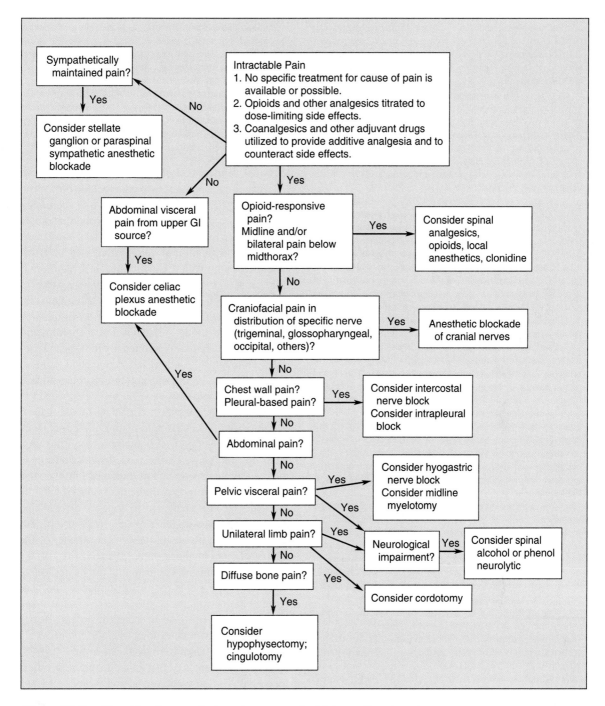

Figure 13–5. Algorithm for anesthetic and neurosurgical interventions in pain control.

atic and other intra-abdominal cancers. Superior hypogastric plexus block may provide effective relief in selected patients with intractable pelvic pain of malignant origin. Stellate ganglion block may be useful in some cases of malignant pain of the upper extremity or head and neck, and lumbar sympathetic block may occasionally be effective for pain associated with pelvic tumors or lumbosacral plexus infiltration. Studies of the comparative efficacy of these procedures relative to aggressive pharmacotherapy are lacking. Such studies would substantially enhance the use of these procedures relatively early in the course of the pain if they can be shown to provide more complete analgesia with fewer side effects than can be achieved with drugs alone.

Neuroablative procedures.   Neuroablative procedures provide pain relief by modifying pain pathways. A neuroablative procedure should be considered in the management of cancer pain when pharmacotherapy is inadequate or associated with unacceptable side effects. These procedures may also benefit patients disabled by incident pain, which is notoriously difficult to manage with drugs. In general, neuroablative procedures are most appropriate for individuals whose life expectancy is short, as delayed recurrence of pain, sometimes more severe than the initial pain, may occur secondary to deafferentation.

Cordotomy, which interrupts the ascending lateral spino-thalamic tract, is the most commonly performed neuroablative procedure and can be performed percutaneously in the cervical region using radiofrequency lesions. Cordotomy is indicated for patients with unilateral lower extremity pain of malignant origin and is less successful in the management of midline or bilateral pain. Nociceptive pain generally responds best to cordotomy whereas neuropathic or deafferentation pain are less reliably relieved. Bilateral cordotomies may result in bladder and sexual dysfunction or respiratory compromise and are therefore not recommended for patients with midline or bilateral pain.

Commissural myelotomy interrupts the fibers of the spinothalamic tracts as they decussate in the midline and may be effective for selected patients with intractable midline or bilateral lower extremity pain of malignant origin. Myelotomy carries a relatively low risk of producing disturbances of bowel, bladder, or motor function and has the disadvantage of requiring an open surgical procedure, generally involving a multilevel laminectomy.

Dorsal rhizotomy involves interruption of the posterior sensory nerve roots, performed either by operative nerve section or chemical neurolysis. This approach may be effective for intractable chest wall pain due to tumor invasion or intractable pain in the head and neck region related to invasive tumors. Like any neuroablative procedure, dorsal rhizotomy is most appropriate for individuals with a limited life expectancy.

Cingulotomy has been used to manage diffuse and midline pain of bony and visceral origin (Hassenbusch et al., 1990). The mechanism of pain relief is unknown although, as described earlier, PET and fMRI imaging studies of experimental and clinical pain demonstrate consistent activation of the anterior cingulate gyrus.

Ablation of the pituitary gland by chemical, radiofrequency, or radiosurgical means may produce widespread analgesic effects in patients with metastatic bone pain, especially when they have not responded to primary chemotherapy, radiation therapy, radiopharmaceutical treatments such as strontium-89, or aggressive analgesic interventions. Although the mechanism of analgesia is unknown, pain relief may be achieved in both hormone-dependent and hormone-independent tumors.

Physical and psychological treatments.   Nonpharmacologic approaches to pain include both physical and psychological modalities. While such treatments are almost always adjunctive to pharmacologic management they are often useful.

Local application of heat or cold may be effective in relieving pain related to muscle spasm. Similarly, massage may help in the management of myofascial pain. Counterstimulation techniques, including transcutaneous electrical nerve stimulation, are thought to modify transmission of painful impulses and may reduce pain intensity in some individuals, although a randomized, controlled trial in chronic low back pain did not demonstrate efficacy (Deyo et al., 1990).

Psychological support is critical for the cancer patient with pain and should be provided to all such patients. Such support takes many forms. Education regarding the cause of the pain, its relationship to the underlying cancer, and its expected future course is crucial. Ensuring that the patient understands the rationale for the analgesic treatments offered and dealing up front with fears related to the use of narcotics will improve compliance. The impact of the degree of emotional or psychological distress on the patient's experience of pain should not be neglected, with selected patients requiring supportive psychotherapy or psychiatric referral for evaluation and treatment of depression or other disorders. Relaxation techniques, mental imagery, and hypnosis are techniques that may be introduced at any stage of pain management as an adjunct to pharmacologic treatment. These psychological and behavioral interventions may serve not only to enhance the effects of analgesics but also to improve the patient's sense of autonomy and control over his or her pain, thus reducing anxiety and emotional distress.

For additional information on the drugs discussed in this chapter, see chapters 23, 24, and 27 in *Goodman & Gilman's The Pharmacological Basis of Therapeutics* (Ninth Edition), McGraw-Hill, New York, 1996.

REFERENCES

Adams JU, Chen X, Deriel JK et al.: Intracerebroventricular treatment with an antisense oligodeoxynucleotide to kappa-opioid receptors inhibited kappa-agonist-induced analgesia in rats. *Brain Res* 1994;667:129–132.

Akil H, Mayer DJ, Liebeskind JC: Antagonism of stimulation-produced analgesia by naloxone, a narcotic antagonist. *Science* 1976;191:961–962.

Ardati A, Henningsen RA, Higelin J et al.: Interaction of [^{3}H]orphanin FQ and ^{125}I-Tyr14-orphanin FQ with the orphanin FQ receptor: kinetics and modulation by cations and guanine nucleotides. *Mol Pharmacol* 1997;51:816–824.

Bare LA, Mansson E, Yang D: Expression of two variants of the human μ opioid receptor mRNA in SK-N-SH cells and human brain. *FEBS Lett* 1994;354:213–216.

Basbaum AI, Fields HL: Endogenous pain control systems: brainstem spinal pathways and endorphin circuitry. *Ann Rev Neurosci* 1984;7:309–338.

Beecher HK: Pain in men wounded in battle. *Ann Surgery* 1946;123:96–105.

Bonica JJ: The treatment of cancer pain: current status and future needs, in Fields HL (ed): *Advances in Pain Research and Therapy.* New York, Raven Press, 1985, pp 589–616.

Breitbart W, McDonald MV, Rosenfeld B et al.: Pain in ambulatory AIDS patients. I: Pain characteristics and medical correlates. *Pain* 1996;68:315–321.

Brown GP, Yang K, King MA et al.: 3-Methoxynaltrexone, a selective heroin/morphine-6β-glucuronide antagonist. *FEBS Lett* 1997;412:35–38.

Bunzow JR, Saez C, Mortrud M et al.: Molecular cloning and tissue distribution of a putative member of the rat opioid receptor gene family that is not a μ, δ or kappa opioid receptor type. *FEBS Lett* 1994;347:284–288.

Casey KL: Pain and central nervous system disease: a summary and overview, in Casey KL (ed): *Pain and Central Nervous System Disease: The Central Pain Syndromes.* New York, Raven Press, 1991, pp 1–11.

Cervero F: Sensory innervation of the viscera: peripheral basis of visceral pain. *Physiol Rev* 1994;74:95–138.

Chakrabarti S, Sultana M, Portoghese PS, Takemori AE: Differential antagonism by naltrindole-5'-isothiocyanate on [^{3}H]DSLET and [^{3}H]DPDPE binding to striatal slices of mice. *Life Sci* 1993;53:1761–1765.

Chang K-J, Cooper BR, Hazum E, Cuatrecasas P: Multiple opiate receptors: different regional distribution in the brain and differential binding of opioids and opioid peptides. *Mol Pharmacol* 1979;16:91–104.

Chang K-J, Hazum E, Cuatrecasas P: Possible role of distinct morphine and enkephalin receptors in mediating actions of benzomorphan drugs (putative k and δ agonists). *Proc Natl Acad Sci USA* 1980;77:4469–4473.

Chavkin C, James IF, Goldstein A: Dynorphin is a specific endogenous ligand of the k-opioid receptor. *Science* 1982;215:413–415.

Chavkin C, Goldstein A: Specific receptor for the opioid peptide dynorphin: structure-activity relationships. *Proc Natl Acad Sci USA* 1981;78:6543–6547.

Chen Y, Fan Y, Liu J et al.: Molecular cloning, tissue distribution and chromosomal localization of a novel member of the opioid receptor gene family. *FEBS Lett* 1994;347:279–283.

Cheng J, Roques BP, Gacel GA et al.: Kappa$_3$ opiate receptor binding in the mouse and rat. *Eur J Pharmacol* 1992;226:15–20.

Cheng J, Standifer KM, Tublin PR et al.: Demonstration of kappa$_3$-opioid receptors in the SH-SY5Y human neuroblastoma cell line. *J Neurochem* 1995;65:170–175.

Chien C-C, Brown G, Pan Y-X, Pasternak GW: Blockade of U50,488H analgesia by antisense oligodeoxynucleotides to a kappa-opioid receptor. *Eur J Pharmacol* 1994;253:R7–R8.

Chien C-C, Pasternak GW: (-)-Pentazocine analgesia in mice: interactions with a σ receptor system. *Eur J Pharmacol* 1995;294:303–308.

Clark JA, Liu L, Price M et al.: Kappa opiate receptor multiplicity: evidence for two U50,488-sensitive kappa$_1$ subtypes and a novel kappa$_3$ subtype. *J Pharmacol Exp Ther* 1989;251:461–468.

Cleeland CS, Gonin R, Hatfield AK: Pain and its treatment in outpatients with metastatic cancer. *N Engl J Med* 1994;330:592–596.

D'Honneur G, Gilton A, Sandouk P et al.: Plasma and cerebrospinal fluid concentrations of morphine and morphine glucuronides after oral morphine: the influence of renal failure. *Anesthesiology* 1994;81:87–93.

Deyo RA, Walsh NE, Martin DC et al.: A controlled trial of transcutaneous electrical nerve stimulation (TENS) and exercise for chronic low back pain. *N Engl J Med* 1990;322:1627–1634.

Deyo RA: Magnetic resonance imaging of the lumbar spine: terrific test or tar baby? *N Engl J Med* 1994;331:115–116.

Dooley CT, Houghten RA: Orphanin FQ: receptor binding and analog structure activity relationships in rat brain. *Life Sci* 1996;59:PL23–PL29.

Dray A, Patel IA, Perkins MN, Rueff A: Bradykinin-induced activation of nociceptors: receptor and mechanistic studies on the neonatal rat spinal cord-tail preparation *in vitro. Br J Pharmacol* 1992;107:1129–1134.

DuPen SL, Kharasch ED, William A: Chronic epidural bupivacaine-opioid infusion in intractable cancer pain. *Pain* 1992;49:293–300.

Eisenach JC, DuPen SL, Dubois M: Epidural clonidine analgesia for intractable cancer pain. *Pain* 1995;61:391–399.

Eppler CM, Hulmes JD, Wang J-B et al.: Purification and partial amino acid sequence of a μ opioid receptor from rat brain. *J Biol Chem* 1993;268:26447–26451.

Evans CJ, Hammond DL, Frederickson RCA: The opioid peptides, in Pasternak GW (ed): *The Opiate Receptors.* Clifton, NJ, Humana Press, 1988, pp 23–74.

Evans CJ, Keith DF, Morrison H et al.: Cloning of the delta opioid receptor by functional expression. *Science* 1992;258:1952–1955.

Fields HL, Basbaum AI: Brainstem control of spinal pain-transmission neurons. *Ann Rev Physiol* 1978;40:217–248.

Fine PG, Marcus M, De Boer J, Van de Oord J: An open-label study of oral transmucosal fentanyl citrate (OTFC) for the treatment of breakthrough pain in cancer. *Pain* 1991;45:149–153.

Foddi MC, Mennini T: [^{125}I][Tyr^{14}]orphanin binding to rat brain: evidence for labeling the opioid-receptor-like 1 (ORL1). *Neurosci Lett* 1997;230:105–108.

Foley KM: Changing concepts of tolerance to opioids: what the cancer patient has taught us, in Chapman CR, Foley KM (eds): *Current and Emerging Issues in Cancer Pain: Research and Practice.* New York, Raven Press, 1993, pp 331–350.

Foley KM: Pain syndromes in patients with cancer, in Portenoy RK, Kanner RM (eds): *Pain Management: Theory and Practice.* Philadelphia, FA Davis Co., 1996, pp 191–215.

Fukuda K, Kato S, Mori K et al.: cDNA cloning and regional distribution of a novel member of the opioid receptor family. *FEBS Lett* 1994;343:42–46.

Gebhart GF: Visceral nociception: consequences, modulation and the future. *Eur J Anesthesiol Suppl* 1995;10:24–27.

Gistrak MA, Paul D, Hahn EF, Pasternak GW: Pharmacological actions of a novel mixed opiate agonist/antagonist, naloxone benzoylhydrazone. *J Pharmacol Exp Ther* 1990;251:469–476.

Goldstein DJ, Ropchak TG, Keiser HR et al.: Bradykinin reverses the effect of opioids in the gut by enhancing acetylcholine release. *J Biol Chem* 1983;258:12122–12124.

Grace D, Fee JPH: A comparison of intrathecal morphine-6-glucuronide and intrathecal morphine sulfate as analgesics for total hip replacement. *Anesth Analg* 1996;83:1055–1059.

Grisel JE, Mogil JS, Belknap JK, Grandy DK: Orphanin FQ acts as a supraspinal, but not a spinal, anti-opioid peptide. *Neuroreport* 1996;7:2125–2129.

Hahn EF, Carroll-Buatti M, Pasternak GW: Irreversible opiate agonists and antagonists: the 14-hydroxydihydromorphinone azines. *J Neurosci* 1982;2:572–576.

Hara N, Minami T, Okuda-Ashitaka E et al.: Characterization of nociceptin hyperalgesia and allodynia in conscious mice. *Br J Pharmacol* 1997;121:401–408.

Harris La: Nuprin Pain Report, in Anonymous, New York, 1985.

Hassenbusch S, Pillay PK, Barnett GH: Radiofrequency cingulotomy for intractable cancer pain using stereotaxis guided by magnetic resonance imaging. *Neurosurgery* 1990;27:220–223.

Heyman JS, Williams CL, Burks TF et al.: Dissociation of opioid antinociception and central gastrointestinal propulsion in the mouse: studies with naloxonazine. *J Pharmacol Exp Ther* 1988;245:238–243.

Houde RW, Wallenstein SL: Clinical studies of morphine-nalorphine combinations. *Fed Proc* 1956;15:440–441.

Hughes J: Isolation of an endogenous compound from the brain with pharmacological properties similar to morphine. *Brain Res* 1975;88:295–308.

Hughes J, Smith TW, Kosterlitz HW et al.: Identification of two related pentapeptides from the brain with potent opiate agonist activity. *Nature* 1975;258:577–579.

Iwamoto ET, Martin WR: Multiple opioid receptors. *Med Res Rev* 1981;1:411–440.

Jacox A, Carr DB, Chapman CR: *Acute Pain Management: Operative or Medical Procedures and Trauma.* Rockvillle, MD, US Department of Health and Human Services, 1992.

Jacox A, Carr DB, Payne R: *Management of Cancer Pain: Clinical Practice Guidelines.* Rockville, MD, US Department of Health and Human Services, 1994.

Janik J, Callahan P, Rabii J: The role of the mu$_1$ opioid receptor subtype in the regulation of prolactin and growth hormone secretion by beta-endorphin in female rats: studies with naloxonazine. *J Neuroendocrinol* 1992;4:701–708.

Jiang Q, Takemori AE, Sultana M et al.: Differential antagonism of opiate delta antinociception by [D-Ala^2,Cys^6]enkaphalin and naltrindole-5′-isothiocyanate: evidence for subtypes. *J Pharmacol Exp Ther* 1991;257:1069–1075.

Kaiko RF, Foley KM, Grabinski PY et al.: Central nervous system excitatory effects of meperidine in cancer patients. *Ann Neurol* 1983;13:180–185.

Kamei J, Iwamoto Y, Kawashima N et al.: Possible involvement of μ$_2$-mediated mechanisms in μ-mediated antitussive activity in the mouse. *Neurosci Lett* 1993;149:169–172.

Keith D Jr, Maung T, Anton B, Evans C: Isolation of cDNA clones homologous to opioid receptors. *Regul Pept* 1994;54:143–144.

Kieffer BL, Befort K, Gaveriaux-Ruff C, Hirth CG: The δ-opioid receptor: isolation of a cDNA by expression cloning and pharmacological characterization. *Proc Natl Acad Sci USA* 1992;89:12048–12052.

King MA, Rossi GC, Chang AH et al.: Spinal analgesic activity of orphanin FQ/nociceptin and its fragments. *Neurosci Lett* 1997;223:113–116.

Knapp RJ, Malatynska E, Collins N et al.: Molecular biology and pharmacology of cloned opioid receptors. *FASEB J* 1995;9:516–525.

Kolesnikov YA, Jain S, Wilson R, Pasternak GW: Peripheral morphine analgesia: synergy with central sites and a target of morphine tolerance. *J Pharmacol Exp Ther* 1996;279:502–506.

Kozak CA, Filie J, Adamson MC et al.: Murine chromosomal location of the μ and kappa opioid receptor genes. *Genomics* 1994;21:659–661.

Lachowicz JE, Shen Y, Monsma FJ Jr, Sibley DR: Molecular cloning of a novel G protein-coupled receptor related to the opiate receptor family. *J Neurochem* 1995;64:34–40.

Lai J, Bilsky EJ, Bernstein RN et al.: Antisense oligodeoxynucleotide to the cloned delta opioid receptor selectively inhibits supraspinal, but not spinal, antinociceptive effects of [D-Ala^2, Glu^4]deltorphin. *Regul Pept* 1994;54:159–160.

Laneuville O, Breuer DK, DeWitt DL: Differential inhibition of human prostaglandin endoperoxide H synthetase-1 and -2 by nonsteroidal anti-inflammatory drugs. *J Pharmacol Exp Ther* 1994;271:927–934.

Lasagne L, Beecher HK: Analgesic effectiveness of nalorphine and nalorphine-morphine combinations in man. *J Pharmacol Exp Ther* 1954;112:356–363.

Li CH, Chung D: Primary structure of human β-lipotropin. *Nature* 1976;260:622–624.

Ling GSF, Spiegel K, Nishimura S, Pasternak GW: Dissociation of morphine's analgesic and respiratory depressant actions. *Eur J Pharmacol* 1983;86:487–488.

Ling GSF, Spiegel K, Lockhart SH, Pasternak GW: Separation of opioid analgesia from respiratory depression: evidence for different receptor mechanisms. *J Pharmacol Exp Ther* 1985;232:149–155.

Ling GSF, Simantov R, Clark JA, Pasternak GW: Naloxonazine actions in vivo. *Eur J Pharmacol* 1986;129:33–38.

Liu H-C, Lu S, Augustin LB et al.: Cloning and promoter mapping of mouse kappa opioid receptor gene. *Biochem Biophys Res Commun* 1995;209:639–647.

Lord JAH, Waterfield AA, Hughes J, Kosterlitz HW: Endogenous opioid peptides: multiple agonists and receptors. *Nature* 1977;267:495–499.

Lötsch J, Stockmann A, Kobal G et al.: Pharmacokinetics of morphine and its glucuronides after intravenous infusion of morphine and morphine-6-glucuronide in healthy volunteers. *Clin Pharmacol Ther* 1996;60:316–325.

Lutz RA, Cruciani RA, Costa T et al.: A very high affinity opioid binding site in rat brain: demonstration by computer modeling. *Biochem Biophys Res Commun* 1984;122:265–269.

Lutz RA, Cruciani RA, Munson PJ, Rodbard D: Mu$_1$: a very high affinity subtype of enkephalin binding sites in rat brain. *Life Sci* 1985;36:2233–2338.

Maciewicz R: Organization of pain pathways, in Asbury AK, McKhann GM, McDonald WI (eds): *Diseases of the Nervous System: Clinical Neurobiology.* Philadelphia, PA, W B Saunders, 1992, pp 849–857.

Malmberg AB, Yaksh TL: Hyperalgesia mediated by spinal glutamate or substance P receptor blocked by spinal cyclooxygenase inhibition. *Science* 1992;257:1276–1279.

Manfreidi PL, Ribeiro S, Chandler SW, Payne R: Inappropriate use of naloxone in cancer patients with pain. *J Pain Symp Manag* 1996;11:131–134.

Martin WR: Opioid antagonists. *Pharmacol Rev* 1967;19:463–521.

Martin WR, Eades CG, Thompson JA et al.: The effects of morphine and nalorphine-like drugs in the nondependent and morphine-dependent chronic spinal dog. *J Pharmacol Exp Ther* 1976;197:517–532.

Mathis JP, Ryan-Moro J, Chang A et al.: Biochemical evidence for orphanin FQ/nociceptin receptor heterogeneity in mouse brain. *Biochem Biophys Res Commun* 1997;230:462–465.

Matthes HWD, Maldonado R, Simonin F et al.: Loss of morphine-induced analgesia, reward effect and withdrawal symptoms in mice lacking the μ-opioid-receptor gene. *Nature* 1996;383:819–823.

Mattia A, Vanderah T, Mosberg HI, Porreca F: Lack of antinociceptive cross tolerance between [D-Pen^2,D-Pen^5]enkephalin and [D-Ala^2]deltorphin II in mice: evidence for delta receptor subtypes. *J Pharmacol Exp Ther* 1991;258:583–587.

Max MB: Antidepressants as analgesics, in Fields HL, Liebeskind JC (eds): *Pharmacological Approaches to the Treatment of Chronic Pain: New Concepts and Critical Issues.* IASP Press, 1995, pp 229–246.

Mersky H: Classification of chronic pain: description of chronic pain syndromes and definitions of pain terms. *Pain* 1986;3:S217.

Meunier JC, Mollereau C, Toll L et al.: Isolation and structure of the endogenous agonist of the opioid receptor like ORL$_1$ receptor. *Nature* 1995;377:532–535.

Min BH, Augustin LB, Felsheim RF et al.: Genomic structure and analysis of promoter sequence of a mouse μ opioid receptor gene. *Proc Natl Acad Sci USA* 1994;91:9081–9085.

Minami M, Toya T, Katao Y et al.: Cloning and expression of a cDNA for the rat kappa-opioid receptor. *FEBS Lett* 1993;329:291–295.

Mogil JS, Grisel JE, Reinscheid KK et al.: Orphanin FQ is a functional anti-opioid peptide. *Neuroscience* 1996a;75:333–337.

Mogil JS, Grisel JE, Zhangs G et al.: Functional antagonism of μ-, δ- and kappa-opioid antinociception by orphanin FQ. *Neurosci Lett* 1996b;214:1–4.

Mollereau C, Parmentier M, Mailleux P et al: ORL-1, a novel member of the opioid family: cloning, functional expression and localization. *FEBS Lett* 1994;341:33–38.

Nishimura S, Recht LD, Pasternak GW: Biochemical characterization of high affinity ^{3}H-opioid binding: further evidence for mu$_1$ sites. *Mol Pharmacol* 1984;25:29–37.

Paakkari P, Paakkari I, Vonhof S et al.: Dermorphin analog Tyr-D-Arg^2-Phe-sarcosine-induced opioid analgesia and respiratory stimulation: the role of Mu$_1$-receptors. *J Pharmacol Exp Ther* 1993;266:544–550.

Pan Y-X, Cheng J, Xu J, Pasternak GW: Cloning, expression and classification of a kappa$_3$-related opioid receptor using antisense oligodeoxynucleotides. *Regul Pept* 1994;54:217–218.

Pan Y-X, Cheng J, Xu J et al: Cloning and functional characterization through antisense mapping of a kappa$_3$-related opioid receptor. *Mol Pharmacol* 1995;47:1180–1188.

Pan Y-X, Xu J, Pasternak GW: Structure and characterization of the gene encoding a mouse kappa$_3$-related opioid receptor. *Gene* 1996a;171:255–260.

Pan Y-X, Xu J, Ryan-Moro J et al.: Dissociation of affinity and efficacy in KOR-3 chimeras. *FEBS Lett* 1996b;395:207–210.

Pasternak GW, Goodman R, Snyder SH: An endogenous morphine like factor in mammalian brain. *Life Sci* 1975;16:1765–1769.

Pasternak GW, Childers SR, Snyder SH: Naloxazone, long-acting opiate antagonist: effects in intact animals and on opiate receptor binding in vitro. *J Pharmacol Exp Ther* 1980a;214:455–462.

Pasternak GW, Childers SR, Snyder SH: Opiate analgesia: evidence for mediation by a subpopulation of opiate receptors. *Science* 1980b;208:514–516.

Pasternak GW, Bodnar RJ, Clark JA, Inturrisi CE: Morphine-6-glucuronide, a potent mu agonist. *Life Sci* 1987;41:2845–2849.

Pasternak GW: Pharmacological mechanisms of opioid analgesics. *Clin Neuropharmacol* 1993;16:1–18.

Pasternak GW, Snyder SH: Identification of a novel high affinity opiate receptor binding in rat brain. *Nature* 1975;253:563–565.

Pasternak GW, Standifer KM: Mapping of opioid receptors using antisense oligodeoxynucleotides: correlating their molecular biology and pharmacology. *Trends Pharmacol Sci* 1995;16:344–350.

Patt RB: Anesthetic procedures for the control of cancer pain, in Arbit E (ed): *Management of Cancer-Related Pain*. Mont Kisco, NY, Futura Press, 1993, pp 381–407.

Paul D, Standifer KM, Inturrisi CE, Pasternak GW: Pharmacological characterization of morphine-6β-glucuronide, a very potent morphine metabolite. *J Pharmacol Exp Ther* 1989;251:477–483.

Paul D, Levison JA, Howard DH et al.: Naloxone benzoylhydrazone (NalBzoH) analgesia. *J Pharmacol Exp Ther* 1990;255:769–774.

Paul D, Pick CG, Tive LA, Pasternak GW: Pharmacological characterization of nalorphine, a kappa$_3$ analgesic. *J Pharmacol Exp Ther* 1991;257:1–7.

Paul D, Pasternak GW: Differential blockade by naloxonazine of two μ opiate actions: analgesia and inhibition of gastrointestinal transit. *Eur J Pharmacol* 1988;149:403–404.

Payne R: Role of epidural, intrathecal narcotics and peptides in the management of cancer pain. *Med Clin North Am* 1987;71:313–328.

Payne R: Pathophysiology of cancer pain, in McDonald N, Doyle D, Hanks G (eds): *Oxford Textbook of Medicine*. London, Oxford University Press, 1997.

Payne R, Pasternak GW: Pain, in Johnston MV, Macdonald RL, Young AB (eds): *Principles of Drug Therapy in Neurology*. Philadelphia, FA Davis, 1992, pp 268–301.

Pela IR, Rosa AL, Silva CAA, Huidobro-Toro JP: Central B$_2$ receptor involvement in the antinociceptive effect of bradykinin in rats. *Br J Pharmacol* 1996;118:1488–1492.

Perl ER: Characterization of nociceptors and their activation of neurons in the superficial dorsal horn: first steps for the sensation of pain, in Kruger L, Liebeskind JC (eds): *Advances in Pain Research and Therapy*. New York, Raven Press, 1984, pp 23–52.

Pert CB, Snyder SH: Opiate receptor: demonstration in nervous tissue. *Science* 1973;179:1011–1014.

Pick CG, Paul D, Pasternak GW: Comparison of naloxonazine and β-funaltrexamine antagonism of μ$_1$ and μ$_2$ opioid actions. *Life Sci* 1991;48:2005–2011.

Pick CG, Paul D, Pasternak GW: Nalbuphine, a mixed kappa$_1$ and kappa$_3$ analgesic in mice. *J Pharmacol Exp Ther* 1992;262:1044–1050.

Portenoy RK: Nonopioid and adjuvant analgesics, in Portenoy RK, Kanner RM (eds): *Pain Management: Theory and Practice*. Philadelphia, FA Davis, 1996, pp 219–276.

Portoghese PS, Lipkowski AW, Takemori AE: Binaltorphimine and nor-binaltorphimine, potent and selective κ-opioid receptor agonists. *Life Sci* 1987;40:1287–1292.

Price M, Gistrak MA, Itzhak Y et al.: Receptor binding of ^{3}H-naloxone benzoylhydrazone: a reversible kappa and slowly dissociable μ opiate. *Mol Pharmacol* 1989;35:67–74.

Rainville P, Duncan GH, Price DD et al.: Pain affect encoded in human anterior cingulate but not somatosensory cortex. *Science* 1997;277:968–971.

Reinscheid RK, Nothacker HP, Bourson A et al.: Orphanin FQ: a neuropeptide that activates an opioidlike G protein-coupled receptor. *Science* 1995;270:792–794.

Reisine T, Pasternak GW: Opioid analgesics and antagonists, in Hardman JG, Limbird LE (eds): *Goodman & Gilman's: The Pharmacological Basis of Therapeutics*. New York, McGraw-Hill, 1996, pp 521–556.

Reynolds DV: Surgery in the rat during electrical analgesia induced by focal brain stimulation. *Science* 1969;162:444–445.

Rossi G, Leventhal L, Boland E, Pasternak GW: Pharmacological characterization of orphanin FQ/nociceptin and its fragments. *J Pharmacol Exp Ther* 1997;282:858–865.

Rossi GC, Pan Y-X, Cheng J, Pasternak GW: Blockade of morphine analgesia by an antisense oligodeoxynucleotide against the mu receptor. *Life Sci* 1994;54:PL375–379.

Rossi GC, Pan Y-X, Brown GP, Pasternak GW: Antisense mapping the MOR-1 opioid receptor: evidence for alternative splicing and a novel morphine-6β-glucuronide receptor. *FEBS Lett* 1995;369:192–196.

Rossi GC, Brown GP, Leventhal L et al.: Novel receptor mechanisms for heroin and morphine-6β -glucuronide analgesia. *Neurosci Lett* 1996a;216:1–4.

Rossi GC, Leventhal L, Pasternak GW: Naloxone-sensitive orphanin FQ-induced analgesia in mice. *Eur J Pharmacol* 1996b;311:R7–R8.

Rossi GC, Leventhal L, Pan YX et al.: Antisense mapping of MOR-1 in rats: distinguishing between morphine and morphine-6β-glucuronide antinociception. *J Pharmacol Exp Ther* 1997a;281:109–114.

Rossi GC, Su W, Leventhal L et al.: Antisense mapping DOR-1 in mice: further support for δ receptor subtypes. *Brain Res* 1997b;753:176–179.

Rothman RB, Jacobson AE, Rice KC, Herkenham M: Autoradiographic evidence for two classes of μ opioid binding sites in rat brain using [^{125}I]FK33824. *Peptides* 1987;8:1015–1021.

Sherry S: Low-dose heparin for the prophylaxis of pulmonary embolism. *Am Rev Resp Dis* 1976;114:661–666.

Shimomura K, Kamata O, Ueki S et al.: Analgesic effect of morphine glucuronides. *Tohoku J Exp Med* 1971;105:45–52.

Simon EJ, Hiller JM, Edelman I: Stereospecific binding of the potent narcotic analgesice [^{3}H]Etorphine to rat-brain homogenate. *Proc Natl Acad Sci USA* 1973;70:1947–1949.

Simonin F, Gavériaux-Ruff C, Befort K et al.: Kappa-opioid receptor in humans: cDNA and genomic cloning, chromosomal assignment, functional expression, pharmacology, and expression pattern in the central nervous system. *Proc Natl Acad Sci USA* 1995;92:7006–7010.

Sora I, Takahashi N, Funada M et al.: Opiate receptor knockout mice define μ receptor roles in endogenous nociceptive responses and morphine-induced analgesia. *Proc Natl Acad Sci USA* 1997;94:1544–1549.

Spiegel K, Kalb P, Pasternak GW: Analgesic activity of tricyclic antidepressants. *Ann Neurol* 1983;13:462–465.

Standifer KM, Chien C-C, Wahlestedt C et al.: Selective loss of δ opioid analgesia and binding by antisense oligodeoxynucleotides to a δ opioid receptor. *Neuron* 1994;12:805–810.

Stanton-Hicks M, Janig W, Hassenbusch S et al.: Reflex sympathetic dystrophy: changing concepts and taxonomy. *Pain* 1995;63:127–133.

Steranka LR, DeHaas CJ, VaaVrek RJ et al.: Antinociceptive effects of bradykinin antagonists. *Eur J Pharmacol* 1987;136:261–262.

Swerdlow M: Anticonvulsant drugs and chronic pain. *Clin Neuropharmacol* 1984;7:51–82.

Tal M, Bennet G: Dextorphan relieves neuropathic heat-evoked hyperalgesia in the rat. *Neurosci Lett* 1993;151:107–110.

Terenius L: Characteristics of the "receptor" for narcotic analgesics in synaptic plasma membrane from rat brain. *Acta Pharmacol Toxicol* 1973;33:377–384.

Thompson PI, Joel SP, John L et al.: Respiratory depression following morphine and morphine-6-glucuronide in normal subjects. *Br J Clin Pharmacol* 1995;40:145–152.

Thompson RC, Mansour A, Akil H, Watson SJ: Cloning and pharmacological characterization of a rat μ opioid receptor. *Neuron* 1993;11:903–913.

Tian JH, Xu W, Fang Y et al.: Bidirectional modulatory effect of orphanin FQ on morphine-induced analgesia: antagonism in brain and potentiation in spinal cord of the rat. *Br J Pharmacol* 1997;120:676–680.

Tian M, Broxmeyer HE, Fan Y et al.: Altered hematopoiesis, behavior, and sexual function in μ opioid receptor-deficient mice. *J Exp Med* 1997;185:1517–1522.

Tiseo PJ, Thaler HT, Lapin J et al.: Morphine-6-glucuronide concentrations and opioid-related side effects: a survey in cancer patients. *Pain* 1995;61:47–54.

Tive LA, Ginsberg K, Pick CG, Pasternak GW: Kappa₃ receptors and levorphanol analgesia. *Neuropharmacology* 1992;31:851–856.

Toll L, Keys C, Plogar W, Loew G: The use of computer modeling in describing multiple opiate receptors. *Neuropeptides* 1984;5:205–208.

Torebjork HE, Hallin RG: Microneurographic studies of peripheral pain mechanisms in man, in Bonica JJ (ed): *Advances in Pain Research and Therapy*. New York, Raven Press, 1979, pp 121–131.

Treede RD, Meyer RA, Raja SN, Cambell JN: Peripheral and central mechanisms of cutaneous hyperalgesia. *Prog Neurobiol* 1992;38:397–421.

Turk DC, Melzak R (eds): *Handbook of Pain Assessment*. New York, Guilford, 1992.

Uhl GR, Childers S, Pasternak GW: An opiate-receptor gene family reunion. *Trends Neurosci* 1994;17:89–93.

Vanderah T, Takemori AE, Sultana M et al.: Interaction of [D-Pen²,D-Pen⁵]enkephalin and [D-Ala², Glu⁴]deltorphin with δ-opioid receptor subtypes in vivo. *Eur J Pharmacol* 1994;252:133–137.

Vane JR: Inhibition of prostaglandin synthesis as a mechanism of action for aspirin-like drugs. *Nature* 1971;234:231–238.

Verdugo RJ, Ochoa JL: Sympathetically maintained pain. I. Phentolamine block questions the concept. *Neurology* 1994;44:1003–1010.

Von Roenn JH, Cleeland CS, Gonin R, Pandy KJ: Physician attitudes and practice in cancer pain management: a survey from the Eastern Cooperative Oncology Group. *Ann Intern Med* 1993;119:121–126.

VonVoightlander PF, Lahti RA, Ludens JH: U50,488: a selective and structurally novel non-mu (kappa) opioid agonist. *J Pharmacol Exp Ther* 1983;224:7–12.

Wang JB, Johnson PS, Imai Y et al.: cDNA cloning of an orphan opiate receptor gene family member and its splice variant. *FEBS Lett* 1994;348:75–79.

Wick MJ, Minnerath SR, Lin X et al.: Isolation of a novel cDNA encoding a putative membrane receptor with high homology to the cloned μ, δ, and kappa opioid receptors. *Mol Brain Res* 1994;27:37–44.

Wick MJ, Minnerath SR, Roy S et al.: Expression of alternate forms of brain opioid "orphan" receptor mRNA in activated human peripheral blood lymphocytes and lymphocytic cell lines. *Mol Brain Res* 1995;32:342–347.

Willis WD: *The Pain System: The Neural Basis of Nociceptive Transmission in the Mammalian Nervous System*. Basel, Switzerland, 1985.

Wolfe CJ: The dorsal horn: state-dependent sensory processing and the generation of pain, in Wall PD, Melzak R (eds): *Textbook of Pain*. Edinburgh, Churchill Livingston, 1994, pp 101–112.

Xu XJ, Hao JX, Wiesenfeld-Hallin Z: Nociceptin or antinociceptin: potent spinal antinociceptive effect of orphanin FQ/nociceptin in the rat. *Neuroreport* 1996;7:2092–2094.

Yasuda K, Raynor K, Kong H et al.: Cloning and functional comparison of kappa and δ opioid receptors from mouse brain. *Proc Natl Acad Sci USA* 1993;90:6736–6740.

Yeung JC, Rudy TA: Multiplicative interaction between narcotic agonisms expressed at spinal and supraspinal sites of antinociceptive action as revealed by concurrent intrathecal and intracerebroventricular injections of morphine. *J Pharmacol Exp Ther* 1980;215:633–642.

Yoshimura H, Ida S, Oguri K, Tsukamoto H: Biochemical basis for analgesic activity of morphine-6β-glucuronide I: Penetration of morphine-6β-glucuronide in the brain of rats. *Biochem Pharmacol* 1973;22:1423–1430.

Zadina JE, Hackler L, Ge LJ, Kastin AJ: A potent and selective endogenous agonist for the μ-opiate receptor. *Nature* 1997;386:499–502.

Zimprich A, Bacher B, Höllt V: Cloning and expression of an isoform of the rmu-opioid receptor (rmuOR1B). *Regul Pept* 1994;54:347–348.

EPILEPSY

Robert S. Fisher

Epilepsy is the most prevalent and serious neurologic disorder affecting all age groups. Although great strides have been made in defining, diagnosing, and treating this condition, many patients are still poorly controlled or suffer from medication side effects. A seizure results from an imbalance between excitatory and inhibitory systems in brain. Different types of seizures are mediated by different physiologic mechanisms and affect different areas of the brain. Some antiepileptic medications enhance inhibitory influences in the central nervous system by facilitating γ-aminobutyric acid (GABA) neurotransmission, whereas others reduce excitatory input by inhibiting glutamic acid transmitter activity. Some antiepileptic medications block rapid firing of neurons by interacting with neuronal sodium channels. Since the introduction of phenobarbital in 1912, several dozen antiepileptic medications have been developed. To date, no single medication has demonstrated an overriding advantage over others because none are effective against all seizure types under all circumstances. Selection of medications, therefore, continues to be based on accurate diagnosis and clinical response.

Many of the problems associated with epilepsy are psychosocial as well as medical. In cases where seizures are not controlled by medication, other treatments, such as neurosurgery, may be of value. The ultimate goal of any treatment for epilepsy remains elimination of seizures and enhancement in the quality of life.

CLINICAL FEATURES

A seizure is a sudden, stereotyped episode with a change in motor activity, sensation, behavior, or consciousness that is due to an abnormal electrical discharge in the brain. Epilepsy is a condition of recurrent, spontaneous seizures. Therefore, a seizure is the event and epilepsy the disorder. One seizure is not diagnostic for epilepsy, nor are a series of seizures if they are due to precipitating factors such as alcohol withdrawal or brain tumors. Rather, seizures must be spontaneous and recurrent to be considered epilepsy.

Seizures result from an electrochemical disorder in brain. Because neurons either excite or inhibit adjacent neurons, most types of epilepsy are due to a disruption in the balance between these two actions. Although it is likely that virtually every brain neurotransmitter and neuromodulator is involved in epilepsy, glutamic acid and GABA play prominent roles because they are the major excitatory and inhibitory transmitters in brain, respectively. Thus, antiepileptic medications have been designed to block glutamate-induced excitation. Although this action terminates seizures, inhibition of glutamate, which is found throughout the central nervous system, is associated with a number of undesirable side effects, limiting this pharmacologic approach. As the most abundant inhibitory neurotransmitter in brain, GABA has also been a target for the development of antiepileptic medications, with a number of these approved for use in the treatment of this disorder.

There has been extensive debate as to whether a seizure results from a dysfunction of an entire neuronal system or just a few diseased neurons, with data suggesting that systems disorders are more prevalent. Thus, although seizures use the preexisting anatomy, physiology, and neurochemistry of the brain, they extend neuronal firing to excessive amounts in a hypersynchronous fashion, with intracellular recordings from a seizure focus disclosing a paroxysmal depolarization shift (PDS).

Shown in Fig. 14-1 is a paroxysmal depolarization shift in a hippocampal neuron exposed to kainic acid, a glutamate receptor agonist that also blocks GABA-mediated inhibitory circuits. Although the PDS appears to be a giant excitatory postsynaptic potential, it also displays a voltage-dependent increase in calcium conductance, which provides a boost as the cell begins to depolarize. With normal GABA-mediated inhibition, the neuron remains sufficiently hyperpolarized that most depolarization-dependent calcium channels are closed, which would support the "epileptic neuron" theory. It is the enhanced synchronous drive from circuits of neurons, however, that ultimately provokes the abnormal depolarization.

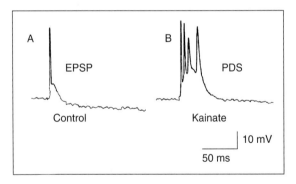

Figure 14–1. *An intracellularly recorded excitatory postsynaptic potential (EPSP) produced in a hippocampal pyramidal cell by stimulation of the afferent fibers. A. Tracing in control bath of artificial cerebrospinal fluid. B. Response to a similar stimulus in perfusate containing the excitatory glutamate analogue kainate. The EPSP has converted to a paroxysmal depolarizing shift. Polarity is displayed with positive upgoing.*

Inhibitory influences in brain appear to be selectively vulnerable to certain types of insults. The inhibitory circuitry is polysynaptic, requiring connections with interneurons that employ GABA and other inhibitory neurotransmitters. These pathways appear to be more sensitive to stresses such as hypoxia, hypoglycemia, or mechanical trauma than are excitatory, monosynaptic pathways. When excitatory synapses are functional and inhibitory synapses impaired, seizures ensue. If the insult is severe enough to block excitatory transmission as well, seizures cease, followed by coma or death.

Neuronal inhibition in brain is not a single process, but rather a hierarchy of processes. The inhibitory postsynaptic potential (IPSP) generated by the $GABA_A$ receptor is the most important of these. As noted previously, this receptor is selectively vulnerable to insults and to $GABA_A$ receptor antagonists, such as penicillin, picrotoxin, or bicuculline. Some neurons also possess a $GABA_B$ receptor, which is selectively activated by the antispasticity drug baclofen. Although $GABA_B$ receptor antagonists have been developed, none has yet been approved for clinical use. The $GABA_B$ receptor appears to be especially important for generating the wave as part of spike-wave absence epilepsy. A third level of inhibition involves calcium-mediated potassium currents, sometimes referred to as postburst after-hyperpolarizations. Thus, an increase in intracellular calcium activates a potassium channel that allows potassium ions to exit the neuron, resulting in hyperpolarizations that last approximately 200 to 500 ms. A fourth level of inhibition involves activation of metabolic pumps, with ATP as the energy source. These pumps exchange three intracellular sodium ions for two extracellular potassium ions, increasing intracellular negativity. Although such pumps are activated by intensive neuronal firing and serve to restore the steady-state balance of ions, they may leave neurons hyperpolarized for many minutes. The existence of this hierarchy is important because disruption of one inhibitory process does not completely eliminate others that protect the brain from excessive excitation.

Absence (petit mal) seizures are an exception to the rule that seizures result from a decrease in inhibitory influences because these probably occur following an increase in, or hypersynchronous, inhibition. Thus, clinical absence seizures reflect primarily a lack of behavioral activity rather than exaggerated movement or automatic behaviors as seen with other types of seizures.

During an absence attack the electroencephalogram (EEG) shows recurrent sequences of spikes and waves (Fig. 14-2). Three forces are required for this pattern: an excitatory stimulus to generate the spike, an inhibitory stimulus to generate the wave, and a pacemaker for rhythmicity. It appears the spike is due to glutamate-mediated EPSPs, the wave to GABA$_B$-mediated IPSPs, and the rhythmicity to calcium currents in certain thalamic nuclei. These insights could provide new approaches for the treatment of absence epilepsies.

There is no simple theory to explain why most seizures are self-limiting because neurons can be made to fire after a seizure. Some factors that may be responsible for this postictal state include neuronal hyperpolarization, which is probably due to the action of metabolic pumps, and decreased cerebral blood flow, which may contribute to the relative inactivity of neuronal circuits. The excessive release of neurotransmitters and neuromodulators during seizure-induced discharges may also contribute to the postictal state. For example, it appears that endogenous opioid peptides are released during a seizure and that these inhibit brain function after the event because the opioid receptor antagonist, naloxone, arouses stuporous rodents after an electroshock seizure. Moreover, adenosine, which is released during a seizure, activates adenosine A$_1$ receptors to partially block further excitatory synaptic transmission; nitric oxide, a second messenger with effects on blood vessels and neurons in brain, also appears to play a role in the postictal state. Whereas physiologic mechanisms responsible for the postictal state are critical for terminating seizures, they create clinical problems, with some patients being more disabled by the aftermath of a seizure than by the seizure itself. For this reason, treatments that reduce the duration of the postictal state would be a boon.

Because epilepsy is characterized by recurrent seizures, a complete explanation of the mechanisms of this disorder must account for chronic changes in brain that allow for

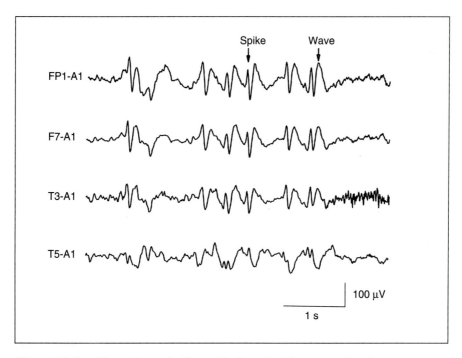

Figure 14–2. *Illustrations of spikes and aftergoing slow waves in a human electroencephalogram. Electrode abbreviations here and in subsequent figures are those of the International EEG system. Polarity is displayed with negative upgoing.*

such seizures. Thus, a wide variety of brain injuries, such as perinatal hypoxia, head trauma, cerebral hemorrhage and stroke, may lead to recurrent seizures, often after a delay of weeks or years. Research has focused on injury-induced changes in brain that lead to chronic hyperexcitability. A useful model for this purpose is the hippocampus after chemical injury with kainic acid, a relatively selective neurotoxin, or it is damaged by excessive afferent electrical stimulation, both of which cause a selective loss of certain neurons. This cell death results in the axonal expansion (sprouting) of other neurons that attempt to connect with the deafferented cells. Such sprouting is analogous to changes that occur in motor units that results in fasciculations. In this sense some seizures may be viewed as brain fasciculations caused by neuronal reorganization. The aim of the reorganization is, of course, not to produce seizures, but to restore the neuronal circuitry. The price paid, however, is increased neuronal excitability.

It is known that seizures do not originate from any single place in brain but rather result from an interactive circuitry that behaves as an abnormal network. Removal of a focal region, however, may be effective in stopping some types of seizures. Such surgery is effective, just as cutting a phone cable interrupts a conversation even if it occurs at a great distance from the callers.

Certain regions of the brain are believed to be particularly important in the generation of seizures. The nonspecific thalamic nuclei, particularly the nucleus reticularis thalamus, is crucial in the generation of spike-wave absence epilepsy, with the hippocampus and amygdala in the mesial temporal lobes being of prime importance in the generation of complex partial seizures. The area tempestas, a region in the prepyriform frontal cortex, is known to be a focal point in rodents, cats, and primates for temporal lobe seizures (Piredda et al., 1987). In rodents, the substantia nigra pars reticularis facilitates the spread and generalization of epileptiform activity. In humans it appears that the cerebral cortex is the most important structure for the generation of seizures, with focal seizures typically resulting from an injury or dysfunction of the neocortex, or of the archicortex and paleocortex in the case of the mesial temporal lobes. Although the primary manifestations of these seizures are evident in neocortex, subcortical systems are also involved, although the precise regions and pathways are unknown.

Basic research on the epilepsies has provided new insights about the condition, particularly with respect to focal seizure disorders. Many questions remain unanswered, however, including which systems are involved in generalized seizures, why seizures start and stop when they do, what mechanisms govern development of epileptogenic brain tissue after an injury, what accounts for a genetic predisposition to seizures, why there is a developmental profile for different types of epilepsy, and why abnormal electrical excitability manifests as different seizure types.

Manifestations of Seizures

The manifestations of a seizure depend on several factors, one of the most important being the site in brain where the abnormal electrical discharge originates. Shown in Fig. 14-3 are the types of seizures in relation to functional neuroanatomy. Thus, neural control centers for strength and sensation are arrayed along the border of the frontal and parietal lobes, with strength more toward the rostral (frontal) and somatosensory perception more toward the caudal (parietal) regions of the strip. Moving from the superior regions laterally and down the brain are representations of the trunk, arms, hands, fingers, face, and lips, with the tongue represented most laterally and inferiorly on the motor-sensory strip. Electrical activity during a seizure can travel through this area, activating each muscle group in sequence over seconds to minutes (Jacksonian march). Broca's motor speech area is usually in the left frontal lobe in front of the motor strip, with a Wernicke's speech comprehension area in the temporal-parietal region. Visual perception is governed in the posterior poles of the occipital lobes. Focal seizure activity in these regions produces impairment of the involved modality or disordered fragments of sensation.

A particularly important brain region for seizures is the undersurface of the temporal lobes. The temporal lobes include the amygdala and hippocampus, the most seizure-prone structures in the brain and the regions most commonly involved in adult epilepsy. For this reason, the amygdala and hippocampus, which are involved in emotionality and memory consolidation, are important surgical targets in the treatment of epilepsy.

Thus, if an abnormal electrical discharge originates in the motor cortex, the patient experiences a motor seizure; if in the sensory cortex, a sensory perception; if in the visual cortex, lights and elemental visual perceptions. Seizures in the deep temporal lobe structures present with arrest of activity, memory, and awareness, along with automatic behaviors. If a seizure spreads to all brain regions, the typical tonic-clonic convulsion results with loss of consciousness, stiffening, and jerking.

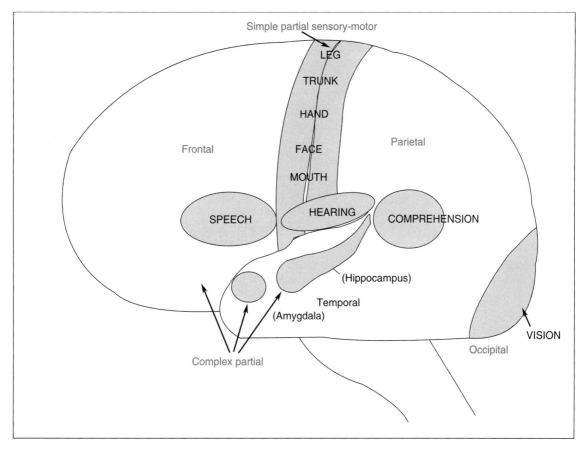

Figure 14–3. *Diagrams of selected functional regions of brain important for partial seizures. Structures in parentheses are located in mesial temporal lobe.*

Seizure Classification

Because seizures are classified primarily on the basis of a committee-generated convention of terminology rather than any fundamental properties, the classification scheme will undoubtedly change as knowledge about epilepsy grows (Table 14-1).

Seizures are divided into two broad categories, partial (focal) and generalized. Partial seizures originate in a restricted area of the brain, resulting in focal symptomatology such as twitching in the extremities or face, a sensory change, or even an alteration in memory, such as occurs with temporal lobe seizures. Generalized seizures apparently originate throughout the brain. Although some believe these seizures emanate from structures deep in the brain and project to the cortical surface, with manifestations appearing almost simultaneously, the pathophysiology of generalized seizures is poorly understood.

Partial seizures are subdivided further into simple partial, with no loss of consciousness or memory, and complex partial, with loss of consciousness or memory. Simple partial seizures manifest as motor seizures with twitching, abnormal sensations, abnormal visions, sounds, or smells, and distortions of perception. When seizure activity spreads to the autonomic nervous system, there is flushing, tingling, or nausea. With all such simple partial seizures, the

Table 14-1

Simplified International Classification of Seizures

Partial Seizures (initiated in one place)
  Simple (no loss of consciousness or memory)
    Sensory
    Motor
    Sensory-Motor
    Psychic (abnormal thoughts or perceptions)
    Autonomic (heat, nausea, flushing, etc.)
  Complex (consciousness or memory impaired)
    With or without aura (warning)
    With or without automatisms
  Secondarily generalized

Generalized Seizures
(appear to be initiated over wide area of brain)
  Absence (petit mal)
  Tonic-clonic (grand mal)
  Atonic (drop seizures)
  Myoclonic

Unclassified seizures

patient will be conscious and will fully recall the event. If the patient becomes confused, or cannot remember what happened during the episode, then it is classified as a complex partial seizure.

Complex partial seizures were previously called psychomotor seizures, temporal lobe seizures, or limbic seizures. Complex partial seizures may have an aura, a warning for the seizure, which is typically a familiar feeling (déjà vu), nausea, heat, tingling, or distortion of sensory perceptions. About 50% of patients with complex partial seizures do not remember an aura. During a complex partial seizure patients may fumble or perform automatic fragments of activity, such as lip smacking, picking at their clothes, walking around aimlessly, or repeating nonsense phrases. Such purposeless activities are called automatisms, which are displayed by about 75% of those with complex partial seizures.

Generalized seizures are divided into several categories (Table 14-1). Absence seizures, previously

called petit mal, usually have their onset in childhood. These present with brief staring spells lasting several seconds, perhaps with some eyelid fluttering or head nodding. Absence seizures can be difficult to distinguish from complex partial seizures, which may also result in staring, although absence seizures are usually briefer than complex partial seizures, and there is a more rapid recovery from absence seizures. An EEG is quite useful in distinguishing between the two (see the following).

Generalized tonic-clonic seizures, previously called grand mal seizures, begin with a sudden loss of consciousness and stiffening (tonic activity) of the limbs, followed by rhythmic jerking (clonic activity) of the limbs. The patient emits a cry because of contraction of the respiratory muscles against a closed glottis. The seizure, or ictus, usually lasts 1 to 3 min, after which the patient is postictal, which is characterized by sluggishness, sleepiness, and confusion, possibly for hours. Any seizure can have a postictal period.

Focal seizures can spread throughout the brain, in which case a tonic-clonic seizure ensues. It is important, however, to distinguish true grand mal seizures, which are generalized from the start, from those that start focally and then develop secondarily into a grand mal seizure because different drugs are used to treat primary tonic-clonic than are used for secondarily generalized tonic-clonic seizures. Moreover, the secondarily generalized tonic-clonic seizure patient may be a candidate for epilepsy surgery, whereas the primarily generalized tonic-clonic seizure patient is not because there is no definable originating site (focus) to remove.

Atonic seizures typically occur following brain injury. Patients with atonic seizures suddenly become limp and may fall to the ground. In some cases the patient must wear a helmet to protect against serious injuries.

A myoclonic seizure is a brief, unsustained jerk or series of jerks, often less coordinated or organized than a generalized tonic-clonic seizure.

Status epilepticus is a seizure, or a recurring series of seizures, without intervening return of normal function, that persists for at least 30 min. Status epilepticus is a medical emergency because it can be associated with neuronal injury and medical complications. There is a type of status epilepticus that corresponds to every type of seizure. Partial simple status is known as epilepsia partialis continua, whereas complex partial and absence status are known by several names, including nonconvulsive status, spike-wave stupor, absence status, and epileptic twilight state. Guidelines for the diagnosis and treatment of status epilepticus can be found in a summary by the Working Group on Status Epilepticus (Anonymous, 1993).

Patients may have more than one type of seizure, and one type may progress into another as the electrical activity spreads throughout the brain. A typical progression is a simple partial, to a complex partial, to a secondarily generalized tonic-clonic seizure. In some cases, antiepileptic medications enhance the ability of the brain to limit the spread of a seizure.

In adults, the most common type of seizure is complex partial, accounting for about 40% of all cases, with simple partial seen in about 20%, primary generalized tonic-clonic seizures in 20%, absence in 10%, and other seizure types in 10%. In the pediatric population, absence seizures are more prevalent than in adults.

Classification of the Epileptic Syndromes

The seizure classification reveals little about the clinical condition of the patient, or the cause, severity, or prognosis. An additional scheme, therefore, has been developed to classify epileptic syndromes. This is a broader classification, which includes not just a description of the seizure type, but information on its clinical features. A few of these additional syndromes are described in the following.

INFANTILE SPASMS/WEST'S SYNDROME

Infantile spasms occur in children 3 months to about 3 years of age and are associated with sudden epileptic flexor spasms and a high risk for mental retardation. During flexor spasms the child may suddenly extend his limbs, flex forward at the trunk, and emit a cry. The episode is over within seconds, but may occur several times each hour. An associated electroencephalographic pattern is hypsarrhythmia, with high-voltage spikes and a disordered high-voltage background. Early and vigorous treatment is thought to minimize the risk for lifelong mental retardation. Although valproic acid and benzodiazepines are treatments of choice, they are not very effective. Among the newer medications, vigabatrin, felbamate, and, possibly, lamotrigine and topiramate appear to be the most promising for this condition.

LENNOX-GASTAUT SYNDROME

The Lennox-Gastaut syndrome is a relatively rare (except in epilepsy centers, where it comprises a significant fraction of the uncontrolled patients) disorder with the following characteristics: 1) multiple seizure types, usually including atonic or tonic seizures; 2) variable degrees of mental retardation; and 3) abnormal EEG, including a slow spike-wave pattern. Although onset is usually in childhood, adults can suffer from this syndrome as well. Lennox-Gastaut epilepsy is very difficult to treat, with only 10 to 20% of patients showing a satisfactory response to therapy. Because the seizures almost always are multifocal, surgery is of little value in this condition, although corpus callosotomy may reduce the sudden onset of seizures and prevent injuries. Although valproate, benzodiazepines, lamotrigine, vigabatrin, topiramate, and felbamate have been used to treat this condition, the results have not been satisfactory.

FEBRILE SEIZURES

Provoked by fever, febrile seizures tend to present as tonic-clonic convulsions in children from 6 months to 5 years of age. Febrile seizures must be distinguished from a seizure caused by some underlying serious condition, such as meningitis. Although very alarming to parents, febrile seizures are usually benign. Although they are a risk factor for the development of complex partial epilepsy, there is no good evidence that prevention of febrile seizures reduces this risk. Indeed, the majority of children who experience febrile seizures do not progress to lifelong epilepsy. This is important because the effects of antiepileptic medication on a young child's learning and personality can be severe. Phenobarbital is typically used to prevent febrile seizures. However, to be effective, it must be taken daily because by the time of a recognized fever the seizure has normally already occurred. Daily administration of phenobarbital produces hyperactivity and behavioral and learning problems in a significant percentage of children. Many pediatric neurologists believe that treatment of febrile seizures is worse than the occasional seizure, which may never recur, and advise no therapy. A few trials with agents other than phenobarbital have not yielded encouraging results. Thus, treatment of febrile seizures remains controversial.

BENIGN ROLANDIC EPILEPSY

Benign rolandic epilepsy (BRE) is a genetically based seizure type usually appearing in children or adolescents from 6 to 21 years of age. The rolandic region is the area of the brain anterior to the frontal-parietal junction. Seizures originating in this area usually produce twitching or tingling of the face or hand, sometimes with secondarily generalized tonic-clonic seizures. With BRE the EEG usually shows prominent spikes over the central and temporal area, and the seizures are more common when falling asleep. The term "benign" is used, not because individual seizures are minor, but because the long-term prognosis is very good for outgrowing the seizure. Depending on the severity of the seizures, BRE may or may not be treated with antifocal seizure drugs.

JUVENILE MYOCLONIC EPILEPSY

Juvenile myoclonic epilepsy (JME) is the most common generalized seizure syndrome in young adults. Unlike BRE, the prognosis for outgrowing JME is poor. Juvenile myoclonic epilepsy is a genetic epilepsy syndrome with onset in late childhood or the teenage years. The abnormal gene has been linked in some families to chromosome 6. Patients with JME typically have morning myoclonus (limb or head jerking) and occasional generalized tonic-clonic convulsions. The EEG in juvenile myoclonic epilepsy shows a 3 to 6 cycles per s generalized spike-wave pattern. Responsiveness to medications, such as valproic acid or benzodiazepines, is good. If side effects limit the use of these drugs, lamotrigine or topiramate are other possible choices.

Causes of Seizures

Although any injury to the brain can generate a seizure focus, no such injury or other cause can be found in more than 50% of people with epilepsy. It is presumed that in such cases there is a subtle injury or a subtle imbalance of excitatory and inhibitory neurotransmitters in brain. Epilepsy specialists now distinguish between the term "idiopathic," meaning a nonlesional and presumably genetic form of epilepsy, and "cryptogenic," meaning an epilepsy that probably has a specific, nongenetic cause that has yet to be found.

The type of injury that may cause a seizure is age-dependent. Childhood seizures are often caused by birth traumas, infections such as meningitis, or high fevers. Although seizures in the middle years are commonly caused by head trauma, infections, alcohol, cocaine, or prescription medications, in the

elderly, brain tumors and stroke are more important etiologies. The most common etiology at any age, however, remains cryptogenic.

GENETIC CAUSES OF SEIZURES

Basic scientists and clinicians have come to recognize the importance of genetic factors in the origin of epilepsy. Genetics appear to be especially important in generalized disorders, such as absence, generalized tonic-clonic, or myoclonic seizures. Genetic defects do not in themselves appear to cause epilepsy, but rather alter the excitability of the brain so as to predispose the individual to epilepsy. Sometimes epilepsy requires more than one gene abnormality, or a gene abnormality in combination with an environmental factor. Many, perhaps hundreds, of genetic defects will eventually be found to be related to epilepsy. Although only a few genetic defects are now recognized, this is one of the most rapidly growing areas in medical research. Once there is a better definition of the genetic predisposition for seizures, pharmaceutical companies will be able to design new, more effective, and safer antiepileptic medications.

Relatives of patients with primary generalized epilepsies are at higher risk than others for developing seizures. Because the penetrance of the genetic factors is relatively low, most relatives will not have epilepsy. Certain lesional epilepsies that are not genetic may be associated with predisposing genetic risk factors that, for example, increase the likelihood of seizures after head trauma.

HEAD TRAUMA

Head trauma, which is epidemic in society, is a common cause of epilepsy. Nevertheless, most people who experience head trauma do not develop epilepsy because the head trauma must be severe enough to damage the brain permanently. This usually requires a penetrating injury to the brain or blow severe enough to cause coma or amnesia. Being stunned, or experiencing a brief loss of consciousness, usually does not lead to epilepsy. Moreover, seizure at the time of the head trauma does not necessarily mean epilepsy will ensue. In such cases antiseizure medication may be given for a short period or medications may be withheld to see if seizures return. The development of epilepsy after head trauma may not occur for years after the injury. Algorithmic formulae are available to predict the likelihood of epilepsy after head trauma.

BRAIN TUMORS

Although relatively rare, brain tumors are troublesome causes of seizures. Both benign and malignant tumors can produce seizures, including meningiomas, low-grade astrocytomas, anaplastic astrocytomas, glioblastomas, oligodendrogliomas, gangliogliomas, lymphomas, and metastatic carcinomas to the brain. Tumor-induced seizures usually are focal (partial), with a character that depends on where the tumor resides in the brain. With few exceptions, such as gangliogliomas, seizures usually do not originate from tumor cells themselves, but from the irritated brain tissue that surrounds the tumor. Focal seizures from tumors can be very difficult to treat, with inhibition of secondary generalization sometimes the only realistic goal. If the tumor can be successfully treated, seizures usually diminish in number and intensity. Patients should know that removal of all, or most, of a brain tumor by surgery, radiation, or chemotherapy will not necessarily completely cure the epilepsy, requiring that antiseizure medications be taken for a long period of time. In a patient with a brain tumor, an unexplained deterioration in the seizure pattern calls for a re-evaluation of the tumor.

INFECTIONS AND SEIZURES

Infections are common causes of epilepsy, particularly in children or adults with bacterial, fungal, or viral meningitis. The brain may itself become infected with encephalitis or an abscess. All of these infections can lead to recurrent seizures. Herpes simplex encephalitis, with a predilection for the temporal lobes, is especially likely to cause epilepsy. Worldwide, parasitic infections, such as cysticercosis, are the most prevalent infectious causes of epilepsy, with toxoplasmosis increasingly important as a cause of seizures in HIV patients.

STROKE AND SEIZURES

When a stroke injures but does not kill brain cells, the damaged tissue may develop into a seizure focus. Although approximately 5 to 15% of strokes produce seizures acutely, more with embolic or hemorrhagic strokes, less than 50% of these individuals will progress to long-term epilepsy. Seizures from strokes can be focal or secondarily generalized. Many strokes are not obvious because they are small or in functionally silent areas of brain. Small strokes may not be remembered by the patient, and may not be visible on a brain MRI scan. It is common to suspect that a small stroke has occurred in an individual who is having seizures, although it is not possible to visualize where the stroke is located. The converse problem occurs when an elderly individual presents with new-onset seizures and the almost inevitable pattern of small-vessel white-matter disease is seen with an MRI scan. At present, there is no way to determine whether these microinfarcts are related to the seizures.

SEIZURES FROM DYSPLASIAS

A dysplasia is a mass of normal brain cells that resides in an abnormal place in the brain. Other terms for dysplasias are migration abnormalities, heterotopias, and developmental defects. The signals that direct developing neurons to their proper location are not fully understood. Some brain cells appear to receive the wrong instructions and migrate only part of the way to the cortex. Perhaps because these cells are not surrounded by their usual neighbors, they are not subject to the normal controls that inhibit hyper-excitability. Dysplasias are more common than previously believed. Although they are usually not visible on a CT scan, they may be detected with a high-quality MRI. Dysplasias can range in severity from MRI-invisible microdysplasias to the full dysplastic syndrome of tuberous sclerosis.

CHEMICAL IMBALANCES

Not all seizures result from a structural problem in the brain; chemical imbalances can cause seizures in a brain that appears perfectly normal on an MRI scan. Chemical imbalances that result in seizures are caused by a number of substances and insults including alcohol, cocaine, stimulants, antihistamines, ciprofloxatin, metronidazole, aminophylline, phenothiazines, tricyclic antidepressants, hypoglycemia, hypoxia, hyponatremia, hypocalcemia, renal or hepatic failure, and complications of pregnancy.

HORMONES

Some women notice a connection between their seizures and their menstrual cycle, and seizures may worsen, or improve, during pregnancy. Seizures sometime originate, or deteriorate, at the time of puberty, and may improve with menopause. Female hormones, particularly estrogen and related substances, are known to regulate brain excitability, making the link between hormones and seizures quite real. Unfortunately, there is as yet no treatment that alters the hormone balance so as to provide long-term seizure control.

Epidemiology of Epilepsy

Epilepsy is a common condition, with the risk among Americans being 0.5 to 1%. Up to 5% or more of the population may have at least one seizure from any cause in their lifetime, with a 10% cumulative risk for those who live into their 70s (Hauser et al., 1996). Anyone can develop epilepsy, from young babies to the elderly.

Many historical figures had epilepsy, including Julius Caesar, Peter the Great, Napoleon, James Madison, Alexander the Great, Charles V, Joan of Arc, Saint Paul, Dostoevsky, Flaubert, Molière, Jonathan Swift, Lord Byron, Handel, Tchaikovsky, Vincent Van Gogh, Alfred Nobel, Pythagoras, and Socrates.

Circumstances That Provoke Seizures

Although most seizures are spontaneous, there are certain factors that contribute to their occurrence. These include missing seizure medications, times of the menstrual cycle, pregnancy, flashing lights, TV or video games, lack of sleep, illness, and migraine headaches. Less common precipitating factors are certain sounds, foods, sensory inputs, or changes in temperature. Although stress is sometimes thought to be a provoking factor, this relationship is unproven. Because stress is very common in our society, and most of the time it does not provoke seizures, it is unclear why some stress does, and some does not, precipitate a seizure.

Alcohol consumption and alcohol withdrawal are often triggers for seizures, as is withdrawal from prescription sedative/hypnotics such as the barbiturates or benzodiazepines. Although many commonly used medications may cause seizures, there is no convincing evidence that caffeine, cigarettes, or Nutra-Sweet do, although a few people claim individual sensitivity to these substances. There are also reports of highly unusual provoking factors such as a certain smell or kind of music, or certain thoughts. Some factors are falsely blamed for a seizure owing to coincidence. This should be suspected if the seizure occurs more than a day after the supposed trigger, or if the seizure only happened on one occasion after the trigger. The fact is, most seizures do not have a provoking factor.

Social Issues in Epilepsy

Some of the most important issues for patients with epilepsy are social. Although in discussions with patients physicians talk mostly about seizure frequency, medication side effects, and the results of testing, patients may have a different set of concerns, such as how to deal with the embarrassment of a seizure. Moreover, patients want to know how seizures are going to affect their ability to obtain, or retain, a job, or succeed in school, and they want to know what seizures will mean for their social life, marriage, family, and the advisability of having children. Patients are also curious to know how seizures will affect their ability to obtain a driver's license and influence their independence. Overall, there is considerable fear, misinformation, and stigma associated with epilepsy. For obscure historical reasons, epilepsy is viewed by many as a disorder linked to insanity or, in some cases, evil. Successful treatment

therefore requires that these social issues be addressed with the patient.

There is much discussion about driving and epilepsy. Although patients with frequent seizures should not drive, those with infrequent seizures may drive under some conditions. Different states have different requirements for seizure-free intervals, varying from a few months to 2 years. The shorter time intervals allow people with epilepsy to make other arrangements for temporary transportation, theoretically encouraging honesty in reporting. Persons with seizures can obtain exemptions allowing them to drive if the seizures are exclusively nocturnal, or they have a prolonged and consistent warning that would allow time to bring the car to a safe stop. Most, but not all, states make it the responsibility of the patient to notify the motor vehicle division. Required physician reporting encourages dishonesty between the patient and the physician about the occurrence of seizures, preventing appropriate treatment.

EMPLOYMENT

Most people with epilepsy work full time at productive jobs. Occupations that involve driving, operation of life- or limb-threatening machinery, caustic chemicals, or prolonged periods on heights or underwater should not be undertaken by those with uncontrolled seizures. The 1990 *Americans for Disabilities Act* prohibits discrimination on the job against people with epilepsy. If people with epilepsy cannot perform their jobs because of seizures, attempts must be made to accommodate them within the context of their employment.

SCHOOL

Children with epilepsy can perform well in school, although some do not. Failure may be because of social and peer pressure, or poor self-image and lessened expectations. Other children perform poorly because of an underlying brain injury. Another major factor in poor school performance is antiepileptic medication; the barbiturates are particularly problematic in this regard.

PREGNANCY

Women with epilepsy can become pregnant, have normal children, and participate fully in parenthood. Nonetheless, such pregnancies are high risk because of the seizures and the antiepileptic medications. Risks of birth defects are a few percent higher in women with epilepsy; some birth defects are probably due to the seizures, underlying general risk factors, and antiepileptic medications. Thus, monotherapy is preferred during pregnancy, provided it controls the seizures. Although there is a great deal of debate about the best medications for use during pregnancy, there are no controlled clinical studies to provide guidance on this issue. A fetal hydantoin syndrome, however, is known to be associated with phenytoin birth defects linked to barbiturates, and dysraphism syndrome is associated with the use of valproic acid and carbamazepine. The best strategy during pregnancy is to use the single medication that is most effective in treating the seizures. Because folic acid supplementation appears to be of some value in preventing birth defects in those mothers without neurological disease, it may be prudent to recommend 0.4 to1.0 mg of folate per day if a patient is at risk for pregnancy.

INJURIES FROM SEIZURES

Although the goal of therapy is to allow people with epilepsy to live their lives as fully as possible, there must be an appreciation of the potential for injuries resulting from this condition. Patients with infrequent seizures (e.g., small seizures less than every 3 months) may have no need for restrictions, whereas those with frequent seizures should be particularly careful around water, including bathtubs (it may be safer to shower sitting), heights (brief climbs up ladders or stairs are usually safe), some machinery, and other potentially dangerous situations. These risks are present in both the home and the workplace. For the best care, safety precautions should be individualized for each patient.

DIAGNOSIS

The most important diagnostic tools in epilepsy are a careful history and detailed information on the nature of the episodes. A physical and neurological examination should be performed looking for evidence of neurological dysfunction that might provide a clue as to the cause and location of the seizure focus. With epilepsy, however, the history is usually more important than the physical exam.

Blood tests are performed to determine whether there are infectious or chemical causes of the seizures and to establish baseline data on white and red blood cell counts, platelets, and hepatic and renal function before medications are given. A lumbar puncture should be performed if there is a possibility of infectious meningitis.

The physician may obtain a neuroradiologic study to determine whether there is an underlying structural cause for the seizures such as a tumor, hematoma, cavernous angioma, arteriovenous mal-

formation, abscess, dysplasia, or an old stroke. An MRI scan is more detailed and useful for seizure diagnosis than a CT scan because MRI may show subtle lesions or a pattern consistent with mesial temporal sclerosis, with atrophy of the hippocampus and increased hippocampal signal on the T2 images.

Mesial temporal sclerosis (MTS) is often found in association with temporal lobe epilepsy. There has been much discussion about whether it is a cause or the result of seizures. Although laboratory animals develop MTS after a period of recurrent temporal lobe seizures, there are only a few human cases documented with serial MRI scans showing onset and development of MTS with chronic seizures. On the other hand, hypoxia-ischemia can cause hippocampal changes resembling MTS in advance of clinically evident seizures. In any event, MTS is a very useful marker for temporal lobe epilepsy and for establishing the site of a seizure focus. It does not, however, prove that all seizures originate at that site.

The EEG has special importance in the diagnosis of epilepsy. The EEGs are representations of time-varying voltages between two points, usually displayed for 8 to 32 electrode pairs over different regions of the scalp. Recordings typically consist of 15 to 30 min of data, ideally in both the waking and sleeping state because epileptiform activity may only be evident with drowsiness or in light sleep. The electroencephalographer interprets the record with regard to overall voltage, symmetry over homologous regions, a normal frequency spectrum, presence of certain patterns, such as the 8 to 12/s posterior alpha rhythm, and absence of focal and paroxysmal abnormalities. Focal abnormalities may be in the form of slow waves, such as 0 to 3/s delta activity or 4 to 7/s theta activity, or may be noted as a regional loss of EEG voltage. Paroxysmal activities include spikes, sharp waves, spike waves, and electroencephalographic seizure patterns.

Shown in Fig. 14-4 is an interictal spike. Sharp waves are similar to spikes but have longer duration, with spikes lasting less than 70 ms and sharp waves 70 to 200 ms. The spike is the regional manifestation of the paroxysmal depolarization shift of synchronously firing neurons. Spikes usually are interictal, that is, between seizures, and have little or no behav-

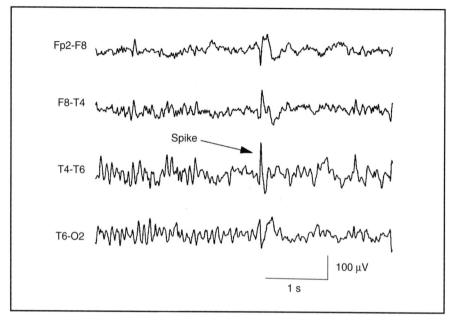

Figure 14–4. A clinical EEG demonstrating an interictal spike. Polarity is displayed with negative upgoing.

ioral correlate. These EEG spikes help diagnose and classify epilepsy and localize the seizure focus. Approximately 50 to 80% of individuals with epilepsy display interictal spikes, although repeat recordings may be necessary to observe them.

Shown on Fig. 14-2 is a spike-wave pattern associated with absence epilepsy, and in Fig. 14-5 is the EEG pattern at the start of a temporal lobe complex partial seizure. Partial seizures show several types of scalp EEG patterns. The most common is a focal pattern of rhythmic 2 to 10/s slow waves with an evolution of frequency and amplitude over seconds to minutes, and which spreads to other areas of the scalp. Seizures may also begin with rhythmic spikes, spike-waves, or low-voltage, fast activity. Very focal neocortical seizures, and deep frontal or temporal seizures with no projection to cortex, may not be visible on a scalp EEG. Over 90% of seizures, however, have an EEG correlate.

Routine EEGs rarely capture seizures. Thus, when seizures must be recorded, for example, to localize a seizure focus for possible ablative surgery,

prolonged EEG recording may be necessary. Video and audio recording can be synchronized to the EEG to correlate behaviors and electrical patterns. Some candidates for seizure surgery require invasive recording with intracranial electrodes.

The EEG alone is never used to make a diagnosis of epilepsy because it is only an adjunctive test to support a clinical history consistent with epileptic seizures. Thus, some individuals may display abnormal EEG spikes but never have a seizure and therefore should not be diagnosed as having epilepsy. Conversely, the EEG may be normal between seizures in people with epilepsy.

Imitators of Epilepsy

Several conditions can result in abnormal movements, sensations, or loss of awareness but are not associated with the abnormal electrical discharge in the brain (Table 14-2). Thus, syncope may incorrectly be considered seizures, although, typically, there is not a prolonged period of jerking with this

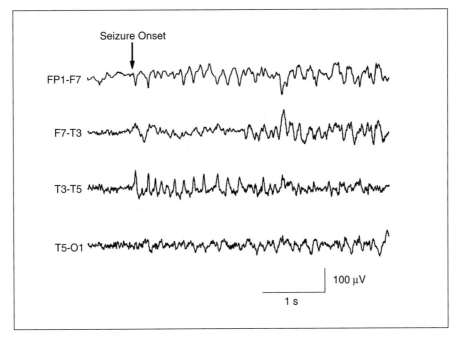

Figure 14–5. *A clinical EEG demonstrating onset of rhythmical sharp activity in the left temporal region at the start of a complex partial seizure. Polarity is displayed with negative upgoing.*

Table 14-2
Imitators of Epilepsy

Syncope
Transient ischemic attacks (TIAs)
Cardiac arrhythmias
Hypoglycemia
Hypoxia
Confusional migraine
Transient global amnesia
Sleep disorders (e.g., narcolepsy, cataplexy, excessive daytime hypersomnolence)
Vertigo
Tremors, tics, dystonias
Panic attacks
Hyperventilation spells
Night terrors
Nonepileptic seizures (psychogenic seizures, pseudoseizures)

condition. Interruptions of brain circulation produce symptoms similar to epilepsy. Moreover, hypoglycemia or hypoxia can cause confusional episodes that resemble seizures, and some patients have confusional spells with severe migraine headaches. Transient global amnesia, which presents as an acute and self-limited loss of the ability to register new memories, can be distinguished from complex partial seizures by its duration (a few hours) and by the preservation of all other cognitive functions. Sleep disorders, such as narcolepsy, cataplexy, or excessive daytime sleepiness, resemble seizures. Patients sometimes present with tremors, tics, dystonic posturing, or other forms of abnormal movement such as with Huntington's disease that are sometimes confused with simple partial motor seizures.

Psychological imitators are the most difficult to differentiate from epilepsy. These include panic attacks, hyperventilation, episodic dyscontrol syndrome (rage attacks, intermittent explosive disorder), and psychogenic seizures that provide real diagnostic difficulties. With breath-holding spells, which are variants of temper tantrums in children, the child becomes angry, holds his or her breath, turns blue, loses consciousness, and exhibits some jerking. Night terrors are screaming episodes during sleep that are typically seen with children. Although breath-holding spells and night terrors are alarming, they are benign. Psychological seizures are also called psychosomatic seizures, pseudoseizures, psychogenic seizures, or nonepileptic seizures where subconscious stress causes the patient to have seizure-like episodes. In most cases a nonepileptic seizure does not reflect a conscious effort to fake a seizure, but a subconscious psychosomatic stress reaction. The treatment for psychogenic seizures is psychological counseling and behavior modification therapy, not antiepileptic medications. Video-EEG monitoring is usually needed to confirm a diagnosis of psychogenic seizures because the expected EEG changes associated with a seizure will be absent. Because imitators of epilepsy are so difficult to distinguish from seizures, some patients have been treated inappropriately for years with antiepileptic medications. A detailed history of the event is the key to diagnosing imitators of epilepsy, with consideration given to prodrome, stereotypy, duration, setting, triggers, and behavior during the episode (Fig. 14-6).

PHARMACOTHERAPY

Bromide salts were the first effective antiepileptic medications. Discovered in 1850, the bromides were employed on the mistaken notion that by reducing sexual drive they would reduce seizures. Although bromides inhibit seizures, they are toxic and were abandoned when phenobarbital was introduced 60 years later. Phenobarbital was first used as a sedative/hypnotic; it was serendipity that led to discovery of its antiepileptic potential. Many seizure medications were developed that are chemical derivatives of phenobarbital, an example of which is phenytoin, developed in 1938 as the first nonsedating antiepileptic. By contrast, carbamazepine was developed in the 1950s as a medication for treating depression and pain and valproic acid was a solute found by chance

to be antiepileptic when it was used for dissolving compounds to be tested as antiepileptic agents.

Potential antiepileptic medications are screened in animal models, such as maximal electroshock (MES). In this case drugs are tested for their ability to inhibit tonic convulsions in a mouse or rat exposed to an electric shock, with protection against MES predicting efficacy against partial and secondarily generalized seizures. Phenytoin was discovered using this approach.

In the early 1950s, ethosuximide was found to be of value in absence (petit mal) epilepsy. Interestingly, although this drug has no protective value in MES it inhibits seizures produced by pentylenetetrazol (PTZ). This led to the use of PTZ seizures as a model to predict efficacy in petit mal seizures. Seizures induced by other convulsants such as a strychnine, picrotoxin, allylglycine, and N-methyl-D-aspartic acid are sometimes used to screen for antiepileptic drugs. Occasionally, a medication will protect against one but not another type of convulsant, suggesting a selectivity of action for particular types of seizures.

More recently, the kindling model has been used as a screen for antiepileptics and a model of complex partial epilepsy. In this model electrical shocks are transmitted by electrodes implanted into deep structures of the brain. Although the shocks have no residual effect initially, when repeated over a few days or weeks they cause complex electrical discharges to persist, resulting in a convulsive seizure. Under this circumstance the animal is said to be "kindled." Kindled seizures have been used to study drugs that may be of use in treating temporal lobe epilepsy. Because kainic acid, an analogue of glutamic acid, appears to be preferentially toxic to the deep temporal lobes, it is sometimes used to create a model of temporal lobe seizures. Moreover, particular strains of rats and mice have been bred for tendencies toward different types of seizures. Of particular value in this regard are the rat absence models.

Although different animal models are thought to test the utility of a drug for different types of seizures, the correspondence between effects in animal models and seizure protection in humans is poor. In general, drugs that are effective in more than one animal model of epilepsy at relatively nontoxic doses are better clinical candidates than others. Thus, although demonstrated efficacy in animal models is a necessary first step toward human testing, it by no means guarantees a drug candidate will be safe and effective in patients.

Antiepileptic drug development has passed through several stages (Table 14-3). Bromides represented the era of wrong theory, phenobarbital the era of serendipity, primidone and mephobarbital the phenobarbital imitation era, and phenytoin the MES screening era. Most newer medications were designed for their ability to selectively modify neurochemical systems in brain. Thus, vigabatrin and tiagabine increase the synaptic availability of GABA, the former by blocking GABA metabolism and the latter by blocking the reuptake of GABA into neurons and glia. Lamotrigine and remacemide work, in part, by blocking the release of, or the receptor for, glutamic acid. Phenytoin, carbamazepine, valproic acid, felbamate, lamotrigine,

Table 14-3
History of Antiepileptic Drug Therapy

Decade of introduction	Era	Mechanism	Example
1850	Wrong theory	Reduce sex drive	Bromides
1910	Serendipity	Sedatives	Phenobarbital
1930	Imitation	Barbiturates	Primidone
1940	Screening	Maximal electroshock Pentylenetetrazol Other models	Phenytoin Ethosuximide
1990	Physiochemistry	GABA Glutamate Ion channels	Vigabatrin Remacemide Several others
2000	Genetics	Replace gene products Repair gene	?

and several other medications appear to prolong the time during which the neuronal sodium channel is closed after inactivation. This prolongation prevents the axon from generating another action potential too quickly, diminishing the rapidity of firing.

Future therapies are likely to result from the identification of the genes responsible for epilepsy. Replacement of the missing gene products, or repair of the gene itself, will provide an opportunity to cure epilepsy, not just suppress seizures.

Several issues must be considered when selecting an antiepileptic medication (Table 14-4). The first is to decide whether to treat with drugs at all. Thus, some simple partial seizures presenting only with tingling or minor motor activity might not re-

Table 14-4
Principles of Antiepileptic Drug Therapy

Decide whether to treat
Decide how long to treat
Use monotherapy when possible
Use simple regimens
Encourage compliance
Choose the best drug for the seizure type

quire therapy. Even absence seizures or partial complex seizures might not require treatment provided they do not bother the patient, they don't cause falls or injuries, and there is no need for the patient to drive or work near dangerous types of machinery. Also, a single seizure might not demand treatment because 50% of individuals who experience an idiopathic generalized tonic-clonic seizure and who have a negative EEG, MRI, and blood test will not have another seizure. A second seizure, however, usually demands the initiation of treatment.

Antiepileptic therapy is not necessarily for life because, under some conditions, medications can be tapered and withdrawn. This is particularly true if a patient has been seizure free for at least 2 to 5 years, has no underlying structural lesion, does not have an identifiable genetic condition, such as juvenile myoclonic epilepsy, that predisposes to ongoing seizures, has not had problems with status epilepticus, and shows no seizure activity on a routine EEG. Even under these circumstances, however, there is still a one in three chance of a seizure within 1 year of withdrawing medication. Patients should be advised not to drive, or at least to minimize driving, for 3 months while tapering the dose of their seizure

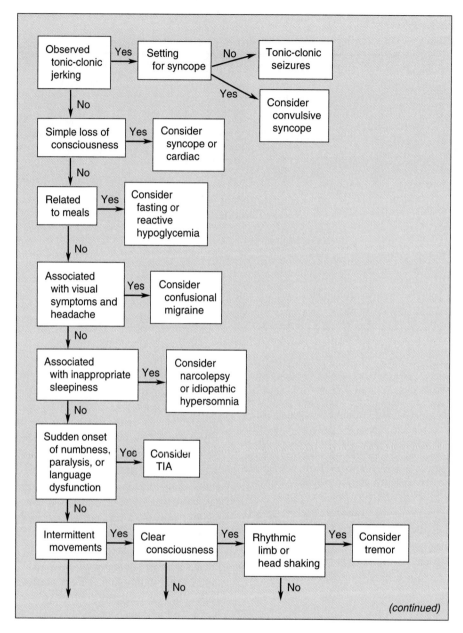

Figure 14-6. *A flowchart for diagnosis of epilepsy and its imitators.*

medicine. Unfortunately, this driving restriction discourages many from terminating therapy.

When prescribing drugs the medication regimen should be as simple as possible because complex regimens are not followed by the patient. Thus, a once-daily dosage is more often followed correctly than a two-, three-, or four-times-per-day schedule. The worst regimens involve the use of different drugs on different time schedules. Thus, monotherapy, which is successful in some 80% of epileptic patients,

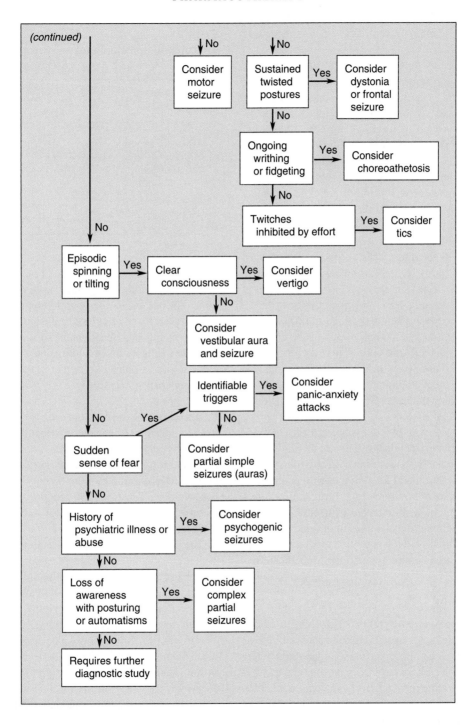

is simpler than polypharmacy and avoids drug interactions.

Some drugs must be initiated slowly to avoid side effects. Whereas the doses of carbamazepine, valproic acid, lamotrigine, primidone, topiramate, felbamate, and vigabatrin must be increased gradually over a period of weeks or months, phenytoin, phenobarbital, and gabapentin can be initiated at therapeutic doses. Dosing schedules must be prepared in advance and given to the patients and their families in writing. In addition, it is important to be in contact with patients, especially at the beginning of therapy, to deal with possible side effects.

Changing from one medication to another can be difficult. If the dose of the second medicine must be increased slowly, it is usually not advisable to taper the first until the new medication is given at the full therapeutic dose. Without this precaution the patient may have seizures because of inadequate protection during the changeover period, although there is a greater likelihood of toxicity during the time of overlapping medications. Patients must be warned to expect a temporary period of side effects, and possible withdrawal seizures, when changing medications.

Although serum blood levels are useful in guiding the treatment of epilepsy, they are probably overused. If a patient is seizure free and experiencing no toxicities, serum blood level monitoring is unnecessary. When two or more drugs are administered, measurement of serum levels is useful for determining which one may be causing a toxic response. Shown in Table 14-5 are recommended serum blood levels for some common antiepileptic medications.

Antiepileptic Drug Selection

Carbamazepine or phenytoin are the drugs of choice for partial seizures, whereas valproic acid is preferred for primary generalized seizures, being slightly less effective than carbamazepine for partial seizures. Because most of the medications have comparable efficacy, a selection can be made on the basis of side effects, ease of use, and cost (Table 14-6). It should be noted that the recommendations shown here reflect the opinions of the author. Indeed, not all of these medications have been approved for use in some of these

Table 14-5
Therapeutic Serum Levels of Antiepileptic Drugs

Medication	Optimal serum level ($\mu g/mL$)
Phenytoin	10–20
Carbamazepine	6–12
Phenobarbital	15–35
Valproic acid	50–125
Gabapentin	2–10 (not predictive)
Lamotrigine	2–10 (not predictive)

seizure types. Displayed in Table 14-7 are names and dosage forms of the new, widely used seizure medications. The best reference on antiepileptic medications is the review text by Levy and colleagues (1995). This book is useful as a referral source for additional details on these medications, including data from individual clinical trials. Figure 14-7 depicts a therapeutic strategy flow chart for seizures.

Partial seizures. The usual drugs of choice for partial seizures are phenytoin or carbamazepine. If one of these is not effective, the other is typically tested in monotherapy, with some switching to valproic acid alone if a third round of monotherapy is necessary. If neither phenytoin nor carbamazepine is effective, then therapy with either phenytoin or carbamazepine in combination with valproic acid, gabapentin, lamotrigine, vigabatrin, or topiramate may be attempted. Although phenobarbital or primidone are used as add-ons, or second-line monotherapy, they present a significant risk for sedation. Felbamate can be effective as an alternative monotherapy, but may cause aplastic anemia and hepatic injury.

In a major clinical study, phenytoin, carbamazepine, phenobarbital, and primidone were compared in the treatment of partial seizures (Mattson et al., 1985). Efficacy was similar for the four medications, although more patients randomized to primidone withdrew from the trial because of sleepiness. Overall, carbamazepine displayed the best seizure control, a finding that was subsequently confirmed in a second trial.

Table 14-6
Medications of Choice

Seizure type	First monotherapy	Second monotherapy	Add-on
Partial seizures with or without secondary generalization	CBZ PHT VPA	PBB FLB	GPN LTG VPA TPM VGB
Absence seizures	ESM	VPA LTG	BDZ TPM
Primary generalized tonic-clonic seizures	VPA	PHT CBZ PBB LTG TPM	BDZ
Myoclonic seizures	VPA BDZ	LTG TPM	BDZ ACZ
Atonic seizures	VPA BDZ	FLB	LTG TPM ACZ

ACZ = Acetazolamide (Diamox); BDZ = Benzodiazepines (Valium, Ativan, Klonopin, Tranxene); CBZ = Carbamazepine (Tegretol); ESM = Ethosuximide (Zarontin); FLB = Felbamate (Felbatol); GPN = Gabapentin (Neurontin); LTG = Lamotrigine (Lamictal); PBB = Phenobarbital (Luminal); PHT = Phenytoin (Dilantin); TPM = Topiramate (Topamax); VPA = Valproic acid (Depakene, Depakote)

Secondarily generalized seizures. Secondarily generalized seizures respond to the same regimens as partial seizures.

Absence seizures. The drug of choice for absence (petit mal) seizures is ethosuximide, whereas mixed absence and tonic-clonic seizures, and patients who are unresponsive to ethosuximide, are treated with valproic acid. Because of its potential hepatotoxicity and expense, valproic acid is not the drug of choice for simple absence. Neither phenytoin nor carbamazepine have any role in the treatment of absence seizures and occasionally may make them worse. Lamotrigine is useful for absence, but has not been approved for this indication in the United States. Although benzodiazepines are useful for the treatment of generalized seizures, they are sedating and their effectiveness declines over time (tolerance).

Primary generalized tonic-clonic seizures. Valproic acid is the drug of choice for primary generalized tonic-clonic seizures, particularly if there is a myoclonic component. Phenytoin, carbamazepine, phenobarbital, lamotrigine, and topiramate may all be used to treat this condition.

Myoclonic seizures. Although myoclonic seizures respond best to valproic acid, other drugs, such as benzodiazepines, lamotrigine, and topiramate, are also effective in this disorder.

Atonic seizures. Atonic seizures are often difficult to treat, but valproic acid and benzodiazepines such as clonazepam can be used to manage this condition.

Table 14-7

List of Selected Medications and Available Dosages

Acetazolamide (Diamox) (125, 250 mg and 500 mg sequels)

Carbamazepine (Tegretol) (100, 200 mg and 100, 200, 400 mg extended release)

Clonazepam (Klonopin) (0.5, 1, 2 mg)

Clorazepate (Tranxene) (3.75, 7.5, 15 mg and 11.25 and 22.5 mg single dose)

Diazepam (Valium) (2, 5, 10 mg)

Ethosuximide (Zarontin) (250 mg)

Ethotoin (Peganone) (250, 500 mg)

Felbamate (Felbatol) (400, 600 mg)

Gabapentin (Neurontin) (100, 300, 400 mg)

Lamotrigine (Lamictal) (25, 50, 100, 150, 200 mg)

Lorazepam (Ativan) (0.5, 1, 2 mg)

Mephenytoin (Mesantoin) (100 mg)

Mephobarbital (Mebaral) (32, 50, 100 mg)

Oxcarbazepine (Trileptal) (in preparation)

Phenacemide (Phenurone) (250, 500 mg)

Phenobarbital (Luminal) (15, 30, 60, 100 mg)

Phenytoin (Dilantin) (30, 50, 100 mg)

Primidone (Mysoline) (50, 250 mg)

Tiagabine (Gabatril) (in preparation)

Topiramate (Topamax) (25, 100 mg)

Valproic acid (Depakote) (125, 250, 500 mg)

Vigabatrin (Sabril) (500 mg)

Some of the newer drugs, including lamotrigine, vigabatrin, and topiramate, may be effective as well. Although felbamate has been found to be useful in atonic seizures, its potential toxicity limits its utility.

Antiseizure Medications

Phenytoin. Phenytoin (Fig. 14-8) was introduced in 1938 as the first nonsedating antiepileptic. Its anticonvulsant properties were identified on the basis of its effect on maximal electroshock in laboratory animals. Phenytoin is presently the most widely used drug in the United States for the treatment of partial and secondarily generalized seizures.

Phenytoin appears to act at multiple sites within the central nervous system, the net result being a limit in the spread of epileptiform activity from a place of origin in the cerebral cortex and a decrease in maximal seizure activity. The ability of phenytoin to block maximal electroshock seizures in laboratory animals is an index of its effectiveness in treating partial and secondarily generalized seizures. Phenytoin is ineffective in the pentylenetetrazol animal model of seizures, which predicts its lack of efficacy in absence epilepsy.

Phenytoin blocks posttetanic potentiation, which represents an increase in the output of a neuronal system after high-frequency stimulation. Although posttetanic potentiation may be involved in neuronal plasticity, an important property of the cell, it may also contribute to the enhancement and propagation of epileptiform discharges. Phenytoin is thought to block posttetanic potentiation by interfering with calcium ion influx into the neuron, or by increasing the refractory period of the neuronal sodium channel. The latter effect is most likely a key action of phenytoin because it has been shown to decrease sustained high-frequency firing in several neuronal systems (MacDonald and McLean, 1982).

Although phenytoin does not decrease the amplitude or configuration of individual action potentials, it reduces the rate at which neurons generate action potentials in response to brief periods of depolarizing stimulation. The effect, which represents blockade of neuronal sodium channels, occurs only with depolarized neurons and is negated by hyperpolarization. Thus, the precise mechanism of action of phenytoin is thought to be stabilization of the inactive form of the neuronal sodium channel. Because this blockade is use dependent, it does not occur on neurons that are not firing rapidly.

Phenytoin also depresses synaptic transmission by inhibiting the release of certain neurotransmitters, probably by blocking L type calcium channels in the presynaptic nerve terminal. Calcium regulatory systems in brain cells involving calmodulin are also influenced by therapeutically relevant concentrations of phenytoin.

Phenytoin has remained popular as a treatment for partial and secondarily generalized seizures despite the fact it is associated with a number of adverse reactions that may be divided into dose related, idiosyncratic, and chronic.

Dose-related toxicities associated with phenytoin are primarily neurological, possibly resulting from its ability to block the rapid firing of neurons. Many cells in brain fire rapid bursts of action potentials normally, making them liable to impairment by therapeutic concentrations of phenytoin. Thus, the vestibular nuclei responsible for rapid adjustments in balance and posture represent such a system, with effects on these cells being responsible for some of the ataxia associated with this drug. Because eye movement centers in the pons also fire rapidly to maintain eccentric gaze against the elastic forces of the orbit, a reduction of rapid firing in this system results

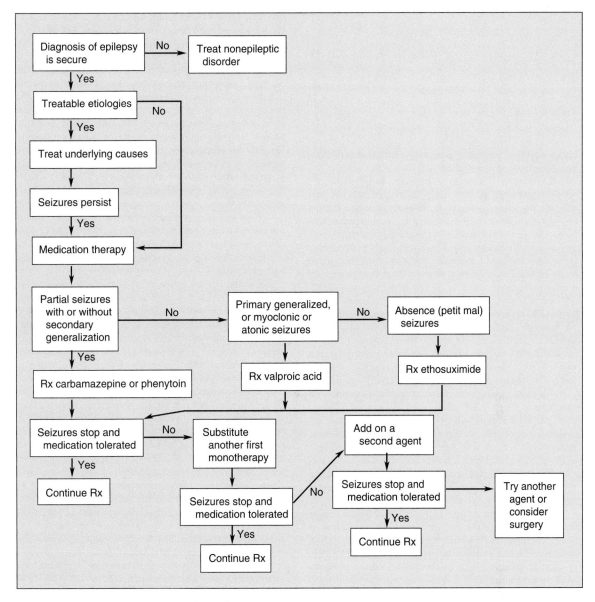

Figure 14–7. *A flowchart for epilepsy therapy.*

in nystagmus. Somnolence, confusion, and dizziness are other dose-related side effects associated with phenytoin. These side effects may be observed with doses yielding therapeutic blood levels (10 to 20 μg/mL) or less in patients who are particularly susceptible to these effects, or in those receiving multiple medications. Ataxia, dysarthria, somnolence, confusion, and nystagmus become more likely as phenytoin serum levels increase to 20 to 40 μg/mL; very high blood levels, typically those above 40 μg/mL, produce significant encephalopathy or even coma, sometimes coupled with ophthalmoplegia.

Movement disorders are an infrequent, although sometimes disabling, side effect of phenytoin. These may take the form of dystonia, dyskinesia, choreoathetosis, tremor, or asterixis. Such effects may be categorized either as idiosyn-

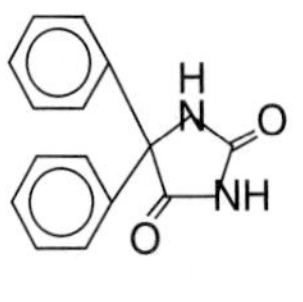

Phenytoin

Figure 14–8. *Structural formula of phenytoin.*

cratic or dose-related reactions because a reduction in medication sometimes provides relief.

The effect of phenytoin on cognitive functions has received considerable attention. Although it is generally believed to be less impairing than the barbiturates in this regard, there is less agreement about its effects in comparison with carbamazepine. Although initial studies suggested that carbamazepine impaired cognition less than phenytoin, reanalysis of patients with serum levels in comparable portions of the therapeutic range suggests no difference between these two drugs with respect to cognitive activities (Dodrill and Troupin, 1991).

Because phenytoin has effects on atrioventricular conduction and ventricular automaticity, rapid parenteral administration causes cardiac arrhythmias and hypotension, although some of these effects are undoubtedly due to the propylene glycol vehicle. Although dose-related gastrointestinal upset is rare, some patients experience nausea, vomiting, epigastric discomfort and weight loss, or weight gain, while taking this drug.

The most notable idiosyncratic reaction associated with phenytoin is allergy, which usually manifests as a morbilliform skin rash. More serious forms of rash noted with this drug are exfoliative dermatitis, Stevens-Johnson syndrome, and toxic epidermal necrolysis, with their frequency estimated to be 1 in 10,000 to 50,000. Fever, arthralgias, lymphadenopathy, and a flu-like syndrome may occur in isolation or in association with a skin rash. Lymphadenopathy is sometimes severe enough to raise suspicion of underlying lymphoma.

Phenytoin is metabolized in the liver, and hepatotoxicity can appear with its acute or chronic use. Mild elevations of SGOT (AST) or SGPT (ALT) are observed in some 10% of patients. Although a cholestatic picture with a mild elevation of alkaline phosphatase is common, an increase in serum bilirubin is seen less often. Induction of the cytochrome P450 enzyme γ-glutamyltranspeptidase (GGTP) can be anticipated with either subacute or chronic phenytoin treatment and is not indicative of liver injury. A decision to discontinue phenytoin must be made on the basis of the clinical picture and serial measurements of hepatic enzymes, rather than on any one laboratory test.

Adverse hematopoietic reactions are relatively uncommon with phenytoin, but may be serious, or even fatal, when they occur. These reactions include leukopenia, thrombocytopenia, agranulocytosis, disseminated intravascular coagulation, and pure red cell aplasia. Chronic administration of phenytoin sometimes causes macrocytosis and megaloblastic anemia, which may respond to folic acid therapy. Phenytoin

may also cause an immunologic picture of a lupus-like syndrome with elevated ANA, interstitial nephritis, polyarteritis nodosa, and other manifestations of immune dysfunction. Phenytoin rarely decreases levels of serum immunoglobulins.

The chronic toxicity of phenytoin can limit its use, with the most troublesome effects being cosmetic. Thus, phenytoin induces proliferation of subcutaneous tissue that may lead to thickening of the skin on the bridge of the nose, coarsening of facial features, gum hyperplasia (sometimes requiring orthodontic surgery), and growth of hair on the face and body. Gingival hyperplasia may occur in 25 to 50% of patients, particularly those with poor oral hygiene, although the cosmetic side effects are most noticeable in females and children. The proliferation of connective tissue rarely causes Dupuytren's contracture, Peyronie's disease, or pulmonary fibrosis.

Phenytoin can produce a peripheral neuropathy, usually manifest as a loss of the Achilles reflexes and a mild slowing of peripheral conduction velocities. Clinically significant neuropathies with weakness and sensory changes are seldom noted with phenytoin.

Chronic administration of phenytoin can cause a ricketslike condition, with interference of the conversion of vitamin D precursors to the metabolically active form. Although nearly half of those taking phenytoin for years have measurable changes in bone density and in serum levels of 25-hydroxy cholecalciferol, very few experience fractures or bone discomfort. Nonetheless, some physicians advocate administration of vitamin D with phenytoin.

The endocrine system is frequently affected in individuals taking phenytoin chronically because the drug is extensively bound to serum proteins, increasing the clearance of thyroid hormones. Although most patients are euthyroid, with normal levels of serum thyroid-stimulating hormone, a few will become hypothyroid. Phenytoin can also impair insulin secretion in patients at risk for diabetes and, in extreme cases, cause a phenytoin-induced hyperglycemia. Phenytoin can increase circulating ACTH and cortisol levels, decrease release of antidiuretic hormone, increase the secretion of luteinizing hormones, and enhance the metabolism of testosterone and estradiol. These actions, and the effects on epileptiform discharges, may combine to alter sexual physiology.

Patients on long-term phenytoin therapy often have cerebellar atrophy, with a decrease in the number of Purkinje cells. There has been much debate as to whether this atrophy is due to the seizures or the drug. Both appear to contribute, because the drug causes cerebellar atrophy in normal dogs when given chronically. The clinical significance of this finding remains uncertain.

A fetal hydantoin syndrome, in its broadest form, includes cleft lip or palate, hypertelorism, atrial or ventricular septal defects, skeletal and central nervous system abnormalities, hypospadia, intestinal malformation, failure to thrive, fingernail and finger hypoplastic changes, and mental defects. This syndrome should more properly be called the fetal anticonvulsant syndrome because many of the these infants were exposed to a number of antiepileptics *in utero*.

Phenytoin is formulated as the free acid or sodium salt. The most commonly used form, Dilantin, is available in 30- or 100-mg capsules of phenytoin sodium, the latter of which is equivalent to 92 mg of the free acid per capsule. Other forms of phenytoin sodium, including a 50-mg Dilantin Infatab and generic forms of the drug, may have a shorter half-life than Dilantin. Suspensions of phenytoin for oral administration are also available because it is well absorbed by this route, with a plasma half-life of approximately 22 h. Over 95% of absorbed phenytoin is metabolized in the liver, mainly by glucuronidation. The CYP2C isoform of the P450 enzyme family is primarily responsible for phenytoin metabolism.

The usual therapeutic blood level for phenytoin is 10 to 20 μg/mL. A key feature of phenytoin metabolism is nonlinear kinetics, with increasing oral doses of the drug producing linear increases in serum levels within a relatively narrow range, after which the levels increase dramatically with small increases in dose. This occurs when the liver ceases to metabolize phenytoin at a rate proportional to serum concentration (first-order kinetics) and begins to metabolize it at a constant rate (zero-order kinetics). As blood levels approach the lower limit of the therapeutic range further increases should be made in weekly increments of 30 mg to avoid serious toxicity.

Phenytoin is extensively bound to serum proteins, primarily albumin, with the amount of free drug equal to approximately 10% of the total. Because only unbound phenytoin penetrates the blood-brain barrier, alterations in serum binding can affect the therapeutic response. This is especially important in circumstances such as hypoproteinemia from malnutrition or chronic illness and with serum protein changes that occur during pregnancy. Although during pregnancy the total serum concentration of phenytoin declines, the level of free phenytoin does not change.

Phenytoin is found in virtually all body fluids, including the cerebrospinal fluid, saliva (which can serve as a source for measuring the concentration of free phenytoin), breast milk, and bile. Because of its extreme lipid solubility, phenytoin concentrates in brain, where 100 to 300% of total serum levels may be found.

Phenytoin interacts with a number of other drugs. Thus, it may affect, or be affected by, other agents with regard to absorption, binding to serum proteins, metabolism, and pharmacodynamic effects (Table 14-8).

Interactions among antiepileptic medications are complex and variable. For example, phenobarbital induces the hepatic enzymes that metabolize phenytoin, but also displaces phenytoin from serum proteins and competes with it for metabolizing enzymes. Therefore, plasma phenytoin levels may either rise or fall when phenobarbital is taken at the same time. Although the interactions between phenytoin and carbamazepine or valproic acid are also variable, in most cases phenytoin increases the metabolism of these drugs, requiring an increase in the dose of these medications. In contrast, carbamazepine inhibits the metabolism of phenytoin, increasing its serum levels. The interaction between phenytoin and primidone is even more complex, with decreases in serum levels of primidone itself but increases in circulating concentrations of phenobarbital, its metabolite. Whereas felbamate and topiramate increase serum levels of phenytoin, vigabatrin decreases blood levels. Such changes typically range from 10 to 30%.

Phenytoin is indicated for the treatment of partial and secondarily generalized seizures, including status epilepticus. Included are those seizures previously categorized as focal motor, focal sensory, complex partial, and secondarily generalized tonic-clonic. Although phenytoin may also be of benefit in treating primarily generalized tonic-clonic seizures, efficacy against absence, myoclonic, and atonic seizures is quite variable.

For individuals with status epilepticus, phenytoin treatment should begin with an intravenous loading dose of 18 to 20 mg/kg or, more preferably, a loading dose of the fosphenytoin form (see the following section) at 18 to 20 mg/kg. In other circumstances, when serum levels must be attained within 1 to 24 h, oral loading with a dose of 400 mg three times per day for three doses usually suffices in a typical adult. Gastrointestinal intolerance usually limits oral administration of more than 500 mg in a single dose to a drug-naive patient. In less urgent cases, phenytoin is initiated at 300 mg per day, or more precisely, 3 to 5 mg/kg. Because the half-life

Table 14-8
Phenytoin Drug Interactions

Drugs that may increase phenytoin serum levels

Acute alcohol use
Amiodarone
Chloramphenicol
Benzodiazapines
Coumadin
Disulfiram
Estrogens
Histamine$_2$ receptor antagonists
Halothane
Isoniazid
Methylphenidate
Miconazole
Propoxyphene
Phenothiazines
Phenylbutazone
Salicylates
Succinimides
Sulfonamides
Tolbutamide
Trazodone

Drugs that may decrease phenytoin levels

Carbamazepine
Chronic alcohol use
Reserpine
Sulcrafate
Certain antacids

Drugs whose efficacy is potentially impaired by phenytoin

Corticosteroids
Coumadin
Digoxin
Estrogen
Furosemide
Oral contraceptives
Quinidine
Rifampin
Tetracyclines
Theophylline
Vitamin D

---

is 22 h, this dose will yield a steady-state in serum in 5 to 7 days. Although Dilantin Kapseals can be administered as a single daily dose, other forms may require twice-daily administration because of differences in bioavailability. Phenytoin doses can be increased by 100 mg per week until the therapeutic effects, toxicity, or recommended therapeutic serum range of 10 to 20 µg/mL is attained. As the therapeutic range is approached, increases should be made at 30-mg increments to avoid entering the nonlinear portion of the metabolic curve and the associated risk of sudden toxicity. The 50-mg capsules do not have a half-life sufficient to ensure efficacy for a single daily dosing regimen. Phenytoin oral suspension contains 125 g of phenytoin per 5 cc teaspoon, with up to 0.6% alcohol. A 30 mg/5 mL suspension form is also available. As children may metabolize phenytoin more rapidly than adults, twice daily dosing may be preferred in the younger age group.

If phenytoin is administered intravenously it should not be mixed with dextrose because this affects its solubility, and it should be infused no faster than 50 mg per minute, with blood pressure and cardiac conduction monitored to avoid heart block or hypotension. Phenytoin may be employed on a daily basis for decades, and indeed for a lifetime if necessary, provided it is effective and well tolerated. Some patients have taken phenytoin for over 50 years. Although, in general, the drug maintains its effectiveness, a few individuals may show tachyphylaxis. Tapering of phenytoin can be performed over a 1- to 3-month period, unless adverse events require a more rapid rate of withdrawal.

Phenytoin is recommended in doses of 3 to 7 mg/kg per day initially, 5 mg/kg per day in two or three divided doses for a total of 300 mg per day in the average adult. This may be attained with the 100-mg and 30-mg long-acting capsules or the oral suspension containing 125 mg or 30 mg per 5 mL. Generic or shorter-acting phenytoin should be administered on a two or three times daily schedule. Parenteral phenytoin is supplied in ready-mixed solutions containing 50 mg/mL of phenytoin sodium in 2-mL sterile disposable syringes or vials. Parenteral phenytoin sodium is not recommended for intramuscular use because it is irritating to tissues.

Fosphenytoin. Fosphenytoin is a phosphate ester analogue of phenytoin that is much more water-soluble than the parent compound. Fosphenytoin is cleaved by phosphatases in lung and blood vessels to yield phenytoin with a conversion half-life of approximately 10 min. Because fosphenytoin is more soluble in aqueous solution than phenytoin, the propylene glycol and ethanolamine compounds required to solubilize the latter are not required for the ester analogue. Some of the adverse effects of intravenous phenytoin are believed due to these vehicles.

Fosphenytoin produces less pain and irritation at the injection site than does intravenous phenytoin. There is also the expectation that fosphenytoin will be less likely than phenytoin to cause hypotension, cardiac arrhythmias, and necrotic tissue reactions with extravasation. These benefits remain to be documented by clinical trials and experience.

Although the fosphenytoin molecule weighs 50% more than a phenytoin molecule, fosphenytoin is labeled in phenytoin equivalents. Therefore, injection of 1000 mg of fosphenytoin yields the same serum concentration of phenytoin as does injection of 1000 mg of phenytoin. Fosphenytoin can safely be injected at a rate of 150 mg per min, which is three times faster than the recommended upper limit for phenytoin. This more rapid rate of injection, and some favorable characteristics related to protein binding, result in free phenytoin blood levels rising as quickly with fosphenytoin as with phenytoin itself. Fosphenytoin is also well tolerated when injected intramuscularly. Side effects of fosphenytoin are generally the same as those associated with phenytoin, although possibly to a lesser degree. An exception to this is the face, body, or genital pruritus associated with the rapid injection of fosphenytoin, which is probably related to its formic acid metabolite. Other issues of importance with respect to fosphenytoin pertain to its higher cost as compared with phenytoin, its limited availability, and the risk of inadvertently substituting phenytoin for fosphenytoin with a dangerously rapid intravenous infusion rate.

Other hydantoins. Hydantoins are characterized by a phenyl ring linked to a five-membered ring with alternating keto groups and nitrogen groups at four of the corners. Substitution of side chains at the five nitrogen position (between the keto groups) has a substantial effect on the activity of the compound. Besides phenytoin, three other hydantoins have been used as antiepileptics. The first, 5-ethyl-5-phenyl-hydantoin, preceded the introduction of phenytoin. It was used as an anticonvulsant and sedative to treat movement disorders. A high incidence of drug allergy has, however, restricted its use.

Ethotoin, which has been available since 1956, may be useful in instances where phenytoin is efficacious but toxic. Ethotoin almost never causes cosmetic changes, and there is usually less ataxia with ethotoin than with phenytoin. The disadvantages of ethotoin are its short half-life, requiring three or four daily doses, and the sense that it is less efficacious than phenytoin. Ethotoin is available in 250-mg and 500-mg tablets. Its mechanism of action is assumed to be similar to phenytoin. Dosing can be initiated at 250 mg four times each day (1 g daily) or substituting 250 to 500 mg of ethotoin for each 100 mg of phenytoin on a daily basis. The dose of ethotoin may be increased by 250 to 500 mg per week, as tolerated, to a therapeutic effect, or to a total dosage of 2 to 3 g per day. Although ethotoin blood levels can be ascertained by high-performance liquid chromatography, a therapeutic range is not defined. Ethotoin produces side effects similar to phenytoin, but with a lower incidence. One relatively unique side effect of ethotoin is a visual distortion reported as an increased brightness of lights. Gum hyperplasia and cosmetic changes induced by phenytoin may subside as patients are converted to ethotoin.

The other clinically important hydantoin is mephenytoin, 3-methyl-5-ethyl-5-phenylhydantoin. Mephenytoin is demethylated to its active metabolite, 5-phenylhydantoin. Mephenytoin has properties similar to hydantoins and barbiturates and is active against both maximal electroshock and pentylenetetrazol-induced seizures in laboratory animals. Introduced in 1945, it was used for the treatment of partial and secondarily generalized seizures. Mephenytoin is supplied in 100-mg scored tablets, with a typical daily dose being 200 to 800 mg. Because the active metabolite of mephenytoin has a half-life of approximately 3 to 6 days, it can be administered once daily. Mephenytoin appears to be effective against partial and secondarily generalized seizures, but has never been considered a drug of choice because of its toxicity. In addition to all the adverse effects associated with phenytoin, mephenytoin has a higher incidence of rash, adenopathy, fever, and serious, or even fatal, blood dyscrasias.

Barbiturates. Phenobarbital (Fig. 14-9) was the most widely used antiepileptic medication for several decades following its introduction in 1912. Today, it is still the drug of choice for some types of seizures in countries where cost and ease of administration are major determinants. In the United States, phenobarbital use has declined because of its sedative properties and effects on cognition. Chemically, phenobarbital is 5-ethyl-5-phenylbarbituric acid. Because

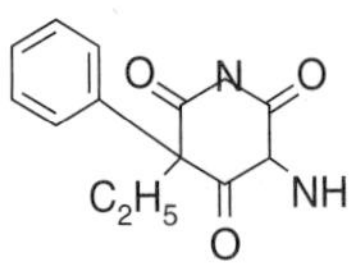

Phenobarbital

Figure 14–9. *Structural formula of phenobarbital.*

of different physicochemical properties, different barbiturates have widely differing actions. In general, the long-acting barbiturates, such as phenobarbital, are antiepileptic, whereas shorter-acting members of this class, such as thiopental and methohexital, tend to be ineffective in this regard, or even enhance epileptiform activity. Phenobarbital and primidone are the two most widely used barbiturates for the treatment of epilepsy.

Phenobarbital is active in a number of animal models of epilepsy, including maximal electroshock and pentylenetetrazol-induced seizures. Despite its broader spectrum of action in animal models than phenytoin or carbamazepine, phenobarbital is most useful for the same types of seizures, namely, partial and secondarily generalized.

Phenobarbital enhances $GABA_A$ receptor-mediated inhibitory postsynaptic potentials by increasing the duration of the receptor-related chloride channel opening in response to GABA. Besides enhancing inhibitory postsynaptic potentials, phenobarbital reduces excitatory responses to glutamate in cultured neuronal systems, blocks the rapid firing of neurons, probably by an action on the neuronal sodium channel, and reduces calcium ion influx into neurons under certain circumstances.

Phenobarbital is well absorbed after oral or intramuscular administration. The therapeutic blood levels of phenobarbital range from 5 to 40 μg/mL, with 10 to 30 μg/mL being fairly typical. Approximately 45% of the phenobarbital in blood is bound to serum proteins, with only the free fraction (55%) penetrating into brain. It is metabolized by the hepatic cytochrome P450 enzyme system. Although phenobarbital induces hepatic microsomal metabolism, it does not produce a significant degree of autoinduction. A significant fraction (25%) of unchanged phenobarbital is eliminated by the kidneys, with the remainder metabolized in liver, primarily to *p*-hydroxyphenobarbital. Elimination of phenobarbital and its metabolites is linear, with the drug having a half-life of 72 to 120 h. In neonates, the half-life may be as high as 150 h, progressively shortening over the first years of life. Because of its long half-life, phenobarbital can be administered once per day, with little except habit to recommend the traditional three times daily dosing regimen. Without a loading dose phenobarbital requires several weeks of continuous administration to achieve steady-state serum levels.

Addition of valproic acid rapidly increases phenobarbital blood levels by 20 to 50%, although coadministration of phenytoin has a variable effect on phenobarbital blood levels, and carbamazepine, topiramate, and benzodiazepines are generally without effect. Because phenobarbital induces hepatic microsomal enzymes, the metabolic transformation of other antiepileptics is increased when phenobarbital is added. Although phenobarbital enhances the metabolism of phenytoin, serum levels of the hydantoin may not change because both drugs compete for similar metabolic pathways. Phenobarbital may cause a slight decrease in the blood level of carbamazepine and variable changes in the 10,11-carbamazepine-epoxide metabolite, and it only mildly decreases the blood levels of valproic acid. Other medications that may affect phenobarbital blood levels include propoxyphene and phenothiazines, both of which increase the blood levels of the barbiturate. Conversely, phenobarbital may reduce serum levels of theophylline, tetracyclines, coumadin, phenothiazines, and vitamin D. Like phenytoin and carbamazepine, phenobarbital may reduce levels of endogenous estrogens, which can render low-dose oral contraceptives ineffective. In combination with other sedative/hypnotics, such as alcohol and the benzodiazepines, phenobarbital can cause life-threatening respiratory depression.

Phenobarbital is used for acute and chronic treatment of partial and secondarily generalized seizures. Although it occasionally provides benefit for primary generalized seizures, atonic seizures, absence seizures, and myoclonic seizures, its efficacy is variable. Daily doses of phenobarbital of 1 to 1.5 mg/kg in adults, and 1.5 to 3 mg/kg in children are usually required to yield therapeutic serum concentrations. With status epilepticus, patients can be treated with a loading dose of 18 to 20 mg/kg intravenously, administered no faster than 100 mg/min. Without a loading dose, achievement of a steady-state blood level requires many weeks.

Phenobarbital is about as effective as phenytoin and carbamazepine in the control of partial seizures (Mattson et al., 1995) and is a drug of choice for seizures in neonates and prevention of febrile seizures in children. In the latter instance, there is a high incidence of hyperactivity and learning impairment with phenobarbital use.

One of the primary dose-related side effects of phenobarbital is sedation, being most prominent during the first month or two of treatment. Thus, those who have taken phenobarbital for years are often unaware of their degree of sedation or fatigue until the drug is slowly withdrawn. Other central nervous system side effects, such as ataxia, dysarthria, dizziness, nystagmus, and cognitive impairment, are relatively common with phenobarbital, particularly at higher serum levels.

Children and the elderly taking phenobarbital sometimes experience a paradoxic hyperactivity rather than sedation. All patients may experience some depression with phenobarbital, enhancing the risk for suicide.

Idiosyncratic side effects associated with phenobarbital include hypersensitivity, rash, and, infrequently, hematologic or hepatic reactions. Men taking phenobarbital may report sexual dysfunction, and women loss of libido. Hepatic necrosis, cholestasis, and gastrointestinal disturbances are rare.

Phenobarbital-induced hepatic microsomal enzyme activity can influence vitamin D metabolism, causing osteomalacia, and can cause a folate deficiency and produce megaloblastic anemia. Moreover, chronic administration of phenobarbital can induce proliferation of connective tissue, although the cosmetic effects are generally not as noticeable as with phenytoin. Connective tissue proliferation from phenobarbital can lead to Dupuytren's contracture in the hand, Peyronie's disease, frozen shoulder, and diffuse joint pains, with or without plantar fibromatosis (Ledderhose's syndrome).

Phenobarbital causes cognitive impairment, an effect that may persist even after discontinuation of the drug. Farwell et al. (1990) found that children administered phenobarbital suffered an 8.4 point drop in their IQ, and remained 5.2 points lower than controls 6 months after discontinuation of the medication.

Although phenobarbital has been recommended by the American College of Obstetrics and Gynecology for treatment of epilepsy during pregnancy, there is little definitive evidence indicating it is safer than most other antiepileptic drugs in this circumstance. Phenobarbital administration during pregnancy is associated with birth defects, including tracheoesophageal fistulas, small bowel hypoplasia, pulmonary hypoplasia, digital malformations, ventricular-septal cardiac defects, hypospadias, meningomyelocele, mental retardation, and microcephalus. There are no data directly linking these malformations to phenobarbital itself, however, as opposed to other antiepileptic drugs that may have been used concurrently, or as opposed to epilepsy or some other underlying disorder.

Phenobarbital and other drugs that induce the activity of hepatic enzymes, such as phenytoin and carbamazepine, increase the metabolism of coagulation factors, including prothrombin, leading to hemorrhagic disease of the newborn. This is prevented by maternal ingestion of vitamin K, 10 mg orally each day for the week before birth. Because the precise date of birth cannot be predicted, vitamin K administration should be initiated after the eighth month of pregnancy.

Phenobarbital is available in 15-, 30-, 60-, and 100-mg dosage forms. Caution must be exercised because all of these dosages may be viewed by patients as "little white pills," making it easy for them to be mistaken for one another. A typical adult starting dose, without a load, is 90 to 120 mg per day. Although the 100-mg tablet is more convenient, it may be best to begin with three or four of the 30-mg tablets to allow titration. The 15-mg tablet may be useful for fine titration or for tapering of phenobarbital, which should be accomplished over several months provided there are no critical adverse events requiring more rapid tapering. Phenobarbital for intravenous injection is available in several dosage forms. The drug should be infused no more rapidly than 100 mg per min while being alert for cardiorespiratory depression. Some preparations of phenobarbital now contain propylene glycol, which can be irritating to tissues.

Primidone. Primidone, a 2-deoxy analogue of phenobarbital, is effective against seizures as are its two metabolites, phenylethylmalonic acid (PEMA) and phenobarbital. In animal tests primidone is equivalent to phenobarbital against maximal electroshock seizures, but is less effective against pentylenetetrazol seizures. It is superior to phenobarbital in myoclonic models of epilepsy.

Primidone itself and PEMA are relatively short-acting, with half-lives of 5 to 15 h. Approximately half of a primidone dose is excreted unchanged in the kidney. At steady state the phenobarbital in serum is most likely to be responsible for the response to primidone. Primidone is well absorbed following oral administration and approximately 25% is bound to serum proteins. Drug interactions with primidone are similar to those for phenobarbital.

Primidone is used to treat partial seizures, secondarily generalized seizures, and, occasionally, myoclonic seizures. Although most studies comparing phenobarbital and primidone have demonstrated equivalent efficacy, retention rates are lower for primidone than for phenobarbital, carbamazepine, or phenytoin (Mattson et al., 1985). The reason for this is that sedation, nausea, vomiting, or dizziness are more prominent with primidone, particularly during the first week of therapy. Those patients continuing on primidone for 1 month showed a similar rate of retention as with the other agents, with adverse events and efficacy being similar to the others at this time as well. Some 63% of the patients given primidone were seizure free after 1 year of treatment, as compared with 58% given phenobarbital, 55% given carbamazepine, and 48% given phenytoin.

The key to the use of primidone is slow initiation of the medication. Some patients develop a hypersomnolence reaction after an initial dose, with uncontrollable sleepiness for several days. A 50-mg test dose is useful as an initial trial. If the patient tolerates this dose, then the 125-mg dosage form can be given at bedtime for 3 to 7 days, with increments of 125 mg every 3 to 7 days, to a target dose in adults of 250 to 500 mg orally three times daily. The divided dosage is demanded by the relatively short half-lives of primidone and PEMA. If the goal is control of nocturnal seizures the total dose can be administered at bedtime. Phenobarbital levels will, however, persist throughout the day even with this dosing regimen.

The therapeutic blood level of primidone varies between 4 and 15 μg/mL, with a typical level of 12 μg/mL. Its short half-life requires that this concentration be present at trough periods. Some physicians ignore primidone blood levels and simply measure the steady-state concentration of phenobarbital, which is not critically dependent on the time of blood sampling in relation to dose because of its longer half-life.

It is extremely difficult to taper the dose of primidone because of the high risk for withdrawal seizures. Taper, unless mandated otherwise by serious adverse reactions, should be performed over several months, switching at the end to 125- or 50-mg dosage forms for the final tapering.

Side effects associated with primidone are similar to those for phenobarbital, including sedation, ataxia, cognitive impairment, depression, irritability, hyperactivity, and gastrointestinal disturbances. Idiosyncratic and chronic side effects are identical to phenobarbital.

Primidone is available in 50-, 125-, and 250-mg tablets, and as an oral suspension (250 mg per 5 mL). Parenteral primidone is not available in the United States. Patients unable to take primidone orally can be administered phenobarbital parenterally as a temporary measure. A conversion factor of 250 mg of primidone being approximately equivalent to 30 mg of phenobarbital can be applied in this circumstance.

Other barbiturates. Mephobarbital (methylphenobarbital) is indicated for the treatment of partial and secondarily generalized seizures, and possibly primary generalized seizures. It is not thought to be effective against absence seizures.

Absorption of orally administered mephobarbital may not be as complete as for phenobarbital, with required dosages being generally 50 to 300% higher than for phenobarbital. Moreover, the absorption, efficacy, and metabolism are different for the two racemic forms of the drug. Approximately 66% of mephobarbital is protein bound in serum, with a terminal half-life for the pooled enantiomers being approximately 48 h. Mephobarbital is metabolized in the liver and the metabolites are excreted in the urine. Much of the drug is demethylated in the liver to phenobarbital, making it possible to measure therapeutic blood levels of phenobarbital after achieving a steady state with mephobarbital. Although there are other metabolites of mephobarbital resulting from aromatic hydroxylation, it is unknown whether they provide any therapeutic benefit. Therapeutically effective serum concentrations of mephobarbital range from 0.5 to 2.0 μg/mL, although the phenobarbital concentration in blood is a better clinical target.

Use and side effects of mephobarbital are identical to phenobarbital. Although some physicians believe that occasional patients are less sedated with mephobarbital than phenobarbital, this has not been substantiated by clinical trials. Mephobarbital is habit forming, as are all of the barbiturates.

The typical adult dose of mephobarbital is 400 to 600 mg per day, with tablets supplied in 32-, 50-, and 100-mg doses. Children under 5 years of age are administered 50 to 100 mg per day; those over 5 years of age are administered 100 to 300 mg per day. Dosing is usually initiated with about one quarter of the target final dosage, and is increased weekly, or as tolerated. Because mephobarbital has a duration of action of 10 to 16 h, it is usually given in three divided doses daily.

Other barbiturates, such as pentobarbital or secobarbital, are occasionally used acutely to treat seizures. The barbiturates with half-lives shorter than phenobarbital are not as effective as antiepileptic agents and therefore have never achieved popularity as chronic therapies.

Carbamazepine. Carbamazepine (Fig. 14-10) is a drug of choice for the treatment of partial and secondarily generalized tonic-clonic seizures. Although it may be effective in primary generalized seizures, it has little or no role in the treatment of absence, myoclonic, and atonic seizures. Although carbamazepine was developed in the 1950s as a chemical analogue of the tricyclic antidepressants, it is categorized as an iminostilbene. Carbamazepine was initially tested as an antidepressant, then in pain syndromes associated with depression, and then trigeminal neuralgia. Because of its efficacy in trigeminal neuralgia it was tested as an antiepileptic, which is also a condition characterized by rapid, uncontrolled neuronal firing.

Carbamazepine is effective in maximal electroshock, mildly effective against pentylenetetrazol seizures, and is more effective than phenytoin in blocking amygdala-kindled seizures in laboratory animals. Because carbamazepine blocks rapid firing of neuronal bursts in hippocampal slices it probably inhibits neuronal sodium channels in a manner similar to phenytoin (McLean and Macdonald, 1986). Thus, it has been hypothesized that carbamazepine binds to inactive sodium channels, delaying their recovery to the active state. Carbamazepine also has effects on neuronal response to excitatory amino acids, monoamines, acetylcholine, and adenosine. Blockade of presynaptic fibers secondary to the action on sodium channels may reduce neurotransmitter release from, and calcium transport into, the neuron.

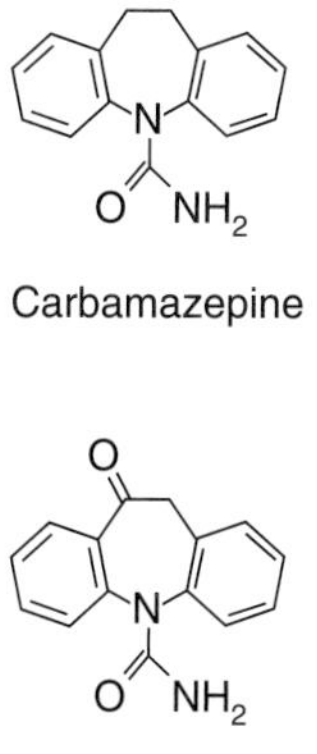

Carbamazepine is slowly and erratically absorbed following oral administration. Peak plasma concentrations are usually attained 4 to 8 h after ingestion, but can be delayed as long as 24 h, which is of particular importance in cases of carbamazepine overdosage. About 80% of carbamazepine is bound to plasma proteins, with the brain concentration being proportional to the free fraction in blood. Carbamazepine is transformed into several metabolites, the most important of which is the 10,11-epoxide, which probably contributes to efficacy and toxicity. Concurrent administration of other drugs tends to increase the proportion of carbamazepine converted to the epoxide, which may account for toxicity even when serum levels of carbamazepine are quite low. If necessary, the serum levels of the 10,11-epoxide can be measured.

Therapeutic blood levels of carbamazepine range from 4 to 12 μg/mL, although some patients may require levels as high as 8 to 12 μg/mL. Although serum levels reflect total carbamazepine, both bound and unbound, levels of unbound drug can be assayed separately. The epoxide metabolite represents 10 to 25% of the blood levels of carbamazepine, and may be higher when other drugs are given concurrently.

Carbamazepine induces hepatic microsomal enzymes, with autoinduction evident during the first few weeks of administration. The CYP3A4 enzyme system is the major metabolic pathway for both carbamazepine and the 10,11-epoxide.

Drug interactions with carbamazepine are complex because some may affect the ratio of the 10,11-epoxide without altering the serum levels of carbamazepine itself. Although carbamazepine decreases serum phenytoin levels to an inconsistent extent, a greater fraction of primidone is converted to phenobarbital when carbamazepine is added. Carbamazepine also increases the metabolic clearance of valproic acid, decreasing its steady-state serum concentration. Carbamazepine reduces blood levels of benzodiazepines and other medications, including phenothiazines, fentanyl, tetracycline, cyclosporin A, tricyclic antidepressants, coumadin, and oral contraceptives. Because of its effects on contraceptives, administration of carbamazepine can result in unexpected pregnancies in women taking less than the equivalent of 50 μg of ethinyl estradiol per day.

Serum levels of carbamazepine are affected by a number of other medications, the most significant of which are erythro-

Carbamazepine

Oxcarbazepine

Figure 14–10. Structural formula of carbamazepine and oxcarbazepine.

mycin, propoxyphene, cimetidine, isoniazid, and selective serotonin reuptake inhibitor antidepressants. The experimental antiepileptic stiripentol significantly inhibits the clearance of carbamazepine and the 10,11-epoxide, thereby increasing the blood levels of carbamazepine. A similar effect is noted with concurrent use of valproic acid or acetazolamide with carbamazepine. Drugs that induce hepatic microsomal enzymes, such as phenytoin, phenobarbital, primidone, and felbamate, enhance the metabolism of carbamazepine, decreasing its plasma levels 10 to 30%.

Carbamazepine is effective against partial and secondarily generalized seizures and is one of the drugs of choice for these conditions. In a major clinical study comparing various antiepileptics, complete seizure control was achieved by a significantly greater fraction of those individuals taking carbamazepine than was the case with other drugs (Mattson et al., 1985). Although primary generalized tonic-clonic seizures are also reduced by carbamazepine, absence and myoclonic seizures are rarely affected, and carbamazepine is relatively ineffective against febrile seizures (Loiseau and Duché, 1995). Carbamazepine has a formal indication in the United States for use in children 6 years of age and older, although it is used off-label for the treatment of partial seizures in even younger patients.

Carbamazepine therapy must be initiated slowly because of gastrointestinal and central nervous system side effects. A starting dosage of 100 mg three times per day, with increases of 100 to 200 mg every 3 to 7 days is used to attain a target dose of 400 mg three times per day (1200 mg daily). Although doses up to 1600 mg per day or more are sometimes recommended, these higher doses are used by experienced physicians for people with intractable seizures. Sequential increases in the dose of carbamazepine may be required over the first few weeks because of hepatic autoinduction. The drug may be employed as a monotherapy or with other antiepileptic medicatons. Common combinations are carbamazepine and phenytoin, although this often produces unacceptable ataxia, carbamazepine with valproic acid, carbamazepine with gabapentin, carbamazepine with lamotrigine, and occasionally, carbamazepine with phenobarbital.

Although carbamazepine itself is usually associated with few side effects, idiosyncratic, dose-related, and chronic side effects typical of antiepileptics do occur. The most significant idiosyncratic effect of carbamazepine is a hypersensitivity reaction with skin rash. Although the rash is usually maculopapular, erythema multiform, Stevens-Johnson syndrome, and toxic epidermal neurolysis can occur. Lymphadenopathy, a vasculitis-like syndrome, including a lupus picture, and nephritis occur rarely with carbamazepine. Hematologic side effects are significant, with from 5 to 10% of patients given carbamazepine experiencing a decrease in granulocyte count, and white blood cell counts sometimes falling to 2000 to 4000 per mm^3. Moreover, platelet count can also decline with carbamazepine therapy. Such hematologic changes are usually transient over the first weeks of therapy and are responsive to a reduction of carbamazepine dose or the rate of titration. Aplastic anemia, occurring in from 1 in 50,000 to 1 in 200,000 exposures, is a very rare side effect and should not be confused with the more common transient leukopenia.

Acute side effects associated with carbamazepine are primarily gastrointestinal and neurological, including nausea, diarrhea, ataxia, dizziness, diplopia, somnolence, and cognitive impairments, and are minimized by a slow increase in dosage. Diplopia is a characteristic, although not unique, adverse event with carbamazepine. Moreover, carbamazepine has significant anticholinergic effects, including dry mouth, dry eyes, tachycardia, urinary retention, and constipation. Elderly individuals are especially vulnerable to these side effects.

Although elevation of serum liver enzymes is common with carbamazepine, hepatotoxicity is rare. Such toxicity may take the form of a hypersensitivity-induced granulomatous hepatitis with cholestasis, or direct hepatitis and hepatic necrosis without cholestasis. This usually occurs within the first month of therapy. Carbamazepine also enhances the secretion of antidiuretic hormone, resulting in low serum sodium levels.

Blood monitoring is recommended for patients taking carbamazepine. Because of early anecdotal experience with leukopenia, initial recommendations were for frequent monitoring, although less frequent and more individualized blood monitoring is now recommended. A possible regimen might include baseline assessment, measurement at 1 month and 3 months, and then as needed. Serum assays should include complete blood and platelet counts, serum sodium, hepatic enzymes, and total carbamazepine blood levels.

Carbamazepine may produce a subclinical or, rarely, a clinically evident peripheral neuropathy. Chronic alterations of thyroid hormone resulting in chemical or, rarely, clinical hypothyroidism occurs in some patients. When administered chronically, carbamazepine increases free cortisol levels and decreases the level of luteinizing hormones and the free concentrations of sex hormones, which may be responsible for the occasional reports of sexual dysfunction with the drug. Carbamazepine renders low-dose oral contraceptives ineffective and alters the metabolism of vitamin D, although there are only a few reports of clinical osteomalacia. Cardiac conduction can be affected by carbamazepine with either its acute or chronic use. This may take the form of sinus tachycardia because of the anticholinergic effect, bradyarrhythmias, or heart block. Cardiac problems are most likely to occur in elderly patients or those with an underlying cardiac disease.

The extent to which carbamazepine produces cognitive impairment has been a matter of controversy. There is general agreement that carbamazepine is less deleterious in this regard than barbiturates or benzodiazepines. Although early studies suggested that carbamazepine impaired cognitive function less than phenytoin, reevaluation of these results indicated a comparable effect for the two agents. Encephalopathy, delirium, and paranoid psychosis have been noted following either acute or chronic administration of carbamazepine.

Carbamazepine is teratogenic, having been reported to occasionally induce so-called minor malformations consisting of facial or digital distortions. These tend to resolve during the first few years of life. Spinal dysraphism may occur in 1% or less of children born to mothers on carbamazepine. Although administration of folic acid (0.4 to 1 mg) may be of benefit in preventing the teratogenic effects of carbamazepine on the spine, this has not been demonstrated in controlled clinical trials.

Carbamazepine is available in the United States in 100-mg chewable tablets, 200-mg tablets, and a suspension of 100 mg per 5 mL. An extended release form, suitable for twice daily dosing with 100-, 200-, and 400-mg capsule sizes, has recently become available. Other forms of oral carbamazepine must be administered three or four times daily. The recommended initiation schedule is 100 mg three times daily, increased by 100 to 200 mg each day every 3 to 7 days as tolerated, to a target daily dose of 1200 mg in three divided doses. Dosage may be increased to 1600 mg per day or higher in special instances by individuals experienced with the use of this agent. Although a parenteral form of carbamazepine has been developed, it is not yet available for clinical use.

Oxcarbazepine.
Oxcarbazepine is structurally related to carbamazepine (Fig. 14-10). In this case the keto group on the molecule prevents its metabolism to the 10,11-epoxide, which may lessen the incidence of side effects as compared with carbamazepine. Clinical studies have shown that oxcarbazepine was as effective, and better tolerated, in patients having

difficulties with carbamazepine. Although, in general, the adverse effects of oxcarbazepine are similar to carbamazepine, they occur less often. An exception to this is hyponatremia, which may be more common with oxcarbazepine than carbamazepine.

A recent inpatient presurgical study demonstrated that oxcarbazepine prolongs the time to the fourth seizure as compared with placebo. Although oxcarbazepine is available in Europe, it has not yet been approved for use in the United States.

Valproic acid.
Valproic acid, or valproate, is 2-propylpentanoic acid, a fatty acid analogue with a terminal carboxyl group (Fig. 14-11). Valproic acid was discovered by serendipity when it was used as a solvent for dissolving putative antiepileptic agents. When all of the test agents proved effective, which was implausible, the investigators correctly surmised that the active ingredient was the solvent. The first clinical trials were performed in Europe in 1964; the drug was marketed in France in 1967 and released in the United States in 1978. The enteric-coated formulation, sodium divalproex, became available in 1983, and a sprinkle formulation for use in children in 1990. The intravenous form was only recently released in the United States.

Although valproic acid is a broad-spectrum antiepileptic in animal models and in humans, it is a low-potency medication, requiring high-milligram doses for efficacy. It inhibits both maximal electroshock and pentylenetetrazol seizures in laboratory animals, with a therapeutic index of 4 to 8, which is roughly equivalent to phenytoin, carbamazepine, and phenobarbital. Valproic acid is somewhat more effective against pentylenetetrazol than maximal electroshock seizures, predicting its utility in absence epilepsy. It also inhibits chemically induced seizures and is effective against expression of kindled seizures.

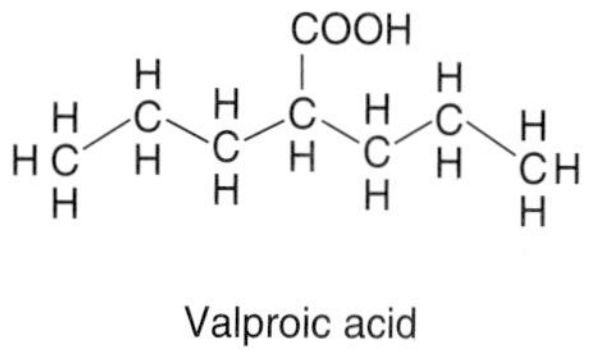

Valproic acid

Figure 14–11. *Structural formula of valproic acid.*

In high doses valproic acid inhibits succinic semialdehyde dehydrogenase, an enzyme involved in the metabolism of GABA. This effect, however, requires concentrations of valproate much higher than those normally achieved in the brain. Variable effects have been found on its ability to potentiate GABA$_A$ receptor-mediated IPSPs, and valproate has an effect similar to phenytoin and carbamazepine in inhibiting rapid, repetitive firing of depolarized neurons, possibly through an interaction with the neuronal sodium channel. An interaction with the low-threshold calcium currents responsible for repetitive firing of thalamic pacemakers may account for some of its efficacy in absence seizures. Other possible actions on calcium currents, and potential blockade of excitatory amino acid transmission, remain under investigation.

Sodium valproate and divalproex are readily absorbed following oral administration, with peak plasma levels occurring 1 to 2 h after ingestion. Although absorption occurs with food, there is a 4- to 5-h delay in the peak. The ease of absorption makes it possible to load valproic acid through a nasogastric tube in critically ill patients. In this case doses of approximately 20 mg/kg are used. Rectal valproic acid, at the same dose, is also well absorbed. After absorption, sodium valproate is 85 to 95% bound to plasma proteins, with only the unbound form penetrating into brain. The serum half-life of valproate is 5 to 16 h, with therapeutic serum levels typically in the 50 to 100 μg/mL range, although patients with severe seizures may require blood levels as high as 150 μg/mL.

Valproic acid is metabolized by glucuronic acid conjugation in the liver, with subsequent excretion in urine. The parent compound is also conjugated with carnitine, glycine, and coenzyme A. A portion of valproic acid undergoes oxidative metabolism in mitochondria with two of the oxidative metabolites, 2-propyl-2-pentenoic acid and 2-propyl-4-pentenoic acid, displaying anticonvulsant activity. The former, also known as 2-N-valproic acid, is thought to be partially responsible for the therapeutic action and toxicity of valproate. Although the efficacy of valproate often persists for a week or two after the parent compound has disappeared from serum, it is unknown whether this is due to accumulated 2-N-valproic acid, tissue binding of valproic acid or its metabolites, or some prolonged physiologic change.

Valproic acid differs from most traditional antiepileptics in being an inhibitor of hepatic microsomal enzymes rather than an inducer, increasing the risk for certain types of drug interactions. Thus, valproate administration increases serum levels of phenobarbital, unbound phenytoin, lamotrigine, and, sometimes, ethosuximide. Because the interaction with phenobarbital is significant, consideration should be given to reducing the dose of the barbiturate by about one third when initiating add-on therapy with valproic acid. At steady state valproate decreases serum levels of carbamazepine and total phenytoin and increases the fraction of carbamazepine metabolized to the 10,11-epoxide. Most other antiepileptic medications increase the hepatic clearance of valproate, reducing its blood levels. Therefore, addition of phenytoin, phenobarbital, primidone, carbamazepine, or felbamate may be accompanied by a decline in the serum level of valproic acid.

Valproic acid is a broad-spectrum antiepileptic, with indications for absence and partial seizures, with or without secondary generalization, and for some myoclonic and atonic seizures. It is the drug of choice in the treatment of generalized seizures associated with juvenile myoclonic epilepsy. Valproic acid may be used as a monotherapy, or as an adjunctive agent, typically with phenytoin or carbamazepine.

Therapy with valproic acid must be initiated gradually, primarily because of gastrointestinal side effects that are severe with large initial doses. Although the recommended initial dose is 15 mg/kg divided into three doses, it is more practical with available dose forms to begin with 125 mg twice or three times per day. Increases are then made by 125- to 250-mg increments every 3 to 7 days, depending on the severity of the seizures and side effects. A target dose for adults is 250 to 500 mg given orally three times per day, or approximately 30 mg/kg per day. The recommended upper limit of dosing is 60 mg/kg per day. Target serum concentrations are 50 to 100 μg/mL, although they may go as high as 150 μg/mL in severely affected patients.

Valproate produces a rash in 1 to 5% of patients, sometimes with accompanying fever and lymphadenopathy. Hepatic toxicity, a more worrisome idiosyncratic effect, typically develops within 3 months of drug initiation. Although an increase in hepatocellular serum enzymes is common, hepatic toxicity is rare. A review of hepatic fatalities associated with valproic acid found an incidence of 1 in 50,000 per year (Dreifuss et al., 1987). Although this incidence is low, patients less than 3 years of age taking multiple drugs have a 1 in 600 risk of developing a fatal hepatic complication. This must be taken into account when using valproate in this age group. In contrast, adults given monotherapy with valproic acid experienced no hepatic fatalities.

Sporadic acute hemorrhagic pancreatitis and pseudocysts have also occurred with valproic acid therapy. Acute, idiosyncratic hematologic effects consist primarily of thrombocytopenia or inhibition of platelet aggregation. Neutropenia and suppression of the bone marrow is a rare side effect of valproic acid.

The primary acute side effects associated with valproic acid administration are gastrointestinal disturbances including nausea, vomiting, epigastric discomfort, and diarrhea. A lower incidence of these side effects is associated with the enteric-coated formulation, as is taking the medication with food. Central nervous system side effects are less prominent than with phenobarbital, phenytoin, or carbamazepine, although some patients experience sedation, ataxia, diplopia, dizziness or, rarely, encephalopathy or hallucinations. Postural tremor is more prominent with valproic acid than with other antiepileptic medications.

The main limiting chronic toxicity is a tendency for weight gain, with weight loss being a less common side effect. The mechanism responsible for weight gain is uncertain; some physicians speculate that decreased beta oxidation of fatty acids and increased appetite may play a role. The chronic use of valproate can also produce peripheral edema and alopecia. Amenorrhea and altered sexual function have been reported by some patients during chronic therapy.

Valproic acid commonly produces hyperammonemia, which need not reflect hepatic dysfunction because valproate inhibits nitrogen metabolism. Carnitine, which assists in transporting fatty acids across mitochondrial membranes, can restore nitrogen balance, although there is no proof that administration of carnitine helps individuals who are not carnitine deficient.

Valproic acid appears to be teratogenic, with reports of neural tube defects first surfacing in 1981. The incidence of a dysrhaphic syndrome is 1 to 2% of children born to mothers taking sodium valproate during the first trimester. Folic acid has been proposed to be effective in reducing this risk. Other minor malformations of face and digits also occur in a small percentage of offspring.

In the United States valproic acid is available in 125-, 250-, and 500-mg tablets as divalproex sodium, various sizes with nonenteric-coated valproic acid, valproic acid syrup containing the equivalent of 250 mg of valproic acid per 5 mL as the sodium salt, and a recently released parenteral form. The parenteral form is administered by infusion at 20 mg per min, in a dosage equivalent to the desired oral dose.

Ethosuximide. Ethosuximide, which is chemically related to phenytoin, is a drug of choice for absence (petit mal) seizures (Fig. 14-12).

Ethosuximide is effective against pentylenetetrazol, but not maximal electroshock or amygdala kindled seizures, in laboratory animals. It is relatively ineffective in blocking seizures induced by bicuculline, N-methyl-D-aspartic acid, strychnine, or allylglycine.

The spectrum of action of ethosuximide is narrower than for most antiepileptics, with effectiveness against absence seizures and, to a lesser extent, myoclonic or atonic seizures, but little efficacy against other forms of epilepsy. This selectively suggests that ethosuximide may have a predominant effect on the thalamocortical regulatory system that underlies generation of rhythmic spike waves. The neurons of the thalamic system have a special type of calcium channel, the low-threshold (T-type) calcium channel, that causes neurons to fire when the membrane potential shifts from a hyperpolarized to a relatively depolarized state. Ethosuximide partially blocks this low-threshold calcium ion current and may therefore have an inhibitory effect on thalamocortically generated spike waves.

Although many mechanisms of action have been proposed for the antiabsence action of ethosuximide, none have been proved. Thus, ethosuximide may inhibit the synthesis of γ-hydroxybutyrate in brain and sodium-potassium-ATP activity in plasma membranes, although these effects are observed only at concentrations greater than those normally found in brain. Modifications of GABA, glutamate, or dopamine synaptic transmission do not appear sufficient to explain the actions of ethosuximide.

Ethosuximide is a water-soluble substance that is readily absorbed after oral administration. Peak plasma concentrations are attained 1 to 4 h after administration, with the syrup providing slightly

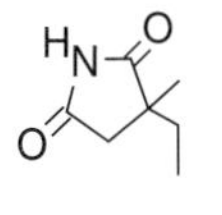

Ethosuximide

Figure 14–12. *Structural formula of ethosuximide.*

faster absorption than the capsule. Ethosuximide distributes in a space equivalent to total body water, with less than 10% of the drug bound to serum proteins. It readily crosses the blood-brain barrier, with the concentration in CSF being similar to that in serum. In children, ethosuximide has a serum half-life of 30 to 40 h, and in adults 40 to 60 h. About 20% of ethosuximide is excreted unchanged in the urine; the remainder is metabolized, mainly by oxidative metabolism. Four metabolites, formed by the hepatic CYP3A enzyme system, have been identified, all of which are thought to be pharmacologically inactive. Drug interactions with ethosuximide are fewer than with some other antiepileptics because it is not bound to a significant extent to plasma proteins. Variable interactions have been reported between ethosuximide and phenytoin, phenobarbital, carbamazepine, and valproic acid, but with few consistent or clinically important patterns. The product package insert notes the possibility of increased phenytoin serum levels with concurrent ethosuximide.

Ethosuximide is indicated for the treatment of absence seizures. Although no formal age range is provided for this indication, such seizures typically occur in young children. Previously ethosuximide was used in patients with mixtures of absence and tonic-clonic seizures, usually together with phenytoin. This combination has been replaced by monotherapy with valproic acid. Because of potential hepatotoxicity in young children with valproate, and its relatively higher cost, ethosuximide remains a drug of choice for isolated absence epilepsy. Valproic acid is the drug of choice for mixed absence seizure types, or atypical absence.

For patients 3 to 6 years old, the typical starting dose of ethosuximide is 250 mg per day as a single dose, given as a capsule or in a syrup. Doses can be increased at a rate of 250 to 500 mg every 3 to 7 days to the usual maintenance dose of 20 mg/kg. Serum concentrations in the range of 40 to 100 μg/mL are sought, although refractory patients may require levels up to 150 μg/mL. This range is conveniently similar to that reported for valproic acid. Because of its long serum half-life, ethosuximide can be administered once per day. It is prudent, however, to administer the drug in two to four divided doses if side effects, such as nausea and vomiting, limit

single daily dosing. Multiple daily dosing can be useful for initiation of therapy, to minimize side effects. The most common dose-related side effect of ethosuximide is gastrointestinal discomfort, with the medication occasionally producing anorexia and weight loss, sleepiness, dizziness, irritability, ataxia, fatigue, and hiccups. A few children experience psychiatric side effects with behavioral changes, aggression, and, rarely, hallucinations, delusions, or severe depression. Only a few studies have been performed to measure the effect of ethosuximide on cognition, which is believed to be much less than that of the barbiturates.

Idiosyncratic side effects associated with ethosuximide administration include skin rash, erythema multiforme, and Stevens-Johnson syndrome. A lupus-like reaction has rarely been described, as with other seizure medications. Among the most worrisome, but rare, side effects of ethosuximide are blood dyscrasias, including bone marrow suppression, aplastic anemia, and thrombocytopenia. Because of this possibility, periodic laboratory assessment of the blood count is recommended. A decrease in granulocyte count more likely reflects a dose- or time-related reduction than an ethosuximide-induced aplastic anemia, but monitoring is warranted under this condition.

Side effects associated with the chronic use of ethosuximide are fewer than with other antiepileptics. There have been occasional reports of thyroiditis, immune renal disease, suppression of serum corticosteroid levels, and movement disorders. Ethosuximide has also been reported to worsen seizures in some patients. Although this may occur with atypical absence seizures, including emergence of new generalized tonic-clonic seizures, the exacerbation is more likely with myoclonic or partial seizures.

Ethosuximide has the potential to cause teratogenic effects because of its lack of protein binding and its hydrophilicity, which enhance its penetration into placenta and breast milk. Although hard evidence is lacking for ethosuximide-induced teratogenesis in isolation from other medications and causes, this drug should be used during pregnancy only when the benefits clearly outweigh the risk.

Ethosuximide should be withdrawn gradually to avoid exacerbation of absence seizures or precipitation of absence status epilepticus.

In the United States, ethosuximide is supplied as 250-mg capsules and as a syrup containing 250 mg per 5 mL. The initial dosage is 250 mg per day for a child 3 to 6 years old, or 500 mg per day for individuals over 6 years of age. The daily dosage is increased by 250 mg every 3 to 7 days to clinical effect, toxicity, or a maximum of 1.5 g per day. Although the dosage is usually initiated in two or three divided doses, it can be given in a single daily dose if tolerated. The optimal dose is usually in the range of 20 mg/kg per day.

Other succinimides. In addition to ethosuximide, two other succinimides are available for clinical use, methsuximide and phensuximide. Ethosuximide is somewhat more effective than the others against pentylenetetrazol seizures in laboratory animals and is more effective against absence seizures in humans. In contrast, methsuximide is the most effective of the succinimides against maximal electroshock seizures in laboratory animals. This accounts for its use as a second-line drug in the treatment of partial seizures.

Methsuximide is well absorbed after oral administration, attaining its peak concentration in plasma 1 to 4 h later. The drug is rapidly metabolized in the liver and excreted in urine. An active metabolite, N-desmethylmethsuximide, has a half-life of 40 to 80 h. Several other metabolites may also have some clinical effects. The mechanism of action of methsuximide is believed to be similar to ethosuximide.

Methsuximide is indicated for the treatment of absence seizures and is used as a second- or third-line drug in this setting. Methsuximide may also be used for the treatment of refractory complex partial seizures. The usual initial dose of methsuximide is 300 mg per day, increased by 150 or 300 mg every 1 to 2 weeks to a maximum 1200 mg per day or until a clinical effect or toxicity is encountered at a lower dose. The serum concentration of methsuximide is almost too low to measure, but the target serum concentration of N-desmethylmethsuximide is about 10 to 50 μg/mL. Methsuximide increases serum levels of concurrently administered phenytoin and phenobarbital and increases the conversion of carbamazepine to the 10,11-epoxide.

Side effects associated with methsuximide are relatively common, consisting of drowsiness, dizziness, ataxia, gastrointestinal upset, reduction in blood counts, skin rash including serious rashes, and presumably, all of the side effects associated with ethosuximide.

Phensuximide is indicated for control of absence seizures, but may occasionally be used as a second- or third-line agent in other seizure types. The capsules are supplied in dosages of 500 mg, with the starting dose typically being 500 mg per day, increased every 3 to 7 days to a maximum in adults of 3 g per day in three divided doses. Adverse reactions are similar to those described for ethosuximide and methsuximide.

Felbamate. Felbamate, 2-phenyl-1,3-propanediol dicarbamate, was the first major new antiepileptic introduced in the United States since the approval of valproic acid in 1978 (Fig. 14-13). Although it was initially a very popular medication, postmarketing surveillance during the first year after its approval indicated several cases of aplastic anemia and hepatotoxicity associated with its use, diminishing enthusiasm for this drug. Nevertheless, marketing continued with requirements for strict warnings and informed consent. Since then, the drug has experienced a minor resurgence in popularity.

Felbamate was developed as an analog of meprobamate, a tranquilizer used before the introduction of the benzodiazepines. Felbamate is active against maximal electroshock seizures in mice and rats, and against pentylenetetrazol-induced convulsions, although at a lower potency. Felbamate also blocks seizures caused by a variety of other convulsants, inhibits amygdala kindling, and reduces focal motor seizures in monkeys produced by applying aluminum hydroxide on the cerebral cortex. Felbamate was remarkably safe in animal toxicology studies, leading to a false sense of security about its tolerability in patients.

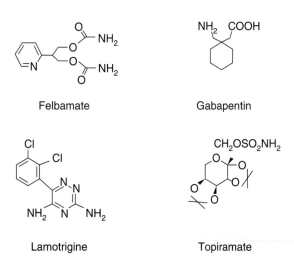

Felbamate   Gabapentin

Lamotrigine   Topiramate

Figure 14–13. *Structural formula of the four newly released antiseizure medications.*

Felbamate interacts with the neuronal sodium channel and receptors for excitatory amino acids. The sodium channel effect is similar to that of carbamazepine and phenytoin, with blockade of sustained repetitive firing of neurons, presumably because the drug prolongs the inactive state of the channel. Felbamate also appears to block the glycine binding site, which regulates the activity of the NMDA subclass of glutamic acid receptor in brain. Felbamate also may directly block the quisqualate subtype of the glutamate receptor system. These actions suggest felbamate may be neuroprotective as well as an anticonvulsant.

Felbamate is well absorbed after oral administration, despite its limited aqueous solubility. Its lipophilicity enables it to readily penetrate the blood-brain barrier, with CSF levels approximating those in serum. Approximately 25% of the total drug is bound to serum proteins, with the serum half-life ranging from 1 to 22 h. Although it does not appear to induce enzymes responsible for its own metabolism, the terminal elimination half-life decreases from 20 h to about 14 h in the presence of drugs that induce microsomal enzymes. The apparent volume of distribution for felbamate is about 0.8 L/kg. Although serum levels of felbamate have not been well established in relation to efficacy, clinical trials suggest they are in the range of 40 to 80 μg/mL.

Felbamate undergoes first-order metabolism by the hepatic cytochrome P450 system. It induces the hepatic microsomal enzyme system, enhancing the metabolism of other drugs that are substrates for the same enzymes. Metabolites of felbamate include the monocarbamate and conjugated felbamate, and other less abundant substances. Approximately 50% of the absorbed dose of felbamate is excreted unchanged in the urine.

Felbamate is responsible for very significant drug interactions. In general, it increases by 20 to 50% the serum levels of other antiepileptics, particularly phenytoin, valproic acid, and barbiturates. With carbamazepine, the levels of the parent compound are decreased, although the concentration of the 10,11-epoxide is usually increased by felbamate. Some of these interactions occur at the level of the enzyme epoxide hydrolase, which is involved in the metabolism of the carbamazepine 10,11-epoxide and phe-

nytoin. Conversely, phenytoin and carbamazepine increase the metabolism of felbamate, resulting in a 15 to 30% decrease in blood levels. Circulating concentrations of some other medications are also influenced by felbamate, particularly if they compete for the same microsomal enzymes. Of particular note is the fact that felbamate slows the metabolism of coumadin, increasing the response to a given dose of the anticoagulant.

Felbamate has been studied primarily as a treatment for partial seizures, with and without secondary generalization. It was the first antiepileptic to use the presurgical trial design, in which it was administered to patients alone at the end of a presurgical monitoring (Bourgeois et al., 1993). A responder rate of 40 to 45% with partial seizures was recorded. Felbamate was also shown to be effective against partial seizures in an outpatient study in comparison with valproic acid, and against seizures associated with Lennox-Gastaut syndrome. This latter trial was of particular importance because these seizures, including tonic, atonic, and others, were previously resistant to medication. Small-scale clinical trials suggest that felbamate might also be useful in absence and juvenile myoclonic epilepsy, rendering it a broad-spectrum antiepileptic.

Felbamate is available in 400-mg and 600-mg scored tablets. The medication should be initiated only after consideration of alternatives given its potential for serious toxicity. A typical starting dosage, depending on the urgency of the treatment, is 300 to 600 mg twice daily. The dosage may be increased in 300-mg to 600-mg increments every 1 to 2 weeks to a target dose of 3600 mg daily in three divided doses. Lower doses may suffice in some patients, and others may benefit from doses as high as 4800 mg per day or to individual tolerability. Children are started at 15 mg/kg per day, increased weekly by 30 to 45 mg/kg per day, to a maximum of 3000 mg per day. Administration with meals reduces gastrointestinal side effects. Regular hematologic and hepatic monitoring is warranted for patients given felbamate.

In toxicity studies in rats, the lethal dose of felbamate could not be determined because massive quantities could be administered without serious incident. Nevertheless, the drug can cause serious side effects in patients. Dose-related side effects include gastrointestinal upset, weight loss, headaches, insomnia, and behavioral changes in children. Felbamate appears to have fewer deleterious effects on cognition and overall energy levels than other antiepileptic medications, and may in fact have a positive effect on learning and memory. Whereas weight loss is welcome for some patients, it is unwelcome for others, and insomnia often requires the drug be taken no later than dinner time. Nausea necessitates concomitant administration of felbamate with food or sulcrafate, and headache is treated with common analgesics. The incidence of adverse events with felbamate is much higher when the drug is used as an add-on than as monotherapy, reflecting the potential for significant drug interactions.

Approximately 1500 patients were involved in clinical trials with felbamate before its release, including 366 in two monotherapy studies. The mean exposure time to felbamate in these trials was approximately 1 year per patient. In the clinical trials, 12% of patients withdrew because of adverse events. Moreover, there were no significant changes in hematologic or hepatic parameters with felbamate, except for a few cases of transient leukopenia, thrombocytopenia, or anemia, and there were no cases of aplastic anemia in the clinical trials. To date, however, a total of 31 cases of aplastic anemia have been associated with felbamate use, all in 1994. For the period 1995 to 1997 the manufacturer was not informed of any additional cases. The mean time for diagnosis of aplastic anemia following initiation of felbamate therapy was 6 months, with a range of 2.5 to 12 months. The majority of these 31 cases had preexisting immunologic problems, other serious underlying illnesses, or previous episodes of hematologic changes with antiepileptic medications. Nevertheless, no specific predictive factor for aplastic anemia has been identified. Of the 31 reported cases, 8 died from the condition.

Fourteen patients were reported to have developed severe hepatotoxicity after treatment with felbamate for 0.5 to 10 months. Although most of these individuals were taking several medications at once, a few were receiving felbamate alone.

The risk for aplastic anemia and hepatic injury vastly curtailed the use of felbamate and nearly caused its withdrawal from the market. Patients and advocacy groups argued that felbamate was the only effective or tolerated medication for some people, and therefore should be available. Because of the risks, patients are required to sign a consent form before using felbamate. The manufacturer suggests monitoring of complete blood counts and hepatic screening every 1 to 2 weeks while taking felbamate, although this is impractical for most patients. There is a sense that the risk for complications lessens after 1 year of treatment, and therefore perhaps the need for monitoring declines after this time. Furthermore, there is no evidence that hematologic monitoring will reduce the incidence of aplastic anemia or hepatotoxicity. Thus, clinicians and patients should tailor a monitoring program that meets their needs. The patient and his or her family must be warned to watch for unusual infections, bruising, bleeding, pallor, or jaundice.

Felbamate is supplied in 400-mg and 600-mg scored tablets and an oral suspension containing 600 mg per 5 mL.

Gabapentin. Gabapentin, 1-aminomethyl-cyclohexaneacetic acid, was introduced in the United States in late 1993 (Fig. 14-13). A GABA analogue, the cyclohexane ring structure is designed to aid penetration into brain. Gabapentin is used as add-on therapy for partial and secondarily generalized seizures and, anecdotally, for a variety of other nonepileptic conditions such as pain and bipolar illness.

Although designed as a GABA analog, gabapentin has a very low affinity for GABA receptors and the enzymes responsible for the synthesis or degradation of this neurotransmitter. It also has a minimal effect on inhibitory postsynaptic potentials mediated by GABA. Rather, it is believed gabapentin may increase intracellular concentrations of GABA by influencing an amino acid transport system. This system, which transports large, neutral amino acids such as L-phenylalanine and leucine, is found on neuronal and glial membranes. The manner in which gabapentin interacts with the transporter in intestines and brain remains under study. Brain membrane binding sites for radiolabeled gabapentin are distinct from those for the usual neurotransmitters and neuromodulators, with the highest binding in superficial layers of the neocortex, in the dendritic regions of the hippocampus and the molecular layer of the cerebellum (Hill et al., 1993). The peak anticonvulsant action in animal models is delayed for several hours after intravenous administration of gabapentin, suggesting it is converted to another molecule or there is a need for time for it to accumulate in a critical cellular compartment. Although gabapentin has some effects on neuronal sodium channels, monoamine release, and calcium ion channels in brain, these are not likely to be responsible for its actions. It has been speculated that gabapentin may interact with Krebs cycle amino acids, influencing the amount of glutamate available for neuronal release. It has also been suggested that gabapentin may be a neuroprotectant under some circumstances (Rothstein et al., 1993).

In animal models, gabapentin blocks maximal electroshock seizures with a potency similar to phenytoin. Although it is mildly effective against pentylenetetrazol seizures, it is ineffective in rat models of absence seizures, and in the myoclonic seizure model in photosensitive baboons. Gabapentin increases seizure threshold and decreases mortality associated with N-methyl-D-aspartic acid administration in rodents. Kindled limbic seizures in rodents are also attenuated by gabapentin. This profile suggests gabapentin is likely to be useful against partial and secondarily generalized seizures.

Although the absorption of gabapentin increases with increasing doses, its fractional absorption declines. This nonlinearity is thought to result from saturation of the system L transport mechanism in the gastrointestinal tract that is responsible for the absorption of the drug. Thus, doses above about 4800 mg per day produce only small increases in the serum levels of the drug. Gabapentin is not bound significantly to plasma proteins and is cleared virtually unchanged in the urine and feces. Because gabapentin is not metabolized, it does not induce or inhibit hepatic microsomal enzymes. These characteristics suggest a low potential for drug interactions, which is borne out by pharmacokinetic studies and clinical experience. Other antiepileptic medications do not substantially affect gabapentin blood levels and vice versa. Although concurrent administration of antacids reduces the absorption of gabapentin by about 20%, and there is a 10% increase in gabapentin levels when it is given with cimetidine, these interactions are not usually clinically significant. Gabapentin does not alter the metabolism of estrogens, suggesting it is unlikely to interfere with the action of contraceptives.

The elimination half-life of gabapentin ranges from 5 to 8 h, requiring it be administered three or four times per day. Serum levels of gabapentin have not yet been precisely correlated with clinical efficacy, although they are thought to be in the range of 2 to 4 μg/mL. In some cases the range may be as much as 2 to 10 μg/mL, or to individual tolerability.

There have been five controlled efficacy studies with gabapentin, with daily doses ranging from 600 to 1800 mg, and several long-term safety follow-up studies. The responder rates (percentage of patients experiencing 50% or better reduction in seizures as compared with baseline) were 20 to 30% when gabapentin was used as an add-on therapy in those with refractory seizures. Subsequent clinical experience, yet to be

documented by controlled trials, suggests that daily doses of 2400 to 4800 mg may be associated with a higher responder rate while preserving the favorable therapeutic ratio. Small-scale clinical trials have failed to demonstrate any efficacy for gabapentin in the treatment of absence, myoclonic, or atonic seizures. Although the drug is not approved for monotherapy in the United States, two monotherapy trials have been completed. One was an inpatient trial with rapid titration to 3600 mg per day using a presurgical monitoring design. In comparison with placebo, gabapentin in monotherapy was effective against partial and secondarily generalized seizures. An outpatient monotherapy study, however, failed to show significant efficacy. This is believed due to a flaw in the trial design whereby a significant fraction of patients had increased seizures when tapered from carbamazepine, contaminating the seizure counts in the gabapentin portion of the trial.

Gabapentin is available in 100-, 300-, and 400-mg doses. There is no liquid form for oral or parenteral use, nor sprinkle form for pediatrics. The manufacturer recommends initiation of gabapentin treatment with 300 mg once on the first day, twice on the second day, and three times each day thereafter. More rapid titration, for example, initiation at a dose of 300 mg three times per day is usually well tolerated. Dosage can be increased by 300 mg every 3 to 7 days as tolerated to clinical effect, or to 1800 mg per day. Clinical experience suggests that 3600 mg per day or more may be beneficial in some patients. Although serum levels are not helpful in managing patients given gabapentin, they may be used to validate compliance or for other clinical indications. The range of therapeutic serum levels varies from 2 to 10 μg/mL. The addition of gabapentin does not, in general, require the adjustment of dosage of other antiepileptic medications, although this should be individualized. Occasional pharmacodynamic interactions, for example, increased dizziness in conjunction with carbamazepine or increased somnolence with most other antiseizure medicines, may occur when gabapentin is added, even though serum levels of the medications do not change. Frequent hematologic monitoring is not necessary for gabapentin, although some physicians prefer to conduct occasional blood monitoring of the CBC and liver enzymes after initiating gabapentin therapy.

Animal toxicology studies showed that gabapentin is well tolerated in rodents in acute doses up to 8 g/kg, and in monkeys up to 1.25 m/kg. Although male Wistar rats evidenced pancreatic acinar cell tumors, which variably were considered to be hyperplasia or low-grade malignancies, these tumors did not affect mortality, and it appears they are species specific. No evidence of increased pancreatic cancer has been reported in patients taking gabapentin.

Dose-related side effects include somnolence, ataxia, dizziness, and fatigue, and there are occasional gastrointestinal disturbances associated with this drug. The rate of withdrawal from double-blind clinical trials was only slightly higher ($<5\%$) for the gabapentin group as compared with the placebo group, indicating excellent tolerability.

To date, there have been over 450,000 patient-years of exposure to gabapentin. Although there have been occasional reports of idiosyncratic side effects, including rash and depression of blood counts, serious allergic reactions are extremely rare. The level of safety of this drug in pregnancy is unknown. Overall, the tolerability and safety of gabapentin appears to be unusually favorable in comparison with other antiepileptic medications.

Lamotrigine. Lamotrigine, 3,5-diamino-6-2,3-dichlorophenyl-1,2,4-triazine, is another of the more recently developed antiepileptic medications (Fig. 14-13). Initially it was designed as an inhibitor of folic acid synthesis, although this is no longer believed to be its primary mechanism of action.

Lamotrigine inhibits maximal electroshock and kindled and photosensitive seizures in laboratory animals. It is efficacious, but weak, in inhibiting pentylenetetrazol-induced convulsions.

Lamotrigine blocks the sustained rapid firing of neurons in a manner similar to phenytoin and carbamazepine. This is thought to be due to an interaction with a voltage-dependent neuronal sodium ion channel, prolonging the refractory period of the cell. Lamotrigine also inhibits the release of glutamate, an excitatory amino acid neurotransmitter, which may also suggest it possesses neuroprotective properties. It does not appear to affect chloride ion currents, or GABA, dopaminergic, noradrenergic, muscarinic, or adenosine systems in brain.

Lamotrigine is well absorbed when taken orally, with or without food, with almost complete bioavailability. Peak concentrations in serum appear 2 to 3 h after administration. Plasma protein binding for lamotrigine is approximately 55%, with a volume of distribution of 0.9 to 1.3 L/kg. Lamotrigine is metabolized in the liver, mainly by conjugation with glucuronic acid, with the primary metabolite being the 2-N-glucuronic acid conjugate that is excreted in urine. The elimination of lamotrigine is linear with dose, indicating first-order kinetics.

Although lamotrigine has only minor effects on the blood levels of other antiepileptics, drugs that enhance or inhibit hepatic enzyme activity have substantial effects on its metabolism. Thus, although in monotherapy lamotrigine has a terminal serum half-life of approximately 24 h, when taken with hepatic enzyme inducers such as phenytoin, carbamazepine, or phenobarbital, its half-life is only 12 h. In contrast, valproic acid, an inhibitor of the hepatic microsomal enzyme system, prolongs the half-life of lamotrigine to approximately 60 h. The dosing frequency of lamotrigine, therefore, depends on the context of its use. Although lamotrigine induces its own metabolism, it is unclear whether this has any clinical significance.

Lamotrigine was introduced in the United States in 1994, although it had already been in use in other countries for many years. Definitive clinical trials in the United States examined its effect as an add-on therapy for partial and secondarily generalized seizures. In three major studies there was at least a 50% reduction in seizures compared with baseline in 20 to 30% of subjects, with a mean seizure reduction of 25 to 35% for dosages of 300 to 500 mg per day. Several recent clinical trials suggest lamotrigine may be useful in monotherapy. Small-scale clinical studies and clinical experience support its use for treating a wide variety of seizures, including absence, myoclonic, atonic, and mixed, in addition to its documented efficacy against partial and secondarily generalized seizures. A clinical study has also shown that lamotrigine is of benefit in seizures associated with Lennox-Gastaut syndrome, and there are ongoing studies to determine its efficacy against infantile spasms. Although indicated for partial and secondarily generalized seizures, some physicians find lamotrigine of greatest value as an alternative for treating intractable primarily generalized seizures. There are also anecdotal reports of its usefulness in treating nonepileptic disorders, including chronic pain, bipolar depression, movement disorders, and neurodegenerative conditions. Formal documentation of its efficacy and safety in these cases, however, is lacking.

Lamotrigine is available in the United States in 25-, 100-, 150-, and 200-mg scored tablets. When used as monotherapy, the target dose of lamotrigine is 300 to 500 mg daily. In conjunction with valproic acid, which may double the serum levels of lamotrigine, the dosage should be kept at the lower end of this range. Nevertheless, there is as yet no definite upper dosage range for lamotrigine. Some have used more than 1 g per day, or even more, in certain cases. Although serum levels of lamotrigine correlate poorly with clinical efficacy or toxicity, experience suggests these should be in the 2 to 10 μg/mL (some say 2 to 20 μg/mL) range.

Initiation of treatment with lamotrigine must be slow because of a risk for rash. The manufacturer recommends beginning treatment in patients over 16 years of age with 50 mg each day for 2 weeks, followed by 50 mg twice per day for 2 weeks, and then rapid titration to the target dose. If the titration rate is too fast it may provoke a rash. A slower titration regimen begins with 25 mg per day for 1 week, increased by 25 mg every week to 100- or 200-mg per day, followed by a switch to 100-mg tablets and more rapid titration to the desired clinical effect. If a patient is also taking valproic acid, a titration rate for lamotrigine as slow as 25 mg per day, with increases every other week, may be required. Typically, other antiepileptic medications are continued during the titration with lamotrigine until a nearly therapeutic dose, in the range of 200 to 300 mg per day, is achieved, whereupon the dose of the other drugs may be adjusted or tapered. In monotherapy, or with valproic acid, lamotrigine may be given in a single daily dose. Typically, lamotrigine is usually given twice per day in divided doses when used in conjunction with phenytoin, phenobarbital, carbamazepine, felbamate, or other agents known to induce hepatic microsomal enzymes.

The primary adverse reaction to lamotrigine is rash. The rash can take the form of a simple morbilliform or maculopapular rash, or extend in seriousness to erythema multiforme, Stevens-Johnson syndrome, or toxic epidermal neurolysis. In controlled clinical trials the incidence of rash in adults was approximately 10%, versus 5% in the placebo group. Notably, this incidence is similar to that reported in some trials with carbamazepine or phenytoin. Recently, a warning was issued about the possibility of serious rash in the pediatric population because children may be more susceptible to the effect of lamotrigine, with cases of Stevens-Johnson syndrome or toxic epidermal neurolysis having been reported. In some small-scale clinical trials the incidence of serious rash has been as high as 1 in 40 children or, with pooled results, 1 in 200. Therefore, it is important to obtain informed consent for the use of this medication in patients under 16 years of age and provide warnings about the possibility of rash. The risk for rash appears to be higher when the drug is used concurrently with valproic acid. In adults, the rash occurs as a function of the rate of dose escalation and sometimes disappears with reduction in dosage and reinitiation with a slower titration.

The primary dose-related toxicity of lamotrigine is neurological, with ataxia, blurred vision, dizziness, confusion, and fatigue being most common. Nausea and vomiting are occasionally reported. In add-on clinical trials, 10% of individuals who withdrew were given lamotrigine, as compared with 8% given placebo. In monotherapy studies in Europe, the drug was well tolerated, except for rash. Hematologic or hepatotoxicity are rare with lamotrigine, although isolated cases have been reported. Other side effects, although rare, include delirium, delusions, choreoathetosis, changes in libido or sexual function, and paradoxic worsening of seizures. In toxicology tests, lamotrigine caused cardiac arrhythmias in dogs, which is attributed to the N-2 methyl conjugate, which does not exist in humans. Although there have been scattered reports of cardiac arrhythmias in patients, the incidence is not high.

Lamotrigine is available in 25-, 100-, 150-, and 200-mg scored tablets. No liquid or parenteral dosage form is available in the United States. Although lamotrigine does not have a formal indication in the United States for children under 16 years of age, it does have pediatric indications in other countries. A child receiving a hepatic enzyme inducer without valproic acid should be administered a starting dose of lamotrigine of 2 mg/kg per day for 2 weeks, followed by 5 mg/kg per day for 2 weeks, advancing to a maintenance dose of 5 to 15 mg/kg per day. For monotherapy the recommended dose is 0.5 mg/kg initially for 2 weeks, followed by 1 mg/kg per day for 2 weeks, advancing to 2 to 10 mg/kg per day. Initiation at about half this dose is recommended when the drug is used in combination with valproic acid in children. These recommendations may require revision in light of the serious rashes recently reported in pediatric trials.

Topiramate. *Topiramate,* 2,3:4,5-bis-O-(1-methylethylidene)-beta-D-fructopyranose sulfamate, has a novel chemical structure in comparison with other antiepileptics (Fig. 14-13). It was developed by the R. W. Johnson Pharmaceutical Research Institute in collaboration with the Epilepsy Branch of the National Institutes of Health. Topiramate is useful for partial and secondarily generalized seizures and, potentially, a wide range of other seizure types. Its use may be limited in some instances by its effects on cognition.

Topiramate is active against maximal electroshock seizures in rodents and, to a lesser extent, convulsions induced by pentylenetetrazol, bicuculline, or picrotoxin. Although topiramate inhibits carbonic anhydrase, this probably does not contribute significantly to its mechanism of action as an antiepileptic. Of greater importance are its ability to increase GABA-mediated influx of chloride ions and its inhibition of subtypes of excitatory amino acid receptors in brain.

Topiramate is well absorbed after oral administration, with or without food, with peak serum levels 2 to 4 h after ingestion, approximately 15% is bound to serum proteins. Although a small amount of topiramate is metabolized in the liver, over 80% is excreted unchanged in the urine. Because its half-life ranges from 18 to 24 h, twice daily dosing is necessary. The clinically relevant serum levels of the medication are not yet established. Both phenytoin and carbamazepine increase clearance, and thereby lower plasma levels, of topiramate. In turn, topiramate increases circulating levels of phenytoin and carbamazepine as much as 20% and reduces estrogen blood levels.

Topiramate has been most studied as a treatment for partial and secondarily generalized seizures. Three multicenter, double-blind, dose-ranging, controlled add-on trials have been executed with doses of topiramate ranging from 200 to 1000 mg per day. In other trials, doses as high as 1600 mg per day have been examined. Results suggest that the efficacy of topiramate increases little above a dose of 400 mg per day (Tassinari et al., 1996), unlike gabapentin and lamotrigine which were tested clinically at doses lower than those believed to be optimal in general practice. Doses of topiramate greater than 400 mg are associated with significant adverse events, such as confusion and slowed speech, without improving efficacy. There are, of course, exceptions to this rule.

Small-scale clinical trials and anecdotal clinical experience suggest that topiramate is a broad-spectrum antiepileptic with possible efficacy in absence, atonic, myoclonic, and tonic seizures. Definitive proof of effectiveness in these conditions awaits controlled clinical trials.

The manufacturer recommends that topiramate be started at 50 mg twice per day. Many physicians believe, however, that this rate is too fast, with a high likelihood of cognitive impairment. Initial doses of 25 mg per day, followed by increases every 1 to 2 weeks of 25 mg, have been advocated. For some adults the target dose may be as low as 100 mg per day, although the recommended final target dose is 200 to 400 mg per day, in two divided doses. Under these circumstances, approximately 40 to 50% of patients with intractable seizures experience at least a 50% reduction in events as compared with baseline. Although topiramate is expected to be effective in monotherapy, clinical trials examining this issue are not yet completed.

Adverse events associated with topiramate are related primarily to the central nervous system, including confusion, somnolence, ataxia, dizziness, and headaches. The incidence of side effects is believed to be higher with multiple drug therapy and with rapid titration of dose. The incidence of cognitive problems with topiramate approaches 30% and consists of slower thinking, increased forgetfulness, slowed speech, poor speech comprehension, disorientation, and other complaints. These effects may improve over time or with a reduction in dose.

There are occasional reports of gastrointestinal upset, rash, renal stones, and serious psychiatric problems associated with topiramate use. Topiramate has not been established as safe during pregnancy and, indeed, has been shown to cause some fetal malformations in laboratory animals.

Topiramate is marketed in the United States in 25-mg and 100-mg tablets. No liquid or injectable form is available in this country.

Benzodiazepines. Benzodiazepines most commonly used in the treatment of seizures are diazepam, clonazepam, lorazepam, and clorazepate. These medicines are effective as fast-acting antiepileptics that do not require a loading dose. Therefore, injectable forms, such as intravenous diazepam or lorazepam, are drugs of choice for treating status epilepticus. Benzodiazepines are not useful as chronic medications because their effectiveness wanes after a few weeks and doses must often be increased to maintain the desired effect. Chronic use of the benzodiazepines is sometimes attempted for the treatment of atonic, myoclonic, or completely intractable seizures, where few alternatives exist. When taken for a day or two, benzodiazepines can be useful as booster therapy for clusters of seizures. This approach is used when patients know one seizure is likely to lead to another, or during the menstrual period. A typical antiepileptic dose of diazepam is 2 to 5 mg every 4 to 6 h. Clonazepam is usually given as 0.5 to 2.0 mg orally three times per day. Lorazepam may be administered in 0.5- to 1.0-mg boosters, repeated as needed to terminate seizures, up to a dose of about 4 mg per day.

Tiagabine. Tiagabine was recently approved in the United States for partial and secondarily generalized seizures, and will probably have a profile similar to phenytoin, carbamazepine, and gabapentin. This drug is not likely to be effective against absence or myoclonic seizures. The responder rate for tiagabine ranges from 20 to 30% among select populations of patients with resistant seizures. The drug is well tolerated, with only a few reports of sedation, abnormal thinking, and dizziness. There have been some reports of worsening of seizures with tiagabine, and a few serious psychiatric complications, but it is unclear whether these are attributable to the medication or simply reflect the background incidence of these conditions in severe epilepsy. Because of its short half-life, tiagabine will likely be administered three or four times per day.

VIGABATRIN

Although vigabatrin is marketed in many countries, it has not yet been approved in the United States. Vigabatrin appears to be most effective against partial and secondarily generalized seizures, although it also has displayed efficacy in certain pediatric syndromes such as infantile spasms, which are difficult to control with other medications. Vigabatrin appears to be efficacious as an add-on in intractable partial seizures, with responder rates approximating 40 to 50%. Overall, it appears to be better tolerated than more established medications.

Although side effects of vigabatrin include dizziness, unsteadiness, sleepiness, and thinking or memory impairments, thought processes appear to be less influenced than with many older drugs. A small percentage of patients develop depression or other serious psychiatric problems while taking vigabatrin, which resolve when the medication is discontinued. Some patients on vigabatrin develop abnormal visual fields. Approval of vigabatrin has been delayed in the United States because of animal toxicology studies indicating it causes edema of brain myelin. Although this occurs at high doses in rodents and dogs, and possibly monkeys, it has so far not been noted in humans. The effect is reversible and is detectable by MRI or evoked potential analysis. No pattern of myelin problems has emerged after about 200,000 patient-years of usage. A typical adult dose of vigabatrin is 2000 to 3000 mg per day, taken in two divided doses. The dose should be increased incrementally over several weeks to attain maximum levels.

OTHER MEDICATIONS

Several antiepileptic medications are being studied at this time, including zonisamide, remacemide, UCB LO59, losigamone, pregabalin, rufinamide, ganaxalone, and stiripentol. It is unlikely all of these drugs will ultimately be used routinely because any new drug must have an obvious benefit over current medications in efficacy, safety, tolerance, ease of use, or cost.

Although none of the drugs approved recently have outstanding advantages over older medications, patients with epilepsy now have a much wider range of treatment options than was the case 5 years ago. As clinical experience grows with these agents, safer and more effective therapies will be developed.

OTHER TREATMENTS

Epilepsy Surgery

Antiepileptic drug therapy is effective in two-thirds to three-fourths of patients. The remainder fail to obtain good seizure control or have unacceptable side effects associated with their medication. The concept of good seizure control is elusive. In many states an individual cannot obtain a driver's license if he or she has had a seizure within the past 12 months. Therefore, good control might represent being seizure free for 1 year. The standard is often set too low, with physicians believing that a seizure or two every month, or even every few months, is acceptable. Any seizure, however, can have a major impact on the quality of life of people with epilepsy. Part of the challenge for epilepsy specialists is to encourage treating physicians and patients to strive for better control, and to not just surrender and accept the limitations imposed by occasional seizures.

Some epilepsy patients who cannot be controlled with medication are candidates for surgery. It has been estimated that up to 100,000 patients may qualify for such surgery in the United States. Because only a few thousand operations are performed each year, surgery for epilepsy appears to be an underused procedure. Although the high cost of the surgery, which can approach $50,000, has dampened enthusiasm for this approach, economic analysis indicates that this cost is recovered in 5 to 10 years after a successful procedure. If individuals can return to work and lead a more normal life, costs are usually recovered more quickly. Although epilepsy surgery is elective, it may be the best way to eliminate seizures in some individuals.

For epilepsy surgery to be successful the seizure focus must be localized. Typically, seizures that can be cured with surgery will arise from either the left or right mesial temporal structures, comprising the amygdala, hippocampus, and parahippocampal cortex. Bilateral temporal lobe seizures are not amenable to surgery because bilateral temporal lobectomy creates severe memory registration and retrieval problems. In seizure surgery, the path of spread of a seizure is not critically important. Rather, the surgical target, the site from which the seizure originates, is the focus. Moreover, secondarily generalized tonic-clonic seizures will cease if the focal point of origin is removed.

The temporal lobe is the usual target of epilepsy surgery. Although it is possible to operate on other lobes of the brain and sometimes cure seizures, the targets and boundaries of extratemporal surgery are less clear. Exceptions to this are lesion areas, such as a cavernous angioma or arteriovenous malformation, posttraumatic cicatrix, brain tumor, prior brain abscess, or dysplasias.

Before considering a patient for temporal lobe surgery it is important to rule out imitators of epilepsy, such as psychogenic seizures. In this regard an EEG can help localize the seizure focus. Although interictal spikes are suggestive, they are not as reliable as the electrical activity at the start of a seizure. For this reason, surgical candidates usually undergo video-EEG monitoring as inpatients to capture several of their typical seizures (usually with discontinuation of medications). The hope is that all seizures originate from the same focus located at the anterior to mid portion of one temporal lobe.

Another important part of the presurgical evaluation is the MRI to rule out causative lesions and document MTS. Although MTS is not always present, its appearance is a strong indication that the temporal lobe is involved in the epilepsy.

The positron emission tomography (PET) scan depicts glucose utilization in brain. For this procedure, ^{11}C-fluoro-deoxyglucose is injected systemically and is accumulated into brain cells. A positron isotope decays at every point in the brain where the glucose molecule is accumulated, and tomographic techniques are used to image the distribution of the radioactive glucose. In about 65% of patients with temporal lobe seizure foci, the lobe on the involved side consumes less glucose during the interictal period than the one on the noninvolved side. If a PET scan is being performed during a partial seizure, the seizure focus will be seen to consume much more glucose during the episode.

Neuropsychological tests are performed to determine whether a patient has impairments in the verbal sphere, usually reflecting injury to the dominant left hemisphere, or in the sphere of picture, face, and shape recognition, usually reflecting right hemisphere damage. Personality testing may also be useful as a screen for depression, which is very prevalent in this population. Psychosocial adjustment after epilepsy surgery is a key to the success of the procedure because the goal is improving the quality of life in addition to attenuation of seizures.

The Wada test, also called the intracarotid amobarbital test, is performed to localize speech and memory functions in candidates for epilepsy surgery. The internal carotid vascular distribution of half of the brain is anesthetized by injection of amobarbital into the internal carotid artery. During the next 5 to 15 min, speech and memory are tested. Although surgery can be performed on the temporal lobe of the speech-dominant side, not as much neocortex can be safely removed as from the nondominant side. Global amnesia after injecting one internal carotid artery is a danger signal because it suggests there may be severe memory problems after the operation.

Although some patients appear to be surgical candidates, the seizure focus may not be adequately localized by scalp EEG monitoring. These individuals may undergo invasive monitoring with electrodes implanted into suspect areas of the brain, or with sheets of electrodes embedded in plastic grids or strips placed over the surface of the brain. Grids are also used to electrically stimulate the area underneath the contact points and map the function of the brain at that region. This somewhat heroic procedure is used when the seizure focus appears to be very close to a speech or sensory-motor area of the brain and precise delineation of boundaries is required. The grid usually remains in place for about 1 week, and when it is removed the surgical procedure to remove the involved brain region is performed at the same time. Only a small number of epileptic patients undergoing surgery need mapping with a grid, although between 10 and 40% will need some type of invasive recording.

Epilepsy surgery is successful in about 75% of the cases. Patients may be completely cured of their epilepsy and be able to discontinue antiepileptic medications, usually within 1 year. Some patients choose to continue taking medication; others, who are free of seizures, may still require some pharmacotherapy. The surgical cure is not always absolute. Some patients may continue to have occasional auras (simple partial seizures) or rare breakthrough seizures. Some 25% of the surgery patients do not respond favorably to seizure surgery, usually because the entire focus could not be removed, or the seizure was multifocal.

Other specialized types of epilepsy surgery are performed less often than partial temporal lobectomy. The corpus callosum resection (known colloquially as the split-brain operation), separates the major band of fibers connecting the left and the right hemispheres of brain. This operation almost never cures seizures, but may slow the onset of the seizure and prevent it from becoming rapidly generalized, giving patients an opportunity to protect themselves from seizures. Corpus callosotomy, therefore, is a procedure to prevent injuries from seizures rather than cure seizures.

Hemispherectomy is removal of the majority of one brain hemisphere. This radical procedure is performed on individuals, usually children, who have severe damage to the hemisphere or Rasmussen's encephalitis, in which the local damage to a hemisphere is progressive over years. Although the child is hemiparetic after the procedure there is usually very good recovery of function if the operation is performed before the age of 10. Such children usually grow up with only a clumsy hand and a mild limp.

Seizure surgery is considered when a patient is diagnosed as having definite epilepsy, there is a reasonable likelihood the seizure onset is focal, and it is possibly limited to one temporal lobe. The candidates must be motivated to have surgery and be able to demonstrate that reduction of seizures will make a difference in their lifestyle. They must understand the risk of serious complications from the surgery, which is about 2%. Surgery should be considered only if pharmacotherapy is ineffective. The definition of a medication failure is, however, changing as more antiepileptic drugs become available. Previously, if a patient failed after taking phenytoin, phenobarbital,

and carbamazepine, he or she was a candidate for surgery. With the advent of new medications, the question arises as to whether the patient should be given a trial with these drugs as well. Should drug combinations be attempted? Because such trials could consume 5 to 10 years it is not reasonable to delay seizure surgery for that length of time. The fact is, most patients with complex partial seizures who fail to respond to carbamazepine or phenytoin may be helped, but will not be made seizure free by the addition of any of the newer agents. Because there are occasional exceptions, many epileptologists try only one or two of the newer medications before recommending surgery.

The Ketogenic Diet

In the early part of the 1900s it was noted that seizures improved during fasts. The *ketogenic diet* is designed to imitate the chemistry of the fasting state by depriving the brain of sugar, being very low in carbohydrates and high in fat and protein. The resulting changes in body chemistry make the brain more resistant to seizures. Although there have been some well-publicized successes with the ketogenic diet, the majority of patients do not benefit from this regimen. Studies suggest it seems to work best with children under the age of 12 with drop (atonic or tonic) seizures and is less effective after puberty. Partial adherence to the diet is not useful as it requires strict compliance to be effective. The long-term safety of this diet is not established because it can raise blood fats and cholesterol, inhibit growth, and decalcify bones. In some cases with a good therapeutic response, the diet can be halted after 2 years. The diet can be used in conjunction with antiepileptic medications, or on its own. The guidance of an experienced medical team is crucial in using this approach.

Biofeedback for Seizures

Several types of biofeedback have been attempted to control seizures. In its simplest form, a machine is used to help patients control their muscle tension or body temperature, which may help some people with seizures. Another form of biofeedback uses EEG to teach patients to change some aspect of their EEG pattern. Although biofeedback is harmless, it has not yet been shown to be effective in controlled clinical studies.

ACKNOWLEDGMENT

The author is supported by the Sandra Solheim Aiken fund for research in epilepsy.

For additional information on the drugs discussed in this chapter, see chapter 20 in *Goodman & Gilman's The Pharmacological Basis of Therapeutics* (Ninth Edition), McGraw-Hill, New York, 1996.

REFERENCES

Anonymous: Treatment of convulsive status epilepticus: recommendation of the Epilepsy Foundation of America's Working Group on Status Epilepticus. *JAMA* 1993;270:854–859.

Bourgeois B, Leppick IE, Sackellaris JC et al.: Felbamate: a double-blind controlled trial in patients undergoing presurgical evaluation of partial seizures. *Neurology* 1993;43:693–696.

Carraz G, Farr R, Chateau R, Bonnin J: First clinical trials of the antiepileptic activity of N-dipropylacetic acid. *Ann Med Psychol* (Paris) 1964;122:577–584.

Dodrill CB, Troupin AS: Neuropsychological effects of carbamazepine and phenytoin: a reanalysis. *Neurology* 1991;41:141–143.

Dreifuss FE, Santilli N, Langer DH et al.: Valproic acid hepatic fatalities: a retrospective review. *Neurology* 1987;37:379–385.

Farwell JR, Lee YJ, Hirtz DG et al.: Phenobarbital for febrile seizures—effects on intelligence and on seizure recurrence. *N Engl J Med* 1990;322:364–369.

Hauser WA, Annegers JF, Rocca WA: Descriptive epidemiology of epilepsy: contributions of population-based studies from Rochester, Minnesota. *Mayo Clin Proc* 1996;71:576–86.

Hill DR, Suman-Chauhan N, Woodruff GN: Localization of [^{3}H] gabapentin to a novel site in rat brain: autoradiographic studies. *Eur J Pharm* 1993;244:303–309.

Levy RH, Mattson RH, Meldrum BS (eds): *Antiepileptic Drugs,* 4th ed. New York, Raven Press, 1995, pp 1–1120.

Loiseau P, Duché B: Carbamazepine: clinical use, in Levy RH, Mattson RH, Meldrum BS (eds): *Antiepileptic Drugs,* 4th ed. New York, Raven Press, 1995, pp 555–566.

Macdonald RL, McLean MJ: Cellular basis of barbiturate and phenytoin anticonvulsant drug action. *Epilepsia* 1982;23:57–18.

Mattson R, Cramer J, Collins J et al.: Comparison of carbamazepine, phenobarbital, phenytoin and primidone in partial and secondarily generalized tonic-clonic seizures. *N Engl J Med* 1985;313:145–151.

McLean MJ, Macdonald RL: Carbamazepine and 10, 11–epoxy–carbamazepine produced use-and voltage-dependent limitation of rapidly firing action potentials of mouse central neurons in cell culture. *J Pharm Exp Ther* 1986;238:727–738.

Piredda S, Pavlick M, Gale K: Anticonvulsant effects of GABA elevation in the deep prepiriform cortex. *Epilepsy Res* 1987;1:102–106.

Rothstein JD, Jin L, Dykes-Hoberg M, Kuncl RW: Chronic inhibition of glutamate uptake produces a model of slow neurotoxicity. *Proc Nat Acad Sci USA* 1993;90:6591–6595.

Tassinari CA, Michelucci R, Chauvel P et al.: Double-blind, placebo-controlled trial of topiramate (600 mg daily) for the treatment of refractory partial epilepsy. *Epilepsia* 1996;37:763–68.

STROKE

James J. Vornov

Acute syndromes of cerebral ischemia are commonly referred to as "stroke." When a cerebral artery that supplies part of the brain is suddenly occluded, function of the affected brain region is immediately lost. If the occlusion persists, the tissue becomes infarcted, leading to a permanent loss of function. Given these facts, the aims of therapy are to reperfuse the affected area, limit injury by increasing the resistance of the brain to ischemia, and prevent future arterial occlusions. Although there are a number of problems associated with achieving these goals, progress has been made in developing effective therapies. Included are drugs to prevent stroke and others to limit the neurological damage associated with the event.

CLINICAL FEATURES

Stroke is a broad term encompassing a number of causes for abrupt loss of brain function. It is more precise to use the term cerebral ischemia to describe what occurs following an arterial occlusion. Venous thrombosis can also lead to ischemia but is much less common than arterial occlusion. Excluded from the following discussion are all types of intracranial hemorrhage, including subdural hemorrhage, subarachnoid hemorrhage, and intracerebral hemorrhage.

Stroke presents as a significant loss of neurologic function with onset over a few minutes or hours. Occasionally, strokes may have a stuttering onset over longer periods of time, sometimes days. Because the ischemic area in the brain may spread over time, the patient may suddenly experience a small neurological deficit, followed by a worsening of symptoms over subsequent hours or days.

The key to identifying cerebral ischemia is to recognize that an acute neurological deficit is a loss of function in the territory of a particular cerebral artery. Although the diagnosis of stroke etiology, and the identification of risk factors, are important considerations, they must follow the vascular diagnosis.

Normally, the clinical course of ischemic injury is improvement in function. Thus, the deficit is maximal near the time of onset if there is no progression, and recovery is most rapid in the first few days following a stroke, with dramatic return of function commonly seen. Although progress slows after the first week, it is still substantial and continues during the months and years following the event. Because patients and their families are often frightened by the loss of mobility, speech, or the use of limbs, it is important to inform them that improvement normally occurs with time, lending hope for a steady recovery.

Many patients recover fully from a stroke after hours or days, perhaps because the arterial occlusion was only temporary. When the deficit lasts less than 24 h, the episode is classified as a transient ischemic attack (TIA). If it lasts longer, but resolves completely, it is considered a reversible ischemic neurological deficit (RIND). These terms are used widely in classifying patients for research databases. The risk for a recurrence is the same whether the patient suffers a temporary or permanent arterial occlusion because the critical feature is the underlying pathology that led initially to the arterial occlusion.

Primary Symptoms of Stroke

Most patients who suffer a stroke develop an obvious loss of motor or sensory function that is usually confined to one side of the body. The motor symptoms may appear as a true weakness, paresis, or as a loss of coordination or ataxia. Often, patients characterize the motor symptoms as "clumsiness" or "heaviness." Although any of the sensory systems may be involved in a stroke, the somatosensory or the visual systems are most commonly affected, with smell, taste, and hearing being normally spared.

Although acute, focal symptoms are the hallmark of a stroke, diffuse, constitutional symptoms are unlikely to be due to focal ischemia. Thus, it is important to search for clear focal symptoms in a patient who presents with vague complaints, such as fatigue, faintness, the legs "giving way," or migratory sensory changes that involve both sides of the body. A diagnosis of stroke should not be made without clear specific complaints.

Monocular visual loss, amaurosis fugax, deserves special mention because it commonly arises from disease in the proximal carotid artery. The ophthalmic artery, which supplies the retina, is the first branch of the internal carotid artery. Because carotid disease may be surgically treatable, evaluation of the carotids should be undertaken immediately when this symptom is present.

Cognitive function is sometimes impaired by cerebral ischemia. The loss of function may be obvious, as with aphasia when the patient loses the ability to produce and/or understand language, or more subtle if association areas of the cerebral cortex are affected in isolation. In the latter case the patient may present with hallucinations or confusion. Occasionally, patients with language difficulties and no obvious motor or sensory deficits are mistakenly diagnosed with a psychiatric disorder. It is rare, however, for cognitive changes to occur in the absence of more typical focal motor or sensory deficits, which usually help establish the diagnosis of cerebral ischemia.

The acute onset of vertigo is a particularly difficult symptom to evaluate because it can arise from loss of either brain function (the brain stem and cerebellum) or the peripheral vestibular apparatus (the semicircular canals or the eighth cranial nerve). The evaluation is complicated further by the fact that the vestibular apparatus is partially supplied by the same vessels that perfuse the brain stem. Thus, ischemia of the inner ear can be caused by the same mechanisms as ischemia of the brain.

Inasmuch as pain, in general, is not a symptom of stroke, limb pain is unlikely to be caused by cerebral ischemia. An exception to this rule is headache, which is quite common with a stroke. No conclusions can be drawn, however, from the presence, severity, or localization of the headache.

Because occasionally seizures or loss of consciousness accompany the onset of a stroke, the simultaneous appearance of a new, persistent focal neurological deficit suggests strongly that the event was not a simple seizure or syncope, but rather a stroke accompanied by these symptoms. Although seizures and loss of consciousness are more common with intracranial hemorrhage, both can occur with arterial occlusion. While they are more common with cardiac emboli to the cerebral circulation, this relationship is not consistent enough to allow an etiology to be inferred from the presence of seizures or loss of consciousness.

DIAGNOSIS

The diagnosis of stroke is divided into two phases. First, the presence of arterial occlusion must be inferred from the time course and presenting symptoms. Second, the etiology of the occlusion must be identified. The second step is not critical for acute therapeutic intervention because most strokes are treated similarly, regardless of etiology, to protect the brain and encourage reperfusion. Rather, the etiology is important for selecting a therapy to prevent further ischemic events.

It is useful to compare cerebral ischemia with cardiac ischemia even though there are profound differences between the two. Although there has been rapid progress in developing treatments for cardiac ischemia, advances in stroke therapy have been slow. It is hoped that by defining the similarities between cerebral and cardiac ischemia it may be possible to design treatments for the former as has been successfully done for the latter.

Methods used for the diagnosis of cardiac ischemia are well known to clinicians as is the clinical syndrome to patients and their families. Thus, crushing retrosternal chest pain, shortness of breath, diaphoresis, and other signs of general circulatory failure readily bring patients to the emergency department. With cardiac ischemia, patients rush for treatment given the complex of symptoms combining severe pain with the feeling that death is imminent. Those who do not feel pain with cardiac ischemia are less likely to have their disease discovered and treated, a situation common, for example, among diabetics.

In contrast, because stroke is painless, patients often fail to recognize the importance of their symptoms. Because this delays the request for medical assistance, acute therapy is difficult to initiate before brain damage is irreversible. Thus, if a patient awakens with a flaccid arm he may not know whether he slept on the arm during the night or has suffered a stroke. Although there may be a suspicion this is more than a nerve compression, patients often delay seeking treatment hoping for spontaneous improvement.

The diagnostic tools available for cardiac ischemia are vastly more powerful than for cerebral ischemia. Thus, the diagnosis of cardiac ischemia is greatly aided by the electrocardiogram (ECG), which entails the use of basic equipment and yields data that are readily interpreted. An ECG can even be obtained by emergency medical technicians as a patient is transported to the hospital. The ECG provides a remarkable amount of information, including the presence of a prior cardiac ischemia, the reversibility of current ischemia, and the location of the old and new ischemia.

In contrast, stroke is diagnosed solely on the basis of clinical observation. In this case the clinician must recognize the neurological syndrome of an acute occlusion of a cerebral artery. Although occlusions of large, named vessels, like the middle cerebral artery, produce an easily recognizable syndrome, blockade of smaller vessels may yield symptoms that make a diagnosis more difficult. Moreover, the presence of a preexisting ischemic injury makes recognition of new lesions more difficult.

There is no simple procedure like the ECG for diagnosing a stroke. Although computed tomography (CT) and magnetic resonance imaging (MRI) are useful for confirming a diagnosis, they are generally normal when patients first present with symptoms, the time when therapy is most important. Thus, it is the responsibility of the clinician to make a diagnosis of stroke by determining that the syndrome corresponds with a loss of function in a specific vascular territory. In the acute situation, imaging studies are most useful in excluding other causes of neurological symptoms such as hemorrhage, tumors, or multiple sclerosis. When there is a major neurological deficit a CT scan should be obtained immediately, with an MRI scan used as a follow-up a day or two later to confirm the diagnosis of stroke if there is a persistent deficit. Magnetic resonance angiography (MRA) can be added as part of the etiologic workup.

Vascular Diagnosis

The stroke syndrome must be acute in onset, display a focal neurological deficit, and be consistent with the occlusion of one cerebral vessel. In most cases, the patient presents with a well-defined complaint of acute loss of central nervous system function that matches a vascular syndrome. The correct diagnosis of a stroke depends on the combined knowledge of functional and vascular brain anatomy because the particular clinical features of the syndrome depend on the vessel involved. The acute therapies that are now becoming available for stroke must all be initiated well before imaging techniques are able to confirm the location and size of the infarct. Thus, the diagnosis must be made rapidly and solely on the basis of clinical symptoms.

A stroke is characterized by a rapid onset because slowly progressing syndromes are not likely to be caused by cerebral ischemia. When onset is slow, one possibility is a sequential occlusion of many small vessels. In this case, close questioning should reveal a stepwise progression characteristic of many, small ischemic events. Multiple small infarcts lead to a vascular dementia that may be distinguished from Alzheimer's disease by the presence of focal neurological deficits and evidence of many discrete stokes with MRI or CT scanning.

With stroke, the size of the involved vessel determines the extent of the brain lesion, with occlusions of large vessels causing large deficits and occlusions of small vessels causing small deficits. Certain deep parts of the brain are supplied by long penetrating vessels that are prone to occlusion, causing characteristic small strokes. These common small-vessel occlusion syndromes are often referred to as lacunar syndromes because little holes (lacunae) are seen in deep brain structures at autopsy. In this case the lesion is called a lacunar stroke.

Although the correct determination of the involved vessel is critical for diagnosis, it is of limited value in determining etiology because the size or location of an occlusion does not predict its cause. Rather, it is necessary to examine the entire vascular tree proximal to the ischemic area to identify the possible source of the emboli. Although a small penetrating vessel may itself be diseased, it may also be blocked by an artery-to-artery embolus arising from its larger parent vessel or by a small embolus from the heart. Indeed, the embolus can even arise in the venous circulation if the heart has a right-to-left shunt.

Vascular Anatomy

The brain is supplied by two pairs of large arteries originating from the aortic arch: the carotid arteries and the vertebral arteries. The vascular territory supplied by the carotids is known as the anterior circulation whereas the vertebral arteries give rise to the posterior circulation (Fig.15-1).

The common carotid bifurcates near the angle of the jaw, giving rise to the internal and external carotid. The internal carotid continues as an unbranched artery until it enters the skull and penetrates the dura, where it gives rise to its first branch, the ophthalmic artery. As noted earlier, amaurosis fugax results from occlusion of this artery, the terminal branch of which is the central retinal artery. Thus, monocular visual loss is diagnostic of a problem in the carotid artery or heart.

The internal carotid bifurcates at the base of the brain into the anterior and middle cerebral arteries. The anterior cerebral artery (ACA) remains medial, supplying part of the cerebral hemisphere. Because the cortical representation of the legs is most medial, ACA occlusions affect the leg more than the hand and face. Because the cortical representation is contralateral to the body, the deficit will be opposite the stroke with, for example, left-sided strokes in the cortex causing right-sided weakness.

The middle cerebral artery (MCA) takes a course through the sylvian fissure on its way from the base of the brain to the lateral surface of the cerebral hemisphere. While passing through the sylvian fissure it gives rise to penetrating vessels, the lenticulostriate arteries, which supply the internal capsule, the basal ganglia, and part of the thalamus. Occlusion of these vessels leads to lacunar syndromes, most notably pure motor stroke from small infarctions of the internal capsule. Small strokes in the basal ganglia are commonly asymptomatic.

As it emerges from the sylvian fissure, the MCA bifurcates or trifurcates into branches that supply the lateral surface of the cerebral hemisphere. Occlusion of these branches causes large, wedge-shaped infarctions of the cortex, with the clinical syndrome depending on whether motor or somatosensory areas are involved. Thus, if the optic radiations are affected, a visual loss will occur. Cognitive syndromes, such as aphasia, are most commonly due to branch occlusions of the MCA.

A proximal occlusion of the MCA will affect the entire vascular distribution, including both deep and cortical structures (Fig. 15-1). This event will be reflected by a loss of both motor and sensory function, with the face, arm, and leg all affected. Even if the ACA territory is spared, infarction of the internal capsule will cause a loss of leg function. Often occlusion of the carotid results in a partial or full MCA distribution stroke because of collateral supply.

The posterior circulation is supplied by the vertebral arteries, which join at the junction of the medulla and pons to form the basilar artery (Fig. 15-1). Accordingly, each half of the medulla (and the caudal cerebellum) is supplied by one vertebral artery. The basilar artery provides the blood supply for the pons. At the level of the midbrain, the basilar artery splits again to form the posterior cerebral artery (PCA) on each side. The PCAs wrap around the midbrain, moving posteriorly along the base of the cortex. Penetrating vessels from the vertebrals, basilar artery, and PCAs supply the brain stem.

Penetrating vessels emanating from the PCA supply much of the thalamus as the PCA courses back to supply the posterior cerebral cortex, specifically the medial temporal lobes and the occipital lobes. The dual blood supply of the central visual cortex protects it from arterial occlusion, creating the tendency for macular sparing in strokes affecting vision.

Syndromes that fail to reflect the vascular anatomy are unlikely to be strokes. Although brain tumors, both metastatic and primary, can present abruptly, there is usually some clue that the acute onset is superimposed on a more prolonged course. Tumors may also hemorrhage or rapidly expand and

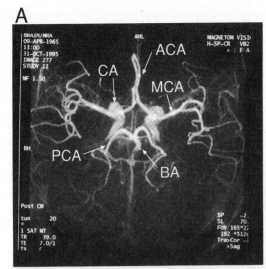

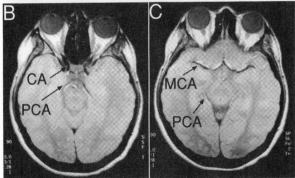

Anterior Circulation:

CA	Carotid Artery
ACA	Anterior Cerebral Artery
MCA	Middle Cerebral Artery

Posterior Circulation:

BA	Basilar Artery
PCA	Posterior Cerebral Artery

Figure 15–1. *Basic vascular anatomy. In panel A, a normal magnetic resonance angiogram (MRA) illustrates the major vessels of the circle of Willis. In the anterior circulation, each large carotid artery (CA) can be seen giving rise to a midline anterior cerebral artery (ACA) and a lateral middle cerebral artery (MCA). In the posterior circulation, a single basilar artery (BA) gives rise to paired posterior cerebral arteries. In panels B and C, successive cuts through the base of the brain illustrate the course of the major vessels. In panel B, the carotids are seen as paired vessels coming up into the brain. At this level in the posterior circulation, the basilar is bifurcating to form the PCAs, which wrap around the midbrain. In panel C, the middle cerebral arteries can be seen arising from the carotids and moving laterally in the sylvian fissure. At this level, the PCAs are seen at the top of the midbrain where they can continue on to supply the medial occipital cortex.*

produce a stroke-like, abrupt onset of symptoms. Moreover, multiple sclerosis can present quite suddenly, mimicking a stroke. With either tumors or multiple sclerosis, imaging studies will identify them as the causes of the abrupt neurologic deficit.

Imaging Studies and the Progression of Histologic Changes

There is no consensus on when an imaging study should be performed on a patient suspected of having had a stroke because, at the onset of symptoms, only tumors or hemorrhage will be revealed. If the syndrome is due to ischemia it will take hours for an MRI or CT to detect any changes in the brain. Indeed, changes of an ischemic event may not be detectable with these techniques for several days. The situation is complicated further by the fact that a significant number of stroke patients never show lesions on a CT or MRI scan.

An understanding of the pathologic changes associated with a stroke helps explain why CT and MRI scans are of limited immediate value. Depending on the level of blood flow it may take many hours for the affected brain region to experience energy failure. When blood flow ceases completely, as occurs in cardiac arrest, energy failure occurs within a few minutes. The mildest levels of ischemia that are capable of causing injury may require 6 h or more to cause energy failure, which must occur for there to be detectable histologic changes in the brain. Even with energy failure, however, histologic changes are minimal, as illustrated by the lack of ischemic changes noted at autopsy. Thus, if ischemic damage occurred instantly, all autopsies would reveal massive changes in brain brought on by death, which is not the case. Rather, the characteristic changes associated with ischemia require perfusion of the affected brain region for several hours.

The degree of ischemia determines the speed and severity of pathologic changes in the infarct. The most severe change is frank necrosis, where tissue structure is lost entirely. Less severe is a selective loss of neurons with preservation of glia and tissue structure. In both cases, as pathologic changes develop, excess water accumulates in the tissue, causing edema. Only later, as the infarcted brain reorganizes, is there a loss of tissue volume.

Thus, on a CT or MRI scan there is unlikely to be any detectable change until 6 to 24 h after the onset of symptoms. Of the two scanning methods, the MRI is more sensitive because, as water accumulates, the area becomes bright on T2-weighted imaging sequences. Older infarctions are marked by decreased densities on T1-weighted images on MRI and CT scans.

Because of the time required to detect changes in brain characteristic of a stroke, MRI or CT scans are of no value in the acute diagnosis of this condition. Because the MRI and CT can rule out other causes for the loss of neurologic function, however, patients with severe deficits should have an imaging study performed acutely. All patients with major neurological findings undergo CT scanning immediately, primarily to rule out etiologies such as intracranial hemorrhage. Because MRI scanning is more sensitive 24 h after the onset of symptoms, it should be delayed for at least 1 day.

Diagnosis of Stroke Etiology

Stroke results from an occlusion in the arterial supply to the brain. The reason for occlusion should be established for every patient to select the most appropriate long-term therapy. To this end it is necessary to examine the vascular tree proximal to the infarction. For example, if the carotid artery is occluded, the only possible sources of the problem are the heart, the aorta, or the artery itself. Occlusion of a small vessel emanating from the carotid could be due to an embolus formed anywhere between the heart and that vessel.

Although it is tempting to believe that the type of onset or the involved vessel can be used to determine etiology, clinical data indicate these clues are unreliable. For example, although stroke of abrupt onset, with a maximal deficit at the time of presentation, is often thought to be embolic, this presentation is also seen in patients with disease at the carotid bifurcation that may require surgery.

The size of the involved vessel is also not diagnostic of any particular etiology. On one hand, a small vessel may be occluded by an embolus coming from the heart, or from a proximal large artery. On the other hand, the vessel may be occluded by atherosclerotic disease at the site of its origin from an intracranial vessel, or the disease may be local. There is also some confusion surrounding the concept of lacunar disease, with the supposition that a distinctive pathology occurs in these small penetrating vessels. Although this process, termed *lipohyalinosis*, certainly exists, it can be used to explain a stroke only after more proximal cardiac and arterial diseases are eliminated.

There is also confusion about the difference between the etiology of a stroke and risk factors. Etiology relates to the pathology directly responsible for the arterial occlusion. These events range from clot formation in the left atrium, to vessel wall atherosclerosis, to hypercoaguable states. In contrast, risk factors are identified conditions that increase the likelihood a stroke will occur. These factors are often multiple and interactive. Thus, smoking is a risk factor for stroke but is not a proximal cause. Thus, because smoking causes many physiologic and biochemical changes there are a number of ways it increases the risk for stroke. Included are smoking-enhanced blood coagulability and risk for developing atherosclerosis.

Given their multiplicity of effects, the influence of risk factors is complex. For example, hypertension is a risk factor for atherosclerotic disease at multiple sites, including small penetrating vessels, larger intracranial vessels, and at the carotid bifurcation. It also is a risk factor for coronary artery disease, which in turn is a cause of atrial fibrillation and myocardial infarction, each of which are potentially embologenic.

Because of this, it is impossible to evaluate a patient and conclude that a stroke was caused by hypertension, diabetes, smoking, or any single risk factor. Rather, the underlying condition that led to the arterial occlusion should be identified. This is not simply an academic exercise, because the therapy chosen is based on the long-term risk of another stroke, which is directly related to the etiology.

Tools to examine the vascular tree.   There are a number of noninvasive techniques used to identify the cardiac or arterial lesion responsible for vessel occlusion. The overall strategy is to quickly identify any likely cause requiring immediate therapy to prevent recurrence, with the drug chosen depending on the risk associated with the abnormality discovered. In general, high-risk conditions are treated with warfarin, whereas aspirin is used to treat lower-risk situations.

Every patient with ischemia in the anterior circulation should undergo a noninvasive evaluation of the carotid arteries, primarily to determine whether a carotid endarterectomy is indicated. The benefits of surgically removing the atherosclerotic plaque by endarterectomy was debated for years because of the absence of reliable clinical data. The North American Symptomatic Carotid Endarterectomy Trial (NASCET) ultimately demonstrated that patients with symptoms of stroke or TIA from the affected artery greatly benefited from this surgery (Gasecki et al., 1995). Because significant advantage was found only in patients with greater than 70% stenosis, the degree of carotid stenosis must be determined whenever there is ischemia in a carotid distribution.

The standard noninvasive method to study the carotid bifurcation is the duplex ultrasound technique, which provides an accurate evaluation when performed by a well-trained operator (Eliasziw et al., 1995). On one hand, the advent of MRA provides an alternative with several advantages (Kallmes et al., 1996). Thus, although duplex ultrasound only provides information on the carotid bifurcation, MRA images the entire internal carotid, including the siphon. In fact, MRA can provide images of the vertebral arteries and the entire circle of Willis. On the other hand, duplex ultrasonography is less stressful than MRA because the latter requires that the patient remain motionless for many minutes under conditions that frequently induce claustrophobia. Although the accuracy of MRA in identifying carotid bifurcation lesions is comparable to duplex ultrasonography, it has not been verified as extensively. Unlike MRA, duplex ultrasonography also provides velocity information that complements the anatomic data.

Because duplex ultrasonography can often be obtained rapidly it should be undertaken soon after admission in those with anterior circulation symptoms. If negative, MRA may be performed later to identify lesions in the rest of the vasculature. There is often a delay in using MRA to increase the sensitivity of the MRI in detecting the ischemic area.

Angiography remains the gold standard for evaluating the cerebral vasculature. It does, however, carry a measurable risk of stroke or death in approximately 0.5% of patients. Given the availability of noninvasive ultrasound and magnetic resonance techniques, angiography should be used only to address a specific question, the answer to which would alter therapy.

Transcranial doppler (TCD) is a useful adjunct for detecting intracranial vascular disease. Although TCD does not provide the kind of imaging detail obtained with duplex ultrasonography, by measuring flow velocity and pulsatility it provides further information about atherosclerotic disease in the circle of Willis. For example, when the basilar artery, or a middle cerebral artery, appears abnormal on MRA imaging, TCD can provide additional information that may be important in justifying a cerebral angiogram.

Although ultrasound and MRA provide information about the vasculature in the neck and within the skull, echocardiography is best for identifying cardiac embolic sources. Echocardiography is indicated in two very different groups of patients. The first consists of those who have a clinical history or exam suggestive of cardiac abnormalities such as cardiac valvular disease or a murmur. The second is composed of those with no identified cause for the stroke. Although as many as 50% of patients were previously categorized as having "cryptogenic stroke," many of these patients have now been found to have unappreciated cardiac sources or an abnormality of coagulation. With an intensive workup vascular disease will generally be discovered, especially when using MRA to noninvasively examine the larger intracranial vessels.

Several studies have demonstrated that transthoracic echocardiography is unlikely to identify a cause of stroke in patients without a history of cardiac disease or an abnormal cardiac examination, making it an inappropriate procedure for patients with cryptogenic stroke. This is especially true in obese patients or those with emphysema, in which case a new technique, transesophageal echo (TEE), is much more useful. Indeed, TEE is the method of choice for patients with no vascular abnormality. With transthoracic echocardiography the ultrasound probe is passed into the esophagus to view the heart without the obstruction of the ribs or lungs. The aorta can also be imaged in this way, allowing for identification of thick or protruding aortic atherosclerotic plaque that can serve as an embolic source.

If the heart and vessels are normal, the arterial occlusion may be due to an inherited or acquired coagulation abnormality. Some conditions alone, like Trousseau's syndrome, which is a hypercoaguable state that occurs in some patients with carcinoma, may explain why a patient suffered a stroke with normal heart and cerebral arteries whereas other conditions may be risk factors for stroke. These conditions may include the presence of antiphospholipid antibodies, an abnormality common in the elderly that increases the risk for stroke (Feldmann and Levine, 1995). Like cardioembolic sources, hypercoaguable conditions with a high associated stroke risk are treated chronically with warfarin.

PHARMACOTHERAPY

The 1995 publication of the results of the National Institute of Neurological Disease and Stroke tissue plasminogen activator (t-PA) trial was a historic landmark in stroke therapy because it provided the first unequivocal evidence that stroke damage can be limited by a therapeutic intervention. Because of this finding, stroke is now a neurological emergency. Although at the present time t-PA and subsequent chronic antithrombotic drug administration are the only available treatments for stroke, a number of putative neuroprotective drugs are in late clinical trials. It appears that soon stroke, like cardiac ischemia, will be treated with the combination of reperfusion and cytoprotection.

Historically, ischemic brain injury was thought to occur rapidly because the onset and maximal severity of the deficit is rapid. Even if brain tissue at risk could be salvaged, there was no clinical indication of therapeutic success because the functional deficit does not change. Likewise, there was no information on the amount of time necessary for irreversible brain damage to occur because there was no means of intervention. From clinical signs, the brain injury appears rapid and maximal at the onset of symptoms.

It is possible that this conclusion was conditioned by knowledge of the more clearly defined blood flow changes associated with cardiac arrest. When the heart stops, cerebral perfusion quickly drops to zero, with reperfusion of the brain clearly defined by restoration of blood pressure. The brain can tolerate cessation of blood flow for less than 10 min, after which there is irreversible injury to the most vulnerable regions. Less vulnerable brain regions are capable of withstanding only a few additional minutes of global ischemia. Thus, there is massive damage to the cerebral cortex if a patient is resuscitated after blood flow was halted for 15 min. The other organs of the body are not much more resistant than the brain to ischemic injury; the kidney, liver, and heart are significantly damaged with a cardiac arrest of sufficient duration to cause massive brain injury. The rapid clinical onset of stroke led to the belief that brain damage was rapidly irreversible, which has, until recently, led to the conclusion that acute stroke therapy was unlikely to be of any benefit.

The Ischemic Penumbra

Fortunately, arterial occlusions responsible for ischemic stroke do not stop blood flow in all affected regions of the brain because only some tissue experiences a reduction in flow to the levels seen with cardiac arrest. This tissue, referred to as the ischemic core, is probably damaged irreversibly within minutes and for now, at least, is not amenable to therapy. Most of the affected brain tissue, however, is exposed to an intermediate level of ischemia because the farther the distance from the ischemic core, the greater the blood flow, until a region of normal flow, supplied by another vessel, is reached. Because there is some threshold of blood flow above which brain tissue can survive indefinitely, there may be transient disruption of function, although infarction will never occur (Hossmann, 1994b). When a cerebral artery is occluded the border of the infarction is defined by the outline of the threshold level of blood flow separating tissue that will survive from that which will eventually infarct (Fig. 15-2).

The diminution of blood flow causes an immediate loss of function, explaining the rapid, maximal onset of clinical symptoms. Although symptoms appear rapidly, however, complete infarction takes time. Animal models of brain ischemia have shown that 3 to 6 h of mild ischemia are needed to cause infarction. Indeed, if no infarct develops after 6 h of

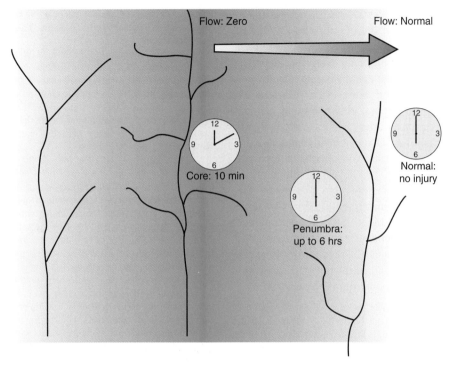

Figure 15–2. The ischemic penumbra. After occlusion of the central artery in the figure, the shaded area denotes the graded decrease in blood flow in the cortex. The period of occlusion needed to cause injury is shown for the core, penumbra, and normal regions.

a mild reduction in blood flow it is unlikely the tissue will ever infarct. The region of intermediate blood flow where infarction takes hours to occur, the ischemic penumbra, is the target of acute stroke therapy. Although an ischemic penumbra, or area that can be rescued after the onset of symptoms, has not been clearly demonstrated in patients, it is inferred from the results obtained with the animal models. Clinically, the experimental tools do not exist that allow for an examination of the blood flow and functional status of the human brain during an ischemic episode.

Stroke Teams and the Concept of Brain Attack

Realizing the difficulties associated with getting patients to the hospital and mobilizing physicians to diagnose and treat stroke, hospitals have been encouraged to establish specialized teams to treat this condition. The term "brain attack" has been promoted as an alternative to "stroke" to emphasize that cerebral ischemia is now a treatable condition like a heart attack.

As acute stroke therapy becomes the standard of care, hospitals will have to provide timely assessment of patients presenting with cerebral ischemia as is done with cardiac ischemia. As with most emergency medical service (EMS) systems, not every community hospital receives patients with acute cardiac ischemia, and it is not anticipated that all will have the resources to rapidly evaluate and treat patients for cerebral ischemia.

The only currently available acute therapy for stroke is t-PA, which must be administered within 3 h of the onset of symptoms. Before t-PA can be given, however, a head CT must be performed to rule out cerebral hemorrhage. These requirements define the resources needed for acute stroke therapy: rapid neurological diagnosis, the availability of t-PA, and head CT (Fig. 15-1).

Therapeutic Strategies

The principles of acute stroke therapy are similar to those for treating cardiac ischemia. Thus, with cardiac ischemia several strategies are used to mini-mize injury to the heart muscle, the first of which, reperfusion, is most critical. Thus, blood flow must be restored when possible to avoid further damage. To this end the most acute therapy is generally throm-bolysis to restore blood flow, often followed by structural repair of arteries, either through balloon angioplasty or coronary artery bypass surgery. Cyto-protection therapies are also instituted to increase the resistance of cardiac muscle to ischemia, allowing it to survive longer with low levels of blood flow. Thus, pharmacologic manipulations that reduce the workload of the heart enable the ischemic tissue to survive periods of low blood flow. In addition, pa-tients with cardiac ischemia are treated with drugs to prevent subsequent episodes. Drugs for this purpose include anticoagulants and antiplatelet agents to pre-vent formation of additional thrombosis.

Reperfusion and thrombolytic therapy. Given the inability to easily and reliably measure blood flow in patients with symptoms of cerebral ischemia, little is known about the time course of the ischemia itself, with available evidence suggest-ing that spontaneous reperfusion is common in cerebral isch-emia. It appears, however, that such reperfusion occurs well after the opportunity to decrease tissue injury has passed.

Thrombolytic therapy for cardiac ischemia was first in-vestigated with intra-arterial injections of clot-lysing enzymes or activators, such as urokinase, streptokinase, and t-PA. Once intra-arterial therapy was shown to be practical, intravenous clot lysis was studied, but with monitoring of the vascular occlusion with coronary arteriography.

The initial studies of thrombolysis in stroke also included intra-arterial injection of thrombolytic agents. The results were often quite dramatic, especially when a large occluded vessel was rapidly freed of a clot, with some patients experiencing remarkable recovery from their deficit. Studies indicated, how-ever, that hemorrhage would be a major complication of thrombolytic therapy, especially when clot lysis was attempted many hours after ischemia.

The National Institutes of Health t-PA study established the therapeutic efficacy of intravenous thrombolysis in stroke, with the trial demonstrating improved outcome at 3 months using any of four assessment scales. The t-PA trial was well designed and emphasized the need to minimize the time be-tween onset of symptoms and treatment. It was also designed to test a clinical protocol that could be used in any hospital where rapid neurological evaluation and CT scanning were available. Because the study was aimed at testing the use of t-PA under normal clinical conditions, angiography was not performed, so the presence of a vascular occlusion was as-sumed only from clinical symptoms and drug efficacy estab-lished on the basis of clinical outcome. No attempt was made to determine whether the drug induced reperfusion under these conditions.

The chief complication of thrombolytic therapy is cere-bral hemorrhage. The rate for cerebral hemorrhage in the t-PA trial was 6.4%, much lower than the 21% in the European streptokinase trial, which failed to show a therapeutic benefit with thrombolysis (Hacke et al., 1995). Even though t-PA caused some fatal cerebral hemorrhages, there was no signifi-cant difference in mortality between treatment and control groups after 3 months.

The clinical use of t-PA follows the study guidelines (Table 15-1), with the dose used being 0.9 mg/kg, not to exceed 90 mg total. Of greatest importance is the requirement that the patient have a clearly defined onset of symptoms within 3 h of drug administration. Those with minor, or rapidly resolving symptoms, should not be treated with t-PA, nor should those with signs of cerebral hemorrhage on CT scan. In the clinical trial patients with blood pressure >185 (systolic) or >110 (diasystolic) were excluded. Some were treated with a mild antihypertensive agent to help them meet the criteria for inclusion in the study. Although this protocol can be fol-lowed, care must be taken to avoid lowering the blood pressure significantly below the levels required for treatment.

It is also prudent to exclude patients with early hypoden-sity on CT scan even though this did not disqualify subjects from the t-PA study. Thus, the data indicated the incidence of CT hypodensity was 9% in patients with symptomatic intracranial bleeding (four were administered t-PA and two placebo), compared with 4% in all patients. Because these early CT changes may indicate an error in timing the onset of symptoms, and the number of these patients is small, it is probably best to withhold t-PA treatment from this group.

Given the results of the t-PA trial, some have been reluc-tant to treat patients with it because of the potential complica-tions. Even with these difficulties, however, overall improve-ment in outcome is significant. It seems likely that as experience grows with the drug its use will become more widespread. At present, efforts are being made to refine the treatment protocol to minimize hemorrhagic complications and determine whether t-PA is effective when given in combi-nation with other drugs, particularly neuroprotective agents.

t-PA AND REPERFUSION

During the t-PA trial the state of blood vessels was not exam-ined. The trial was divided into two parts, however, the first of which entailed an evaluation of the patients 24 h after t-PA administration, a time at which no beneficial effect could be demonstrated using the clinical stroke scale. Rather, the therapeutic effects were most evident during the second phase of the study, 3 months after drug treatment. Some studies using an intra-arterial protocol for t-PA administration have included identification of occluded arteries, making it possible to correlate directly arterial patency with the clinical symptoms.

Table 15-1
T-PA Treatment Checklists

Inclusion Checklist

- Suspected acute ischemic stroke
- Able to treat with rt-PA within 3 h of onset of symptoms
- No acute lesion on CT (including subtle early signs of ischemia)

Exclusion Checklist

- Intracerebral hemorrhage or suspected SAH
- Rapid improvement suggesting TIA
- Minor symptoms (NIH Stroke score less than 5)
- Stroke or serious head trauma within 3 months
- History of intracerebral hemorrhage that is felt to increase the risk of subsequent hemorrhage in this patient
- Major surgery within 14 days
- GI/GU bleeding within the past 21 days
- Noncompressible arterial puncture within the past 7 days
- LP in the previous 7 days
- Systolic BP > 185 or diastolic PB > 110 or requiring aggressive treatment with medications (e.g., nitroprusside)
- Use of warfarin or heparin within the previous 48 h
- Coagulopathy (elevated PTT < PT or platelets < 100,000)—prior use of aspirin or ticlopidine is allowed
- Female who is suspected to be pregnant—must have negative pregnancy test
- Suspected pericarditis
- Hx of significant hepatic disease or end-stage renal disease
- Seizure at onset of stroke
- Coma at the time of admission
- Symptomatic hypoglycemia

Because, in some cases, restoration of blood flow is associated with a dramatic resolution of symptoms, it appears that t-PA may not always directly affect the occluded artery, but may influence primarily collaterals with secondary occlusion due to low blood flow. On the other hand, t-PA must aid in reperfusion of affected brain because a delay in its administration is associated with hemorrhage, suggesting reperfusion.

OTHER STRATEGIES TO IMPROVE REPERFUSION

With rat models of reversible middle cerebral artery occlusion, inhibition of leukocyte adhesion decreases the size of the ischemic lesion. After ischemia, endothelial cells in the affected area increase their expression of the leukocyte adhesion molecule, ICAM-1. Because the size of the ischemic area decreases in animal models when monoclonal antibodies to ICAM-1 are administered during reperfusion, it is presumed that the endothelial response to ischemia slows recovery upon reperfusion. Thus it appears that restoration of blood flow is more complete when leukocyte adhesion is inhibited.

Another factor that may compromise blood flow upon reperfusion is thrombosis in small collateral vessels. Indeed, disruption of such thrombi may be an important component in the action of t-PA. Antithrombotics, such as aspirin or heparin, may also be useful in these cases.

Other strategies to improve blood flow after ischemia have been examined in both experimental animals and patients. Of these, the most extensively studied are hypertension and hemodilution. Induction of hypertension is well established in traumatic brain injury, where elevated intracranial pressure limits cerebral perfusion. Hypertension is also commonly used in the treatment of subarachnoid hemorrhage, where vasospasm of cerebral vessels limits blood flow and may lead to secondary ischemic injury.

Endothelial nitric oxide also plays an important role in reperfusion of brain tissue. Nitric oxide is produced in various tissues, including endothelium, where it serves as an intracellular and intercellular messenger. A potent vasodilator, nitric oxide normally maintains arterial blood flow, although it may also be a mediator of neuronal ischemic injury. Manipulation of nitric oxide levels in animal models of brain ischemia have yielded conflicting results because the outcome depends on the interplay between its effects on blood flow and as a neurotoxin.

Clinically, it is not necessary to control blood pressure within a narrow range during the acute treatment of stroke, except as noted earlier when administering t-PA (Powers, 1993). Although over long periods of time hypertension is a risk factor for stroke, in the acute setting it is likely to improve perfusion. Only when blood pressure is dangerously high is intervention warranted. Although antihypertensive agents are often withheld during the acute treatment period for stroke, this should not be done with those taking β-adrenergic receptor blockers because termination of drug administration could lead to cardiac ischemia.

Prevention of Secondary Recurrence

Stroke studies have consistently demonstrated a relatively high risk of extension of the ischemic area, or of another stroke in a different brain region, over time. This fits with the concept that most strokes are embolic in origin, with the emboli originating in either the heart or on atheromas within vessels. Accordingly, it is believed that early treatment with antithrombotic agents lowers these risks. Information on the effectiveness of this approach is lacking, however, because most published studies focused on late recurrence with patients who were recruited weeks or months after a stroke. Several clinical trials are in progress to examine the utility of early treatment with antithrombotics in preventing extension of the ischemic area and recurrence of the ischemic episode.

The formation and extension of a thrombus results from the action of the platelets and thrombin. Although one or the other of these elements may predominate under different conditions, both prob-

ably contribute to early stroke recurrence. Most of the literature on the effectiveness of antiplatelet agents deals with the long-term use of aspirin or ticlopidine to prevent stroke recurrence in subjects without well-characterized stroke etiologies. These trials are necessarily large because the recurrence risk of stroke in this population is relatively small. More recently, several clinical trials have been undertaken to examine the immediate poststroke period, when the risk of recurrent stroke is highest.

Aspirin. Aspirin (acetylsalicylic acid) irreversibly inhibits cyclo-oxygenase by acetylating a critical serine residue on the enzyme. Cyclo-oxygenase converts arachidonic acid to a variety of eicosanoids including prostaglandins and thromboxanes. Although other effects of aspirin have been described, inhibition of cyclo-oxygenase appears to be critically linked to thrombosis. Because platelets lack a nucleus they are unable to synthesize new enzyme once cyclo-oxygenase has been irreversibly inhibited by aspirin. Thus, the drug need only be administered once daily for this purpose even though its half-life is only about 3 h, because the effect lasts for the lifetime of the platelet.

Aspirin is the most frequently selected therapy for decreasing the risk of recurrent stroke. There have been at least four major clinical trials demonstrating the benefits of aspirin in patients after either TIAs or stroke. A weakness of these trials is that, in general, the end points included events other than recurrent stroke, including death. Thus, the protective effects of aspirin against cardiac ischemia confound the interpretation of some of these studies with respect to recurrent stroke. Nevertheless, aspirin should be used in all patients who are not treated with other antiplatelet or anticoagulant medications.

Although evidence supporting the effectiveness of aspirin in reducing the risk for recurrent stoke is unequivocal, the literature in this area does require some perspective. Thus, the normal risk of recurrent stroke is quite low, only 5 to 10% a year, a figure that is reduced by some 25% with aspirin therapy. Moreover, sometimes the large number of patients needed in these studies is erroneously interpreted as meaning that the clinical significance of aspirin therapy is small. Large groups of patients must be studied even in a relatively high-risk group, however, in case the number of events is small.

On the other hand, there is sometimes the mistaken impression that antiplatelet drugs prevent stroke. Although the drugs decrease the risk for stroke, the rate of recurrent stroke is less than halved in these patients. Those experiencing stroke should be informed of their continuing risk and the relative benefit of aspirin. Because they are at high risk for recurrent stroke they should also be told about new acute therapies that could be used in the event of another stroke.

There is some debate about the optimal dose of aspirin for prevention of secondary strokes (Patrono and Roth, 1996). Clinical data suggest that 75 mg per day might be sufficient to decrease the risk of stroke, just as it is effective in reducing mortality from myocardial infarction. Inasmuch as animal laboratory studies indicate low doses of aspirin are sufficient to completely inhibit cyclo-oxygenase, and the gastrointestinal side effects of this drug are dose-related, questions remain as to whether any additional protection provided by higher doses is outweighed by the risk of side effects. There appears to be a consensus that low doses of aspirin are effective in treating cardiovascular disease, although there is no such consensus concerning the use of aspirin to treat stroke.

Controversy remains about the dose of aspirin necessary to reduce the risk of stroke because there have been no definitive studies on this topic. Thus, higher doses might be of benefit in a subgroup of patients resistant to the antiplatelet effects of aspirin, and it is possible that cyclo-oxygenase inhibition is not the only effect of aspirin that provides benefit in treating cerebrovascular disease because it acetylates a number of proteins. Because low doses of aspirin are effective in preventing cardiac deaths, however, and there are no data suggesting the mechanism of vascular occlusion differs in the cerebral circulation, it seems likely the lower doses should be sufficient for stroke patients as well.

The current practice is to use a low dose (75 mg per day) for reduction of vascular risk in the general population and a medium dose (325 mg per day) in patients at higher risk, lowering it in those experiencing significant side effects. High doses (1300 mg per day) are reserved for patients who continue to have cerebrovascular events despite receiving standard therapy.

The most common side effect of aspirin is gastrointestinal upset, occurring in 2 to 10% of patients at standard analgesic doses. This percentage is much higher (30 to 90%) in those with preexisting ulcer or gastritis. Gastrointestinal side effects include heartburn, nausea, and epigastric distress. These effects are dose-related and are due, at least in part, to local irritation. In general, enteric coated preparations are better tolerated by the majority of patients, even those with chronic ulcer disease or gastritis. It is also best to take aspirin with food or antacids.

Aspirin must be used with caution in patients with active gastrointestinal lesions, such as gastritis or peptic ulcer, and in those with a history of such lesions. It is recommended that these patients be closely monitored, low doses of aspirin be used, and tests for occult gastrointestinal bleeding be performed. Caution should also be exercised when prescribing aspirin to patients who use alcohol or corticosteroids. Aspirin is only absolutely contraindicated in the rare patient with a hypersensitivity to salicylates.

The gastric irritation caused by chronic administration of aspirin can lead to painless occult gastrointestinal bleeding. If the blood loss is significant, iron deficiency anemia can result.

Most toxicities associated with aspirin occur only with doses much higher than those used for stroke prophylaxis, with tinnitus and hearing loss often being the first symptoms of acute or chronic toxicity. These effects usually diminish with a reduction in the dose of aspirin. Acute aspirin overdose causes a metabolic acidosis and is associated with drowsiness, confusion, nausea, and hyperventilation. Death from aspirin overdose can result from multiple organ failure.

Ticlopidine. Ticlopidine blocks platelet aggregation by inhibiting the adenosine diphosphate pathway of platelet aggregation (Murray et al., 1994). Like aspirin, the effects of ticlopidine are irreversible.

In the Ticlopidine Aspirin Stroke Study (TASS), the efficacy of aspirin and ticlopidine were compared for their effectiveness in preventing a second stroke; the results indicated that ticlopidine is superior to aspirin in this regard (Hass et al., 1989). In the 3069 patients studied, the rates of fatal and nonfatal stroke after 3 years were 10% for ticlopine and 13% for aspirin, a 21% greater rate of protection with ticlopidine. The superiority of ticlopidine was maintained throughout the entire 5-year study period.

Diarrhea, often accompanied by abdominal cramps, is the most common side effect of ticlopidine. It can usually be relieved by a temporary reduction in the dose. Bruising, petechiae, epistaxis, and microscopic hematuria were also observed in the clinical trial, although gastrointestinal bleeding was uncommon. Like aspirin, ticlopidine should be discontinued about a week before elective surgery.

Ticlopidine causes hematologic abnormalities in a small percentage of patients, usually within the first 3 months of therapy, with neutropenia being most common, occurring in 2.4% of patients in the clinical trial. Although less common than neutropenia, agranulocytosis may occur and, more rarely, aplastic anemia, pancytopenia, thrombocytopenia, thrombotic thrombocytopenic purpura, and immune thrombocytopenia. Whole blood counts, including platelet counts and white blood cell count differentials, should be monitored every 2 weeks during the first 3 months of ticlopidine therapy. Ticlopidine should be terminated immediately if blood count abnormalities occur, or if the patient develops an infection or bleeding.

Other toxicities associated with ticlopidine include rashes and pruritus, although they are rarely serious. Rash was noted in 5% of the patients in the ticlopidine clinical trial, usually within the first 3 months of treatment. In some cases the drug can be reinstituted without further incident after a drug holiday to allow the rash to resolve.

Like aspirin, ticlopidine should be used with caution in patients with active peptic ulcers or gastritis. Because ticlopidine lacks the irritating effects of aspirin, however, it may be preferred in these subjects. Similarly, ticlopidine must be used with caution in patients with an increased risk of bleeding. Its safety in combination with aspirin, warfarin, and thrombolytics is unknown.

Because ticlopidine is metabolized in the liver it should be used with caution in patients with hepatic disease, and is contraindicated with hepatic failure.

Clopidogrel.   Clopidogrel, which is chemically related to ticlopidine, has a similar mechanism of action. A recent study demonstrated its effectiveness in secondary protection from vascular events (CAPRIE Steering Committee, 1996), and it does not appear to cause hematologic abnormalities. It was recently approved for use in the United States.

Heparin.   Heparin is a naturally occurring family of molecules found in mast cells. The commercial product is generally obtained from lung or gastrointestinal tissue of cattle. A glycosaminoglycan, heparin has an average molecular weight of about 12,000. Because it is administered intravenously and therefore has a quick onset of action, it is the drug of choice when rapid anticoagulation is desired, such as in the acute secondary prevention of stroke. Heparin is used in the highest-risk patients while evaluation proceeds. For chronic treatment, warfarin, an oral anticoagulant, is employed.

Whereas the antiplatelet drugs decrease platelet aggregation and retard the formation and extension of thrombus, heparin and warfarin directly inhibit blood coagulation. In fact, at sufficient doses, heparin can completely inhibit the coagulation process.

Heparin acts as a catalyst to accelerate the rate at which antithrombin III neutralizes thrombin, the enzyme that converts fibrinogen to fibrin. Because fibrin is the major clot-forming plasma protein, blockade of its formation prevents clotting. At lower doses, heparin prevents factor X from converting prothrombin to thrombin.

Although there is little clinical evidence supporting the effectiveness of heparin as an acute therapy in stroke, its use is justified by the data supporting the therapeutic benefits of warfarin because both inhibit coagulation, although by different mechanisms. Because the anticoagulant response to warfarin is delayed, however, and rapid anticoagulation is desirable because the risk of recurrent embolic stroke is highest in the first few days after an event, heparin is used in the acute setting. Thus, heparin is a rapidly acting anticoagulant that is used until the full therapeutic benefit of warfarin is attained.

Because low doses of heparin only prevent thrombin activation, it is probably most useful for preventing thrombus formation, perhaps in the same way that antiplatelet drugs prevent platelet aggregation (International Stroke Trial, 1996). Because high-dose heparin inactivates thrombin, it may be more useful at this dose in those cases where thrombin is already activated and the aim is to prevent thrombus extension. Thus, heparin is theoretically of greater use in preventing a partially thrombosed artery from becoming fully occluded, or in preventing a clot from propagating in an artery.

Because heparin should be particularly useful in situations where thrombus formation has occurred, it is routinely used in fluctuating strokes affecting part of a vascular distribution. Thus, when temporary ischemic symptoms are repetitive and worsening (crescendo TIAs), or fixed and worsening (stroke in evolution), heparin is indicated. If ischemic symptoms are stable, the stroke is considered completed and heparin is not used. Because the vascular events responsible for these conditions cannot be determined, however, and the course of any particular patient is difficult to predict, it is prudent to administer heparin acutely. Thus, stroke extension is quite common following the onset of symptoms and a completed stroke may in fact progress further. Once a stroke suddenly extends to include more of a vascular distribution, it is too late to initiate therapy for secondary prevention.

Low molecular weight heparin may prove to be an important therapeutic option. The low-molecular-weight portion of heparin has been tested in patients with deep venous thrombosis and found to be more effective, and easier to administer, than standard heparin preparations in this condition.

In a small-scale, randomized clinical trial, low-molecular-weight heparin was administered after an acute stroke. The results showed a low risk of hemorrhagic complications with the drug and an improvement in neurological outcome at 6 months as compared with placebo controls. Treatment was initiated within 48 h of the onset of symptoms and continued for 10 days, after which aspirin was administered, even though it is not considered standard care to delay aspirin until 10 to 12 days after the onset of a stroke. Because early aspirin treatment is thought to be effective, it is important to determine how low-molecular-weight heparin compares with aspirin in these patients.

Heparin has no significant effects other than those related to its anticoagulant properties, with hemorrhage being the major adverse effect of this therapy. The hemorrhage can range in severity from bruises to major bouts of bleeding. Of particular concern with heparin is intracranial bleeding associated with hemorrhagic conversion of infarcted brain areas. This has led to some caution in the timing of anticoagulant therapy in patients with cardioembolic stroke. The risk of hemorrhagic conversion is highest in the first 3 days after the onset of symptoms and is correlated with the size of infarction. Thus, it is recommended that anticoagulant administration be delayed in patients with large cardioembolic stroke. Although there is no precise definition of a large stroke, any infarction involving more than a third of a brain hemisphere would be included in this category.

Great caution must be exercised when using heparin in patients with a risk of hemorrhage. This includes postoperative patients and patients with gastrointestinal lesions, such as gastric ulcers, diverticulitis, or colitis. The limited information regarding the therapeutic efficacy of heparin in stroke prevention makes evaluation of risk and benefit difficult. It is suggested that antiplatelet drugs, or low-dose warfarin, be used instead of heparin when there is a significant risk of bleeding.

Heparin can also cause acute, reversible thrombocytopenia by a direct effect on platelets or by stimulating the production of a heparin-dependent platelet aggregating antibody. Because the thrombocytopenia can be mild, even with continued therapy, heparin treatment need only be discontinued if the fall in the platelet count becomes significant (less than 100,000/mm3). Although allergic reactions to heparin occur, they are rare.

Warfarin. Several blood coagulation factors must be carboxylated to be active, an enzymatic process that requires vitamin K. By interfering with the metabolism of vitamin K, warfarin reduces the production of these factors, thereby inhibiting clotting.

It is important to note that warfarin does not directly affect the coagulation process or inactivate functional coagulation factors, with the onset of the anticoagulant effect depending on the time it takes to metabolize activated factors. Thus, warfarin requires several days of continuous administration for maximal efficacy. Increasing the dose during the first few days of therapy does not speed the response and, in fact, may make it more difficult to reach a stable dose.

Warfarin is established as an effective treatment for reducing the risk of cardioembolic stroke. Its effectiveness has been demonstrated for years, with its use in valvular disease and following insertion of artificial valves where stroke risk is high. Until recently, nonvalvular atrial fibrillation was not considered an indication for warfarin treatment. Several recent clinical trials have indicated, however, that warfarin reduces the rate of stroke by 68% in these patients, with no increase in the incidence of major bleeding. In two of these studies warfarin was compared with aspirin. In one study, a 75-mg daily dose of aspirin did not impart any significant benefit; in the other, 325 mg of aspirin per day significantly reduced the risk for stroke in these patients, being particularly beneficial in those with hypertension.

Warfarin has been shown to be more effective than aspirin and the risk of bleeding complications is not as high as commonly assumed (Atrial Fibrillation Investigators, 1994). Indeed, warfarin is the drug of choice for the compliant patient with atrial fibrillation. An exception is younger patients with no other stroke risk factors (i.e. no hypertension, diabetes, smoking history, or cardiac disease). Because the risk for stroke in these patients with "lone atrial fibrillation" is so low the use of warfarin is not justified (Morley et al., 1996).

Warfarin has few significant effects other than those associated with its anticoagulant properties. As with heparin, hemorrhage, ranging from bruises to major episodes of bleeding, is the major adverse effect of warfarin therapy.

The long-term safety of warfarin has been documented in many studies, and with a variety of indications. Hemorrhagic complications are generally associated with excessive plasma levels of the anticoagulant, stressing the need to monitor the patients carefully (The Stroke Prevention in Atrial Fibrillation Investigators, 1996). Complications can occur even with therapeutic blood levels, with excessive hemorrhage associated with ulcers or following a trauma.

Although warfarin-induced necrosis is rare, it can complicate therapy. Most reported cases are in women and occur early in the course of therapy, although not necessarily on the first exposure to the drug. The necrosis involves skin and subcutaneous tissue where fat is abundant, including abdomen, breasts, buttocks, and thighs.

Rarely, allergic reactions and dermatitis occur with warfarin therapy, although a number of gastrointestinal disturbances have been described, including nausea, vomiting, and diarrhea.

Warfarin is contraindicated in pregnancy because multiple fetal malformations and deaths have been documented with the drug under this condition. Because heparin does not cross the placenta it may be preferred during pregnancy if anticoagulant therapy is absolutely necessary.

Extreme caution must be exercised when using warfarin in patients at risk for hemorrhage.

Interactions with other drugs is an important consideration with long-term warfarin therapy because its effectiveness may be increased or decreased by other agents. For example, other drugs could influence the metabolism of warfarin or of coagulation factors. Because such effects can be temporary, adjustments in the dose of warfarin may have to be made repeatedly if other drugs are coadministered.

Because of the potential for life-threatening interactions, patients must inform the physician whenever a new drug is taken. Alcohol and over-the-counter preparations may also have effects, especially preparations containing large amounts of vitamins E or K. Laboratory monitoring should be increased until the effect of the new medication is known and the coagulation values stabilize.

Perspective on Antiplatelet and Warfarin Therapy

Although aspirin decreases the number of strokes in a given population, many patients will still suffer recurrent strokes in spite of the therapy. Nonetheless, the low cost and a favorable side effect profile have made aspirin the drug of choice for chronic therapy in patients at risk for stroke. Patients who are unable to tolerate aspirin should be treated with ticlopidine or clopidogrel (Table 15-2).

For patients who have recurrent stroke or TIA while on aspirin therapy, it is common to escalate the therapy to warfarin. This policy is based on the faulty assumption that aspirin should prevent strokes, an unreasonable conclusion. Because some patients may be resistant to the effects of aspirin, they should be switched to ticlopidine or clopidogrel rather than warfarin.

Neuronal Protection

At present there are no neuroprotectants approved for use in stroke. Although there is strong experimental evidence supporting their efficacy, these drugs are still under clinical investigation.

In cardiac ischemia there are well-developed strategies to simultaneously restore perfusion and protect the myocardium from the injurious effects of an inadequate energy supply. Likewise, neuronal protection strategies are aimed at making brain cells more resistant to ischemia and assisting their recovery once blood flow is restored. Protective therapies for cardiac ischemia lower the workload of the heart. Thus, the energy requirements are lowered by administering drugs that decrease preload and afterload. This treatment enables the heart to pump longer before reaching the point of energy failure and cellular injury. With brain ischemia, a reduction of energy requirements would also be expected to protect the cells and aid in their recovery.

Tissue culture models of brain ischemia have proven valuable in defining the factors that contribute to neuronal vulnerability. Interestingly, these factors are quite similar to those that are important in heart muscle.

Resistance to injury entails preservation and restoration of cellular homeostasis. The major cellular tasks are maintenance of ionic gradients and oxidation of metabolic fuels for energy. Although the neuron maintains gradients for a number of ions, calcium appears to be a critical factor in causing cellular injury (Choi, 1995). Moreover, oxidation must be strictly controlled to maintain the integrity of cellular components; failure to maintain oxidation-reduction homeostasis causes cellular injury (oxidative stress). Although oxidative stress would be expected to be most prominent during reperfusion, cellular homeostasis is also disrupted by the ischemic episode. Free radicals, which mediate oxidative stress, arise not only through mitochondrial oxidative metabolism, but also as a by-product of intracellular signaling mechanisms. Thus, regulation of calcium levels and of the production of free radicals may attenuate the cell damage associated with brain ischemia.

Glutamate and the NMDA receptor. One of the most critical determinants of neuronal vulnerability are excitatory neurotransmitters, glutamic acid being most important in this regard. Other endogenous agents include aspartic acid, N-acetyl-aspartyl-glutamic acid (NAAG), and quinolinic acid.

Table 15-2
Drug List

---

t-PA (recombinant tissue-Plasminogen Activator, Activase). The intravenous dose is 0.9 mg/kg, not to exceed 90 mg.

Aspirin. Administered at 325 mg per day in an enteric coated tablet, reduced to 75 mg per day if gastrointestinal distress is a problem.

Ticlopidine (Ticlid). The usual dose is 250 mg, administered orally, twice daily with food. Complete blood counts (including platelet counts) with leukocyte differentials should be performed before initiation of therapy and every 2 weeks for the first 3 months thereafter. After 3 months, hematologic studies are performed only when clinically indicated.

Heparin. Full-dose intravenous heparin therapy is monitored by measuring the PTT, with a goal of about 2 times control. Continuous infusion by constant-rate infusion pump is strongly recommended for best control of anticoagulation levels. The usual dosage of heparin is about 1000 units per hour.

In patients without cerebral infarction, a bolus of 2500 to 5000 units of heparin is given initially to speed the response. The PTT should be measured every 4 h until a stable value is attained. Because of the risk of intracranial hemorrhage in patients with infarcts, the infusion should be started without an initial bolus in this circumstance. Shortly after a bolus administration the risk of complications is highest. Because the anticoagulant effect of intravenous heparin is immediate, therapy can be closely monitored and individualized for patients to minimize hemorrhagic risk. If there is no therapeutic effect within the first 4 h the infusion rate should be increased to 1200 units per hour.

Warfarin (Coumadin). Therapy is monitored by measuring the INR (international normalized ratio), which is a calibrated version of the prothrombin time. Therapy can be divided into a low range with an INR of 2 to 3 and a high range with an INR of 3 to 5. The higher range is reserved for patients with higher risk, including those with prosthetic heart valves or recurrent systemic embolism. All other patients should be maintained in the lower range.

Therapy should be initiated at 5 mg per day until the INR begins to rise. The INR should be monitored daily until it reaches a stable level, and then checked weekly and then monthly, changing the dosage in small increments to achieve the desired INR.

Pharmacologic and molecular studies have identified four major families of excitatory amino acid receptors. Three of these are ionotropic receptors because they are receptor-gated ion channels. The fourth is a metabotropic receptor coupled to a second messenger system through a G protein.

Of the three ionotropic receptors, the N-methyl-D-aspartate (NMDA) family has been studied most intensively (Fig. 15-3). This receptor is a likely site for mediating cellular injury because its ion channel is permeable to both sodium and calcium. Because calcium plays a critical role in mediating cellular injury, it is not surprising that blockade of NMDA receptors yields a neuroprotective effect in laboratory animal

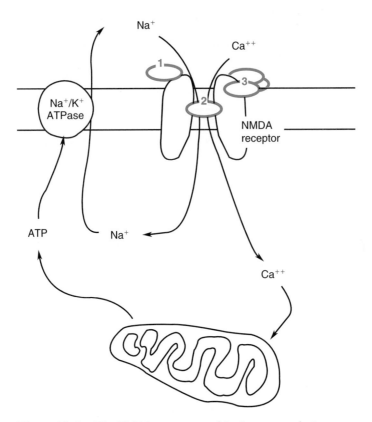

1. Ligand binding site
2. Channel blockade
3. Modulator binding sites

Na⁺

Ca⁺⁺

Na⁺/K⁺ ATPase

NMDA receptor

ATP

Na⁺

Ca⁺⁺

Figure 15–3.   *The NMDA receptor and ionic stresses during ischemia. The NMDA receptor is thought to play a critical role in ischemia because of the large ionic current it conducts when open. Furthermore, as shown, it is permeable to both sodium and calcium ions. Energy demands on mitochondria are indicated by the consumption of ATP by the Na⁺/K⁺ ATPase, which pumps sodium out of the neuron. Mitochondrial buffering of calcium, which may impact energy status, is also shown. The many potential interactions between sodium, calcium, second messenger systems, and energy are not shown for simplicity.*

The complex pharmacology of the NMDA receptor is indicated by the three numbered sites. Site 1 is the agonist binding site where glutamate, the excitatory neurotransmitter, binds. This site can be blocked by competitive receptor antagonists such as APV or CPP. Site 2 is a binding site within the ion channel. When this site is blocked by a noncompetitive agonist, like MK-801 or cerestat, ion movement through the channel is prevented. Site 3 is a collection of modulatory sites that includes binding sites for glycine and polyamines. A site sensitive to oxidation and reduction has also been described. All three of these sites are targets for neuroprotective agents.

models of brain ischemia. Although there is evidence that inhibition of the other ionotropic excitatory amino acid receptors can also yield protective effects in tissue culture and animal models of stroke, only NMDA receptor antagonists are currently being tested in large-scale clinical trials. Given the importance of excitatory amino acids in normal brain function, it would be anticipated that drugs which block the receptors for these substances would have many, and perhaps severe, side effects. Preclinical and clinical studies have shown that although these agents have a negative effect on cognition and are sedating, they appear to be relatively safe, perhaps reflecting the fact that there are few excitatory amino acid receptors outside of the central nervous system. At present, only NMDA receptor antagonists are in advanced clinical trials.

With heart muscle it is sufficient to reduce the workload to make myocytes more resistant to injury. Drastic measures can be taken in this regard, such as those used to preserve hearts for transplantation. There is an upper limit, however, because workload cannot be reduced to a level that would significantly compromise heart function. In brain, it is not necessary to block all excitatory transmission and induce coma to protect neurons from ischemia. Indeed, the goal is not to make neurons impervious to ischemia, only to increase their resistance to the negative effects of low blood flow resulting from arterial occlusion.

There is a great deal of evidence, from both tissue culture and laboratory animal models, that glutamic acid receptor antagonists increase resistance to ischemic injury (Hossmann, 1994a). Initial animal studies focused on global ischemia, mimicking cardiac arrest, in which blood flow is reduced to very low levels for a brief time (less than 30 min). In this case, the injury is confined to the most vulnerable brain regions, most notably the hippocampus. An unusual feature of these models is the delay in the neuronal injury; the hippocampal neurons appear to be normal for several days after the ischemic event, degenerating thereafter. With this delayed time course there is a long period during which neurons can be rescued by blockade of glutamic acid receptors. Indeed, with these models there is a dramatic increase in the amount of extracellular glutamic acid during the ischemic period. Although this glutamic acid may play an important role in triggering neuronal injury, its effects continue during the recovery period because glutamic acid receptor antagonists provide protection even when administered hours after the ischemic event.

Perhaps of greater relevance to stroke therapy are models of focal ischemia in which a single vessel is occluded. Glutamic acid receptor antagonists are effective in this model as well.

It appears that ischemic neuronal injury in the penumbra occurs slowly during the low flow period, with the metabolic and ionic stresses of excitatory neurotransmission increasing tissue vulnerability and speeding the process of energy failure in brain areas experiencing low blood flow. Indeed, repetitive depolarizing events have been recorded in the penumbra, with the associated shifts in ions and pH possibly contributing to the stress on the ischemic tissue.

It is important to determine how much time can pass between the onset of symptoms and initiation of therapy. Thus, it is known that thrombolytic therapy must be initiated promptly, otherwise the risk of cerebral hemorrhage is too great, obviating any advantage of reperfusion. In contrast, the window of opportunity for neuroprotective agents has yet to be defined. In animal studies the time available for decreasing neuronal injury depends on the model, the severity of the ischemic insult, and the drug employed. In some cases, therapy must begin even before the onset of ischemia to be effective. In others, injury can be diminished when drug administration begins as late as 24 h after the insult. The clinical situation is more complex, however, because, unlike the well-defined animal models, vascular occlusion in patients may fluctuate over time. There is also a substantial risk of extension of the ischemic area during the first few days after the stroke (Garcia et al., 1996). Thus, delayed therapy may protect areas that will be exposed to ischemia, rather than rescuing those already damaged.

Neuroprotective Agents

If protection is viewed in the context of metabolic stress, it becomes clear why so many manipulations are capable of reducing ischemic neuronal injury in tissue culture and animal models. Currently, a number of compounds are in late stages of clinical trails as neuroprotectants.

Cerestat. The NMDA receptor antagonist most recently tested in phase III clinical trials, cerestat is a noncompetitive antagonist at this site. This trial has been halted. The chief side effects associated with NMDA receptor blockade are sedation and psychotomimetic effects. Indeed, both phencydidine, a drug of abuse, and ketamine, a dissociative anesthetic, are noncompetitive NMDA receptor antagonists. One of the challenges associated with developing NMDA receptor antagonists has been to define dosage schedules that are neuroprotective but not psychotomimetic.

Cervene (Nalmefene). Cervene is an opiate antagonist that is already used clinically to reverse the effects of opioids. Opioid antagonists display neuroprotective effects in animal models of stroke, perhaps owing to their ability to inhibit glutamic acid release.

Prosynap (Lubeluzole). The mechanism of action of prosynap is unknown, although it has been shown to decrease glutamic acid receptor-mediated injury in tissue culture (Diener et al., 1996; Lesage et al., 1996; Maiese et al., 1997).

Citicoline (Cytidyl diphosphocholine). Citicoline does not seem to act by inhibiting excitatory neurotransmission. An endogenous agent, citicoline is a precursor for lipid synthesis. Pharmacokinetic studies suggest it is largely metabolized to its constituent molecules, cytidine and choline, following oral administration. In rats, orally administered citicoline alters brain lipid composition. In clinical trials, citicoline treatment is being initiated as late as 24 h after the onset of symptoms to test its neuroprotective properties in stroke.

OTHER TREATMENTS

Surgical Therapy

The North American Symptomatic Carotid Endarter-ectomy Trial (NASCET) conclusively showed a benefit of endarterectomy in patients with carotid stenosis of greater than 70% on the symptomatic side. It is important to note that the trial made no distinction between large-vessel or small-vessel occlusion, nor between stroke and TIA. The trial indicated that not only is the risk of stroke recurrence high in these patients, it is highest in the first several weeks after the symptomatic event. This suggests that the maximum benefit of endarterectomy is gained when surgery is performed as soon as possible, within days, after the first event.

For additional information on the drugs discussed in this chapter see chapters 23, 27 and 54 in *Goodman & Gilman's The Pharmacological Basis of Therapeutics* (Ninth Edition), McGraw-Hill, New York, 1996.

REFERENCES

Albers GW: Atrial fibrillation and stroke. Three new studies, three remaining questions. *Arch Intern Med* 1994;154:1443–1448.

Atrial Fibrillation Investigators. Risk factors for stroke and efficacy of antithrombotic therapy in atrial fibrillation. Analysis of pooled data from five randomized controlled trials. *Arch. Intern. Med.,* 1994;154:1449–1457.

Choi DW: Calcium: Still center-stage in hypoxic-ischemic neuronal death. *Trends Neurosci* 1995;18:58–60.

Diener HC, Hacke W, Hennerici M, et al.: Lubeluzole in acute ischemic stroke. A double-blind, placebo-controlled phase II trial. Lubeluzole International Study Group. *Stroke* 1996;27:76–81.

Eliasziw M, Rankin RN, Fox AJ, et al.: Accuracy and prognostic consequences of ultrasonography in identifying severe carotid artery stenosis. North American Symptomatic Carotid Endarterectomy Trial (NASCET) Group. *Stroke* 1995;26:1747–1752.

Feldmann E, Levine SR: Cerebrovascular disease with antiphospholipid antibodies: Immune mechanisms, significance, and therapeutic options. *Ann Neurol* 1995;37(suppl 1):S114–S130.

Garcia JH, Lassen NA, Weiller C, et al.: Ischemic stroke and incomplete infarction. *Stroke* 1996;27:761–765.

Gasecki AP, Eliasziw M, Ferguson GG, et al.: Long-term prognosis and effect of endarterectomy in patients with symptomatic severe carotid stenosis and contralateral carotid stenosis or occlusion: Results from NASCET. North American Symptomatic Carotid Endarterectomy Trial (NASCET) Group. *J Neurosurg* 1995;83:778–782.

Hacke W, Kaste M, Fieschi C, et al.: Intravenous thrombolysis with recombinant tissue plasminogen activator for acute hemispheric stroke. The European Cooperative Acute Stroke Study (ECASS). *JAMA* 1995;274:1017–1025.

Hass WK, Easton JD, Adams HJ, et al.: A randomized trial comparing ticlopidine hydrochloride with aspirin for the prevention of stroke in high-risk patients. Ticlopidine Aspirin Stroke Study Group. *N Engl J Med* 1989;321:501–507.

Hossmann KA: Glutamate-mediated injury in focal cerebral ischemia: The excitotoxin hypothesis revised. *Brain Pathol* 1994a;4:23–36.

Hossmann KA: Viability thresholds and the penumbra of focal ischemia. *Ann Neurol* 1994b;36:557–565.

Kallmes DF, Omary RA, Dix JE, et al.: Specificity of MR angiography as a confirmatory test of carotid artery stenosis. *Am J Neuroradiol* 1996;17:1501–1506.

Lesage AS, Peeters L, Leysen JE: Lubeluzole, a novel long-term neuroprotectant, inhibits the glutamate-activated nitric oxide synthase pathway. *J Pharm Exp Ther* 1996;279:759–766.

Maiese K, TenBroeke M, Kue I: Neuroprotection of lubeluzole is mediated through the signal transduction pathways of nitric oxide. *J Neurochem* 1997;68:710–714.

Morley J, Marinchak R, Rials SJ, Kowey P: Atrial fibrillation, anticoagulation, and stroke. *Am J Cardiol* 1996;77:38A–44A.

Murray JC, Kelly MA, Gorelick PB: Ticlopidine: A new antiplatelet agent for the secondary prevention of stroke. *Clin Neuropharmacol* 1994;17:23–31.

The National Institute of Neurological Disorders and Stroke rt-PA Stroke Study Group. Tissue plasminogen activator for acute ischemic stroke. *N Engl J Med* 1995;333:1581–1587.

Patrono C, Roth GJ: Aspirin in ischemic cerebrovascular disease. How strong is the case for a different dosing regimen? *Stroke* 1996;27:756–760.

Powers WJ: Acute hypertension after stroke: The scientific basis for treatment decisions. *Neurology* 1993;43:461–467.

The Stroke Prevention in Atrial Fibrillation Investigators. Bleeding during antithrombotic therapy in patients with atrial fibrillation. *Arch Intern Med* 1996;156:409–416.

Study design of the International Stroke Trial (IST), baseline data, and outcome in 984 randomized patients in the pilot study. *J Neurol Neurosurg Psychiatry* 1996;60:371–376.

HEADACHE

F. Michael Cutrer, Christian Waeber, and Michael A. Moskowitz

Headache, a common malady experienced by over 90% of the world's population, is among the most frequent reasons for consulting a physician, and among the top three reasons for lost workdays. Rather than a disease, headache is a symptom; which sometimes serves as a valuable warning of hidden pathology. Sometimes the underlying abnormality is readily identified with laboratory and imaging techniques. When the cause is identifiable, the headache often, but not always, responds to effective treatment of the underlying disease. When the origin of the headache is not identifiable, or when treatment of the pathology does not result in resolution of headache, pharmacologic management of the head pain and its associated symptoms is necessary. Pharmacologic treatment of headache is largely empiric and involves many diverse medications. Chronic headaches often require both acute treatments for symptomatic relief and preventive medications that decrease the frequency and severity of attacks. The mechanisms of action of many antiheadache medications are not well defined. As the understanding of the pathophysiology of primary headaches increases, more potent and safer agents may become available.

ANATOMICAL SUBSTRATES OF HEADACHE

A basic understanding of the anatomy of headache has emerged over the past 60 years. The meninges and meningeal and cerebral vessels are key intracranial structures involved in the initial generation of headache. In the late 1930s and 1940s, investigations in awake patients who had undergone craniotomy showed that electrical or mechanical stimulation of meningeal blood vessels produced severe, penetrating, ipsilateral headache (Ray and Wolff, 1940; Penfield, 1935). A similar stimulation of the brain parenchyma caused no pain. Small-caliber pseudounipolar branches of the trigeminal (fifth cranial) nerve and the upper cervical segments innervate the meninges and meningeal vessels and provide most of the somatosensory input that transmits head pain. On activation, these unmyelinated C fibers send nociceptive information from perivascular terminals through the trigeminal ganglia (Mayberg et al., 1981, 1984) and project centrally across synapses onto second-order neurons within the superficial laminae of the medullary trigeminal nucleus caudalis (TNC). These primary afferent neurons co-store substance P, calcitonin gene-related peptide (CGRP), neurokinin A, and other neurotransmitters within their central and peripheral (e.g. meningeal) axon terminals.

The TNC receives inputs from more rostral trigeminal nuclei (Kruger and Young, 1981), the periaqueductal gray, the nucleus raphe magnus (Sessle et al., 1981) and descending cortical inhibitory systems (Sessle et al., 1981; Wise and Jones, 1977) and is an important potential site for the modulation of head pain. Little is known about the role of central trigeminal projections in transmitting nociceptive information. It is believed, however, that second-order neurons within the trigeminal nucleus caudalis transmit nociceptive information to other brainstem and subcortical sites including the more rostral portions of the trigeminal complex (Jacquin et al., 1990), the brainstem reticular formation (Renehan et al., 1986), parabrachial nuclei (Bernard et al., 1989; Hayashi and Tabata, 1990), and the cerebellum (Huerta et al., 1983; Mantle St. John and Tracey, 1987). From the rostral brainstem, nociceptive information is transmitted to limbic areas involved in the emotional and vegetative responses to pain (Bernard et al., 1989). Projections are also sent from the TNC to the ventrobasal (Huang, 1989; Jacquin et al., 1990; Kemplay and Webster 1989; Mantle St. John and Tracey, 1987), the posterior (Peschanski, 1984; Shigenaga et al., 1983) and medial thalamus (Craig and Burton, 1981). From the ventrobasal thalamus, neurons send axonal projections to the somatosensory cortex, where discrimination and localization of pain are thought to occur. The medial thalamus projects to the frontal cortex, where the affective responses to pain are mediated. Evidence indicates, however, that the medial thalamus may participate in the transmission of both the discriminative and affective components of pain (Bushnell and Duncan, 1989). The modulation of nociception may occur at one or more sites from the trigeminal nerve to the cerebral cortex, any of which might be potential targets of drug action.

THEORIES OF HEADACHE PATHOPHYSIOLOGY

Pharmacologic treatment continues to be limited by an incomplete understanding of headache pathophysiology. Testing hypotheses is difficult because headaches are transient and patients are uncomfortable and often vomiting. Animal models mimicking headaches are difficult to develop because of limited knowledge about basic mechanisms and because headache is often part of a symptom complex that begins 24 h before the pain. Activating stimuli may be quite variable. With some patients, an identifiable structural or inflammatory source may be identified using imaging or other techniques. In those who suffer from secondary headaches, treatment of the primary abnormality often results in resolution of the headache. The overwhelming majority of patients, however, suffer from primary headache disorders

like migraine or tension headache in which the physical examination and laboratory studies are normal. Among primary headaches, the research and speculation surrounding migraine pathophysiology have been the most intensive. Traditional theories of migraine fall into two categories:

Vasogenic Theory

In the late 1930s Dr. Harold Wolff and coworkers observed that 1) extracranial vessels become distended and pulsate during a migraine attack in many patients, implying they might be important in migraine; 2) stimulation of intracranial vessels in awake patients causes an ipsilateral headache; and 3) vasoconstrictors, such as ergot alkaloids, abort headache whereas vasodilators, such as nitrates, provoke an attack. Based on these observations, Wolff postulated that intracranial vasoconstriction was responsible for the migraine aura and that headache resulted from a rebound dilation and distention of cranial vessels and activation of perivascular nociceptive axons.

Neurogenic Theory

The alternative hypothesis, the neurogenic theory, holds that the brain is the generator of migraine, and that the susceptibility of any individual reflects thresholds intrinsic to that organ. Supporters of this theory hold that the vascular changes occurring during migraine are the result, rather than the cause, of the attack. They note that migraine attacks are often accompanied by a range of neurologic symptoms that are both focal (in the aura) and vegetative (in the prodrome) in nature and which cannot be explained by vasoconstriction within a single neurovascular distribution.

It is likely that neither of these two theories explains the pathophysiology of migraine or other primary headache disorders. Headaches, including migraine, probably result from a variety of genetic and acquired factors, some of which are intrinsic to brain, others to blood vessels or circulating substances. Thus, Ophoff and colleagues recently reported that point mutations in the gene encoding the alpha 1 subunit of the P/Q calcium channel causes familial hemiplegic migraine (Ophoff et al., 1996).

URGENT EVALUATION AND MANAGEMENT OF SEVERE HEADACHE IN THE EMERGENCY DEPARTMENT

Optimal management of a patient arriving at the emergency department complaining of severe headache (Cutrer, 1995; Edmeads, 1988) requires rapid recognition of whether it represents a severe episode of a primary headache disorder or is secondary to, or symptomatic of, a potentially dangerous underlying abnormality. Several elements of the history and physical exam are crucial in making this distinction.

Elements in the History Suggestive of Headaches of Ominous Cause

1. When the headache is unlike anything experienced previously, the risk of symptomatic headache increases. If it is similar to attacks experienced over many months or years, the probability of a benign process increases. After the age of 40, the probability of a first attack of migraine decreases and the incidence of neoplasm and other intracranial pathology increases.
2. If the headache begins suddenly, reaches maximal intensity within minutes, and persists for several hours, this is cause for concern. Headaches due to subarachnoid hemorrhage have been described as "being hit in the head with a baseball bat." Primary headache disorders like migraine and tension headache usually intensify over 30 min to 1 h. Although cluster headaches intensify rapidly, they generally don't persist beyond 3 h.
3. If there is a history of alteration in consciousness or change in mental status before or accompanying the onset of headache, patients warrant laboratory investigation. Although migraineurs may appear fatigued, especially after prolonged vomiting or analgesic use, obtundation and confusion during the course of the headache are not common. Rather they are more suggestive of intracranial hemorrhage or central nervous system (CNS) infection, although they may occur during poorly understood syndromes such as basilar migraine.
4. If there is recent or coexistent infection in extracranial sites such as lungs, sinuses, or mastoids, the risk of secondary headache increases. Such infections may serve as a nidus for subsequent CNS infections like meningitis or brain abscess.
5. If headache begins during the course of vigorous exercise or exertion, or soon after head or neck trauma, it may suggest subarachnoid hemorrhage or carotid dissection. Effort-induced headache or coital migraine are relatively rare. The rapid onset of headache during strenuous exercise, especially if minor head or neck trauma has occurred, should increase the suspicion of carotid artery dissection or intracranial hemorrhage.
6. Radiation of pain below the neck and into the back is not typical of migraine and may indicate meningeal irritation due to infection or blood.

Other elements of the history that can help in evaluating severe headache include:

1. Family history. While migraine has a strong familial tendency, secondary headaches are usually spontaneous.
2. Current medications. Certain medications cause headache as a side effect and anticoagulants and oral antibiotics place the patient at greater risk for hemorrhage or partially treated CNS infection.
3. History of neurologic abnormality. Old neurologic findings may confuse interpretation of the examination.
4. Location of the headache. Benign headache disorders tend to change sides and locations, at least occasionally.

Important Findings on Physical Examination

1. Nuchal rigidity may indicate either meningitis or subarachnoid hemorrhage.
2. Papilledema reflects an increase in intracranial pressure, increasing the likelihood of tumor or hemorrhage and therefore warranting further investigation.
3. Any impairment of consciousness or orientation must be evaluated urgently.

4. Toxic appearance: Fever is *not* a common occurrence with primary headache disorder. Even low-grade fever, or persistent tachycardia or bradycardia, should be considered as a sign of an underlying infectious cause.
5. Any previously unnoticed neurologic abnormality.

New findings such as a slight pupillary asymmetry, a unilateral pronator drift, or an extensor plantar response increase the probability of intracranial abnormality. It is important to reexamine patients frequently, as the neurologic findings may change. (See Fig. 16-1 for algorithm of acute management of severe headache in the emergency department.)

SECONDARY OR SYMPTOMATIC HEADACHES

Differential Diagnosis, Clinical Features, and Chronic Management of Secondary Headaches

Headaches may result from a host of intracranial and extracranial abnormalities and it is often crucial they be diagnosed quickly and treated appropriately. Treating the underlying cause of most secondary headaches improves the headache as well. Describing the management of secondary headaches is beyond the scope of this chapter. In a few instances, however, drugs may be required for pain control when definitive treatment of the underlying process is either not possible or does not resolve the headache. In these cases, specific management recommendations are made following the clinical features of the syndrome.

Described in the following are some of the more commonly encountered secondary headache disorders.

Posttraumatic headaches.   Chronic headaches may appear after either closed or open head injuries, or following cranial surgery. The severity of the headache often does not correlate with the severity of the injury (Yamaguchi, 1992). The characteristics of posttraumatic headaches may closely resemble primary headache disorders. In one series of 48 patients suffering from chronic posttraumatic headache, 75% experienced headaches classified as tension-type, 21% had headaches clinically indistinguishable from migraine without aura, and 4% had headaches described as "unclassifiable" (Haas, 1996). Quite often in these circumstances a mixed pattern emerges. Headaches occurring daily are usually described as constant and nonthrobbing, punctuated by severe migraine-like attacks and/or frequent brief episodes of sharp, jabbing pain. The International Headache Society classifies headache that disappears within 8 weeks of the injury as acute and those that persist longer as chronic (Headache Classification Committee of IHS, 1988).

Headache following craniotomy is quite variable and may consist of pain and soreness at the incision site; tight, pressure-like discomfort similar to tension-type headache; or throbbing pain usually associated with migraine. Postsurgical headaches are usually not accompanied by nausea, vomiting, or photophobia; however, these migraine-like symptoms are occasionally reported.

Management.   Posttraumatic headaches are managed by several strategies. Cognitive and behavioral methods such as biofeedback and relaxation training are often beneficial, providing patients with strategies for coping with chronic pain. There have been few drug trials for the treatment of posttraumatic headache. One uncontrolled study found that amitriptyline therapy led to improvement in over 90% of patients. (Tyler et al., 1980). There are anecdotal reports of positive responses to doxepin, nortriptyline, imipramine, and selective serotonin reuptake inhibitors (Young and Packard, 1997). Posttraumatic headaches may improve with valproate or gabapentin therapy, either separately or in combination with amitriptyline. These agents are particularly helpful when a posttraumatic seizure disorder is also present. Physical therapy is useful when muscle spasm is persistent and antidepressants are of benefit when depression and anxiety are present.

Infectious.   Headaches may occur with a variety of systemic and intracranial infections. Head pain may accompany trivial febrile illness or may be the harbinger of a potentially fatal CNS infection, making it essential to evaluate the headache within the context of other symptoms. The following is a brief summary of the most important infectious causes of headache that can be treated with antibiotics and/or surgery.

Meningitis, or inflammation of the meninges, is caused by bacterial, viral, mycobacterial, or fungal infection. Meningitis can follow a brief systemic illness or may appear without antecedent infection. The usual symptoms of meningitis are: severe headache, fever, neck pain, photophobia, and stiffness. Additional symptoms may include seizures, rash, or altered mental status. An urgent evaluation including lumbar puncture is crucial if papilledema is not present. When focal findings are present, such as unilateral or focal weakness, eye movement abnormality, pupillary abnormality, or altered mental status, a CT scan, preferably with contrast, should be performed immediately to rule out the presence of a posterior fossa tumor, abscess, or hematoma whose presence would make a lumbar puncture risky. If bacterial meningitis is suspected, however, *waiting for an imaging study should not delay antibiotic treatment* nor should it inordinately delay lumbar puncture.

Meningoencephalitis refers to inflammation in both the meninges and underlying brain parenchyma. It may result from viral infections such as herpes meningoencephalitis. Meningoencephalitis often follows a brief flu-like illness and may be clinically similar to meningitis although its onset is sometimes less sudden. Seizures or mental status changes may occur in the days before presentation. CSF examination may reveal high protein or a lymphocytic pleocytosis. An MRI or CT showing temporal lobe involvement can confirm the diagnosis.

Brain abscess due to bacterial infection is a focal collection of inflammatory and necrotic material within brain. It may develop by direct or hematogenous spread, most commonly including streptococcus, staphylococcus, and anaerobes. Headache, vomiting, focal neurologic signs, and depressed mental status may occur as the result of mass effect and edema.

Subdural empyema is a collection of pus between the brain parenchyma and the dura mater that can manifest as headache, vomiting, altered mental status, and focal neurologic deficits.

AIDS may cause headache during acute and chronic HIV infection and AIDS-related opportunistic infections such as *Cryptococcus* and *Toxoplasma gondii*. In addition, medications for the treatment of both HIV (AZT, 3-TC) and opportunistic infections (fluconazole, amphotericin B) may also cause headache.

Acute sinusitis may cause frontal headache or facial pain. The presence of other features such as sinus opacification on x-ray or transillumination, fever, or purulent nasal discharge should be confirmed before making this diagnosis and beginning antibiotic therapy. Many patients assume that frontal headache means sinusitis. Sphenoid or maxillary sinusitis can mimic migraine.

Upper respiratory or systemic viral infection may cause mild to moderate headache. These minor infections are not associated with neck stiffness, photophobia, or changes in mentation.

Vascular. Severe headaches may be a symptom of occluded intracranial vessels and leakage from weakened or damaged vascular structures. Blood within the subarachnoid space is a potent chemical irritant that may cause severe headache and neck stiffness. Cerebral ischemia may also cause headache. The following vascular abnormalities may be associated with headache.

Subarachnoid hemorrhage, most often the result of leakage from an aneurysmal vessel, is a neurosurgical emergency and can be identified by CT scan or lumbar puncture. The aneurysm itself can be localized by arteriogram.

Clinical features suggesting subarachnoid hemorrhage require urgent evaluation with CT and/or lumbar puncture and include the following:

1. Explosive onset of pain with maximal intensity in seconds
2. Severe intensity of pain, classically described as "the worst headache of my life."
3. Nuchal rigidity or stiff neck as a result of muscle spasm.
4. A rapid decrease in the level of consciousness due to brainstem compression.
5. Other, less specific, features include photophobia and vomiting.

Before a full-blown subarachnoid hemorrhage, small "sentinel bleeds" or warning leaks may occur that are qualitatively similar but of lesser intensity. These warnings must be evaluated promptly as they can be followed by a larger hemorrhage within 2 to 14 days. Minor focal findings may also develop owing to aneurysm expansion and compression of adjacent structures.

Subdural hematoma, a collection of blood between the dura mater and the brain substance, often presents as a dull, continuous headache. Subdural hematomas can occur after minor head trauma but also may occur spontaneously, especially in the elderly or in patients taking anticoagulants.

Cerebellar hemorrhage is a neurosurgical emergency that can present as a posterior headache followed rapidly by signs of brainstem compression such as altered mental status, pupillary or eye movement abnormalities, or focal weakness.

Arteriovenous malformations (AVMs) are congenital vascular anomalies that shunt blood past capillary beds from arterial to venous structures. AVMs can cause ipsilateral headache and in some instances are associated with visual and sensory symptoms similar to the migraine aura. Occasionally an AVM is detected by listening for a bruit over the orbit or head. AVMs can also bleed which results in a more precipitous headache and focal neurologic deficits.

Intracerebral arterial occlusions with infarction can sometimes be accompanied by headache. In general, however, the clinical picture of stroke is dominated by persistent neurologic deficit rather than headache. Cerebral venous sinus occlusion can be associated with headache and neurologic deficits. Cavernous sinus thrombosis is associated with severe ocular pain and injection combined with cranial nerve III, V_1, V_2, and VI abnormalities. Sagittal sinus thrombosis can be manifested as headache, seizures, and focal neurologic signs on examination.

Carotid artery dissection occurs as blood separates muscular layers of the carotid artery following intimal damage. Carotid artery dissection may follow seemingly minor head or neck trauma such as neck turning in taxi-cab drivers, and may cause severe head and neck pain that can be referred to the brow, eye, orbit, or mastoid area. Neurologic signs sometimes occurring with carotid artery dissection may include: 1) tongue paralysis, if cranial nerve XII is affected (presumably via mechanical pressure on ansa cervicalis in the neck); or Horner's syndrome if sympathetic fibers in the pericarotid plexus are involved. Treatment may entail antico-

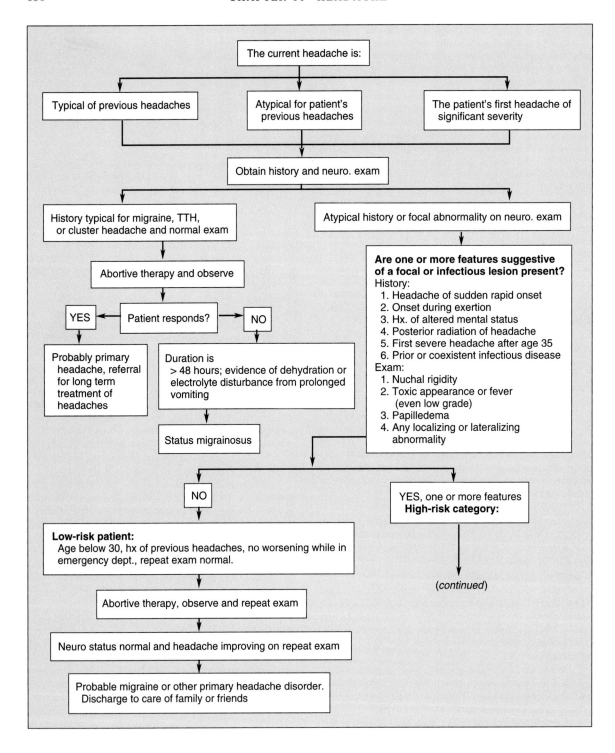

The current headache is:

- Typical of previous headaches
- Atypical for patient's previous headaches
- The patient's first headache of significant severity

Obtain history and neuro. exam

History typical for migraine, TTH, or cluster headache and normal exam

Atypical history or focal abnormality on neuro. exam

Abortive therapy and observe

Patient responds?   →   YES / NO

Are one or more features suggestive of a focal or infectious lesion present?
History:
1. Headache of sudden rapid onset
2. Onset during exertion
3. Hx. of altered mental status
4. Posterior radiation of headache
5. First severe headache after age 35
6. Prior or coexistent infectious disease
Exam:
1. Nuchal rigidity
2. Toxic appearance or fever (even low grade)
3. Papilledema
4. Any localizing or lateralizing abnormality

Probably primary headache, referral for long term treatment of headaches

Duration is > 48 hours; evidence of dehydration or electrolyte disturbance from prolonged vomiting

Status migrainosus

NO

YES, one or more features
High-risk category:

Low-risk patient:
Age below 30, hx of previous headaches, no worsening while in emergency dept., repeat exam normal.

Abortive therapy, observe and repeat exam

Neuro status normal and headache improving on repeat exam

Probable migraine or other primary headache disorder. Discharge to care of family or friends

(continued)

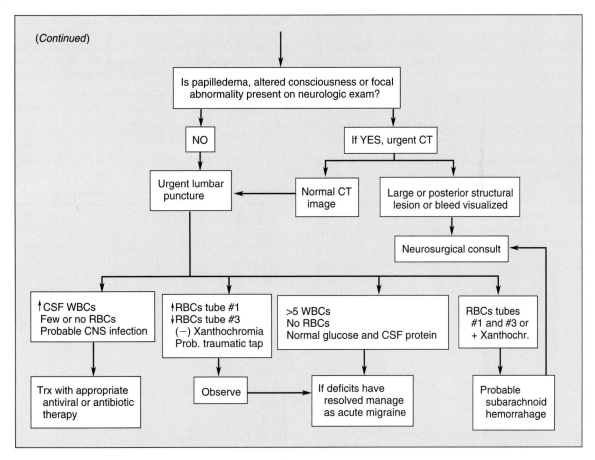

(Continued)

Figure 16–1. *Algorithm for evaluation of severe headache in the emergency department.*

agulation for 3 months followed by antiplatelet therapy for a similar period. Resection of the residual dissecting aneurysm that might be the source of embolization should be considered if technically feasible (Mokri, 1997).

Neoplastic. *Intracranial tumors.* Many patients are concerned they have an undiagnosed intracranial tumor. Fortunately, the overwhelming majority of headache patients do not have an underlying structural lesion. It is, however, important to identify those who do.

In a series of 111 consecutive patients with CT or MRI proven brain tumor, Forsyth and Posner found that 48% reported chronic headache. Tumor-associated headaches were usually dull and bifrontal, although they tended to be worse on the side of the tumor (Forsyth and Posner, 1992). They were

more often qualitatively similar to tension-type headache (77%) than migraine (9%) and tended to be intermittent and of moderate intensity (median of 7 on a 10 point scale). These headaches were accompanied by nausea about half the time. The headaches occurring in patients with increased intracranial pressure were usually resistant to conventional analgesics. "Classic" brain-tumor headache which tends to be progressive beginning in the morning, occurred in only 17% of the patients in this study.

No headache type is specific for a brain tumor. Factors that should increase suspicion of an intracranial tumor include papilledema, new neurologic deficits, first prolonged headache occurring after the age of 45, previous malignancy, cognitive abnormality, or altered mental status.

Treatment of headaches associated with intracranial tumors. With intracranial tumors, headache may improve after surgical resection or radiotherapy. If surgical resection is antic-ipated within a short time, aspirin and other nonsteroidal anti-inflammatory agents should be avoided because they increase the risk of bleeding. For tumors not amenable to surgery, symptomatic treatment is necessary. If headaches are mild to moderate, then routine analgesics are often effective, whereas if the pain is severe, opioids may be useful. Significant edema surrounding the tumor can be treated with steroids (dexamethasone 4 mg orally every 6 h) or mannitol (20% in 200-mL IV every 8 h), both of which may improve the headache secondarily.

Autoimmune/inflammatory.   Temporal arteritis (giant cell arteritis) is an inflammatory vasculitis involving branches of the temporal arteries. It most usually affects individuals over the age of 60 and can result in rapid and permanent loss of vision due to granulomatous occlusion of the posterior ciliary or central retinal arteries. Features suggestive of temporal arteritis are:

1.   Orbital or frontotemporal headaches described as a dull and constant with superimposed jabbing sensations.
2.   Pain aggravated by cold.
3.   Pain in the jaw or tongue, pain on chewing (jaw claudication).
4.   Accompanying constitutional symptoms such as weight loss, anemia, mononeuropathy, and elevated liver function tests.
5.   Decreased visual acuity, visual field cuts, pale or swollen optic disk, retinal splinter hemorrhages (anterior ischemic neuropathy) or pale retina, cherry red spot (central retinal artery infarction).

Proper therapy is crucial as transient visual symptoms can progress rapidly to permanent blindness. When this diagnosis is suspected, prompt treatment with corticosteroids is necessary to avoid visual loss that becomes bilateral in 75% of cases after unilateral loss. Erythrocyte sedimentation rate (ESR) is elevated in 95% of these cases. A definitive diagnosis is made on pathologic findings on temporal artery biopsy that can be obtained within 48 h after initiating steroid treatment. ***Treatment (Adams and Biller, 1990).***   In patients with a positive ESR, intravenous methylprednisolone 500 to 1000 mg every 12 h for 48 h should be followed by oral prednisone 80 to 100 mg per day for 14 to 21 days, followed by a gradual taper over 12 to 24 months. The tapering rate should be guided by serial ESRs.

Tolosa-Hunt syndrome is a granulomatous process within and around the cavernous sinus or superior orbital fissure resulting in painful ophthalmoplegia and sensory loss on the forehead. Treatment includes steroid therapy. ***Autoimmune inflammatory process.***   Headache can be a feature of collagen vascular disorders or autoimmune angiopathies like isolated angiitis of the central nervous system. The headache usually diminishes following treatment of the underlying vasculitis.

Toxic/metabolic.   ***Substance-induced   headache.***   Headaches can occur with acute exposure to some substances or as a result of drug withdrawal after chronic intake (Table 16-1). ***Metabolic abnormalities and headache.***   Several metabolic disturbances may result in headache. These include (Headache Classification Committee of IHS, 1988):

1.   Hypercapnia-induced headache when arterial pCO_2 is above 50 mm Hg without hypoxia.

Table 16-1
Substances Known to Induce Headache

Substances inducing headache with acute exposure
Alcohol
Amphotericin B
Carbon monoxide
Cimetidine
Cocaine/crack
Danazol
Diclofenac
Dipyridamole
Estrogen/oral contraceptives
Fluconazole
Indomethacin
Monosodium glutamate
Nifedipine
Nitrates/nitrites
Ondansetron
Phenylethylamine
Ranitidine
Reserpine
Tyramine
3-TC
Verapamil
Substances inducing headache on withdrawal after chronic use
Alcohol
Barbiturates
Caffeine
Ergotamine
Opioid analgesics

2. Hypoglycemia-induced headache when blood glucose is below 2.2 mmol/L (<60 mg/dL).

3. Dialysis-induced headache during or shortly after hemodialysis. The headache subsides within 24 h after termination of dialysis. To avoid dialysis headache, the rate of dialysis should be decreased.

4. High-altitude headache usually occurs within 24 h after sudden ascent to altitudes above 3000 m. The headache is usually accompanied by at least one of the other symptoms of altitude sickness, which include Cheyne-Stokes respiration at night, marked exertional dyspnea, or desire to overbreathe.

5. Hypoxia-induced headache, usually seen in the context of a low-pressure environment or pulmonary disease causing an arterial $PO_2 < 70$ mm Hg.

6. Sleep apnea-induced headache, probably also related to hypoxia and hypercapnea.

Treatment of the underlying metabolic disturbance results in improvement in headache.

Ocular abnormality. *Glaucoma.* Two forms of glaucoma present with headache:

1. Pigmentary glaucoma, a form of open angle glaucoma, occurs when pigment from the iris is liberated into the aqueous during exercise and subsequently blocks outward flow through the trabecular meshwork. The patients, frequently young myopic males, present with exercise-induced headache and blurred vision.

2. Acute angle closure glaucoma, in which the free flow of aqueous through the pupil is blocked, results in forward bulging of the iris with obstruction of the trabecular meshwork. It presents with a dilated, unresponsive pupil, visual blurring, severe ocular pain, a red injected eye, cloudy cornea, and marked elevation in intraocular pressure. Episodes are precipitated by dilation of the eye, either physiologic or pharmacologic.

Management. Both types of glaucoma require urgent opthalmologic referral. For acute angle-closure glaucoma laser iridotomy is often necessary.

Glaucoma is sometimes confused with cluster headache. In cluster headache, the pupil is small rather than dilated and ptosis is often present.

Hypertensive headache. Extreme elevations in arterial blood pressure (diastolic pressures > 120 mm Hg) can be associated with headache. Hypertensive headaches are often diffuse and tend to peak in intensity in the morning, with gradual resolution over several hours.

Four categories of headache are associated with severe hypertension (Headache Classification Committee of IHS, 1988).

1. Acute pressor response to an exogenous agent. Headache occurs in temporal association with blood pressure rise due to specific toxins or medications and resolves within 24 h after normalization of blood pressure.

2. Preeclampsia or eclampsia. In pregnant and peripartum women, headache may accompany other features of preeclampsia such as elevated blood pressure, proteinuria, and edema. The headache generally resolves within 7 days of reducing blood pressure or terminating the pregnancy.

3. Pheochromocytoma, an epinephrine-secreting adrenal tumor, may cause brief headaches accompanied by sweating, anxiety, or palpitations and extreme hypertension.

4. Malignant hypertension, including hypertensive encephalopathy, causes headache associated with grade 3 or 4 retinopathy and/or altered mental status. In this case the headache is temporally related to the hypertensive episode and disappears within 2 days of reducing blood pressure.

Low-pressure and high-pressure headaches. *Low-pressure headaches.* Decreased intracranial pressure (ICP below 50 to 90 mm H_2O) which is usually caused by a decrease in CSF volume, is commonly associated with dull, throbbing headaches, sometimes of severe intensity. Probably owing to reduced brain buoyancy (Horton and Fishman, 1994) and subsequent traction on pain sensitive meningeal and vascular structures (Campbell and Caselli, 1991), low-pressure headaches become more intense on standing or sitting upright and are relieved with recumbency. The headaches can begin gradually or suddenly and may be accompanied by dizziness, visual symptoms, photophobia, nausea, vomiting, and diaphoresis (Lay et al., 1997). Although low-pressure headaches may begin spontaneously, they most commonly follow a lumbar puncture (LP). Other possible etiologies include intracranial surgery, ventricular shunting, trauma, and various systemic medical conditions such as severe dehydration, postdialysis, diabetic coma, uremia, or hyperpnea. If the headache is prolonged the possibility of a persistent CSF leak may be investigated with radioisotope cisternography or CT myelography.

Postlumbar puncture headaches may be caused by excessive leakage of CSF through the dural tear caused by the LP needle. Headaches follow 10 to 30% of LPs and occur twice as frequently in women as in men. The headache may begin from minutes to several days after the lumbar puncture and can persist from 2 days to 2 weeks (Lay et al., 1997). Treatment strategies may include corticosteroids, oral fluid or salt intake, intravenous fluids, CO_2 inhalation, and methylxanthines such as theophylline (300 mg three times per day) (Feuerstein and Zeides, 1986), caffeine (500 mg IV) (Sechzer and Abel, 1978), or intrathecal autologous blood patch.

Headaches associated with increased intracranial pressure (ICP). Headaches that occur with increased intracranial pressure are caused by deformation of pain-sensitive dural or vascular structures, or direct pressure on cranial nerves involved in nociception, such as the trigeminal nerve (Kunkle et al., 1943). Although the location of these headaches is variable, most commonly the pain is bilateral and in the fronto-temporal region (Wall, 1990). Intracranial pressure may be elevated owing to mass lesion, blockage of CSF circulation, hemorrhage, hypertensive encephalopathy, venous sinus thrombosis, hyperadrenalism or hypoadrenalism, altitude sickness, tetracycline, or vitamin A intoxication, to name only a few. In most instances, the source of headache and raised pressure are identifiable. Treatment of the underlying condition generally improves the headache.

Idiopathic intracranial hypertension (pseudotumor cerebri) is a syndrome comprised of headache, papilledema, and transient visual symptoms that occurs in the absence of CSF abnormalities except for an elevated intracranial pressure. In one series of 12 patients, however, papilledema was not present (Mathew et al., 1996). The syndrome is not associated with hydrocephalus or other identifiable causes. In adults, females have an 8 to 10 times higher incidence of this condition than males (Durcan et al., 1988). The typical patient is an overweight woman of child-bearing age.

The diagnosis of idiopathic intracranial hypertension is made by lumbar puncture (CSF pressure > 250 mm Hg; normal CSF composition) after neuroimaging to exclude a mass lesion. Visual field testing often reveals an enlarged blind spot. While spontaneous recovery is characteristic, treatment to reduce ICP is usually implemented to prevent visual loss. Frequent lumbar punctures may sometimes be effective, although they are not without risks of complications such as postlumbar puncture headache, hindbrain herniation, spinal epidermoid tumor, or infection (Corbet, 1997; Batnitzky et al., 1977). Drug therapies are aimed primarily at reducing CSF production and include acetazolamide and furosemide. Furosemide, a potent loop diuretic, must be given with potassium supplementation and may cause hypotension. Surgical options include optic nerve fenestration and ventricular-peritoneal shunting of CSF.

PRIMARY HEADACHE DISORDERS

Chronic headaches encountered in clinical practice are most commonly the result of headache disorders for which there is no identifiable cause. In fact, the diagnosis of a primary headache disorder is made by excluding other diseases by careful history, physical examination, and judicious laboratory testing. The criteria separating various primary headache syndromes are symptom-based and may or may not reflect differences in pathophysiology (see Fig. 16-2). In 1988 the International Headache Society published a series of guidelines for the classification and diagnosis of the major primary disorders (Headache Classification Committee of IHS, 1988). These IHS criteria are extremely valuable in clinical research, and the essentials of the published criteria are included when describing each of the primary disorders. It must be remembered, however, that these criteria are not absolute. Patients may have features of more than one headache syndrome and may respond to treatment even though they do not meet clinical criteria for a single diagnosis.

Differential Diagnosis and Clinical Features of Primary Headache Disorders

Tension-type headache (TTH). Although tension-type headache is undoubtedly the most common of the primary headache disorders (Rasmussen, 1991), patients infrequently consult a physician. The term "tension-type headache" (TTH) encompasses many syndromes known variously as essential headache, muscle contraction headache, and psycho-myogenic headache and occurs in both episodic and chronic forms. As with all primary headache disorders, details of its pathogenesis and the importance of muscle contraction are poorly understood. Pericranial muscle spasm or tenderness is not consistently present.

The IHS defines TTH as mild to moderate, recurrent bilateral headaches that feel tight or pressing and last minutes to days. Tension-type headaches may be associated with photophobia or phonophobia, but are not made worse by routine physical activity, or associated with nausea or vomiting. (See Table 16-2 TTH for IHS Diagnostic Criteria.) Episodic TTH differs from the chronic form in that the diagnosis may be made with as few as 10 attacks in a lifetime, whereas in the chronic form TTHs are present 15 days per month for at least 6 months and nausea may be present.

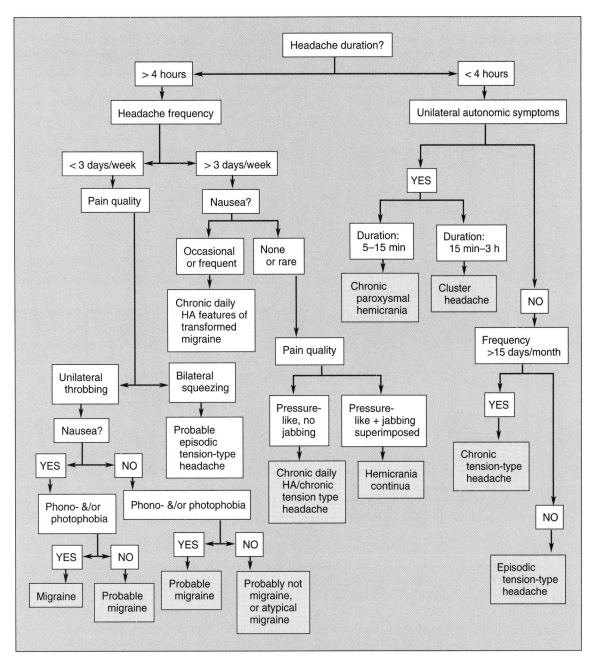

Figure 16–2. *Algorithm for diagnosis of primary headache disorders.*

Table 16-2
Diagnostic Criteria for Tension-Type Headache

A. Headache lasts from 30 min to 7 days.
B. At least two of the following pain characteristics:

1. Pressing/tightening (nonpulsatile) quality
2. Mild or moderate intensity (may inhibit, but
   does not prohibit activities)
3. Bilateral location
4. No aggravation by walking stairs or similar
   routine physical activity

C. Both of the following:

1. No nausea or vomiting (anorexia may occur)
2. Photophobia and phonophobia are absent, or
   one but not the other is present

D. Headaches not correlated to another physical
abnormality

Adapted from IHS criteria

Migraine. Migraine is the second most common
primary headache disorder and has a prevalence of
about 12%. It affects women disproportionately (approximately 17.6% of women vs. 6% of men in the
United States) (Stewart et al., 1992) and afflicts patients commonly during the most productive years
of their life. Migraine falls into two categories: 1)
migraine without aura, previously called common
migraine and 2) migraine with aura, previously called
classic migraine. Patients with aura experience transient episodes of focal neurologic dysfunction 1 to
2 h before the onset of a migraine headache. Patients
with migraine may report prodromal symptoms that
begin 24 to 48 h before a headache attack. These
symptoms can include hyperactivity, mild euphoria,
lethargy, depression, cravings for certain foods, fluid
retention, frequent yawning, and other atypical
symptoms. Prodromal symptoms should not be confused with migraine aura.

Headache features are similar in migraine with

and without aura. Typically they consist of unilateral
throbbing head pain of moderate to severe intensity
that is worsened by routine physical exertion and is
associated with nausea, photophobia, and phonophobia (Table 16-3).

The aura symptoms may be of different types,
and more than a single symptom type may be present
within a given aura. Typical aura symptoms include
the following: 1) homonymous, rarely monocular, visual disturbance, classically an expanding scotoma
with a scintillating margin; 2) unilateral paresthesias
and/or numbness, often affecting the distal extremities
or the perioral region of the face; 3) unilateral weakness; and 4) dysphasia or other language disturbance.

Sometimes aura symptoms localize to the brainstem and may include vertigo, dysarthria, tinnitus,
fluctuating hearing loss, diplopia, bilateral weakness,
ataxia, bilateral paresthesias, and/or a decreased level
of consciousness. Patients in whom brainstem symptoms predominate are given the diagnosis of basilar
migraine. These symptoms can occur with anxiety
and hyperventilation and in many patients basilar
attacks are intermingled with more typical migraine
attacks. Dizziness is frequently reported as a feature
of an otherwise typical attack of migraine with aura.

Familial hemiplegic migraine (FHM), a relatively rare migraine syndrome in which attacks are
sometimes associated with prolonged unilateral
weakness, has been localized to the short arm of
chromosome 19 (19 p 13), although in several families (Ophoff et al., 1996) preliminary data indicate
localization to chromosome 1q as well (Gardener et
al., 1997). FHM is the first identified migraine syndrome caused by mutations in a single gene (Ophoff
et al., 1996). For this diagnosis, a patient must experience recurrent hemiparesis in the context of migraine
attack and have at least one first-degree relative with
identical attacks. Random cases of hemiplegic migraine do not show this genetic mutation.

Complicated migraine, or migraine with prolonged aura, refers to migraine attacks occasionally
associated with persistent aura for more than 1 h,
but less than 1 week, and in which neuroimaging
studies are normal. If symptoms persist for more than
1 week and/or result in neuroimaging abnormalities,
then migrainous infarction is likely. In general, mi-

Table 16-3

Diagnostic Criteria for Migraine With and Without Aura

Diagnostic criteria for migraine without aura

A. At least five headache attacks lasting 4–72 h (untreated or treated unsuccessfully)

B. Headaches have at least two of the following characteristics:

1. Unilateral location
2. Pulsating quality
3. Moderate or severe intensity (inhibit or prohibit daily activity)
4. Aggravation by walking stairs or similar routine physical activity

C. During headache, at least one of the following:

1. Nausea and/or vomiting
2. Photophobia and phonophobia

D. Headaches not correlated to another physical abnormality

Diagnostic criteria for migraine with aura

A. In addition to fulfilling the criteria of migraine without aura, at least two attacks must have had three of the four following characteristics:

1. Attacks were associated with reversible aura symptoms indicating focal cerebral cortical and/or brainstem dysfunction.
2. At least one of the aura symptoms developed gradually over 4 min or two or more symptoms occur in succession.
3. No aura symptom lasted for more than 1 h. (If more than one aura symptom is present, accepted duration is increased accordingly.)
4. Headache followed resolution of aura symptoms within 1 h or less. (Headache can sometimes begin simultaneously with the aura.)

B. Neither the headache nor the aura symptoms can be correlated to another physical abnormality.

Adapted from IHS criteria

---

grainous infarction develops in the context of stereotypical aura symptoms.

Status Migrainosus is the classification given migraine attacks that persist for longer than 72 h despite treatment. During status migrainosus, headache-free periods of less than 4 h (sleep not included) may occur. Status migrainosus is usually associated with prolonged use of analgesics and may require inpatient treatment with detoxification.

Cluster headache.   Cluster headache is an uncommon syndrome that affects men five to six times more often than women. Its name derives from the fact that attacks occur in series lasting for weeks or months, the so-called cluster periods, separated by remissions that usually last for months or years. Cluster headaches consist of extremely severe, throbbing, strictly unilateral orbital, supraorbital, or temporal head pain that lasts from 15 min to 3 h if untreated. The attacks may occur once every other day with up to 8 attacks per day (Table 16-4). Headaches are accompanied by unusual autonomic signs ipsilateral to the head pain. They may include conjunctival injection, eyelid edema, rhinorrhea, miosis, ptosis, nasal congestion, and forehead or facial sweating. Cluster headaches often exhibit an odd cyclicity, with attacks occurring almost to the minute at the same time every day. The cause of this temporal cycling is not known. Cluster headache can be the most devastating among the primary headache disorders because of the excruciating severity and daily fre-

quency of pain and the tendency toward nocturnal occurrence and sleep interruption.

During cluster periods headache attacks are provoked by alcohol, histamine, nitrites, or nitrates. During an attack, cluster patients are often agitated and frequently pace, unlike a migraine patient, who prefers to lie still in a quiet, darkened room. In some instances the clustering pattern can evolve into a nonremitting, chronic form.

Chronic daily headache.   The diagnosis of chronic daily headache (CDH) may apply to headaches lasting more than 15 days per month for at least 1 month. By this definition the term encompasses several clinically distinct syndromes including cluster headache, hemicrania continua, chronic paroxysmal hemicrania, and chronic tension type headache. In the following, chronic daily headache is defined somewhat more narrowly to include headaches that occur on a daily or almost daily basis (> 4 days per week), have features of both migraine and tension-type headache, and are frequently, but not always, associated with overuse of analgesic medications. Patients meeting these criteria account for a significant number of those seen in headache specialty clinics and are often the most difficult to treat. The prototypical CDH sufferer is a woman in the fourth or fifth decade of life with a history of either episodic migraine or tension-type headache beginning in the teens or twenties. Over a period of months to years the patient's headaches gradually increase in severity and frequency to the point where consecutive headache-free days are rare. The headaches are often of two types. The most frequently encountered are headaches of mild to moderate intensity with a pressure-like or mildly throbbing quality but no associated nausea, or vomiting and no, or very mild, photophobia and phonophobia. The duration of these milder headaches is variable, ranging from a couple of hours to constant, although waxing and waning. Superimposed are severe attacks that occur as frequently as three times per week and as infrequently as once or twice per month. The more severe attacks are usually, but not always, throbbing and may be associated with nausea, photophobia, phonophobia, and sometimes vomiting and are sometimes preceded by a migrainous aura. Often

Table 16-4

Diagnostic Criteria for Cluster Headache

A. At least five attacks of severe unilateral orbital or supraorbital and/or temporal pain lasting 15–180 min untreated.

B. Headaches are associated with at least one of the following signs on the ipsilateral side:

1. Conjunctival injection
2. Lacrimation
3. Nasal congestion
4. Rhinorrhea
5. Forehead and facial sweating
6. Miosis
7. Ptosis
8. Eyelid edema

C. Attacks occur with a frequency of at least one attack every other day to eight attacks per day.

D. The headaches are not correlated with any other physical abnormality.

Adapted from IHS criteria.

the patient exhibits features of depression or anxiety and frequently is taking one or more analgesics daily, sometimes in an effort to preempt a headache in anticipation of an important activity.

Chronic daily headaches are referred to as transformed migraine when the migrainous component is prominent. When headaches begin without antecedent migraine or TTH, but with many features of TTH, it is often labeled new daily persistent headache. Medication overuse is the most common exacerbating factor in CDH, with withdrawal of the overused medication usually improving the condition. Medications most often overused include butalbital-containing combinations, ergotamines, oral analgesics containing caffeine in combination with acetaminophen or NSAIDs, and opioids. CDH may develop in the absence of medication, however, and does not always improve after analgesic withdrawal.

CDH is often accompanied by other paroxysmal symptoms that are frequently as distressing as the head pain. These may include dizziness, both vertiginous and nonspecific, tinnitus, extreme phonophobia, fluctuating fatigue or mood alteration, and feelings of depersonalization. It is unclear whether these symptoms are fragments of underlying migraine or a mood disorder. They often, but not always, resolve with improvement in the headaches.

Chronic paroxysmal hemicrania is a relatively uncommon syndrome that shares many features with cluster headache including unilateral orbital/temporal location, severe intensity, and ipsilateral associated autonomic signs such as conjunctival injection, tearing, and rhinorrhea. It differs from cluster headache in its briefer duration (5 to 20 min), higher attack frequency (generally more than five per day), predominance in females, and absolute effectiveness of treatment with indomethacin at 150 mg per day or less (Sjaastad, 1986).

Hemicrania continua is a rare headache syndrome in which unilateral head pain of moderate to severe intensity is present almost constantly. Superimposed on the waxing and baseline pain, patients experience sharp, jabbing pain in a similar location. There appear to be no identifiable triggering factors for this condition (Newman et al., 1993).

Cough headache consists of bilateral head pain of sudden onset that follows coughing or Valsalva's maneuver. In about 90% of cases it is a benign disorder that responds to indomethacin. Because cough headache can sometimes result from posterior fossa tumors or Arnold Chiari malformation, the diagnosis of benign cough headache requires the exclusion of structural lesions by MRI.

Exertional/orgasmic headache, involving bilateral throbbing or pressure-like head pain, is sometimes triggered by exercise or exertion of various types. The headaches may last from several minutes for up to 24 h. Headaches may also result from sexual activity, including coitus and, less likely, masturbation. These headaches usually start as bilateral nonthrobbing pain that escalates as sexual excitement increases. Pain can be extremely intense with orgasm. Both exertional and orgasmic headaches may occur in the absence of intracranial disorders; however, in rare cases coital headache may be associated with unruptured cerebral aneurysms. With coital headache, the possibility of aneurysm should be excluded. Exertional headache may be prevented in many patients by ingestion of ergotamine or indomethacin before the planned exertion.

Idiopathic jabbing headache consists of transient stabbing pain in the orbital, temporal, or parietal regions that lasts for a fraction of a second and occurs either as a single stab or a series of stabs. The stabbing head pain occurs at irregular intervals without evidence of abnormality at the site of the pain or in the distribution of the affected cranial nerve. Jabbing headache is frequently experienced by migraineurs and usually occurs in the location habitually affected by the migraine headaches. Idiopathic jabbing headache usually resolves with 25 mg indomethacin taken orally three times per day.

Pharmacotherapeutics and Clinical Pharmacology of Primary Headaches

Pharmacologic management of primary headache disorders. Although nonpharmacologic treatments such as avoidance of trigger factors, acupuncture, chiropractic manipulation, biofeedback training, stress management, and relaxation techniques may be quite beneficial for some primary headache sufferers, most patients consulting a physician require pharma-cologic intervention. Pharmacologic therapy falls into two broad categories: 1) abortive or symptomatic treatments given during an active attack to shorten or lessen the severity, and 2) prophylactic treatments taken on a daily basis to decrease the frequency of attacks (see Table 16-6). Symptomatic and prophy-lactic treatments are, with few exceptions, discrete groups of medications. Prophylactic medications taken during acute attacks rarely provide significant relief, and abortive agents taken on a daily basis can actually worsen headaches and increase their frequency.

Treatment of tension-type headache. *Tension-type headache: acute treatment* (Fig. 16-3). The majority of episodic tension-type headaches are of mild to moderate intensity. Many patients take conventional nonprescription analgesics such as acetaminophen or NSAIDs quite effectively. As long as headaches are relatively brief (4 h) and their frequency does not exceed 1 per week, this strategy is probably reason-able. When headache frequency is more than 1 per week, analgesics should be used with care because of the risk of analgesic rebound headaches. Although muscle relaxants such as diazepam, baclofen, dantro-lene sodium, and cyclobenzaprine hydrochloride are

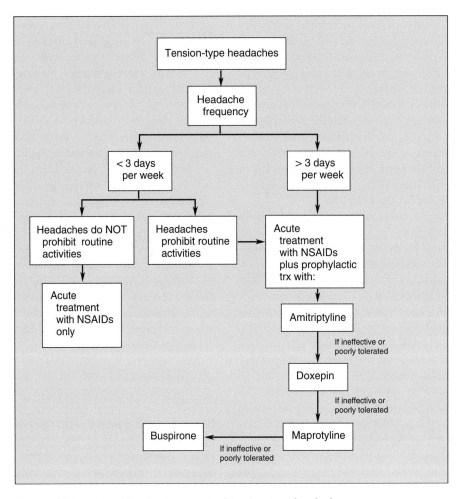

Figure 16–3. *Algorithm for treatment of tension-type headache.*

sometimes used empirically to treat tension-type headache, their efficacy has not been validated by clinical trials. While, theoretically, these agents may reduce pain by relaxing pericranial muscles, these treatments are usually disappointing.

Tension-type headache: prophylactic treatment. When tension-type headaches occur more than 3 days per week, preventive treatment should be considered. Tricyclic antidepressants are the first-line agents in this case. Of these, amitriptyline is the drug of choice (Lance and Curran, 1964). Other types of medications used are NSAIDs, valproic acid, and other antidepressants such as doxepin, maprotyline, and fluoxetine, and the anxiolytic buspirone.

Treatment of Migraine. Migraine: acute treatment. Many patients experience mild to severe headaches and should have access to a hierarchy of treatments appropriate to the severity of their symptoms (Fig. 16-4). In general, agents taken during an attack as symptomatic treatment provide only short-lived benefits and offer little protection against the development of subsequent migraine attacks. The use of analgesic medications more than 3 days per week, including over-the-counter formulations, can increase the frequency and severity of headaches (Mathew et al., 1982; Solomon et al., 1992).

Mild to moderate attacks often respond to treatment with nonprescription analgesics like acetaminophen or NSAIDs like aspirin, ibuprofen, naprosyn, or ketoprofen. During pregnancy mild to moderate attacks should be treated with acetaminophen only. For moderate headaches, a combination of acetaminophen with isometheptene mucate, a mild vasoconstrictor and dichloralphenazone, a mild sedative, is often effective.

Moderate to severe attacks are treated outside the emergency department with a variety of oral and subcutaneous medications, including drugs that bind to serotonin, GABA, and opioid receptors. Ergotamine, the oldest, specifically antimigraine agent, binds to several serotonin receptor subtypes. It is very often effective if the nausea and peripheral vasoconstriction that accompany its use can be tolerated. Ergotamine may be administered by oral or sublingual routes and is most effective if given within the first 15 min of the migraine attack.

Sumatriptan, a relatively selective serotonin receptor agonist, is widely used in the outpatient management of moderate to severe migraine. It is probably the most extensively tested antimigraine agent in history and has exhibited efficacy in multiple clinical trials. The subcutaneous formulation (6 mg) is generally effective within 15 to 45 min. The maximum recommended dose is two injections within 24 h, separated by at least 1 h. The oral formulations of sumatriptan (25 and 50 mg) appear to be effective, but require 60 to 90 min for onset of action. The maximum recommended dose is 300 mg in 24 h. The use of sumatriptan in combination with ergotamine should be avoided because of their potentially additive vasoconstrictive effects.

Several new $5HT_{1B/1D}$ agonists that are chemically similar to sumatriptan may soon be available for the acute treatment of migraine. Included are naratriptan, zolmitriptan, and rizatriptan. The efficacy and side effect profile of these new agents are likely to be similar to sumatriptan, although differences in oral bioavailability, half-life, relative affinity for the human $5HT_{1D}$ and $5HT_{1B}$ receptor subtypes, and blood-brain barrier penetrance may discriminate among them.

Butalbital, a barbiturate, is combined with caffeine, aspirin, and/or acetaminophen and widely prescribed for migraine. Butalbital-containing medications are best suited for the treatment of infrequent moderate-to-severe headaches. Caution is advised when prescribing butalbital because of the potential of dose escalation and increasing headache frequency.

Oral opioids such as codeine, hydrocodone, oxycodone, propoxyphene, and meperidine have little place in the treatment of chronic, recurrent, primary headaches and should be avoided until alternatives have been attempted. During pregnancy and in patients with severe vascular disease, however, opioids may be the only viable option. In this case the drugs must be used with caution. Intranasally administered butorphanol, a synthetic opioid partial agonist, is sometimes used to treat headache. As with the other opioids, its use should be limited to patients with severe, infrequent attacks when there are no alternatives. Even then, the amount prescribed should be

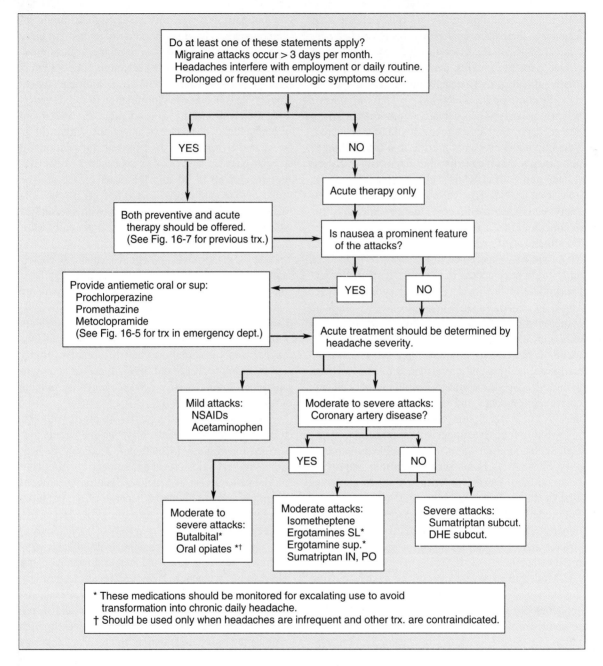

Figure 16–4. *Algorithm for the outpatient management of nonpregnant migraine patients.*

limited. The risks of rebound headaches or dependency associated with opioid use should be discussed with patients before treatment.

Severe attacks. Intense migraine attacks, especially those associated with profound nausea and vomiting, may require subcutaneous or parenteral administration of abortive medication (Fig. 16-5).

Sumatriptan may be administered subcutaneously during such attacks and reportedly continues to be effective for up to 4 h. Onset of relief generally occurs within 30 min. Dihydroergotamine (DHE), an injectable ergot, has less potent peripheral arterial vasoconstrictive effects than ergotamine and is usually quite effective even when administered well into an attack. Dihydroergotamine may be administered subcutaneously or intravenously. When given intravenously, dihydroergotamine causes less nausea than ergotamine, but an antiemetic is still required before intravenous administration (Callaham and Raskin, 1986).

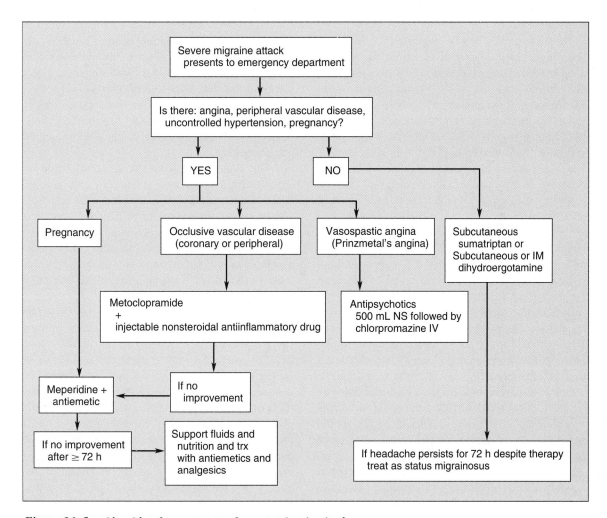

Figure 16–5. *Algorithm for treatment of severe migraine in the emergency department.*

Ketorolac, an injectable NSAID, is sometimes an effective alternative to narcotics in patients who are unable to tolerate vasoactive drugs like sumatriptan or DHE. Meperidine, an opioid analgesic, is frequently administered intramuscularly, especially in combination with an antiemetic, to treat severe migraine attacks. With alternatives now available, the use of parenteral opioids should be limited to patients with infrequent attacks or those for whom other treatments are contraindicated, such as individuals with severe peripheral or cerebrovascular disease, coronary artery disease, or pregnancy.

Antipsychotics can be employed in the emergency department to treat severe or prolonged headache instead of using meperidine or vasoconstrictive medications. The risk of hypotension and the need for intravenous administration, however, limit the use of chlorpromazine. Hypotension can be avoided by administering 500 mL of normal saline intravenously before administering chlorpromazine, which can in turn be repeated once after 1 h. Alternatively, intravenous prochlorperazine can be given without prior saline infusion, and repeated after 30 min.

Therapy of status migrainosus. When a migraine attack persists for more than 3 days, or when efforts to end an attack are unsuccessful, intravenous dihydroergotamine (DHE) is the treatment of choice in the emergency department provided there are no contraindications, such as pregnancy, angina, or coronary artery disease (Fig. 16-6) (Raskin, 1986). The DHE should be given undiluted through an IV heplock. Metoclopramide (10 mg IV) should be administered before DHE to avoid ergot-related nausea, although it may in most cases be discontinued after six DHE doses (Raskin, 1986). In patients who present with status migrainosus, special attention should be given to the amount of analgesic medication taken before admission. Because status migrainosus is frequently associated with an overuse of abortive medications, patients with this condition should be monitored carefully for evidence of barbiturate or opioid withdrawal. If the patient is not currently taking prophylactic medication, initiation of preventive therapy is appropriate.

Migraine: prophylactic therapy. In patients who have rare attacks of migraine, an effective abortive agent is sufficient. If attacks result in disability 3 or more days per month, if they prohibit normal activities, or if dread of the attacks is disabling, then prophylactic therapy should be considered (Fig. 16-7). Prophylactic medications fall into two categories. First-line agents are those likely to be effective without intolerable side effects, whereas second-line agents may be effective when the first-line agents have failed, but carry a risk of more frequent or potentially serious side effects.

First-line agents include β-adrenergic receptor antagonists, NSAIDs, calcium channel blockers, tricyclic antidepressants, and anticonvulsants. A recent multicenter double-blind trial (Schoenen et al., 1997) demonstrated that high-dose riboflavin has prophylactic effects in migraine. As more experience is gained with its use, riboflavin may join the first-line agents. Second-line agents include methysergide and phenelzine.

The choice of a prophylactic agent should be individualized to the patient and take into account concomitant medical problems and other medications that the patient is taking (Table 16-5). Prophylactic medications are largely empirical treatments. Most were originally used for other indications, and their antimigraine effects are likely to be unrelated to the action for which they were originally prescribed.

When prescribing prophylactic therapy, it is important to begin with a low dose and titrate upward every 2 weeks at increments of the dose of the lowest strength available until a significant reduction in headaches occurs, intolerable side effects appear, or the maximum recommended dose is attained. Premature cessation may deprive the patient of an effective and well-tolerated therapy. About midway through the dose escalation it is wise to have the patient continue the same dose for 2 to 3 weeks and communicate any side effects or change in headache frequency or severity. Patients should be warned that the onset of action is gradual, and the full benefit of the drug may not be observed until 3 to 4 weeks after attaining an effective dose. If the first agent proves to be ineffective or poorly tolerated, then

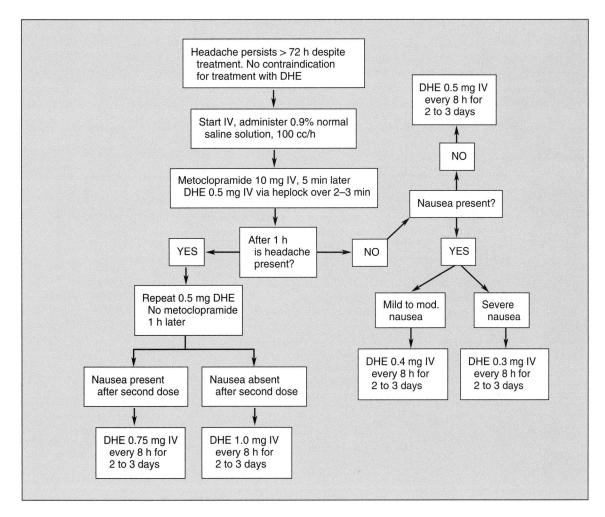

Figure 16–6. *Protocol for repetitive-dose intravenous dihydroergotamine (DHE) treatment of status migrainosus. Adapted in part from Raskin, 1986.*

titrate the patient downward and begin treatment with another of the first-line agents. Before moving to a second-line agent, a representative from each of the noncontraindicated first-line drugs should be tried.

If headaches continue after trying all available first-line agents, then the decision must be made whether to administer second-line agents or to combine two of the first-line drugs. This decision is best made along with the patient after a discussion of the potential side effects. The likelihood of side effects

in general is increased when two agents are used in combination. There are anecdotal reports of synergistic effects such as with combining amitriptyline and divalproex sodium. The increased benefit, if any, has not, however, been rigorously examined.

Another important factor to consider when choosing from the available therapies, and in evaluating treatment response, is patient compliance. If the patient may not comply, then one or two daily dose regimens should be chosen over dosages requiring more complex schedules.

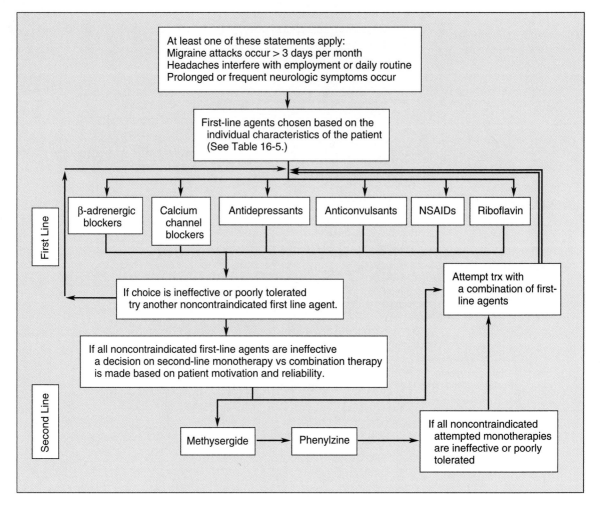

Figure 16–7. Algorithm for the prophylactic treatment of migraine.

Treatment of cluster headache. *Cluster headache: acute treatment.* Acute therapies for cluster headache are geared toward rapid administration and onset of effect. Because the attacks seldom exceed 1 h, slowly absorbed oral remedies generally offer no benefit. Oxygen inhalation is a safe and effective treatment for individual attacks in many patients. Patients most likely to respond are those with episodic-type cluster headaches who are under the age of 50 (Kudrow, 1981). Unlike most other acute treatments effective in cluster headache, oxygen is not contraindicated in patients with coronary artery disease or peripheral vascular disease. Oxygen therapy is given as follows:

Through a loose-fitting face mask, 100% oxygen is delivered at a rate of 8 L per min for 15 min. Nasal biprongs are unlikely to be effective. Patients who respond to oxygen usually do so within 10 min.

Ergotamine tartrate has been used for half a century to treat attacks of cluster headache. The sublingual routes are superior to oral tablets. Inhaled formulations are unfortunately no longer available. Ergotamines are an effective and well-tolerated treatment in many patients. Dihydroergotamine may also

Table 16-5

Comorbid Factors That Influence the Choice of a Prophylactic Treatment of Migraine

Comorbid factors	Consider	Avoid
Coronary artery disease	Verapamil	Methysergide
Heart block	Divalproex	Verapamil, β-adrenergic receptor antagonist
Cardiac tachyarrhythmia	Verapamil, β-adrenergic receptor antagonist	Amitriptyline
Asthma	*	β-Adrenergic receptor antagonist
Peptic ulcer disease	*	NSAIDs
Hypertension	Verapamil, β-adrenergic receptor antagonist	Amitriptyline
Diabetes mellitus	*	β-Adrenergic receptor antagonist
Hyperthyroidism or thyroid replacement	β-Adrenergic receptor antagonist	Amitriptyline
Liver disease	Atenolol, gabapentin	Divalproex
Renal disease	*	Atenolol, gabapentin, NSAIDs
Seizure disorder	Divalproex or gabapentin	Amitriptyline
Depression	Amitriptyline	β-Adrenergic receptor antagonist
Bipolar disorder	Divalproex	β-Adrenergic receptor antagonist Amitriptyline, NSAIDs if on lithium
Menstrually associated migraine	Naprosyn	*

* Follow indications for general treatment.

be of use in an intranasal form (Anderssen and Jespersen, 1986).

Subcutaneous sumatriptan is rapidly becoming the most widely used acute treatment in cluster headache. It is generally effective in reducing both the pain and conjunctival injection within 15 to 20 min. Thus far it appears to be very well tolerated in cluster headache patients. Ergotamine, ergotamine derivatives, and sumatriptan are all contraindicated in patients with coronary artery disease, which is quite common among the middle-aged males who make up a significant portion of cluster headache sufferers.

Cluster headache: prophylactic treatment. Prophylactic treatment for cluster headache is aimed toward early termination of the cluster period. In general, treatment is continued only during the cluster period and is withdrawn a few weeks after resolution of the cluster attacks. In those patients whose cluster headaches return on a seasonal basis, the initiation of a prophylactic regimen a few weeks in advance of the expected cluster is sometimes a successful strategy. The unpredictable course of cluster attacks, however, makes it difficult to know with certainty whether the lack of the expected cluster is owing to treatment.

The prophylactic treatments used in cluster headache are quite variable in their effectiveness. Drugs used include verapamil, ergotamine tartrate, methysergide, lithium, valproate, cyproheptadine, and intravenous and oral steroids (Fig. 16-8).

Treatment of chronic daily headache. Management of patients with chronic daily headache (CDH) is often very challenging as they are sometimes re-

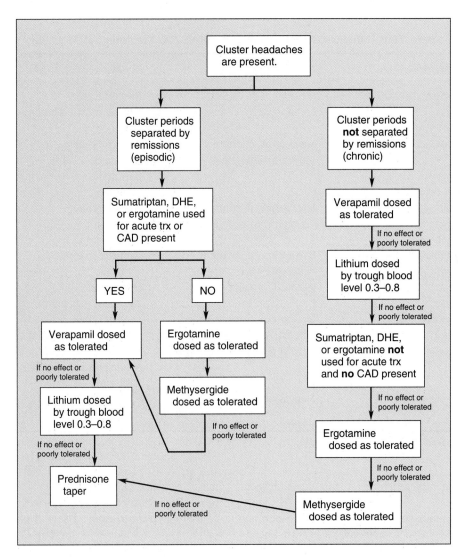

Figure 16–8. *Algorithm for the prophylactic treatment of cluster headache.*

fractory to treatment. Therapy has three major components. First, it is important to exclude a secondary headache disorder or another primary headache disorder that occurs on a daily basis such as cluster headache, hemicrania continua, or chronic paroxysmal hemicrania. When a secondary disorder is present, initiate appropriate treatment. When none is present, provide reassurance to the patient. Second, one must identify and eliminate factors that exacerbate and perpetuate the daily headache cycle. These may include withdrawal and elimination of overused analgesics, detoxification from abused medications, avoidance of known trigger factors, increasing regularity of lifestyle, and identification and treatment of comorbid psychiatric and medical conditions. Third, it is important to begin prophylactic treatment with a medication that suppresses the patient's underlying tendency to develop headache. Even during withdrawal from the overused symptomatic medication, it is important to initiate preventive treatment.

The patient should be forewarned that prophylaxis will not be effective until analgesic overuse has ceased.

It is essential to eliminate any symptomatic medications that are currently overused and substitute another analgesic, preferably an NSAID alone. Naprosyn (500 to 750 mg) or ketoprofen (50 to 100 mg) are frequently effective in this regard. Headaches that appear during withdrawal will probably not respond completely to the new medication but will likely become more responsive once the withdrawal process is complete, usually within 4 to 6 weeks. If barbiturates or benzodiazepines have been overused in great quantities, withdrawal in an inpatient unit may be necessary.

Prophylactic pharmacotherapy in CDH has not been rigorously evaluated in controlled clinical trials. Experience suggests amitriptyline (100 to 150 mg per day) and divalproex sodium (1000 to 1500 mg per day) (Mathew and Ali, 1991) are most effective. Doxepin is also effective if tension-type headache symptoms are especially prominent (Morland et al., 1979). While fluoxetine may also be effective in CDH (Saper et al., 1994), this may not always be the case. If these agents are ineffective, the β-adrenergic receptor antagonists, calcium channel antagonists, methysergide, or selective serotonin reuptake inhibitors (SSRIs) may be attempted.

Other headaches: treatment. Many of the remaining headache syndromes share a common response to indomethacin. It is not known why these headaches respond to indomethacin when others, like migraine, are less responsive. These syndromes include:

1. Chronic paroxysmal hemicrania
2. Hemicrania continua
3. Benign cough headache
4. Effort and coital migraine
5. Idiopathic jabbing headaches

Therapeutic agents used in headache disorders (Table 16-6)

Acetaminophen, an analgesic and antipyretic agent, is often very useful in the treatment of mild migraine and tension-type headache at doses of 650 to 1000 mg. Severe headaches are less likely to respond to this medication alone, and therefore it is frequently combined with barbiturates, caffeine, or opioids for the treatment of more severe attacks. Mild to moderate headache attacks during pregnancy should be treated with acetaminophen. Gastric side effects are much less prominent with acetaminophen than with other NSAIDs. In general, side effects are rare at therapeutic doses. In toxic doses, acetaminophen is associated with hepatic necrosis.

Acetazolamide is a carbonic anhydrase inhibitor used at doses of 500 to 1000 mg twice per day to treat benign intracranial hypertension, presumably by reducing cerebrospinal fluid production. This agent is also sometimes taken in doses of 250 mg twice per day to prevent acute mountain sickness, of which headache is a prominent component. Side effects include paresthesias, renal calculi, anorexia, gastrointestinal disturbance, transient myopia, drowsiness, or fatigue. In a few instances, patients have developed a sulfonamide-like nephropathy. It is contraindicated in patients with a history of nephrolithiasis, hepatic, or renal failure.

Antidepressants of various classes are widely used in the prophylactic treatment of migraine, chronic tension-type, posttraumatic, and chronic daily headaches. Heterocyclic antidepressants such as amitriptyline, imipramine, nortriptyline, clomipramine, doxepin, and trazodone are all used in migraine prophylaxis. The strongest evidence for efficacy is with amitriptyline. Although there are many advocates for the use of selective serotonin reuptake inhibitors such as fluoxetine, sertraline, and paroxetine, evidence supporting their efficacy in headache is scant.

Amitriptyline, a tertiary amine, is an effective treatment for headache as shown in double-blind, placebo-controlled studies (Couch and Hassanein, 1979; Gomersall and Stuart, 1973). In addition, amitriptyline is one of the most effective drug treatments for post-traumatic headache, and the drug of choice for chronic tension-type headache and headache disorders with mixed features of migraine and tension-type headache. For migraine, amitriptyline doses ranges from 10 to 150 mg per day or higher if tolerated. Chronic tension-type headache and post-traumatic headache may require doses up to 250 mg. Beneficial effects may not be observed for 4 to 6 weeks after initiating therapy. In some cases amitriptyline use is limited by its anticholinergic side effects, which include dry mouth, tachycardia, constipation, and urinary retention. Other potential side effects include a lowered seizure threshold, increased appetite, photosensitivity of the skin, and sedation, which is most common. To minimize sedation amitriptyline should be given in a single dose 1 to 2 h before bedtime and should be started at a low dose, such as 10 mg per day, then slowly increased over several weeks in 10-mg increments at intervals of 1 to 2 weeks. Contraindications include recent myocardial infarction, concurrent use of other tricyclic antidepressants or monoamine oxidase inhibitors, narrow angle glaucoma, urinary retention, pregnancy, cardiovascular, and renal or liver disease.

Doxepin, another tricyclic antidepressant, improves headache scores in tension-type headaches (Morland et al., 1979). Dosages of doxepin for this use range from 10 to 150 mg per day. Side effects and contraindications are similar to those of amitriptyline.

Maprotiline is a tetracyclic antidepressant that may be useful in chronic tension-type headache. In a small double-blind, placebo-controlled study, 75 mg per day decreased headache severity by 25% and increased headache-free days by 40%. Dosages of 25 to 150 mg per day are used to treat depression (Fogelholm and Murros, 1985). Low doses should be attempted in headache patients. Side effects include sedation, tachycardia, and lowered seizure threshold. Contraindications include recent myocardial infarction, concurrent use of monoamine oxidase inhibitors and seizure disorders.

Fluoxetine, a selective serotonin reuptake inhibitor, has been reported to improve migraine in doses of 20 to 40 mg per day (Adly et al., 1992). A larger placebo-controlled trial (20 mg per day) showed no effect in migraine, but significant improvement in chronic daily headache patients (Saper et al., 1994). Fluoxetine is also sometimes used empirically in chronic tension-type headache. Side effects associated with its use are insomnia, abdominal pain, and tremor. Contraindications include previous hypersensitivity reaction, concurrent use of monoamine oxidase inhibitors, and liver disease.

Anticonvulsants such as phenytoin and carbamazepine have been used empirically in migraine and facial pain syndromes for years. Strong evidence of efficacy exists, however, for only one anticonvulsant, valproic acid. Preliminary data suggest a possible role for gabapentin in migraine as well.

Valproic acid, a simple branched-chain carboxylic acid, is one of the newest antimigraine prophylactic agents. Valproic acid or divalproex sodium reduced the frequency of migraine in several double-blind clinical trials (Hering et al., 1992; Jensen et al., 1994; Coria et al., 1994; Mathew et al., 1996). Small open trials have also suggested efficacy in cluster headache (Hering and Kuritzky, 1989) and chronic daily (Mathew and Ali, 1991) headache. Treatment with divalproex sodium should begin at 125 to 250 mg per day and increase by 125 mg every 1 to 2 weeks until a marked reduction in headaches occurs or until a dose of 750 to 2000 mg per day, in three divided doses, is achieved. The goal is to obtain maximal

therapeutic effect with few, or tolerable, side effects. The side effects of valproic acid include nausea, sedation, tremor, transient hair loss, weight gain, inhibition of platelet aggregation, and minor elevations in liver function tests. In children, valproic acid treatment has been associated with symptoms similar to Reye's syndrome. Just as with other anticonvulsants, there is a 1 to 2% incidence of fetal neural-tube defects in the infants of women taking valproic acid during the first trimester of pregnancy (Nau, 1994). Contraindications include hepatic disease, anticipated surgery, pregnancy, and clotting abnormality.

Gabapentin, an anticonvulsant, was effective in migraine prophylaxis in preliminary results from a small double-blind (Wessely et al., 1987) and an open trial (Mathew and Lucker, 1996). Larger double-blind clinical trials are under way. Side effects in epileptic patients included only transient sedation and mild dizziness. Indeed, its relatively benign side effect profile makes gabapentin a promising, although as of yet unproven, addition to the antimigraine armamentarium.

β-Adrenergic receptor antagonists have been widely used as antihypertensive agents and five have been found effective against migraine in clinical trials. Included are the nonselective agents propranolol, 40 to 200 mg daily (Frossman et al., 1976), nadolol, 20 to 80 mg daily (Ryan et al., 1983), timolol, 20 to 60 mg daily (Stellar et al., 1984), and the $β_1$-adrenergic receptor blockers atenolol, 25 to 150 mg daily (Frossman et al., 1983), and metoprolol, 50 to 250 mg daily (Kangasneimi et al., 1987). Side effects of these drugs include decreased bronchial dilation, hypotension, bradycardia, fatigue, dizziness, gastrointestinal disturbance (nausea, diarrhea, constipation), depression, sleep disturbance, and memory disturbance. Contraindications include asthma, chronic obstructive pulmonary disease, congestive heart failure, cardiac conduction defects, peripheral vascular disease, and brittle diabetes mellitus.

Buspirone, an azapirone anxiolytic and partial 5-HT_{1A} agonist, has been reported to be as effective as 50 mg amitriptyline in the prophylactic treatment of chronic tension-type headache in doses of 30 mg per day (Mitsikostas, 1997). Side effects associated with buspirone use are dizziness, nausea, headache, nervousness, lightheadedness, and excitement. Contraindications include previous hypersensitivity to the drug and monoamine-oxidase inhibitors.

Butalbital (50 mg) is a barbiturate that is combined with caffeine (40 mg), acetylsalicylic acid

(325 mg), or acetaminophen (325 to 500 mg) in several widely prescribed analgesic medications used for migraine and tension-type headaches. Other preparations include codeine as well. The recommended dosage is two tablets every 4 h not to exceed six tablets per day. When used for the treatment of infrequent, moderate to severe headaches, these combinations can be quite effective. If used to treat headaches occurring more than once per week, overuse and rebound headaches frequently become a problem. When butalbital is employed, patients and physicians should be aware of the potential for escalating use. Side effects include sedation, dizziness, shortness of breath, and gastrointestinal disturbance, and the combination is contraindicated when there has been previous hypersensitivity to any component, history of previous drug addiction, renal, or hepatic impairment.

Calcium channel blockers are used primarily for the treatment of hypertension and vasospasm. They were introduced initially for the treatment of migraine to relieve the vasospastic phase. Flunarizine, the most effective calcium channel blocker in migraine, is not available in the United States. Nimodipine has been tested as a migraine preventive in several clinical trials with mixed results. Of the remaining calcium channel blockers, only verapamil has displayed sufficient efficacy in double-blind clinical trials to warrant its use in headache prophylaxis.

Verapamil is used in the prophylactic treatment of migraine and cluster headache at doses of 160 to 480 mg per day. It has demonstrated superiority to placebo in migraine prophylaxis in two small, controlled, double-blind trials (Solomon et al., 1987; Markley et al., 1984). In the prevention of cluster headache, one open labeled trial reported a response rate to verapamil of 69% (Gabai and Spierings, 1989). Another double-blind trial found verapamil to be as effective as lithium (Bussone et al., 1990). Side effects of verapamil include hypotension, edema, fatigue, nausea, constipation, and, in some cases, headache. The drug is contraindicated if bradycardia, cardiac conduction defects, or sick sinus syndrome are present, and when β-adrenergic receptor antagonists are being taken.

Cyproheptadine is most widely used for its antihistaminic actions. It is also used in migraine prophylaxis in children and adults at 4 to 24 mg per day, and occasionally in cluster headache. There have been no double-blind trials on the effectiveness of cyproheptadine in headache. An open trial in 100 patients found that 15% became headache free and 31% improved substantially at doses of 12 to 24 mg cyproheptadine per day (Curran et al., 1964). Another open trial reported a 65% response rate (Klimek, 1979). Side effects of cyproheptadine are sedation, dry mouth, urinary retention, weight gain, and increased growth in children. Contraindications include glaucoma, previous hypersensitivity, concurrent use of monoamine oxidase inhibitors, peptic ulcer disease, symptomatic prostatic hypertrophy, or pyloroduodenal obstruction.

First available almost half a century ago, ergot alkaloids are widely used in both acute and prophylactic treatment of migraine and cluster headache. The use of these medications is based largely on longstanding clinical experience rather than controlled studies. Potential side effects of these medications are similar, although they are less common and severe with dihydroergotamine than with ergotamine tartrate. Side effects may include nausea, vomiting, muscle cramps, malaise, acral cyanosis, and chest pain. Contraindications include pregnancy, coronary artery disease, angina, peripheral vascular disease, history of thrombophlebitis, Raynaud's phenomenon, uncontrolled hypertension, cardiovascular disease, or severely impaired renal or hepatic function.

Ergotamine tartrate is the classical treatment for both acute migraine and cluster headache. Ergotamine often in combination with other drugs, such as caffeine, phenobarbital, or belladonna alkaloids, is available in the United States in oral, sublingual, and suppository formulations. Dosages in migraine range from 0.25 to 2 mg, depending on the route of administration. Ergotamines are most effective if given early in the migraine attack. Overuse is a potential complication of therapy and may convert intermittent migraine into chronic daily headache. Very rarely, ergotamine overuse, usually over 10 mg per week, leads to ergotism, which is characterized by peripheral cyanosis, intermittent claudication, necrosis of digits, and infarction in various organs.

For acute treatment of cluster headache the sublingual route (1 to 2 mg) is generally preferred to tablets taken orally because of the more rapid onset of action. Ergotamine tartrate was for many years the sole prophylactic agent in cluster headache and was prescribed in doses of 2 to 4 mg per day in either oral or suppository form. In general, ergotamine is well tolerated in cluster headache patients. Any vasoconstrictive medication like ergotamine, however, should be prescribed with caution in males over the age of 40.

Dihydroergotamine (DHE) is an injectable hydrogenated ergot that has less potent peripheral arterial vasoconstrictive effects than ergotamine tartrate. Until recently, DHE was the mainstay of nonopioid treatment of acute severe migraine attacks. Unlike ergotamine tartrate, DHE can be effective even when given well into the attack. It can be administered intravenously with somewhat less nausea than ergotamine; however, an antiemetic is usually required before intravenous treatment.

To give DHE in the acute setting (non-status migrainosus):

1. Early in the attack: Administer DHE 1 to 2 mg IM or subcutaneously; a repeat dose may be given up to 3 mg in 24 h.
2. Well into a severe attack: Administer prochlorperazine 5 mg IV or metoclopramide 10 mg IV followed in 5 to 10 min by DHE 0.75 to 1 mg IV given over 2 to 3 min.
3. If the attack has not subsided after 30 min, an additional 0.5 mg of DHE may be administered IV.

Diarrhea is a common side effect of DHE and can be controlled with oral diphenoxylate. Contraindications to IV DHE include Prinzmetal's angina, pregnancy, coronary artery disease or uncontrolled hypertension, peripheral vascular disease, and severe renal or hepatic disease.

DHE is also used in the acute treatment of cluster headaches (0.5 to 1 mg). In one double-blind cross-over study, intranasal DHE reduced the attack severity but not its duration (Andersson and Jespersen, 1986).

Methysergide, which was introduced in the 1960s, was one of the first drugs used for migraine and cluster headache prophylaxis. Double-blind clinical trials demonstrated the effectiveness of methysergide in reducing the frequency, severity, and duration of migraine attacks (Southwell et al., 1964; Pedersen and Moller, 1966). Recommended doses range from 2 to 8 mg per day. Unfortunately, methysergide use is associated with the serious complications of retroperitoneal, pericardial, or pleural fibrosis. Because of these potentially fatal side effects, methysergide should be reserved for only severe cases that are refractory to the other prophylactic regimens. Because the fibrotic complications are reversible early in the process, methysergide should be discontinued for 6 to 8 weeks every 6 months. The early symptoms of retroperitoneal fibrosis include decreased urine output and leg or back pain.

Methysergide is effective in about 70% of episodic cluster headache patients (Curran et al., 1967). Fibrotic complications are less likely to occur in cluster headache than migraine because the duration of use is generally less than 3 months.

In addition to fibrosis and the typical side effects associated with ergotamines, methysergide may also cause depression, sedation, dizziness, lightheadedness, and peripheral edema.

Furosemide is a loop diuretic sometimes employed at doses of 40 to 160 mg per day in the treatment of benign intracranial hypertension because of its ability to suppress CSF production. Its use should be combined with potassium supplementation. Side effects include nausea, vomiting, anorexia, jaundice, vasculitis, tinnitus, vertigo, blurred vision, anemia, thrombocytopenia, dermatitis, orthostatic hypotension, and hypokalemia. Contraindications include previous hypersensitivity and pregnancy.

Isometheptene mucate, a mild vasoconstrictor (65 mg per capsule), is used in combination with acetaminophen (325 mg) and dichloralphenazone (100 mg), a mild sedative, for the treatment of moderate tension-type and migraine headache. Two tablets should be taken at the onset of headache followed by one each hour until relief occurs or up to a maximum of five capsules within a 12-h period. Side effects include dizziness, tachycardia, and occasional skin rash. Experience suggests that it is less likely than many of the other combination medications to generate a rebound headache syndrome, although daily use of any analgesic is not recommended. Contraindications include glaucoma, severe renal, hepatic or cardiac disease, hypertension, or concurrent use of monoamine oxidase inhibitors.

Lithium carbonate is used in the prophylactic treatment of episodic and chronic cluster headache, with more than 20 open clinical trials demonstrating efficacy in this regard (Ekbom, 1981). Because of its rather narrow therapeutic window, it is important to monitor serum lithium levels 12 h after the last dose. The therapeutic range is from 0.3 to 0.8 mmol/L (trough blood level), and low lithium levels are usually therapeutic. Co-administration of either NSAIDs or thiazide diuretics with lithium may increase the serum levels of the ion. Average daily doses range from 600 to 900 mg but should be titrated according to serum concentrations. Side effects include fine hand tremor, polyuria, thirst, nausea, diarrhea, muscular weakness, ataxia, blurred vision, and giddiness. Contraindications to lithium use are severe debilitation, renal or cardiac disease, dehydration, sodium depletion, concurrent use of diuretics or angiotensin-converting enzyme inhibitors.

Antipsychotics have been used as an alternative to opioids or vasoconstrictive medications in the emergency department setting for the treatment of severe migraine attacks. Possible antimigraine actions include their antiemetic, prokinetic, and sedative effects.

Metoclopramide, a benzamide derivative, is frequently combined with NSAIDs or dihydroergotamine in the acute treatment of severe migraine attacks. One double-blind study showed that metoclopramide alone (10 mg IV) was better than placebo in severe migraine treated in an emergency department (Tek et al., 1990). This is surprising because other trials have failed to demonstrate either additional nausea relief (Tokola et al., 1984) or analgesia with metoclopramide beyond the effect of ergotamine (Slettnes and Sjaastad, 1977). Recommended dosage is 5 to 10 mg IV. Side effects include akathisia, sedation, and dystonic reactions. Contraindications include concurrent use of antipsychotics, breast feeding, pregnancy, and pheochromocytoma.

Chlorpromazine, a phenothiazine antipsychotic agent, is sometimes used in the treatment of acute severe migraine attacks, when vasoactive drugs or opioids are contraindicated or ineffective. In one small parallel double-blind study, pain relief with chlorpromazine did not reach statistical significance (McEwen et al., 1987). In larger blinded comparison studies, chlorpromazine was significantly more effective than IV meperidine (Lane et al., 1989) or dihydroergotamine (Bell et al., 1990). Parenteral administration, hypotension, sedation, and akathisia limit its use. If administered, an IV line should be started and 500 mL of normal saline administered before chlorpromazine. Chlorpromazine can then be administered in a 10-mg dose that can be repeated in 1 h. Patients should have repeated blood pressure measurements in addition to at least 1 h of bed rest after dosing. Alternatively, prochlorperazine, 10 mg IV, can be given without the prior saline infusion and repeated in 30 min. Side effects include orthostatic hypotension, sedation, dry mouth, dystonic reactions, and malignant neuroleptic syndrome. Contraindica-

tions include the concurrent use of CNS depressants and previous hypersensitivity reactions.

Nonsteroidal anti-inflammatory drugs (NSAIDs) exert analgesic, anti-inflammatory, and antipyretic effects by inhibition of cyclooxygenase. Cyclooxygenase inhibition blocks the formation of proinflammatory prostaglandins and the aggregation of platelets. These drugs are useful in both the acute treatment of migraine and tension-type headache and prophylactic treatment of migraine and several other headaches of brief duration. Thus far, it has been difficult to correlate prophylactic efficacy with inhibition of platelet function and there have been few trials that compare the efficacy of different NSAIDs.

NSAIDs are commonly used in the acute treatment of primary headaches such as migraine and tension-type headache.

Medication	Initial Dose (mg)	Repeat Dose (mg)
Aspirin	900–1000	975
Ibuprofen	600–800	600
Ketoprofen	50–75	50
Naprosyn	500–825	500
Naproxen sodium	550	275
Ketorolac (oral)	20	10
Indomethacin (sup)	50	—

In addition, several NSAIDs were effective in migraine prophylaxis. Included are aspirin, 650 mg twice daily (O'Neill and Mann, 1978), naproxen, 250 mg twice daily (Lindegaard et al., 1980), naproxen sodium, 550 mg twice daily (Welch et al., 1985), ketoprofen, 50 mg three times daily (Stensrud and Sjaastad, 1974), and mefenamic acid, 500 mg three times daily (Johnson et al., 1986).

Naproxen sodium was effective in controlled studies for the treatment of migraine associated with menstruation (Sances et al., 1990; Szekely et al., 1989), a subtype of migraine that is particularly refractory to medication.

Side effects of NSAIDs are mainly referable to the gastrointestinal tract, such as dyspepsia, diarrhea, and gastritis, but also include increased bleeding and, with long-term high-dose use, renal abnormalities.

With toxic levels, tinnitus can occur. Contraindications include peptic ulcer disease, hypersensitivity to other NSAIDs, chronic anticoagulation therapy, renal or liver disease, or age under 12 years.

Indomethacin, a methylated indole derivative, is uniquely effective in the treatment of several small headache syndromes including chronic paroxysmal hemicrania, hemicrania continua, benign cough headache, effort and coital induced headache, and idiopathic jabbing headaches.

To treat these syndromes, an initial dose of 25 mg twice per day is increased over several days until the attacks cease. This sometimes requires up to 150 mg per day. After relief is stable for several days, the dose should be titrated downward to the lowest effective maintenance dose which is usually 25 to 100 mg per day. There is great interindividual variation in the required maintenance dose. While headaches often return after maintenance is discontinued, prolonged remissions can occur.

Indomethacin may have potentially serious gastrointestinal side effects when given for long periods of time. These include dyspepsia, peptic ulcer, and gastrointestinal bleeding. Other potential side effects are dizziness, nausea, and purpura. It is important to find the minimum effective dose to reduce the likelihood of these side effects. The elixir and suppository forms appear to be better tolerated than tablets. Contraindications include previous hypersensitivity reaction, asthma, urticaria or rhinnitis after NSAIDs, and peptic ulcer disease.

Ketorolac trimethamine is a potent nonsteroidal anti-inflammatory drug that is available in an injectable form. It can be given IM (60 to 90 mg) for the treatment of severe migraine attacks as an alternative to opioids, especially when nausea and vomiting are present. A single preliminary report indicates this costly treatment is less effective than DHE with metoclopramide (Klapper and Stanton, 1991). Some patients respond well, however, and it may be a viable alternative if intravenous access is a problem or vasoactive agents such as DHE or sumatriptan are contraindicated. Side effects include gastrointestinal disturbance, hypertension, rash, bronchospasm, and increased bleeding with short-term use. As with any NSAIDs, there is a risk of analgesic nephropathy with chronic use. Contraindications are similar to those for other NSAIDs.

Opioid analgesics are widely prescribed as a component of oral combination analgesics for outpatient treatment of moderate to severe migraine, tension-type, and cluster headache. In addition, intramuscular and intravenous opioids such as meperidine are often used to treat severe migraine attacks in emergency departments. Adverse reactions include sedation, dizziness, nausea, vomiting, constipation, ataxia, and dependency. Contraindications to the use of narcotic analgesics include previous hypersensitivity reaction or substance abuse or concurrent use of monoamine oxidase inhibitors. Oral/intranasal narcotic medications should be avoided in the treatment of chronic primary headaches until all other alternatives have been explored. In certain situations, as in pregnancy or when severe vascular disease is present, they are the only viable option. This group includes codeine (15 to 60 mg), hydrocodone (2.5 to 10 mg), oxycodone (5 to 10 mg), propoxyphene (65 to 200 mg), and meperidine (50 to 100 mg), among others. Despite early claims that intranasal butorphanol has a low abuse potential, dose escalation very frequently occurs in migraine patients.

Before treatment of chronic headache with opioids, specific limits should be established for dose, goals, and duration of therapy. The risks of rebound headache syndromes and dependency should be discussed with the patient in detail.

Meperidine in combination with an antiemetic is widely used in the emergency department to treat severe migraine attacks despite the lack of double-blind, placebo-controlled clinical data in support of its efficacy. In one comparison study it was found to be inferior to dihydroergotamine (Belgrade et al., 1989). Meperidine should be used primarily in patients with infrequent, severe attacks, or those in whom other treatments are contraindicated, such as severe peripheral or cerebral vascular disease, coronary artery disease, or pregnancy.

Phenelzine, in doses of 15 to 60 mg per day, is a monoamine oxidase inhibitor sometimes used prophylactically in migraine patients refractory to other treatments. The only evidence of its efficacy in this regard is in an open trial in 25 patients with severe migraine who were unresponsive to other therapies. These patients were treated with 45 mg phenelzine per day for up to 2 years (Anthony and Lance, 1969), with 20 experiencing a greater than 50% reduction in headache frequency. Phenelzine appears safe when used in combination with sumatriptan (Diamond, 1995). The potential for hypertensive crisis after dietary intake of tyramine-containing foods or administration of sympathomimetic drugs limits the use of phenelzine to patients with severe refractory migraine. Other side effects include orthostatic hypotension, urinary retention, gastrointestinal disturbance, hepatotoxicity, and failure of ejaculation. Phenelzine should not be used in combination with sympathomimetic drugs, including over-the-counter antihistamine-decongestants, inhaled asthma treatments, weight reduction pills, monoamine oxidase inhibitors, or dibenzapine-derivative antidepressant medications. Patients taking phenelzine must restrict their intake of tyramine containing foods such as fermented cheeses, alcoholic beverages, broad beans, dry sausages, liver, sauerkraut, etc. and it should not be given in the presence of pheochromocytoma, congestive heart failure, and abnormal liver function tests.

Steroids are frequently used intravenously for the treatment of status migrainosus and refractory cluster headache. With dexamethasone, 12 to 20 mg IV is sometimes effective in this regard (Edmeads, 1988). In both the chronic and episodic forms of cluster headache, tapering doses of oral prednisone are often given both after IV steroids and as an initial therapy in status migrainosus. Thus far, the efficacy of steroids in cluster headache has not been tested in controlled clinical trials (Kudrow, 1991). Prednisone is frequently used in doses of 60 to 80 mg per day for 1 week followed by a taper over 2 to 4 weeks. Doses should be individualized, however. Side effects of steroids include hypernatremia, hypokalemia, osteoporosis, aseptic necrosis of the hip, peptic ulcer disease, gastrointestinal bleeding, hyperglycemia, hypertension, psychiatric symptoms, and weight gain. Steroids are contraindicated in patients with mycobacterial or systemic fungal infections, a history of previous hypersensitivity reactions to the drugs, or ocular herpes.

Sumatriptan is a serotonin receptor agonist that exerts both direct vasoconstrictor and antineurogenic inflammatory effects on meningeal vessels. In large-scale, double-blind clinical trials, 6 mg of sumatriptan injected subcutaneously significantly reduced headache within 1 h in over 80% of patients, versus 22% for placebo (for review see Moskowitz and Cutrer, 1993). Sumatriptan treatment is also associated with lessening of nausea, vomiting, photophobia, and phonophobia. The drug is equally effective when given up to 4 h after the onset of an attack. Oral tablets in 25 and 50 mg doses have a much slower onset of effect. An intranasal formulation recently received FDA approval.

Subcutaneous sumatriptan is rapidly effective in the acute treatment of cluster headache. In a double-blind, controlled study, sumatriptan reduced within 15 min both the pain and conjunctival injection in approximately three quarters of patients (Sumatriptan Cluster Headache Study Group, 1991). Because middle-aged males make up a large proportion of cluster headache sufferers and are at increased risk for coronary artery disease, sumatriptan and other vasoconstrictive treatments should be used with caution in these patients.

Side effects of sumatriptan are generally transient and include pressure-like sensations in the head, neck, and chest, tingling in the neck or scalp, and occasional dizziness. Contraindications include definite or suspected ischemic heart disease, pregnancy, vasospastic angina, or uncontrolled hypertension.

POSSIBLE PHARMACOLOGIC MECHANISMS OF ANTIHEADACHE MEDICATIONS

Serotonergic Drugs

Serotonin (5HT) is the neurotransmitter most frequently mentioned in relation to migraine. Most evidence, however, for its direct role in the pathophysiology of migraine is circumstantial (Ferrari and Saxena, 1993). For example, platelet 5HT levels are reduced 30% during attacks and plasma concentrations are 60% lower. The biogenic amine-depleting drug reserpine causes atypical headaches in migraineurs, probably by inducing 5HT release from intracellular stores. Similarly, m-chlorophenylpiperazine (m-CPP), a major metabolite of the antidepressant trazodone, has been reported to cause migraine-like headaches in humans activating $5HT_{2B}$ or $5HT_{2C}$ receptors. Perhaps the strongest evidence for a role of 5HT in migraine is provided by the fact that some acute, such as ergot alkaloids and sumatriptan, and prophylactic, such as methysergide, pizotifen, and cyproheptadine, antimigraine drugs interact with 5HT receptors.

Currently, 15 different subtypes of 5HT receptors have been identified by pharmacologic and molecular cloning techniques (Hoyer et al., 1994). Because in the case of serotonergic drugs acute and prophylactic antimigraine agents are likely to act by different mechanisms, they will be considered in separate sections.

Acute medications. The efficacy of ergots in migraine was documented in the 1920s, although their ability to interact with 5HT receptors was not known until the 1950s. Pharmacologically, these drugs are highly nonselective, interacting with virtually all monoamine receptor sites. They were initially employed in migraine based on the belief that this condition resulted from an increase in sympathetic activity. Graham and Wolff (1938) proposed that the efficacy of ergotamine was owing to its vasoconstrictive activity on the extracranial vasculature. More recently, sumatriptan was developed by screening for agents that activate vasoconstrictive 5HT receptors (Saxena and Tfelt-Hansen, 1993). The importance of vasoconstriction to the antimigraine efficacy of sumatriptan and ergot alkaloids is controversial, however, with activation of neuronal receptors located on the trigeminal ganglion or in the brain-stem trigeminal nucleus possibly being of equal or greater significance (Moskowitz, 1992).

Neurogenic inflammation has been proposed as a mechanism to explain vascular headache pathogenesis and treatment (Moskowitz, 1992). This process involves vasodilation, plasma protein extravasation and is mediated by the release of vasoactive neuropeptides such as substance P, neurokinin A, and CGRP from trigeminovascular sensory fibers. The tachykinins induce both an endothelium-dependent vasodilation and enhance vascular permeability by acting at receptors located on the endothelium. CGRP induces vasodilation by activating receptors on vascular smooth muscle cells. Several lines of evidence suggest the importance of neurogenic inflammation in acute migraine. Thus, ergotamine and sumatriptan block this process in the dura mater of rodents after electrical stimulation of trigeminal neurons at dosages comparable to those efficacious in relieving migraine headache. These drugs inhibit the inflammatory response even when administered 45 min after electrical stimulation. Moreover, other medications effective in the treatment of migraine attacks such as opioids (Saito et al., 1988), valproic acid (Lee et al., 1995) and aspirin (Buzzi et al., 1989) but which are inactive at $5HT_1$ receptors, block plasma protein extravasation.

The specific receptor subtype responsible for the antimigraine efficacy of ergot alkaloids and sumatriptan has not been identified. Although ergot derivatives are nonselective, sumatriptan activates with high affinity the $5HT_{1B}$, $5HT_{1D}$, $5HT_{1F}$, and, to a lesser extent, the $5HT_{1A}$ receptor subtypes (Saxena and Tfelt-Hansen, 1993). Other newer antimigraine drugs, such as zolmitriptan, have a similar receptor profile (Pauwels et al., 1997). A significant role of $5HT_{1A}$ receptors can be ruled out because these receptors are not involved in the vasoconstrictive actions of these drugs and their inhibitory effects on neurogenic inflammation (see Moskowitz and Waeber, 1997). Functional experiments indicate that $5HT_{1B}$ receptors mediate vasoconstriction. In neurogenic inflammation models it is likely that $5HT_{1B}$ receptors are important in rats and mice, $5HT_{1D}$ in guinea pigs, and possibly $5HT_{1F}$ receptors in rats and guinea pigs.

Reverse transcriptase polymerase chain reaction techniques and *in situ* hybridization experiments have detected similar amounts of the mRNAs for both human $5HT_{1D}$ and $5HT_{1B}$ mRNA in trigeminal ganglia (Bouchelet et al., 1996). The $5HT_{1F}$ receptor mRNA was also found in human trigeminal ganglia, indicating they are located presynaptically. Interestingly, mRNAs for both $h5HT_{1B}$ and $5HT_{1F}$ receptors, but only trace amounts of $h5HT_{1D}$ receptor mRNA, were found on cerebrovascular tissues. Human $5HT_{1B}$ mRNA has been found in one coronary artery. In view of the reported cardiovascular side effects of sumatriptan (MacIntyre et al., 1993), these data suggest that selective $5HT_{1D}$ agonists devoid of effects at $5HT_{1B}$ receptors might alleviate headache with greatly reduced side effects. Antisera specific for $5HT_{1D}$ receptors stained trigeminal axons in the meninges, whereas antisera for $5HT_{1B}$ receptors stained vascular smooth muscle. No selective $5HT_{1D}$ receptor agonists is as yet available for clinical studies.

Prophylactic medications. So-called antiserotonin drugs were the first agents used for migraine prophylaxis and are still important today (Tfelt-Hansen and Saxena, 1993). Methysergide is an ergot derivative that has complex effects on serotonergic and other neurotransmitter systems. Other serotonin antagonists, such as cyproheptadine, pizotifen, and lisuride, are also reportedly effective in migraine prophylaxis. The tricyclic antidepressant amitriptyline is an effective prophylactic agent in migraine. This effect is independent of its antidepressant actions. Interestingly, all of these drugs share the ability to block $5HT_{2A}$ receptors.

It is well known that methysergide potently antagonizes the contractile effects of 5HT on vascular and nonvascular smooth muscles which is mediated by $5HT_{2A}$ receptors. It is, however, unlikely that blockade of these receptors accounts for the efficacy of antiserotonin drugs because other potent $5HT_{2A}$ receptors antagonists, such as mianserin, ketanserin, and ICI 169,369 seem to be without any prophylactic effect in migraine. It has been proposed that the vasoconstrictor action of methysergide, and of its active metabolite methylergometrine, is responsible for its therapeutic activity. Inhibition of neurogenic inflammation after chronic treatment with methysergide has also been invoked as a mechanism of action in migraine prophylaxis.

Fozard and Kalkman (1994) contend that $5HT_{2B}$, or possibly $5HT_{2C}$, receptor activation might be a key factor in the initiation of migraine. This hypothesis is based on the finding that meta-chlorophenyl-piperazine, an agonist at these sites, triggers migraine attacks in control patients and migraineurs, and that the doses of a series of antimigraine prophylactic drugs correlates with their antagonist potencies at $5HT_{2B}$ receptors. The drugs used in this correlation included classical $5HT_2$ receptor antagonists such as methysergide, pizotifen, Org GC 94, cyproheptadine, and mianserin, and agents not primarily considered as such, including amitriptyline, chlorpromazine, and propanolol. An additional argument was that ketanserin and pindolol are inactive as antimigraine agents and are weak $5HT_{2B}$ antagonists. Moreover, $5HT_{2B}$ receptor mRNA is present on all blood vessels investigated and activation of this receptor induces endothelium-dependent vasodilation, presumably as a consequence of nitric oxide release. This, in turn, might activate and sensitize trigeminovascular neurons and initiate the neurogenic inflammation process associated with migraine.

GABAergic Drugs

The simple branched-chain carboxylic acid valproate (n-dipropylacetic acid) has diverse effects on both neurotransmitter-dependent and independent cellular events, as reflected by its efficacy in multiple therapeutic settings (Cutrer et al., 1997). The enhancement of GABAergic neurotransmission is perhaps its best-known action. Valproic acid increases GABA brain levels by stimulating the GABA synthesizing enzyme glutamic acid decarboxylase, and by inhibiting the GABA degrading enzymes. Valproic acid modulates several other neurotransmitter systems, including excitatory and inhibitory amino acids, serotonin, dopamine, and enkephalins, although it is not known whether these effects are due to a direct action of valproic acid itself or are secondary to the increase in GABA. At therapeutically relevant concentrations, valproic acid inhibits sustained repetitive firing induced by depolarization of mouse cortical or spinal cord neurons (McLean and Macdonald, 1986). This effect appears to be mediated by a prolonged recovery of voltage-activated Na^+ channels from inactivation.

The efficacy of valproic acid as an antimigraine drug might be accounted for by an action at different levels of the migraine cascade. For instance, a valproic acid-mediated increase in GABAergic neurotransmission may suppress the abnormal cortical events hypothesized to underlie migraine aura. Valproic acid has also been shown to attenuate plasma protein extravasation in a rodent model of meningeal neurogenic inflammation. This effect is blocked by the $GABA_A$ receptor antagonist bicuculline and mimicked by drugs acting at the $GABA_A$ receptor complex, including muscimol, the benzodiazepines, zolpidem, CL 218,872 and the neurosteroid allopregnanolone. At the level of the trigeminal nucleus caudalis, where meningeal primary afferent fibers terminate, valproic acid has been shown to reduce activation of neurons in laminae I and II after intracisternal administration of capsaicin. This effect also appears to be mediated by $GABA_A$ receptors because it is mimicked by butalbital and allopregnanolone and blocked by the $GABA_A$ receptor antagonist bicuculline.

Structurally, gabapentin is GABA covalently linked to a lipophilic cyclohexane ring (Goa and Sorkin, 1993). Unlike GABA, gabapentin readily crosses the blood-brain barrier. Although it was designed to be a centrally active GABA receptor agonist, gabapentin does not bind to GABA receptors or mimic GABA when applied iontophoretically to neurons in primary culture. Rather, gabapentin appears to act by increasing the release of GABA by some unknown mechanism (Honmou et al., 1995). Its molecular target may be linked, or identical to, a site resembling the L-amino acid transporter protein. Gabapentin has not been found consistently to reduce sustained repetitive firing of action potentials nor to affect significantly any Ca^{2+} channel current (Macdonald and Kelly, 1993). The drug is inactive at neurotransmitter receptor and ion channel binding sites. Because gabapentin seems to increase synaptic GABA levels, its effect is likely to be mediated by GABA receptors and therefore it might resemble valproic acid as a therapy for headache.

Carbamazepine and phenytoin have been used in migraine prophylaxis based on the unproven assertion of an association between migraine and epilepsy. Carbamazepine is an iminostilbene with a structure that resembles tricyclic antidepressants and phenytoin. Its mechanism of action is not fully understood. Carbamazepine is an effective anticonvulsant in several different animal models of epilepsy. It also inhibits synaptic transmission within spinal trigeminal nucleus (Fromm, 1969). Phenytoin inhibits the spread of electroshock-induced seizures by reducing membrane excitability. Its ability to reduce post-tetanic potentiation in the stellate ganglion and spinal cord of cats suggests a possible additional mechanism in the treatment of neuralgias.

Nonsteroidal Anti-inflammatory Drugs

NSAIDs, which display antiinflammatory, analgesic and antipyretic properties, are commonly used for acute and prophylactic treatment of headaches. These drugs block cyclooxygenase, which converts arachidonic acid to prostaglandins and thromboxane, but have little effects on lipoxygenase which is responsible for the production of leukotrienes. Most currently available NSAIDs inhibit both cyclooxygenase 1 and cyclooxygenase 2 activities (Froehlich, 1997). The inhibition of cyclooxygenase 2 is thought to mediate, at least in part, the antipyretic, analgesic, and anti-inflammatory actions of NSAIDs, whereas inhibition of cyclooxygenase 1 causes unwanted side effects, particularly those leading to gastric ulcers, that result from decreased prostaglandin and thromboxane formation. Whereas aspirin, indomethacin, and ibuprofen have a higher affinity for cyclooxygenase 1 than for cyclooxygenase 2, diclophenac and naproxen seem to inhibit both isoform with equal potency. No preferential cyclooxygenase 2 inhibitor is currently used for headache treatment. Meloxicam has been reported to show some selectivity for COX-2 in vitro and is available in several European countries for the treatment of osteoarthritis.

NSAIDs include salicylic acids, such as aspirin, which irreversibly acetylate cyclooxygenase, and several other classes of organic acids, including propionic acid derivatives such as ibuprofen, naproxen, ketoprofen, and flurbiprofen, acetic acid derivatives such as indomethacin and diclofenac, and enolic acids such as piroxicam, all of which compete with arachidonic acid at the active site of cyclooxygenase. Although acetaminophen is a very weak anti-inflammatory agent it is effective as an antipyretic and analgesic agent and lacks some of the side effects of NSAIDs, such as gastrointestinal tract damage and blockade of platelet aggregation.

NSAIDs are usually classified as mild analgesics, but a consideration of the type of pain and its intensity is important in the assessment of analgesic efficacy. For example, in some forms of postoperative pain, NSAIDs can be superior to the opioids. Moreover, they are particularly effective when inflammation has caused sensitization of pain receptors to normally painless mechanical or chemical stimuli. This sensitization appears to result from a lowering of the threshold of the polymodal nociceptor located on C fibers. Increased excitability of central neurons in the spinal cord might also be important (Konttinen et al., 1994). Although the precise mode of action of the central effects of NSAIDs is unknown, these drugs inhibit prostaglandin synthesis in brain neurons, prolong brain catecholamine and serotonin turnover, and block the release of serotonin in response to noxious stimuli (Bromm et al., 1992; Gebhart and McCormack, 1994). Acetylsalicylic acid and ketorolac have also been shown to inhibit central trigeminal nucleus caudalis neurons in cats (Kaube et al., 1993).

Bradykinin, released from plasma kininogen, and cytokines, such as tumor necrosis factor, interleukin-1, and interleukin-8, appear to be particularly important in mediating the pain of inflammation. These agents liberate prostaglandins and probably other substances that promote hyperalgesia. Neuropeptides, such as substance P and CGRP may also be involved in eliciting pain. Indomethacin and acetylsalicylic acid have been reported to block meningeal neurogenic inflammation after trigeminal ganglion stimulation or substance P administration (Buzzi et al., 1989). This inhibitory effect is observed 5 min after trigeminal ganglion stimulation, precluding a significant role of inducible cyclooxygenase 2 in the action of NSAIDs in this model.

Opioids

Opioids decrease the response to noxious stimuli by acting at various sites within the brain, including the periaqueductal gray (μ-receptors), rostral ventral medulla (μ/δ receptors),

substantia nigra (μ-receptors), and dorsal horn of the spinal cord ($\mu/\delta/\kappa$ receptors) (Yaksh, 1997). A number of subclasses of the principal categories of opioid receptors mediate the effects of endogenous ligands. Three distinct families of endogenous peptides have been identified: the enkephalins, the endorphins, and the dynorphins. Each is derived from a distinct precursor and has a characteristic anatomical distribution.

Although morphine is relatively selective for μ-receptors, it can interact with the others, particularly at higher doses. Most of the opioids used clinically, including meperidine, are relatively selective for μ-receptors, reflecting their similarity to morphine. Codeine has a very low affinity for opioid receptors, with its analgesic effect due to its conversion to morphine. Although slightly less selective than morphine, propoxyphene binds primarily to μ-opioid receptors and produces analgesia and other CNS effects similar to those seen with morphine-like opioids. Although highly selective μ-receptor agonists have been developed, antagonists have been most useful in defining μ-receptors. Using these antagonists, investigators have established that morphine elicits analgesia either spinally (μ_2) or supraspinally (μ_1). When administered systemically, however, morphine acts predominantly through supraspinal μ_1-receptors. Both respiratory depression and constipation due to inhibition of gastrointestinal transit are responses believed to be mediated through μ_2-receptors.

In the spinal cord, and probably also the trigeminal nucleus, the opioid effect is mediated by an activation of inhibitory receptors located presynaptically on primary afferent fibers and by a postsynaptic hyperpolarization of projection neurons. Morphine blocks the effects of exogenously administered substance P by exerting postsynaptic inhibitory actions on interneurons and output neurons of the spinothalamic tract that convey nociceptive information to higher centers in the brain. In addition, peripheral μ- and κ-receptors modulate the sensitized state of the small afferent terminals innervating inflamed tissues and reduce hyperalgesia. In the periaqueductal gray, opioid agonists indirectly activate bulbospinal pathways and rostral projections to forebrain areas and modulate afferent input into the brainstem core.

Tricyclic Antidepressants

Antidepressants have been used for many years to treat pain based on the rationale they might relieve concomitant depression. Nevertheless, the fact that amitriptyline is the only antidepressant drug with proven efficacy in migraine prophylaxis suggests that the antimigraine effect is unrelated to antidepressant action (Couch et al., 1976). Tricyclic antidepressants were originally thought to exert their therapeutic effects by increasing the concentrations of norepinephrine and serotonin in the synaptic cleft, leading to adaptive changes in postsynaptic receptors, including β-adrenergic and $5HT_2$ sites. Imipramine and the selective serotonin reuptake inhibitor fluoxetine, however, share this effect with amitriptyline, but have little effect in migraine prophylaxis.

While the possibility that $5HT_{2A}$ receptor blockade might explain the efficacy of amitriptyline, studies suggest that antagonism of this receptor subtype is probably not responsible for the effect of antiserotonin drugs in migraine. Blockade of vascular $5HT_{2B}$ receptors has also been suggested as a possible mechanism of action. Interestingly, amitriptyline has been shown to reverse inflammatory hyperalgesia in rats by a mechanism unrelated to monoamine reuptake inhibition, and more likely due to NMDA receptor antagonism (Eisenach and Gebhart, 1995). The possible relevance of this target is further suggested by the fact that other tricyclic agents such as desipramine, cyproheptadine, and carbamazepine reduce NMDA-induced intracellular $[(Ca^{2+})]$ elevations in neuronal cultures at relevant concentrations (Cai and McCaslin, 1992).

Calcium Channel Antagonists

Calcium channel antagonists, also known as slow channel inhibitors or Ca^{2+} entry blockers, are a heterogenous group of drugs with several classes blocking different types of Ca^{2+} channels (Peters et al., 1991). Calcium channel antagonists have been introduced in migraine prophylaxis because of their vasodilatory effect on cerebral vessels and their protective action against the cerebral hypoxia thought to be present during migraine attacks (Toda and Tfelt-Hansen, 1993). Both phenomena, however, are now thought unlikely to occur in migraine. Nimodipine is more potent than flunarizine at preventing calcium-induced contraction of human cerebral and temporal arteries. This contrasts with the fact that flunarizine is considered to be the best calcium channel antagonist for migraine prophylaxis, whereas the efficacy of nimodipine is only marginal and suggests that flunarizine's site of action is likely to be in the CNS.

Calcium channel blockade is not the only action of flunarizine, which also interacts with central histaminic, dopaminergic, and serotonergic receptors (Greenberg, 1986). It has been suggested that calcium channel antagonists may be effective in migraine prophylaxis via inhibition of cortical spreading depression (CSD), a possible cause of migraine. However, only high doses of flunarizine were able to increase the threshold for CSD, while other studies failed to reproduce this finding. Intracerebroventricular administration of calcium channel antagonists in mice causes analgesia, but nimodipine is more potent than flunarizine in this model (Miranda et al., 1993).

β-Adrenergic Receptor Antagonists

The prophylactic efficacy of β-adrenergic receptor antagonists was discovered serendipitously by Rabkin and colleagues (1966) who reported that migraine improved in a patient with angina pectoris treated with propranolol. Numerous clinical trials have confirmed the efficacy of propranolol and other β-adrenergic receptor antagonists, including nadolol, atenolol, metoprolol, and timolol. By contrast, a number of such drugs,

including acebutolol, oxprenolol, alprenolol, and pindolol do not appear to be effective in migraine therapy. It has been suggested that only silent β-adrenergic receptor antagonists, that is, those devoid of sympathomimetic activity, are effective in migraine prophylaxis.

Some β-adrenergic receptor antagonists interact with $5HT_{1A}$ receptors in both animal and human brains (Peroutka, 1990). Stimulation of these receptors on serotonergic neurons in the raphe nuclei inhibit intrinsic cell firing. The inhibitory effects of $5HT_{1A}$ agonists can be blocked by propranolol. However, β-adrenergic receptor antagonists vary widely in their affinity for the $5HT_{1A}$ receptor. For example, pindolol is the most potent drug studied in this regard and yet has no antimigraine activity. Conversely, a number of β-adrenergic receptor antagonist antimigraine agents, such as propranolol and timolol, display moderate affinity for $5HT_{1A}$ receptors. Therefore, there is no obvious correlation between drug affinity and potency in migraine relief. In addition, atenolol is totally inactive at all 5HT receptor subtypes yet has been reported to be effective against migraine in two independent clinical trials. As a result, the antimigraine efficacy of certain β-adrenergic receptor antagonists cannot derive solely from blockade of 5HT receptors.

There are some indications that β-adrenergic receptor antagonists exert their antimigraine effects on central catecholaminergic systems. The contingent negative variation (CNV), an event-related slow negative cerebral potential recorded over the scalp in a simple reaction time task with warning stimulants, is significantly increased and its habituation reduced in untreated migraine patients in comparison with controls and tension-type headache sufferers. The CNV returns to normal after treatment with β-adrenergic receptor antagonists (Schoenen et al., 1986). This suggests that an action in the CNS might be responsible for the migraine prophylactic effect of these drugs. It should, however, be noted that although atenolol penetrates the CNS poorly, it is an efficient antimigraine prophylactic agent. Thus, the mechanism of action of β-adrenergic receptor antagonists in migraine remains to be established.

Dopamine Receptor Antagonists

Phenothiazines such as chlorpromazine and prochlorperazine possess a three-ring structure in which two benzene rings are linked by a sulfur and a nitrogen atom; a carbon side chain branches off the nitrogen atom. A growing series of heterocyclic antipsychotics are the enantiomeric substituted benzamides, which include the gastroenterologic agent metoclopramide. Phenothiazines and benzamides are dopamine receptor antagonists with a broad spectrum of pharmacologic activity. They also have varying degrees of activity in inhibiting serotonergic, histaminic, adrenergic, and cholinergic receptor systems.

Phenothiazines and benzamides protect against the nausea- and emesis-inducing effects of apomorphine and certain ergot alkaloids, all of which can interact with central dopaminergic receptors in the chemoreceptor trigger zone of the me-dulla. The antiemetic effect of most antipsychotics occurs with low doses. Drugs or other stimuli that cause emesis by an action on the nodose ganglion, or locally on the gastrointestinal tract, are not antagonized by antipsychotic drugs, although potent piperazines and butyrophenones are sometimes effective against nausea caused by vestibular stimulation.

While the mechanism of action of phenothiazines in relieving migraines is unknown, it has been postulated that chlorpromazine might alter serotonergic transmission (Lane et al., 1989). Another possibility is that the relief could be secondary to its antipsychotic effect, causing an indifference to pain.

Other Agents

Lithium.   Lithium, the lightest of the alkali metals, shares some properties of Na^+ and K^+. Although traces of the ion occur in animal tissues, it has no known physiologic role. Both lithium carbonate and lithium citrate are currently available for therapeutic use in the United States. Therapeutic concentrations of lithium ion (Li^+) have almost no discernible psychotropic effects in normal individuals, distinguishing it from other psychotropic agents. Lithium salts were introduced into psychiatry in 1949 for the treatment of mania (Cade, 1949). While its precise mechanism of action is unknown, many of its cellular actions have been characterized. An important property of Li^+ is the relatively small gradient of distribution across biological membranes, unlike Na^+ and K^+; although it can replace Na^+ in supporting a single action potential in a nerve cell, it is not an adequate substrate for the Na^+ pump and therefore cannot maintain membrane potentials. It is uncertain whether important interactions occur between Li^+ and the transport of other monovalent or divalent cations by nerve cells.

Lithium may interfere with neurotransmission by influencing transmitters, receptors, and second messengers (Jefferson, 1990). For instance, it has been suggested that the antidepressant, antimanic, or prophylactic effects of lithium involve serotonergic transmission. Lithium may also alter the concentration of peptides in different regions of the rat brain (Hong et al., 1983). Thus, it has been shown that chronic administration of lithium increases substance P-like immunoreactivity in the corpus striatum, nucleus accumbens and frontal cerebral cortex, but not in the hypothalamus, hippocampus, or brain

stem (Hong et al., 1983; Sivam et al., 1989). Lithium has also been found to inhibit substance P and vasoactive intestinal peptides, but not CGRP-induced relaxations of isolated porcine ophthalmic artery (Vincent, 1992).

Phenelzine.   The first monoamine oxidase (MAO) inhibitors to be used in the treatment of depression were derivatives of hydrazine, a highly hepatotoxic substance. Phenelzine is the hydrazine analog of phenethylamine, a substrate for MAO. Hydrazine compounds are site-directed, irreversible MAO inhibitors which act by attacking and inactivating the flavin prosthetic group following the oxidation of the drug to reactive intermediates by MAO. Monoamine oxidase inhibitors were introduced in migraine prophylaxis because of their ability to increase levels of endogenous serotonin. An open trial of phenelzine did not show any correlation between its prophylactic effect in migraine and increases in platelet 5HT levels. Modulation of central nervous system monoaminergic neurotransmission is more likely to be responsible for the effect of phenelzine in migraine. As with other antidepressants, MAO inhibitors produce a gradual downregulation in $5HT_2$ and β-adrenergic receptors in brain (Heninger and Charney, 1987).

Steroids.   Glucocorticoids can prevent or suppress inflammation in response to multiple events, including radiant, mechanical, chemical, infectious, and immunologic stimuli. The suppression of inflammation results, at least in part, from the inhibition of phospholipase A_2 activity, leading to a decrease of both prostaglandin and leukotriene synthesis, and may underlie the antimigraine efficacy of these drugs. Multiple mechanisms are involved in the suppression of inflammation by glucocorticoids. It is now clear that glucocorticoids inhibit the production of factors that are critical in generating the inflammatory response. As a result, there is decreased release of vasoactive and chemotactic factors, diminished secretion of lipolytic and proteolytic enzymes, and decreased extravasation of leukocytes. Glucocorticoids also inhibit the production of interleukins (IL-1, IL-2, IL-3, IL-6) and tumor necrosis factor a (TNF-a).

Dexamethasone has recently been shown to selectively inhibit expression of cyclooxygenase 2 suggesting this enzyme might be an additional target for steroid drugs (Masferrer et al., 1994). Moreover, dexamethasone and other glucocorticoids are antiemetics, although the mechanisms of this effect is unknown.

Table 16-6
Drug List

Class	Generic name	Trade name	Dose
Para-aminophenol derivative	Acetaminophen	Tylenol tablets, gelcaps, capsules	325, 500, 650 mg
		Tylenol suspension	500 mg/15 mL;
		Feverall suppositories	120, 325 mg
		APAP drops	80 mg/2.5 mL
Carbonic anhydrase inhibitor	Acetazolamide	Diamox	125, 250 mg
Antidepressants	Amitriptyline	Elavil, Endep	10, 25, 50, 75, 100, 150 mg
	Desipramine	Norpramine	10, 25, 50, 75, 100, 150 mg
	Nortriptyline	Pamelor	10, 25, 50, 75 mg
	Doxepin	Adapin, Sinequan	10, 25, 50 , 75, 100, 150 mg;
		Zonalon creme	5%
	Maprotiline	Ludiomil	25, 50, 75 mg
	Fluoxetine	Prozac	10, 20 mg
Anticonvulsants	Valproic acid	Depakene	250 mg
	Divalproex sodium	Depakote	125, 250, 500 mg
	Gabapentin	Neurontin	100, 300, 400 mg
β-adrenergic receptor blockers	Propranolol	Inderal	10, 20, 40, 60, 80 mg
		Inderal LA	60, 120, 160 mg
	Nadolol	Corgard	20, 40, 80, 120, 160 mg
	Timolol	Blockadren	5, 10, 20 mg
	Atenolol	Tenormen	25, 50, 100 mg
	Metoprolol	Lopressor	50, 100 mg
Azapirone anxiolytic	Buspirone	Buspar	5, 10 mg
Barbiturate	Butalbital	Axotal	Butal. 50 mg + ASA 650,
		Fiorinal	Butal. 50 mg + ASA 325 + caffeine 40 mg
		Esgic, Fencet, Fioricet, Medigesic, Pacaps, Repan	Butal. 50 mg + acetaminophen 325 mg, caffeine + 40 mg
		Esgic plus	Butal. 50 mg + acetamin. 500 mg + caffeine 40 mg
		Phreneline	Butal. 50 mg + acetaminophen 325 mg
		Phreneline forte, sedapap, bupap, repan-cf, tecon	Butal. 50 mg + acetaminophen 650 mg

(*continued*)

Table 16-6
Drug List (*continued*)

Class	Generic name	Trade name	Dose
Calcium channel blocker	Verapamil	Calan, Isoptin, Verelan	40, 80, 120, 180, 240 mg
Serotonin antagonist	Cyproheptadine	Periactin	4-mg tab; 2 mg/5 mL syrup
Ergotamine derivatives	Ergotamine tartarate	Cafergot, Wigraine	1 mg + caffeine 100 mg tab; sup ergot. 2 mg + caffeine 100 mg
		Ergomar	Ergot 2 mg tab
		Ergostat	Ergot 2 mg sublingual
	Dihydroergotamine	DHE 45	1 mg/mL injectable
	Methysergide	Sansert	2-mg tab
Diuretic	Furosemide	Lasix	20, 40, 80 mg tabs; 10 mg/mL; oral solution; 10 mg/mL injectable solution, 2-, 4-, 10-mL ampules
Sympathomimetic amine	Isometheptene mucate	Midrin, Duradrin	Isometheptene 65 mg + dichloralphenazone 100 mg + acetamin. 325 mg
		Migralam	Isometheptene 65 mg + caffeine 100 mg + acetaminophen 325
Lithium salts	Lithium carbonate	Eskalith	300 mg
		Eskalith CR	450 mg
		Lithonate	300 capsule and tabs
Antipsychotics/ prokinetics	Metoclopramide	Reglan	5, 10 mg tabs; 5 mg/5 mL syrup; 5 mg/mL injectable 2-, 10-, 30-mL ampules
	Chlorpromazine	Thorazine	10, 25, 50, 100, 200 mg tabs; 30, 75, 150 mg SR caps; 25 mg/mL injectable 1-, 2-, 10-mL ampules; 10 mg/5 mL syrup; 25-, 100-mg sup.
	Prochlorperazine	Compazine	5, 10, 25 mg tabs, 10-, 15-mg caps. 5 mg/mL injectable 2, 10 mg ampules; 2.5-, 5-, 25-mg sup; 5 mg/5 mL syrup
	Promethazine	Phenergan	12.5, 25, 50 tabs, and sup; 10 mg/5 mL syrup

(continued)

Table 16-6
Drug List (*continued*)

Class	Generic name	Trade name	Dose
Nonsteroidal anti-inflammatory drugs	Aspirin	Bufferin, Excedrin	ASA 250 mg + acetaminophen 250 mg + caffeine 65
		Norgesic	Orphenadrin 25 mg + ASA 385 mg + caffeine 30 mg
		Ecotrin, Ascriptin	81, 325, 500 mg
	Ibuprofen	Advil, Motrin, Nuprin, IBU-TAB	200, 300, 400, 600, 800 mg
	Ketoprofen	Orudis	25, 50, 75 mg
	Naproxen	Naprosyn	250, 375, 500 mg
	Naproxen sodium	Aleve, Anaprox, Aflaxen	220, 275, 550 mg
	Ketorolac trimethamine	Toradol	10-mg tabs; 1 mg/mL IM injectable
	Indomethacin	Indocin, Indomethacin	25-, 50-mg capsules; 5 mg/mL elixir; 50-mg sup.
Opioid analgesics	Codeine	Empirin with codeine	Aspirin 325 + codeine 30 or 60 mg
		Tylenol with codeine	Acetaminophen 300 mg + codeine 15, 30 or 60 mg
		Fiorinal with codeine	Butalbital 50 mg + aspirin 325 mg + caffeine 40 mg + codeine 30 mg
		Fioricet with codeine	Butalbital 50 mg + acetaminophen 325 mg + caffeine 40 mg + codeine 30 mg
	Hydrocodone	Lortab	Hydrocodone 5 mg + ASA 500 mg
		Anexsia, Hydrocet, Lorcet, Vicodin	Hydrocodone 5 mg + acetaminophen 500 mg
		Anexsia, Lorcet plus	Hydrocodone 7.5 mg + acetaminophen 650 mg
		Vicodin plus	Hydrocodone 7.5 mg + acetaminophen 750 mg
	Oxycodone	Percodan, Roxiprin	ASA 325 mg + oxycodone 5 mg

(*continued*)

Table 16-6

Drug List (*continued*)

Class	Generic name	Trade name	Dose
Opioid analgesics	Oxycodone	Percocet, Roxicet	Acetaminophen 325 mg + oxycodone 5 mg
		Tylox	Acetaminophen 500 mg + oxycodone 5 mg
	Propoxyphene	Darvon	65 mg
		Wygesic	Acetaminophen 650 mg + propoxyphene 65 mg
	PC-CAP	Darvocet	Acetaminophen 325 or 650 + propoxyphene 50 or 100 mg
	Meperidine	Demerol	50-, 100-, 500-mg tabs, 10 mg/mL syrup; 25, 50, 75 100 mg/mL injectable
		Mepergan	Meperidine 25 mg + promethazine 25 mg/mL
	Butorphanol	Stadol NS	2 mg/mL; 10-mL multidose vial
Monoamine oxidase inhibitor	Phenelzine	Nardil	15 mg
Steroid medications	Dexamethasone	Decadron	4 mg/mL in 1-, 5-, 25-mL vials; 24 mg/mL in 5-, 10-mL vials
	Prednisone	Deltasone, Prednisone, Sterapred, Prednicen-M	2.5, 5, 10, 20, 50 mg
Triptans	Sumatriptan	Imitrex	25, 50 tabs; 6-mg injectable ampules
	Naratriptan	Amergo	2.5 mg tab
	Zolmitriptan	Zomig	2.5, 5 mg tab
	Rizatriptan	Maxalt	Not yet available

For additional information on the drugs discussed in this chapter see chapters 10, 11, 17, 18, 19, 20, 21, 23, 27, 29, 32, and 59 in *Goodman & Gilman's The Pharmacological Basis of Therapeutics* (Ninth Edition), McGraw-Hill, New York, 1996.

REFERENCES

Adams HP, Biller J: Temporal arteritis and vasculitis of the central nervous system, in Johnson R (ed): *Current Therapy in Neurologic Disease*-3. Philadelphia, B.C. Decker, 1990, pp 198–199.

Adly C, Straumanis J, Chession A: Fluoxetine prophylaxis of migraine. *Headache* 1992;32:101–104.

Andersson PG, Jespersen LT: Dihydroergotamine nasal spray in the treatment of cluster headache: a double-blind trial versus placebo. *Cephalalgia* 1986;6:51–54.

Anthony M, Lance JW: Monoamine oxidase inhibition in the treatment of migraine. *Arch Neurol* 1969;21:263–268.

Batnitzky S, Kencher TR, Mealey J Jr, Campbell RL: Iatrogenic intraspinal epidermoid tumors. *JAMA* 1977;237:148–151.

Belgrade MJ, Ling LJ, Schleevogt MB et al.: Comparison of single-dose meperidine, butorphanol and dihydroergotamine in the treatment of vascular headache. *Neurology* 1989;39:590–592.

Bell R, Montoya D, Shuaib A, Lee MA: Comparative trial of three agents in the treatment of acute migraine. *Ann Emerg Med* 1990;19:1079–1082.

Bernard JF, Peschanski M, Besson JM: A possible spino-(trigemino)-ponto amygdaloid pathway for pain. *Neurosci Lett* 1989;100:83–88.

Bouchelet I, Cohen Z, Case B et al.: Differential expression of sumatriptan-sensitive 5–hydroxytryptamine receptors in human trigeminal ganglia and cerebral blood vessels. *Mol Pharmacol* 1996;50:219–223.

Bromm B, Forth W, Richter E, Scharein E: Effects of acetaminophen and antipyrine on non-inflammatory pain and EEG activity. *Pain* 1992;50:213–221.

Bushnell MC, Duncan GH: Sensory and affective aspects of pain perception: is medial thalamus restricted to emotional issues? *Exp Brain Res* 1989;78:415–418.

Bussone G, Leone M, Peccarisi C: Double blind comparison of lithium and verapamil in cluster headache prophylaxis. *Headache* 1990;30:411–417.

Buzzi MG, Sakas DE, Moskowitz MA: Indomethacin and acetylsalicylic acid block neurogenic plasma protein extravasation in rat dura mater. *Eur J Pharmacol* 1989;165:251–258.

Cade JFJ: Lithium salts in the treatment of psychotic excitement. *Med J Aust* 1949;2:349–352.

Cai Z, McCaslin PP: Amitriptyline, desipramine, cyproheptadine and carbamazepine, in concentrations used therapeutically, reduce kainate- and N-methyl-D-aspartate-induced intracellular $Ca2+$ levels in neuronal culture. *Eur J Pharmacol* 1992;219:53–57.

Callaham M, Raskin NH: A controlled study of dihydroergotamine in the treatment of acute migraine headache. *Headache* 1986;26:168–171.

Campbell JK, Caselli RJ: Headache and other craniofacial pain, in Bradley WG, Daroff RB, Fenichel GM, Marsden CD (eds): *Neurology in Clinical Practice*. Stoneham, MA, Butterworth, 1991, pp 1510–1511.

Corbett JJ: Headache due to idiopathic intracranial hypertension, in Goadsby PJ, Silberstein SD (eds): Headache. Boston, Butterworth-Heinemann, 1997, pp 279–283.

Coria F, Sempere AP, Duarte J et al.: Low-dose sodium valproate in the prophylaxis of migraine. *Clin Neuropharmacol* 1994;17:569–573.

Couch JR, Hassanein R: Amitriptyline in migraine prophylaxis. *Arch Neurol* 1979;36:695–699.

Couch JR, Ziegler DK, Hassanein R: Amitriptyline in prophylaxis of migraine: effectiveness and relationship of antimigraine and antidepressant effects. *Neurology* 1976;26:121–127.

Craig AD Jr, Burton H: Spinal and medullary lamina I projection to nucleus submedius in medial thalamus: a possible pain center. *J Neurophysiol* 1981;45:443–466.

Curran DA, Hinterberger H, Lance JW: Methysergide. *Res Clin Stud Headache* 1967;1:74–122.

Curran DA, Lance JW: Clinical trial of methysergide and other preparations in the management of migraine. *J Neurol Neurosurg Psychiat* 1964;27:463–469.

Cutrer FM: Headache, in Borsook D, LeBel A, McPeek B (eds): *The Massachusetts General Hospital Handbook of Pain Management*. Boston, Little Brown, 1995 pp 270–302.

Cutrer FM, Limmroth V, Moskowitz MA: Possible mechanisms of valproate in migraine prophylaxis. *Cephalalgia* 1997;17:93–100.

Diamond S: The use of sumatriptan in patients on monoamine oxidase inhibitors. *Neurology* 1995;45:1039–1040.

Mathew NT, Ravishankar K, Sanin LC: Coexistence of migraine and intracranial hypertension without papilledema. *Neurology* 1996;46:1226–1230.

Durcan FJ, Corbett J, Wall M: The incidence of pseudotumor cerebri: population studies in Iowa and Louisiana. *Arch Neurol* 1988;45:875–877.

Edmeads J: Emergency management of headache. *Headache* 1988;27:675–679.

Eisenach JC, Gebhart GF: Intrathecal amitriptyline acts as an N-methyl-D-aspartate receptor antagonist in the presence of inflammatory hyperalgesia in rats. *Anesthesiology* 1995;83:1046–1054.

Ekbom K: Lithium for cluster headache: review of the literature and preliminary results of long-term treatment. *Headache* 1981;21:132–139.

Ferrari MD, Saxena PR: On serotonin and migraine: a clinical and pharmacological review. *Cephalalgia* 1993;13:151–165.

Feuerstein TJ, Zeides A: Theophylline relieves headache following lumbar puncture. *Klin Wochenschr* 1986;64:216–218.

Fogelholm R, Murro K: Maprotyline in chronic tension headache: double-blind cross over study. *Headache* 1985;25:273–275.

Forsyth PA, Posner JB: Headaches in patients with brain tumors: a study in 111 patients. *Neurology* 1993;43:1678–1683.

Fozard JR, Kalkman HO: 5–hydroxytryptamine (5-HT) and the initiation of migraine: new perspectives. *Naunyn-Schmiedeberg's Arch Pharmacol* 1994;350:225–229.

Froehlich JC: A classification of NSAIDS according to the relative inhibition of cyclooxygenase isoenzymes. *Trends Pharmacol Sci* 1997;18:30–34.

Fromm GH: Pharmacological consideration of anticonvulsants. *Headache* 1969;9:35–41.

Frossman B, Henriksson KG, Johansson et al.: Propranolol for migraine prophylaxis. *Headache* 1976;16:238–245.

Frossman B, Lindblad CJ, Zbornikova V: Atenolol for migraine prophylaxis. *Headache* 1983;23:188–190.

Gabai IJ, Spierings ELH: Prophylactic treatment of cluster headache with verapamil. *Headache* 1989;29:167–168.

Gebhart GF, McCormack KJ: Neuronal plasticity: implication for pain therapy. *Drugs* 1994;47(suppl 5):1–47.

Goa KL, Sorkn EM: Gabapentin, a review of its pharmacological properties and clinical potential in epilepsy. *Drugs* 1993;46:409–427.

Gomersall JD, Stuart A: Amitriptyline in migraine prophylaxis: changes in pattern of attacks during a controlled clinical trial. *J Neurol Neurosurg Psychiat* 1973;36:684–690.

Graham JR, Wolff HG: Mechanism of migraine headache and action of ergotamine tartrate. *Arch Neurol Psychiat* 1938;39:737–763.

Haas DC: Chronic post-traumatic headache classified and compared with natural headache. *Cephalalgia* 1995;16(7):486–493.

Hayashi H, Tabata T: Pulpal and cutaneous inputs to somatosensory neurons in the parabrachial area of the cat. *Brain Res* 1990;511:177–179.

Headache Classification Committee of the International Headache Society: Classification and diagnostic criteria for headache disorders, cranial neuralgias and facial pain. *Cephalalgia* 1988;8(suppl 7):1–96.

Heninger GR, Charney DS: Mechanism of action of antidepressant treatments: implications for the etiology and treatment of depressive disorders, in Meltzer HY (ed): *Psychopharmacology: The Third Generation of Progress.* New York, Raven Press, 1987, pp 535–544.

Hering R, Kuritzky A: Sodium valproate in the treatment of cluster headache: an open clinical trial. *Cephalalgia* 1989;9:195–198.

Hering R, Kuritzky A: Sodium valproate in the prophylactic treatment of migraine: a double-blind study versus placebo. *Cephalalgia* 1992;12:81–84.

Hong JS, Tilson HA, Yoshikawa K: Effect of lithium and haloperidol administration on rat levels of substance P. *J Pharmacol Exp Ther* 1983;224:590–593.

Honmou O, Kocsis JD, Richerson GB: Gabapentin potentiates the conductance increase induced by nipecotic acid in CA1 pyramidal neurons in vitro *Epilepsy Res* 1995;20:193–202.

Horton JC, Fishman RA:Neurovisual findings in the syndrome of spontaneous intracranial hypotension from dural cerebrospinal fluid leak. *Ophthalmology* 1994;101:244–251.

Hoyer D, Clarke DE, Fozard JR et al.: VII. International Union of Pharmacology classification of receptors for 5-hydroxytryptamine (serotonin) *Pharmacol Rev* 1994;46:157–203.

Huang L-YM: Origin of thalamically projecting somatosensory relay neurons in the immature rat. *Brain Res* 1989;495:108–114.

Huerta MF, Frankfurter A, Harting JK: Studies of the prinicipal sensory and spinal trigeminal nuclei of the rat: projections to the superior colliculus, inferior olive, and cerebellum. *J Comp Neurol* 1983;220:147–167.

International Headache Society, Headache Classification Committee: Classification and diagnostic criteria for headache disorders, cranial neuralgias and facial pain. *Cephalalgia* 1988;8(suppl 7):1–90.

Jacquin MF, Chiaia NL, Haring JH, Rhoades RW: Intersub-nuclear connections within the rat trigeminal brainstem complex. *Somatosen Motor Res* 1990;7:399–420.

Jefferson JW: Current and potential uses of lithium. *J Clin Psychiat* 1990;51:392–399.

Jensen R, Brinck T, Olesen J: Sodium valproate has a prophylactic effect in migraine without aura: a triple-blind, placebo-cross-over study. *Neurology* 1994;44:647–651.

Johnson RH, Hornabrook RW, Lambie DG: Comparison of mefenamic acid and propranolol with placebo in migraine prophylaxis. *Acta Neurol Scand* 1986;76:96–98.

Kangasneimi P, Andersen AR, Andersson PG et al.: Classic migraine: effective prophylaxis with metoprolol. *Cephalalgia* 1987;7:231–238.

Kaube H, Hoskin KL, Goadsby PJ: Intravenous acetylsalicylic acid inhibits central trigeminal neurons in the dorsal horn of the upper cervical spinal cord in the cat. *Headache* 1993;33:541–544.

Kemplay S, Webster KE: A quantitative study of the projections of the gracile, cuneate and trigeminal nuclei and of the medullary reticular formation to the thalamus in the rat. *Neuroscience* 1989;32:153–167.

Klapper JA, Stanton JS: Ketorolac versus DHE and metoclopramide in the treatment of migraine headaches. *Headache* 1991;31:523–524.

Klimek A: Cyproheptadine (Peritol) in the treatment of migraine and related headache. *Ther Hungarica* 1979;27:93–94.

Konttinen YT, Kemppinen P, Segerberg M et al.: Peripheral and spinal neural mechanisms in arthritis with particular reference to treatment of inflammation and pain. *Arthritis Rheum* 1994;37:965–982.

Kruger L, Young RF: Specialized features of the trigeminal nerve and its central connections, in Samii M, Janetta PJ (eds): *The Cranial Nerves.* Berlin, Springer-Verlag, 1981, pp 273–301.

Kudrow L: Diagnosis and treatment of cluster headache. *Med Clin North Am* 1991;75(3):579–594.

Kudrow L: Response of cluster headache attacks to oxygen inhalation. *Headache* 1981;21:1–4.

Kunkle EC, Ray BS, Wolff HG: Studies on headache: an analysis of the headache associated with changes in intracranial pressure. *Arch Neurol Psychiat* 1943;49:323–333.

Lance JW, Curran DA: Treatment of chronic tension-type headache. *Lancet* 1964;1:1236–1239.

Lane PL, McLellan BA, Baggoley CJ: Comparative efficacy of chlorpromazine and meperidine with dimenhydrate in migraine headache. *Ann Emerg Med* 1989;18:360–365.

Lay CL, Campbell JK, Morki B: Low cerebrospinal fluid pressure headache, in Goadsby PJ, Silberstein SD (eds): *Headache*. Boston, Butterworth-Heinnemann, 1997, pp 355–367.

Lee WS, Limmroth V, Ayata C et al.: Peripheral GABA$_A$ receptor mediated effects of sodium valproate on dural plasma extravasation to substance P and trigeminal stimulation. *Br J Pharmacol* 1995;116:1661–1667.

Lindegaard K-F, Ovrelid L, Sjaastad O: Naproxen in the prevention of migraine attacks: a double blind placebo-controlled cross-over study. *Headache* 1980;20:96–98.

MacIntyre PD, Bhargava B, Hogg KJ et al.: Effect of subcutaneous sumatriptan, a selective 5-HT$_1$ agonist, on the systemic pulmonary and coronary circulation. *Circulation* 1993;87:401–405.

Mantle St John LA, Tracey DJ: Somatosensory nuclei in the brainstem of the rat: independent projections to the thalamus and cerebellum. *J Comp Neurol* 1987;255:259–271.

Markley H, Cheronis J, Piepho R: Verapamil prophylactic therapy of migraine. *Neurology* 1984;34:973–976.

Masferrer JL, Zweifel BS, Manning PT et al.: Selective inhibition of inducible cyclooxygenase 2 in vivo is antiinflammatory and nonulcerogenic. *Proc Natl Acad Sci USA* 1994;91:3228–3232.

Mathew NT, Ali S: Valproate in the treatment of persistent chronic daily headache: an open-label study. *Headache* 1991;31:71–74.

Mathew NT, Lucker C: Gabapentin in migraine prophylaxis: a preliminary open-label study. *Neurology* 1996;46(suppl 2):A169.

Mathew NT, Saper JR, Silberstein SD et al.: Migraine prophylaxis with divalproex. *Arch Neurol* 1995;52(3):281–286.

Mathew NT, Stubits E, Nigam MP: Transformation of episodic migraine into daily headache: analysis of factors. *Headache* 1982;22:66–68.

Mayberg MA, Langer RS, Zervas NT, Moskowitz MA: Perivascular meningeal projection from cat trigeminal ganglia: possible pathway for vascular headache in man. *Science* 1981;213:228–230.

Mayberg MR, Zervas NT, Moskowitz MA: Trigeminal projections to supratentorial pial and dural blood vessels in cats demonstrated by horseradish peroxidase histochemistry. *J Comp Neurol* 1984;223:46–56.

McEwen J, O'Connor H, Dinsdale H: Treatment of migraine with intramuscular chlorpromazine. *Ann Emerg Med* 1987;16:758–763.

McLean MJ, Macdonald RL: Sodium valproate, but not ethosuximide, produces use- and voltage-dependent limitation of high frequency repetitive firing of action potentials of mouse central neurons in cell culture. *J Pharmacol Exp Ther* 1986;237:1001–1011.

Miranda HF, Pelissier T, Sierralta F: Analgesic effects of intracerebroventricular administration of calcium channel blockers in mice. *Gen Pharmacol* 1993;24:201–204.

Mitsikostas DDD, Gatzonis S, Thomas A, Ilias A: Buspirone, amitriptyline, chronic tension-type headache, treatment. *Acta Scand Neurol* 1997;96:247–251.

Mokri B: Headache in spontaneous carotid and vertebral artery dissections, in Goadsby PJ, Silberstein SD (eds): *Headache*. Boston, Butterworth-Heinemann, 1997, pp 327–353.

Morland TJ, Storli OV, Mogstad TE: Doxepin in the prophylactic treatment of mixed "vascular" and tension headache. *Headache* 1979;19:382–383.

Moskowitz MA: Neurogenic versus vascular mechanisms of sumatriptan and ergot alkaloids in migraine. *Trends Pharmacol Sci* 1992;13:307–311.

Moskowitz MA, Cutrer FM: Sumatriptan: a receptor-targeted treatment for migraine. *Ann Rev Med* 1993;44:145–154.

Moskowitz MA, Waeber C: Neuronal pathophysiology of migraine as a basis for acute treatment with 5HT receptor ligands, in Baumgarten HG, Gothert M (eds): *Handbook of Experimental Pharmacology*. Vol 129: Serotoninergic neurons and 5HT receptors in the CNS. Berlin, Springer Verlag, 1997, 613–636.

Nau H: Valproic acid-induced neural tube defects. Ciba Foundation Symp 1994;181:144–152.

Newman LC, Lipton RB, Solomon S: Hemicrania continua: 10 new cases and a literature review. *Neurology* 1994;44(11):2111–2114.

O'Neill BP, Mann JD: Aspirin prophylaxis in migraine. *Lancet* 1978;2:1179–1181.

Ophoff RA, Terwindt GM, Vergouse MN et al.: Familial hemiplegic migraine and episodic ataxia type-2 are caused by mutations in the Ca2 + channel gene CACNL1A4. *Cell* 1996;87:543–552.

Pauwels PJ, Tardif S, Palmier C et al.: How efficacious are 5HT$_{1B/D}$ receptor ligands: an answer from GTPgS binding studies with stably transfected C6-glial cell lines. *Neuropharmacology* 1997;36:499–512.

Pedersen E, Moller CE: Methysergide in migraine prophylaxis. *Clin Pharmacol Ther* 1966;7:520–526.

Penfield W: A contribution to the mechanism of intracranial pain. *Assoc Res Nerv Ment Dis* 1935;15:399–416.

Peroutka SJ: The pharmacology of current anti-migraine drugs. *Headache* 1990;30(suppl):5–11.

Peschanski M, Roudier F, Ralston HJ III, Besson JM: Ultrastructural analysis of the terminals of various somatosensory pathways in the ventrobasal complex of the rat thalamus: an electron-microscopic study using wheat germ agglutinin conjugated to horseradish peroxidase as an axonal tracer. *Somatosens Res* 1985;3:75–87.

Rabkin R, Stables DP, Levin NW, Suzman MM: Propranolol and prophylaxis of angina pectoris. *Am J Cardiol* 1966;18:370–380.

Raskin NH: Repetitive intravenous dihydroergotamine as therapy for intractable migraine. *Neurology* 1986;36:995–997.

Ray BS, Wolff HG: Experimental studies on headache: pain-sensitive structures of the head and their significance in headache. *Arch Surg* 1940;41:813–856.

Renehan WE, Jacquin MF, Mooney RD, Rhoades RW: Structure-function relationship in rat medullary and cervical dorsal horns. II. Medullary dorsal horn cells. *J Neurophysiol* 1986;55:1187–1201.

Ryan RE Sr, Ryan RE Jr, Sudilovsky A: Nadolol: its use in the prophylactic treatment of migraine. *Headache* 1983;23:26–31.

Saito K, Markowitz S, Moskowitz MA: Ergot alkaloids block neurogenic extravasation in dura mater: proposed action in vascular headaches. *Ann Neurol* 1988;24:732–737.

Sances G, Martignoni D, Fioroni L et al.: Naproxen sodium in menstrual migraine prophylaxis: a double-blind placebo controlled study. *Headache* 1990;30:705–709.

Saper JR, Silberstein SD, Lake AE, Winters ME: Double-blind trial of fluoxetine: chronic daily headache and migraine. *Headache* 1994;34:497–502.

Saxena PR, Tfelt-Hansen P: Sumatriptan, in Olesen J, Tfelt-Hansen P, Welch KMA (eds): *The Headaches.* New York, Raven Press, 1993, pp 329–341.

Schoenen J, Jacquy J, Lenaerts M: High-dose riboflavin as a novel prophylactic antimigraine therapy: results from double blind, randomized, placebo-controlled trial. *Cephalalgia* 1997;17:244.

Schoenen J, Maertens de Hoordhout A, Timsit-Berthier M, Timsit M: Contingent negative variation and efficacy of beta-blocking agents in migraine. *Cephalalgia* 1986;6:229–233.

Sechzer PG, Abel L: Post-spinal anesthesia headache treated with caffeine: evaluation with demand method. Part 1. *Curr Ther Res* 1978;24:307–312.

Sessle BJ, Hu JW, Dubner R, Lucier GE: Functional properties of neurons in trigeminal subnucleus caudalis of the cat. II. Modulation of responses to noxious and non-noxious stimulation by periaqueductal gray, nucleus raphe magnus, cerebral cortex and afferent influences, and effect of nalaxone. *J Neurophysiol* 1981;45:193–207.

Shigenaga Y, Nakatani A, Nishimori T et al.: The cells of origin of cat trigeminothalamic projections: especially in the caudal medulla. *Brain Res* 1983;277:201–222.

Sivam SP, Krause JE, Takeuchi K et al.: Lithium increases rat striatal beta- and gamma-preprotachykinin messenger RNAs. *J Pharmacol Exp Ther* 1989;248:1297–1301.

Sjaastad O: Chronic paroxysmal hemicrania, in Rose FC (ed): *Handbook of Clinical Neurology,* vol 48. Amsterdam, Elsevier Science Publishing, 1986, pp 257–266.

Slettness O, Sjaastad O: Metoclopramide during attacks of migraine, in Sicuteri F (ed): *Headache: New Vista.* Florence: Biomedical Press, 1977, pp 201–204.

Solomon GD, Steel JG, Spaccavento LJ: Verapamil prophylaxis of migraine: a double-blind, placebo-controlled study. *JAMA* 1983;250(18):2500–2502.

Solomon GD, Scott AFB: Verapamil and propranolol in migraine prophylaxis: a double-blind placebo-controlled trial. *JAMA* 1986;26:235.

Solomon S, Lipton RB, Newman LC: Clinical features of chronic daily headache. *Headache* 1992;32:325–329.

Southwell N, Williams JD, Mackenzie I: Methysergide in the prophylaxis of migraine. *Lancet* 1964;1:523–524.

Stellar S, Ahrens SP, Meibohm BR, Reimes SA: Migraine prevention with timolol. *JAMA* 1984;252:2576–2579.

Stensrud P, Sjaastad O: Clinical trial of a new anti-bradykinin, anti-inflammatory drug, ketoprofen in migraine prophylaxis. *Headache* 1974;14:96–100.

Stewart WF, Lipton R, Celentano DD, Reed ML: Prevalence of migraine headache in the United States. *JAMA* 1992;267:64–69.

Szekely B, Merryman S, Croft H, Post G: Prophylactic effects of naproxen sodium on perimenstrual headache: a double-blind, placebo controlled study. *Cephalalgia* 1989;9(suppl 10):452–453.

Tek DS, McClellan DS, Olshaker JS et al.: A prospective, double-blind study of metoclopramide hydrochloride for the control of migraine in the emergency department. *Ann Emerg Med* 1990;19:1083–1087.

Tfelt-Hansen P, Saxena PR: Antiserotonin drugs, in Olesen J, Tfelt-Hansen P, Welch KMA (eds): *The Headaches.* New York, Raven Press, 1993, pp 373–382.

The Sumatriptan Cluster Headache Study Group: Treatment of acute cluster headache with sumatriptan. *N Engl J Med* 1991;325:322–326.

Toda N, Tfelt-Hansen P: Calcium antagonists, in Olesen J, Tfelt-Hansen P, Welch KMA (eds): *The Headaches.* New York, Raven Press, 1993, pp 383–390.

Todd PA, Benfield P: Flunarizine: a reappraisal of its pharmacological properties and therapeutic use in neurological disorders. *Drugs* 1989;38:481–499.

Tokola RA, Kangasneimi P, Neurvonen PJ, Tokola O: Tolfenamic acid, metoclopramide, caffeine and their combinations in the treatment of migraine attacks. *Cephalalgia* 1984;4:253–263.

Tyler GS, McNeely HE, Dick MS: Treatment of post-traumatic headache with amitriptyline. *Headache* 1980;20:213–216.

Vincent MB: Lithium inhibits substance P and vasoactive intestinal peptide-induced relaxations on isolated porcine ophthalmic artery. *Headache* 1992;32:335–339.

Wall M: Headache profile of idiopathic intracranial hypertension. *Cephalalgia* 1990;10:331–335.

Welch KMA, Ellis DJ, Keenan PA: Successful migraine prophylaxis with naprosyn sodium. *Cephalalgia* 1989;9:(suppl 10):452–453.

Wessely P, Baumgartner C, Klingler D et al.: Preliminary results of a double blind study with the new migraine prophylactic drug gabapentin. *Cephalalgia* 1987;7(suppl 6):476–477.

Wise SP, Jones EG: Cells of origin and trigeminal distribution of descending projections of the rat somatic sensory cortex. *J Comp Neurol* 1977;175:129–158.

Yaksh TL: Pharmacology and mechanisms of opioid analgesic activity. *Acta Anaesthesiol Scand* 1997;41:94–111.

Yamaguchi M: Incidence of headache and severity of head injury. *Headache* 1992;32:427–431.

Young WB, Packard RC: Post-traumatic Headache and Post-traumatic Syndrome, in Goadsby PJ, Silberstein SD (eds): *Headache.* Boston, Butterworth-Heinemann, 1997, pp 253–277.

INDEX

Page numbers followed by *f* indicate figures; page numbers followed by *t* indicate tables.